Atlas of Technics in Surgery

General and Abdominal

By JOHN L. MADDEN, M.D., F.A.C.S.

Director of Surgery, St. Clare's Hospital, New York City;
Clinical Professor of Surgery, New York Medical College

With 91 Contributing Authors
Discussing the Illustrated Surgical Technics

Illustrations By

Alfred Feinberg & Robert Wabnitz

With

Frank Robinson   Neil Hardy   Don Johnson

Elizabeth H. Brödel   Harriet E. Phillips

William Didusch   Leonard Dank

APPLETON-CENTURY-CROFTS

Division of Meredith Publishing Company

New York

JOHN L. MADDEN'S

Atlas of Technics

In Surgery

Second Edition

Volume 1: General and Abdominal

To my wife
Birdie
and children
Pam
John
Brian
Michael
Tommy
Kathy

CONTRIBUTING AUTHORS

FREDERICK H. AMENDOLA
Chief of Surgery, Roosevelt Hospital; Director of Surgery, Lincoln Hospital; Associate Clinical Professor of Surgery, Columbia University, College of Physicians and Surgeons

OLIVER H. BEAHRS
Head of a Section of Surgery, Mayo Clinic; Associate Professor of Surgery, The University of Minnesota, Rochester, Minnesota

BRYAN N. BROOKE
Professor of Surgery within the University of London; Honorary Consultant, St. George's Hospital, London, England

JOHN ROBINSON BROOKS
Senior Associate in Surgery, Peter Bent Brigham Hospital; Assistant Clinical Professor in Surgery, Harvard Medical School

ALEXANDER BRUNSCHWIG
Attending Surgeon, Memorial Hospital for Cancer and Allied Diseases and James Ewing Hospital; Professor of Clinical Surgery, Cornell University Medical College

CON AMORE V. BURT
Assistant Professor of Surgery, Columbia University, College of Physicians and Surgeons; Attending Proctologic Surgeon, Department of Surgery, St. Clare's Hospital, New York

DANIEL F. CASTEN
Director of Surgery, Sydenham Hospital; Attending Surgeon, St. Clare's Hospital, New York

CHARLES G. CHILD, III
Professor and Chairman, Department of Surgery, The University of Michigan Medical School; Surgeon-in-Chief, University Hospital, Ann Arbor

ROBERT J. COFFEY
Professor and Director, Department of Surgery, Georgetown University School of Medicine; Surgeon-in-Chief, Georgetown University Hospital, Washington, D.C.

ISIDORE COHN, JR.
Professor and Chairman, Department of Surgery, Louisiana State University School of Medicine; Surgeon-in-Chief, Louisiana State University Surgical Service, Charity Hospital of Louisiana, New Orleans

WARREN H. COLE
Professor and Head, Department of Surgery, The University of Illinois College of Medicine; Chief Surgeon, Illinois Research and Educational Hospitals, Chicago

* BRADLEY COLEY
Consulting Surgeon, Hospital for Special Surgery and Bellevue Hospital; Associate Professor of Clinical Surgery, Cornell University Medical College

RALPH COLP
Consulting Surgeon, Surgeon Emeritus, Mt. Sinai Hospital; Consulting Surgeon, Harlem, French, Beth Israel, Long Beach, and Columbus Hospitals

DENTON A. COOLEY
Professor of Surgery, Baylor University College of Medicine; Chief, Cardiovascular Service, Texas Children's Hospital; Attending Surgeon, Methodist, St. Luke's Episcopal, and Ben Taub General Hospitals, Houston

PHILIP COOPER
Chief, Surgical Service, Veterans' Administration Hospital, Bronx, New York; Professor of Clinical Surgery, Albert Einstein College of Medicine

GEORGE CRILE, JR.
Head, Department of General Surgery, Cleveland Clinic, Cleveland

JAMES T. DANIELS
Chief of Neurological Surgery, St. Clare's Hospital; Associate Professor, New York University Post-Graduate Medical School

MICHAEL R. DEDDISH
Attending Surgeon, Rectal and Colon Service, Memorial Hospital for Cancer and Allied Diseases; Associate Professor of Clinical Surgery, Cornell University Medical College

* Deceased

vii

CLARENCE DENNIS
Professor and Chairman, Department of Surgery, State University of New York, Downstate Medical Center; Chief of Surgery, Kings County Hospital, Brooklyn

EDWARD J. DONOVAN
Associate Professor of Surgery, Columbia University, College of Physicians and Surgeons; Consulting Surgeon, Presbyterian Hospital; Formerly: Director of Surgery, Babies Hospital, New York

* HENRY DOUBILET
Associate Professor of Surgery, New York University College of Medicine; Visiting Surgeon, Bellevue Hospital (Third Division)

LESTER R. DRAGSTEDT
Thomas D. Jones Distinguished Service Professor of Surgery Emeritus, The University of Chicago; Research Professor of Surgery, University of Florida, Gainesville

J. ENGLEBERT DUNPHY
Professor and Chairman, Department of Surgery, The University of California School of Medicine, San Francisco Medical Center; Surgeon-in-Chief, University of California Hospitals, San Francisco

JOHN H. ECKEL
Visiting Surgeon (Second Division), Bellevue Hospital; Associate Attending Surgeon, The New York Hospital; Director of Surgery, North Shore Hospital, Manhasset; Associate Professor of Clinical Surgery, Cornell University Medical College

CHARLES ECKERT
Professor and Chairman, Department of Surgery, Albany Medical College of Union University; Surgeon-in-Chief, Albany Medical Center Hospital

EDWIN H. ELLISON
Professor and Chairman, Department of Surgery, Marquette University School of Medicine; Director of Surgery, Milwaukee County General Hospital; Senior Consultant in Surgery, Wood Veterans' Administration Hospital, Milwaukee

JACK MATTHEWS FARRIS
Associate Professor of Surgery, The University of California School of Medicine; Consultant in Surgery, Veterans' Administration Hospital, Long Beach; Senior Staff Surgeon, The Hospital of the Good Samaritan, The California Hospital, and Methodist Hospital of Southern California

GEORGE A. FIEDLER
Chief of Urology, St. Clare's Hospital, New York;

* Deceased

Assistant Clinical Professor of Urology, Cornell University Medical College

EDGAR L. FRAZELL
Attending Surgeon and Chief of the Head and Neck Service, Memorial Hospital for Cancer and Allied Diseases, New York

FRANK GLENN
Lewis Atterbury Stimson Professor of Surgery, Cornell University Medical College; Surgeon-in-Chief, The New York Hospital

J. C. GOLIGHER
Professor of Surgery, University of Leeds; Surgeon, The General Infirmary, Leeds, England

C. ROLLINS HANLON
Professor and Director, Department of Surgery, St. Louis University School of Medicine; Surgeon-in-Chief, St. Louis University Hospitals, St. Louis

JAMES D. HARDY
Professor and Chairman, Department of Surgery, and Director of Surgical Research, The University of Mississippi Medical Center; Surgeon-in-Chief, Hospital of the University of Mississippi; Chief Surgical Consultant, Jackson Veterans' Hospital and Mississippi Tuberculosis Sanatorium

HENRY N. HARKINS
Professor and Chairman, Department of Surgery, The University of Washington School of Medicine; Surgeon-in-Chief, University Hospital, Director of Surgery, University Teaching Hospitals, Seattle

MARK A. HAYES
Professor of Surgery, Yale University; Attending Surgeon, New Haven Hospital

MARTIN J. HEALY
Consultant Surgeon, St. Joseph's Hospital, Yonkers, New York; Associate Clinical Professor of Surgery, Albert Einstein College of Medicine

ROBERT B. HIATT
Assistant Professor of Surgery, Columbia University, College of Physicians and Surgeons; Associate Attending Surgeon, Columbia Presbyterian Medical Center; and Francis Delafield Hospital

J. WILLIAM HINTON
Professor of Surgery Emeritus, New York University Post-Graduate Medical School; Attending Surgeon, Doctors Hospital

STANLEY O. HOERR
Staff Surgeon and Chairman of the Division of Surgery, Cleveland Clinic, Cleveland

WILLIAM D. HOLDEN
Oliver H. Payne Professor and Director of the Department of Surgery, Western Reserve University School of Medicine; Director of Surgery, University Hospitals of Cleveland

EDMUND HORGAN
Attending Surgeon, Winchester Surgical Clinic, Winchester, Virginia; Formerly: Professor of Surgery, The George Washington University School of Medicine, Washington, D.C.

ARTHUR G. JAMES
Attending Staff, University Hospital, Associate Professor of Surgery, Director, The Columbus Cancer Clinic, The Ohio State University School of Medicine, Columbus

THOMAS H. JOHNSON
Attending Surgeon, Department of Urology, St. Clare's Hospital, New York

EDWARD S. JUDD
Staff Surgeon, Mayo Clinic and Affiliated Hospitals; Professor of Surgery, The University of Minnesota, Rochester, Minnesota

GEORGE A. KEATING
Formerly: Director of Anesthesiology, St. Clare's Hospital, New York

PAUL C. KIERNAN
Associate Professor of Surgery, Georgetown University School of Medicine; Section of General Surgery, Washington Clinic; Attending Surgeon, Georgetown University Hospital; Consultant in Surgery, National Institutes of Health, Washington, D.C.

AMOS R. KOONTZ
Surgeon, Johns Hopkins Hospital; Consultant in Surgery to the Surgeon General of the United States Army; Emeritus Assistant Professor of Surgery, The Johns Hopkins University School of Medicine

J. WILLIAM LITTLER
Associate Attending Surgeon, Plastic and Reconstructive Surgery, Roosevelt Hospital, New York

S. ARTHUR LOCALIO
Visiting Surgeon, Bellevue Hospital; Attending Surgeon, University Hospital; Professor of Clinical Surgery, New York University Post-Graduate Medical School

HUGH B. LYNN
Head of a Section of Pediatric Surgery, Mayo Clinic; Assistant Professor of Surgery, The University of Minnesota, Rochester, Minnesota

W. J. LYTLE
Lecturer in Surgery and Director of Postgraduate Clinical Studies, University of Sheffield; Honorary Consultant Surgeon, Royal Infirmary, Sheffield, England

WILLIAM F. MacFEE
Chief of Surgery, Veterans' Administration Hospital, New York, New York

HOWARD MAHORNER
Surgeon, Baptist Hospital; Clinical Professor of Surgery, Louisiana State University School of Medicine, New Orleans

ROLAND L. MAIER
Consulting Surgeon, Hospital for Special Surgery, and Bellevue Hospital; Associate Professor of Clinical Surgery, New York Medical College

CHARLES MARKS
Associate Professor of Surgery, Marquette University School of Medicine; Attending Surgeon, Milwaukee County General Hospital, Wood Veterans' Hospital, St. Luke's Hospital, St. Mary's Hospital, West Allis Memorial Hospital and Milwaukee Hospital, Milwaukee; Formerly: Hunterian Professor, Royal College of Physicians and Surgeons

JAMES PRATT MARR
Senior Attending Obstetrician and Gynecologist, St. Clare's Hospital; Consulting Obstetrician and Gynecologist, Woman's Hospital, Division of St. Luke's Hospital, New York

AUBRE de L. MAYNARD
Director of Surgery, Harlem Hospital, New York

CHESTER B. McVAY
Clinical Professor of Surgery and Associate Professor of Anatomy, The State University of South Dakota School of Medicine, Chief of Surgery, Sacred Heart Hospital, Yankton, South Dakota

MAURICE MERCADIER
Professeur Agrégé de la Faculté de Médicine de l'Université de Paris; Chirurgien de l'Hôpital Bichat; Attending Surgeon, The American Hospital, Paris, France

WALTER L. MERSHEIMER
Professor and Chairman, Department of Surgery, New York Medical College; Director of Surgery and Attending Surgeon, Flower and Fifth Avenue Hospitals, New York

S. W. MOORE
Attending Surgeon, The New York Hospital; Clinical Professor of Surgery, Cornell University Medical College

JOHN H. MULHOLLAND
George David Stewart Professor and Chairman, Department of Surgery, New York University School of Medicine, Director, Third (N.Y.U.) Surgical Division, Bellevue Hospital

KOMEI NAKAYAMA
Professor of Surgery, Nakayama Surgical Department, School of Medicine, Chiba University; Chief of Surgery, Chiba University Hospital, Japan

CHARLES GEORGE NEUMANN
Visiting Surgeon, Fourth Surgical Division, Bellevue Hospital; Associate Attending Surgeon, University Hospital; Associate Professor of Clinical Surgery (Plastic Surgery), New York University Post-Graduate Medical School

GEORGE T. PACK
Attending Surgeon, Memorial Hospital for Cancer and Allied Diseases; Associate Professor of Clinical Surgery, Cornell University Medical College

HOWARD A. PATTERSON
Chief of Surgery, Roosevelt Hospital, New York; Clinical Professor of Surgery, Columbia University, College of Physicians and Surgeons

RUSSEL H. PATTERSON
Professor of Clinical Surgery Emeritus, Cornell University Medical College; Visiting Surgeon, Bellevue Hospital; Consulting Surgeon, The New York Hospital

GERALD W. PESKIN
Associate in Surgery, The University of Pennsylvania School of Medicine; Surgical Staff, Hospital of the University of Pennsylvania, Philadelphia

HENRY THOMAS RANDALL
Professor of Surgery, Cornell University Medical College; Clinical Director and Chairman, Department of Surgery, Memorial Center for Cancer and Allied Diseases

I. S. RAVDIN
John Rhea Barton Professor of Surgery, and Director, Harrison Department of Surgical Research, The University of Pennsylvania School of Medicine; Surgeon-in-Chief, Department of Surgery, The University of Pennsylvania

MARK M. RAVITCH
Associate Professor of Surgery, The Johns Hopkins University School of Medicine; Surgeon, Johns Hopkins Hospital

PAUL C. SAMSON
Associate Clinical Professor of Surgery, Stanford University School of Medicine; West Coast Area Consultant in Thoracic and Cardiac Surgery, Veterans' Administration

THOMAS V. SANTULLI
Chief of Pediatric Surgical Service, Babies Hospital, Columbia-Presbyterian Medical Center; Associate Professor of Clinical Surgery, Columbia University, College of Physicians and Surgeons

H. WILLIAM SCOTT, JR.
Professor and Chairman, Department of Surgery, Vanderbilt University School of Medicine; Surgeon-in-Chief, Vanderbilt University Hospital, Nashville

LAWRENCE W. SLOAN
Attending Surgeon, Presbyterian Hospital; Professor of Clinical Surgery, Columbia University, College of Physicians and Surgeons

WILLIAM H. SNYDER, JR.
Chief, Department of Surgery, Children's Hospital of Los Angeles; Clinical Professor of Surgery, The University of Southern California, Los Angeles

ROBERT S. SPARKMAN
Attending Surgeon, Baylor University Medical Center, Parkland Memorial Hospital, Dallas; Clinical Professor of Surgery, University of Texas

ROWENA SPENCER
Associate Professor of Surgery, Louisiana State University School of Medicine; Senior Visiting Surgeon, Charity Hospital of Louisiana, New Orleans

E. LEE STROHL
Senior Attending Surgeon, Presbyterian-St. Luke's Hospital, Chicago; Clinical Associate Professor of Surgery, The University of Illinois College of Medicine

* RAYMOND P. SULLIVAN
Director of Surgery, Emeritus, St. Vincent's Hospital, New York; Consultant Surgeon, St. Joseph's Hospital, Yonkers, New York

* Deceased

* RICHARD H. SWEET
    Visiting Surgeon, Massachusetts General Hospital;
    Associate Clinical Professor of Surgery, Harvard
    Medical College

ORVAR SWENSON
    Professor of Surgery, Northwestern University
    Medical School; Surgeon-in-Chief, The Children's
    Memorial Hospital, Chicago

ROBERT TURELL
    Attending Surgeon, Bronx Municipal Hospital
    Center; Associate Clinical Professor of Surgery
    (Proctology), Albert Einstein College of Medicine

PIETRO VALDONI
    Professor of Surgery, University of Rome; Di-
    rector of the Surgical Clinic, Policlinico Hospital,
    Rome, Italy

KENNETH W. WARREN
    Surgeon, Lahey Clinic, New England Baptist and
    New England Deaconess Hospitals, Boston

JOSEPH A. WEINBERG
    Chief, Surgical Service, Veterans' Administration
    Hospital, Long Beach; Clinical Professor of Sur-
    gery, The University of California, Los Angeles

JOHN S. WELCH
    Head of Section of Surgery, Mayo Clinic; As-
    sistant Professor of Surgery, The University of
    Minnesota, Rochester, Minnesota

* WILLIAM CRAWFORD WHITE
    Consulting Surgeon, Roosevelt Hospital, St. Luke's
    Hospital, New York; Clinical Professor of Sur-
    gery, Columbia University College of Physicians
    and Surgeons

JAMES M. WINFIELD
    Attending Surgeon, St. Clare's Hospital, New York

KAZUO YANAGISAWA
    Attending and Chief of Orthopedic Service, St.
    Clare's Hospital, New York; Attending Orthopedic
    Surgeon, St. Giles and Seaview Hospitals, New
    York

ROBERT M. ZOLLINGER
    Professor and Chairman, Department of Surgery,
    The Ohio State University College of Medicine;
    Chief of the Surgical Service, Ohio State Univer-
    sity Hospitals

* Deceased

PREFACE

In the preparation of the Second Edition of the *Atlas of Technics in Surgery,* it was thought desirable to separate the contents into two volumes. This was done for two reasons: 1. To facilitate handling by lessening the bulk. 2. To apportion closely allied subject matter into individual volumes for ease of reference. Volume 1 is comprised of general and abdominal operative technics, and in Volume 2 thoracic and cardiovascular operations are illustrated.

An added feature is the inclusion in Volume 1 of thirteen colored photographs done by John M. Loré, M.D., of fresh cadaver specimens injected with colored dyes and two plates of black and white artist illustrations which depict in detail the anatomy of the portal system. These are considered a distinct aid in clarifying the surgical anatomy of this important area.

In keeping with the policy established in the first edition of the *Atlas* each of the operations illustrated was seen by the artist as performed by the author. This is believed the best way to obtain the anatomic realism of the operation room and to depict most accurately the sequential steps of an operation.

The reference lists, which are considered a most important part of the *Atlas,* were selected on the basis of historic and current interest. Although many references have been added to those contained in the first edition, none has been deleted. The use of references is a tangible way for the author to express gratitude to the many individuals whose efforts have contributed to the progress of surgery.

I am exceedingly grateful to the many surgeons in the United States and abroad who have contributed materially to the *Atlas* by their excellent discussions. It is by reading such discussions that the young surgeon, either in training or in practice, may receive guidance in the conduct of a particular operation. The discussions also serve to emphasize the important fact that there are other ways of accomplishing a desired result than the method illustrated.

I am similarly grateful to the artists, whose names are listed elsewhere, for their excellent portrayals of the varied operative technics. In particular I should like to mention Alfred Feinberg and Robert Wabnitz as the artists who made the major contributions.

I should like also to express my sincere thanks and gratitude to Sister M. Columcille, O.S.F., the Administrator of St. Clare's Hospital, for her expressed kindness and consideration; to Sister M. Francis Aloysius, O.S.F , for her patience and kindness in the performance of the secretarial work which made these volumes possible; to Mary B. McDermott, the medical librarian of St. Clare's Hospital; and the medical library staff of the New York Academy of Medicine for their inestimable aid in securing references; to Miss Catherine O'Regan, an exemplary "scrub" nurse; to Mrs. Paula Arnuk, a most conscientious circulating nurse; and to Dr. Joseph Lawrence, Director of Anesthesiology at St. Clare's Hospital, and the members of his staff for their valued cooperation. I am grateful to the memory of Mother M. Alice, O.S.F., for her inspiration.

Finally, I am indebted to the publishers, Appleton-Century-Crofts, for their advice, guidance, patience, understanding, and unstinting cooperation throughout the preparation of this Second Edition of the *Atlas of Technics in Surgery.*

JOHN L. MADDEN

CONTENTS

Contents

Contents xix

Contents

FOREWORD

The purpose of this volume is to present clearly and concisely a correlation of the anatomy, physiology, and understanding of pathology necessary to the technical "art of surgery." Such a book should be based on the cumulative experience of surgeon-investigators and should include the more recent technical advances.

The author is eminently qualified to meet this challenge and has overcome the obvious difficulties. He has produced a record of certain proved procedures valuable for quick reference for any experienced surgeon and especially stimulating to the thoughtful, inquiring mind in the formative phase of surgical training.

The illustrations are precise, beautifully executed, and presented in an orderly, balanced fashion. The carefully edited legends accompanying the illustrations enhance the visual perfection of this work.

There can be no doubt that this Atlas is outstanding among the volumes portraying a workable anatomic–surgical approach to the practical problems of clinical surgery.

JAMES M. WINFIELD

Atlas of Technics in Surgery

General and Abdominal

Surgical Anatomy of the Portal System

SURGICAL ANATOMY OF THE PORTAL SYSTEM

A, B, C, D, E. Artist illustrations of the anatomic findings in five fresh cadaver specimens, showing the origin and branches of the hepatic artery and their relation to the portal vein and bile ducts. Usually the celiac axis terminated by bifurcation into the hepatic and splenic arteries. However, in two (40 per cent) of the five specimens the hepatic artery had its origin from the superior mesenteric artery (D, E). In one (E) the origin was direct, and in the other (D) it arose from a common stem with an intestinal artery. Michels, in a dissection of 200 cadavers, observed that in 20 (10 per cent) the hepatic artery was a branch of the superior mesenteric artery rather than the celiac axis.

In the isolation of the hepatic artery, the gastroduodenal artery, in juxtaposition to the posterior aspect of the first portion of the duodenum, is first identified as a landmark. It is then traced cephalad to its parent trunk, the hepatic artery. This anatomic relation was constant whether or not the hepatic artery had its origin from the celiac axis or from the superior mesenteric artery.

In one specimen (A) a superior duodenal branch (artery of Wilkie) of the gastroduodenal artery was present. Sites of origin of the right gastric artery were the left hepatic artery (A, C, D, E) and the hepatic propria (B). Its average diameter was 2 mm.

The left gastric or coronary vein was a tributary of the splenic vein in four specimens (A, C, D, E) and a tributary of the portal vein in one (B). Its site of entry into the splenic vein was never more than 2 cm. from the junction of the splenic and superior mesenteric veins to form the portal vein. In a study of the specimens, the inconstancy in the relation of the splenic vein to the splenic artery is immediately apparent.

In its ascent toward the liver, the portal vein, with one exception (E), where it was anterior, coursed in an oblique direction beneath the arch formed by the gastroduodenal artery and the hepatic artery (A, B, C, D). This anatomic relation has proved a valuable landmark for the identification of the portal vein.

Plate I xxix

A

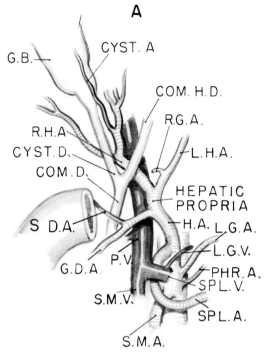

B

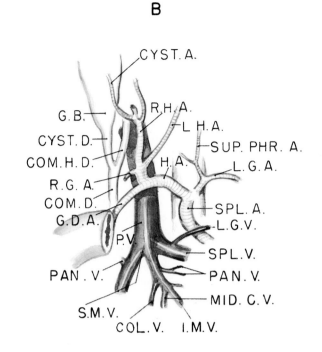

C

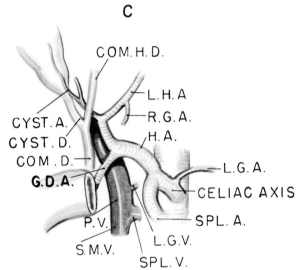

D

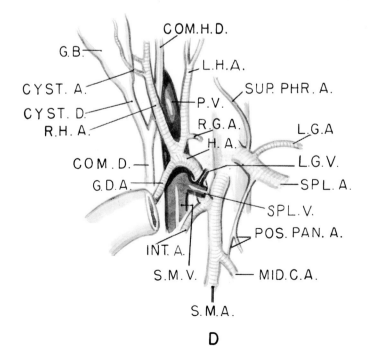

E

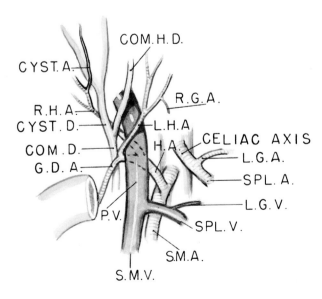

A. Drawing of a fresh postmortem specimen that has been dissected to show the celiac axis and its arterial branches with their final terminations. The relation of the branches of the hepatic artery to the liver, bile ducts, and the portal vein is depicted. The superior duodenal artery (the artery of Wilkie), a branch of the gastroduodenal artery, is visible. The portal vein may again be seen beneath the arch formed by the gastroduodenal artery and its parent trunk, the hepatic artery.

B. In this dissected specimen the portal vein and its tributaries are demonstrated. The superior mesenteric vein is formed by two trunks, right and left. The right trunk receives as tributaries the right colic, the ileocolic, the intestinal, the right gastroepiploic, the anterior superior and the anterior inferior pancreaticoduodenal veins.

The pancreaticoduodenal veins assume a particular surgical significance in the performance of a pancreaticoduodenectomy. The ligation of these multiple tributaries is demonstrated in the illustrated technic for this operation. Failure to isolate and ligate these veins is a cause of troublesome bleeding during the operation. The posterior pancreatic tributaries of the splenic and superior mesenteric veins are also important surgically in the removal of the pancreas. The same applies to the left gastric vein, a tributary of the splenic.

The tributaries of the left trunk of the superior mesenteric vein are the pancreatic, the inferior mesenteric, the middle colic, and colic veins. Prior to its union with the common tributary of the colic veins to form the left trunk of the superior mesenteric vein, the inferior mesenteric receives the middle colic and pancreatic veins as tributaries.

The gastroduodenal vein and the posterior pancreaticoduodenal veins are of surgical importance in the mobilization of the portal vein preparatory to the performance of a portacaval shunt. The location of the portal vein just beneath the arch formed by the hepatic artery and its gastroduodenal branch is again demonstrated as an excellent surgical anatomic landmark for the identification of the portal vein.

REFERENCE

1. Michels, N. A. Blood Supply and Anatomy of the Upper Abdominal Organs, Philadelphia, J. B. Lippincott Company, 1955.

Plate II xxxi

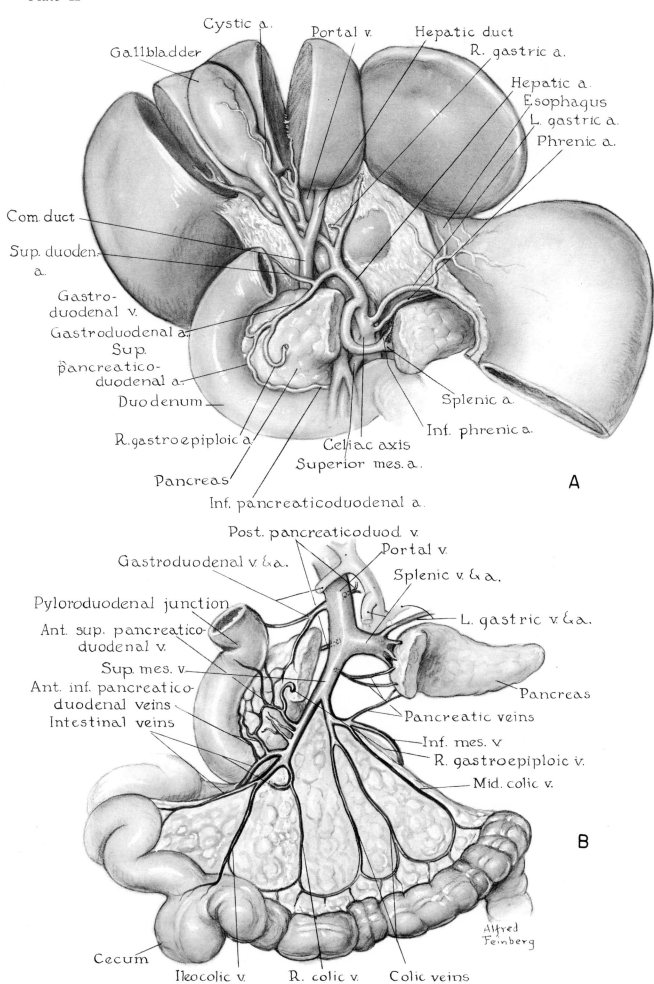

Cystic a.

Gallbladder

Portal v.

Hepatic duct

R. gastric a.

Hepatic a.

Esophagus

L. gastric a.

Phrenic a.

Com. duct

Sup. duoden. a.

Gastro-duodenal v.

Gastroduodenal a.

Sup. pancreatico-duodenal a.

Duodenum

R. gastroepiploic a.

Pancreas

Celiac axis

Superior mes. a.

Inf. pancreaticoduodenal a.

Splenic a.

Inf. phrenic a.

A

Post. pancreaticoduod. v.

Gastroduodenal v. & a.

Portal v.

Splenic v. & a.

Pyloroduodenal junction

Ant. sup. pancreatico-duodenal v.

L. gastric v. & a.

Sup. mes. v.

Ant. inf. pancreatico-duodenal veins

Intestinal veins

Pancreas

Pancreatic veins

Inf. mes. v.

R. gastroepiploic v.

Mid. colic v.

Cecum

Ileocolic v.

R. colic v.

Colic veins

Alfred Feinberg

B

Plate A. In this close-up view of the gallbladder and its related structures, the cystic artery, encircled by a guy suture of blue cotton, arises from the convex arch of the right hepatic artery just proximal to its bifurcation in the hilum of the liver. The cystic vein, a tributary of the long extrahepatic tributary of the portal vein, arches over the cystic artery just proximal to its bifurcation. The cystic vein, clearly demonstrable in this specimen, is rarely seen during a cholecystectomy. The small caliber of the cystic artery in relation to its parent trunk is apparent.

The right hepatic artery is located anterior to the common duct, which is a relatively common anatomic finding. The determination of the relation of the hepatic artery to the common duct as an early step in the performance of a cholecystectomy is believed a practical technical aid. The left hepatic artery and its bifurcation are visible, paralleling the left border of the specimen.

The cystic duct and its junction with the common hepatic duct to form the common bile duct are visible low and to the left of center. The vascularity of the suface of the common ducts is particularly noteworthy. In performing a cholecystectomy, it is believed mandatory to demonstrate the exact relation between the cystic, the common hepatic, and the common bile duct, in order to preclude common duct injury.

Plate B. This is a close-up view of the hepatic artery and its branches. In this specimen there is no hepatic propria. The hepatic artery arose from the superior mesenteric artery and divided into three branches—right and left hepatic arteries and gastroduodenal artery. The right gastric artery (anchored by a guy suture) arose from the point of trifurcation of the hepatic artery. The right gastric vein coursed parallel to the artery and emptied directly into an extrahepatic tributary of the portal vein. The common duct and the related artery and vein on its surface are seen in the lower left-hand corner, just beyond and below the tip of the clamp. The clamp lies beneath the gastroduodenal artery and overlies the portal vein at the site of entrance of its extrahepatic tributary. To the right of center and below, the celic axis and the left gastric artery are visible. The site of origin of the splenic artery is partially obscured by the overlying left gastric vein (coronary vein).

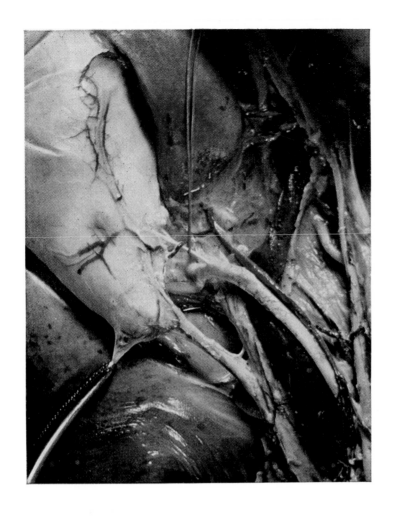

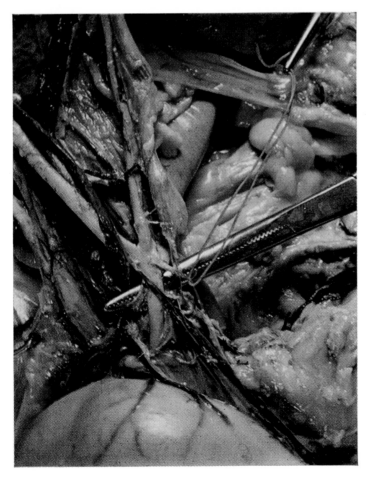

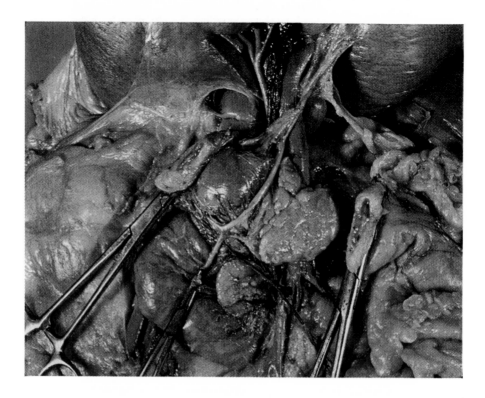

Plate C. The transected ends of the pyloric antrum, held in clamps, are retracted to expose the neck of the pancreas and the portal vein cephalad to its superior border. The vena cava is visible to the right and deep to the portal vein. Along the inferior border of the neck of the pancreas, the pancreatic and intestinal tributaries of the superior mesenteric vein are visible. The relation of the head and neck of the pancreas to the C loop of the duodenum may also be seen. Beneath the angle formed by the junction of the second and third portions of the duodenum, and between the handles of the clamps, a segment of the spermatic vein tributary of the inferior vena cava is demonstrable.

In this injected, fresh necropsy specimen, the hepatic artery arose from the superior mesenteric artery, rather than from the celiac axis. This obtained in 2 (40.0 per cent) of 5 dissected specimens. Michaels noted this origin in 5 (2.5 per cent) of 200 dissections. The right hepatic artery, visible between the vena cava and portal vein, and the left hepatic artery crossing the portal vein obliquely upward and to the left, each arose separately from the arch formed by the hepatic artery, which then coursed downward between the duodenum and pancreas as the gastroduodenal artery. At the inferior border of the pyloroduodenal junction, the gastroduodenal artery bifurcates into its right gastroepiploic and superior pancreaticoduodenal branches. Only a short segment of the superior pancreaticoduodenal artery is visible before it disappears beneath the pancreas. The transected ends of the right gastroepiploic artery and vein are occluded in a clamp. Two branches, the infraduodenal and the pancreatic, arise from the right gastroepiploic just distal to its origin from the gastroduodenal. The infraduodenal is the more proximal and courses to the right to supply the inferior border of the duodenum and segments of its anterior and posterior surfaces. The pancreatic arises opposite and slightly distal to the infraduodenal and passes to the left to enter the substance of the pancreas.

The right kidney lies beneath the handle of the large clamp that occludes the distal segment of the transected gastric antrum.

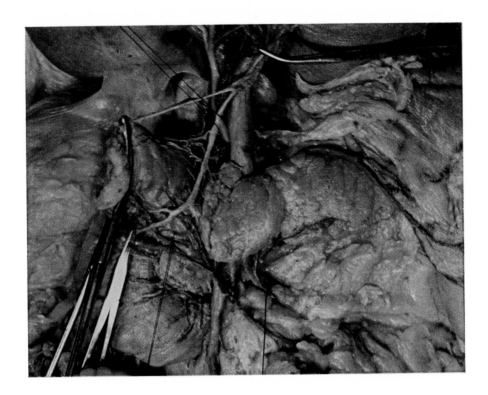

Plate D. This is another view of Plate C. The proximal transected segment of the stomach is retracted to the left to show a broad expanse of the anterior surface of the pancreas and its related blood vessels. In this exposure, the numerous tributaries of the superior mesenteric vein are more clearly seen. Knowledge of the location of these tributaries assumes particular significance in the performance of a pancreaticoduodenectomy. Accordingly, in the illustrated technic for this operation, the surgical management of these tributary veins is stressed.

In the lower central portion of the specimen, a guy suture encircles the inferior mesenteric vein tributary. The left gastric or coronary vein arches above the superior border of the pancreas and passes obliquely across its anterior surface to the lesser curvature of the stomach. Immediately cephalad to this vein along the superior border of the pancreas, a portion of the left gastric artery may be seen.

In the upper portion of the specimen and to the right of center, a guy suture encircles the arch of the hepatic artery proximal to its bifurcation into an ascending left hepatic and a descending gastroduodenal artery. As stated previously, in this specimen the right and left hepatic arteries each arose separately from the arch formed by the hepatic artery. The right gastric artery, a branch of the left hepatic artery, is readily visible as it courses in an obliquity downward to the pyloroduodenal junction. The duodenal and pancreatic branches of the gastroduodenal artery may also be clearly seen.

The first branch of the gastroduodenal artery bifurcates at the superior border of the duodenum to supply portions of its anterior and posterior surfaces. This artery was first described in 1911 by Professor D. P. D. Wilkie of Edinburgh, Scotland, who named it the "supraduodenal artery." It is frequently referred to as the "artery of Wilkie." Its counterpart to the inferior border of the duodenum, which might logically be named the "infraduodenal artery," is visible as a relatively larger branch that arises from the right gastroepiploic artery. Between these two arteries, multiple retroduodenal branches from the gastroduodenal artery are visible, but there is no one main branch like that which Wilkie described and referred to as the "retroduodenal artery."

Below and to the right of center, a guy suture encircles the superior pancreaticoduodenal artery. The tortuosity of this vessel after its origin from the gastroduodenal artery is apparent. This artery courses between the duodenum and pancreas and anastomoses with the inferior pancreaticoduodenal artery, a branch of the superior mesenteric artery.

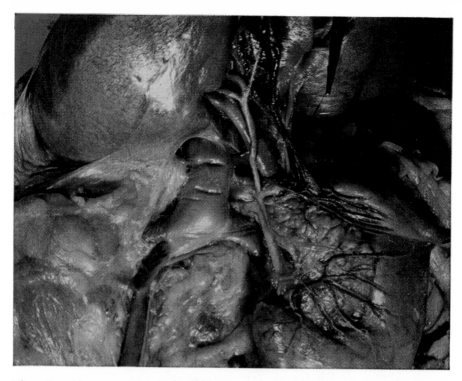

Plate E. The duodenum and head of the pancreas are mobilized and rotated toward the midline to show their relation to the surrounding structures. The inferior vena cava and its renal tributary veins are readily seen. The spermatic vein tributary empties into the inferior vena cava just caudad to the right renal vein. It is accompanied by the spermatic artery, which arises from the right renal artery and not directly from the aorta. The hepatic artery, which in this specimen arose from the superior mesenteric artery, courses cephalad, anterior to the left renal vein, and then arches over the superior border of the pancreas in front of the portal vein. The posterior pancreatico-duodenal vein empties into the portal vein just above this arch. From the arch, the right and left hepatic arteries arise separately. The right hepatic artery, more clearly visible, bifurcates anterior to the bifurcation of the portal vein into its right and left hepatic tributaries. The cystic artery is seen as a branch from the convex border of the right hepatic artery and extends upward to the gallbladder.

The cystic duct, to the left of and paralleling the cystic artery, unites with the common hepatic duct to form the common bile duct. The common bile duct is encircled by a guy suture of 000 silk, the ends of which are held in a clamp. The common bile duct passes between and beneath a venous arcade to enter first the substance of the pancreas and then the duodenum. The relation of the head and neck of the pancreas and its associated blood vessels to the rotated duodenal loop is clearly visible.

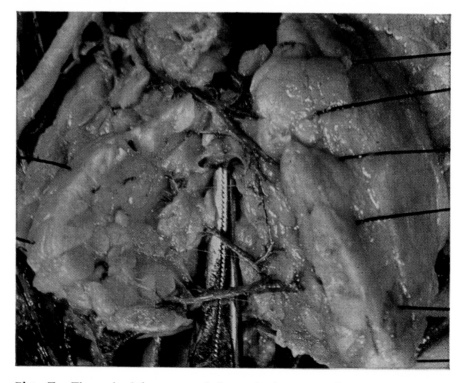

Plate F. The neck of the pancreas is incompletely transected and the respective segments are retracted with guy sutures of silk to show the vessels traversing the parenchyma of the pancreas. Overlying the tip of the clamp, the partially severed and eccentrically located pancreatic duct is visible. In the upper left-hand corner, a segment of the gastroduodenal artery and its branches to the pancreas may be seen.

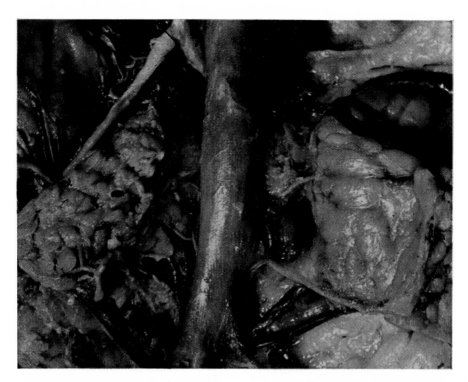

Plate G. The neck of the pancreas is transected and the distal segment is retracted to the left to show the origin of the portal vein by the junction of the superior mesenteric and the splenic veins. The two major venous trunks that form the superior mesenteric vein and their accompanying pancreatic tributary veins are partially visible in the lower central portion of the specimen.

At the left, the cut surface of the proximal segment of the pancreas and the open lumen of the eccentrically placed pancreatic duct are visible. Cephalad to this segment of the pancreas, the angulated arch formed by the hepatic artery and its gastroduodenal branch may be seen. A segment of the black silk guy suture that encircles the gastroduodenal artery at its origin is also visible. At the distal end of the gastroduodenal artery, a segment of one of its branches, the right gastroepiploic, which arises at a right angle from its parent trunk, may be seen.

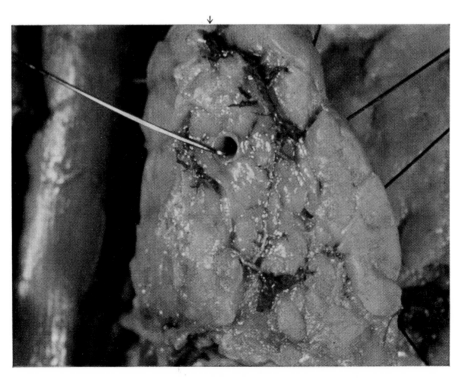

Plate H. The neck of the pancreas is completely transected, and the rich vascularity of its parenchyma is evident. A probe is in the patulous and eccentrically located pancreatic duct. The vein that parallels the posterior cut margin of the transected pancreas is the superior mesenteric vein in its caudad portion and the portal vein cephalad to the entrance of the splenic vein. A small segment of the superior border of the splenic vein is indicated by the arrow.

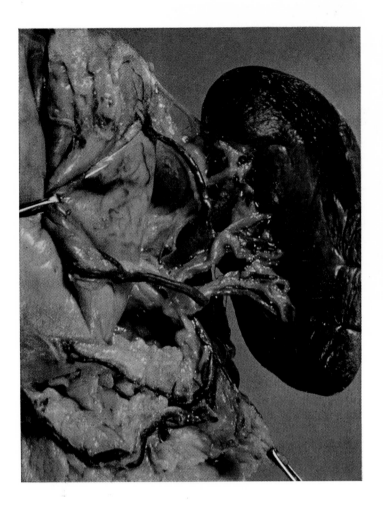

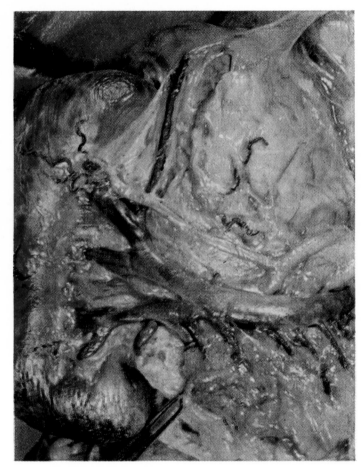

Plate I. This is an anterior view of the splenic hilum after excision of the gastrosplenic ligament. The intact vasa brevia and their relation to the greater curvature of the fundus of the stomach (grasped in clamp) and the splenic pedicle are visible. The left gastroepiploic branch of the splenic artery and its accompanying vein (the lowermost vessels) course in the fatty areolar layer of the gastrocolic ligament and give arterial branches and receive venous tributaries from the greater curvature of the stomach. The tortuosity of splenic arterial branches in the hilum is particularly well demonstrated.

Plate J. This is a close-up view of the splenic hilum posteriorly, and of its relation to the surrounding structures. The posterior aspect of the fundus of the stomach is visible in the upper right-hand quadrant and the tail of the pancreas in the lower right-hand quadrant. The interrelation of the splenic artery and vein and their respective branches and tributaries is clearly shown. The highest of the vasa brevia, which usually is the shortest and the largest, ascends vertically between the superior pole of the spleen and the fundus of the stomach. The identification of these vessels assumes particular surgical significance in the performance of a splenectomy. Also noteworthy are the multiple and obliquely directed pancreatic tributaries of the splenic vein. The isolation, ligation, and severance of these veins is an essential step in obtaining a sufficient length of the splenic vein for the performance of a splenorenal shunt.

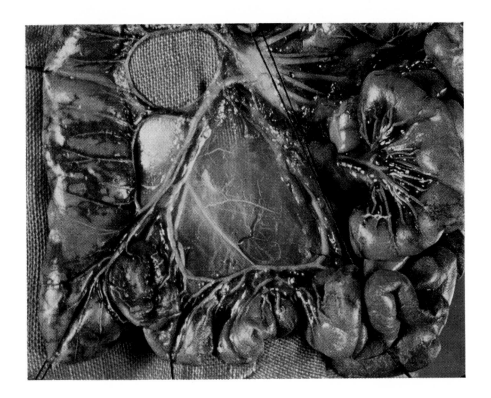

Plate K. This is an injection study in a fresh cadaver specimen to show the vascular supply of the small intestine and the right side of the colon. The specimen was obtained from a newborn infant, which accounts for the absence of fat in the mesentery of both the small and large bowel. The superior mesenteric artery is in the upper central portion of the specimen, and its multiple intestinal branches radiate in a fan-shaped pattern into the mesentery of the small intestine. The lowermost branch on the opposite side of the superior mesenteric artery is the ileocolic artery. This artery arches upward and then descends in an obliquity to the ileocolic region. The right colic artery arises at a right angle from the proximal third of the ileocolic artery and bifurcates into ascending and descending branches, which form anastomotic arcades with the ileocolic artery below and a colic artery above. Terminally, the ileocolic artery, through its long ileal arcade, reanastomoses with its parent trunk, the superior mesenteric artery, within the mesentery of the terminal ileum. From the ileal arcade, multiple branches are given off to supply the terminal ileum.

The guy suture of silk encircles the middle colic artery just distal to its origin from the superior mesenteric artery. Between the middle colic and the ileocolic arteries, a colic branch arises from the superior mesenteric and anastomoses with the right branch of the middle colic and the ascending branch of the right colic. This artery, though commonly present, is not frequently depicted in standard texts and atlases of anatomy. The right colic artery may arise directly from the superior mesenteric rather than from the ileocolic artery as depicted. Even when this obtains the colic branch previously described persists. Accordingly, it is not a compensatory artery that is only present when the right colic artery originates from the ileocolic artery.

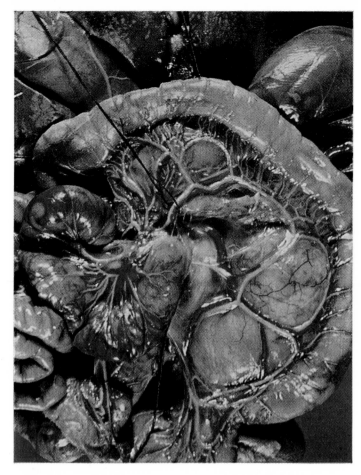

Plate L. The blood supply of the transverse and left side of the colon is demonstrated. The guy suture just along the center of the field encircles the middle colic artery and accompanying vein. This artery bifurcates into right and left branches. The right branch forms anastomotic arcades with the colic branches of the right side of the colon. The left branch unites with the ascending branch of the left colic to form the anastomotic magna of Riolan. The lower boundary of this space is formed by the inferior mesenteric vein, which may be seen arching cephalad behind the ligament of Treitz and beneath the middle colic vessels to empty ultimately into the splenic vein. The arterial pattern formed by the descending branch of the left colic artery and the sigmoidal vessels is visible.

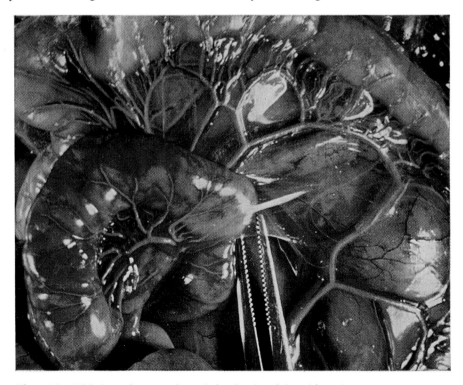

Plate M. This is a close-up view of the duodenojejunal junction and the base of the transverse mesocolon. This specimen, from a newborn, because of its absence of fat deposits, shows clearly the vascular structures. The tip of the open clamp is beneath the suspensory ligament (Treitz) of the duodenum. It lies in juxtaposition to the duodenum and inferior mesenteric vein. The middle colic artery is seen immediately cephalad to the tip of the clamp and the superior border of the first portion of the jejunum. Its anastomosing arcade with the ascending branch of the left colic artery, to form the anastomotic magna of Riolan, is also clearly shown. The body of the pancreas may be seen through the transparent mesocolon immediately below the arcade described earlier.

INTRODUCTION

JOHN H. MULHOLLAND

THERE ARE MANY methods to help a student learn *about* technical operative surgery; the only way he can learn to *perform* operations is by doing them. The creation of a complete surgeon is much more a matter of the development of thought processes than it is training in manual dexterity. Any help in the whole process must provide for the thinking element in a primary way. Offhand, it is difficult to picture how this requirement is met in a book illustrating operative technic, yet Dr. Madden has done so in this book. ·

The ideal author of such a work would be either an artist who is a surgeon, or a surgeon who is an artist. No such fortunate combination in one individual has come forth. The closest analogous person was the anatomist and artist combined in Leonardo. When an artist attempts to portray an operation without the thought processes of the surgeon, the result may be fine art but runs the risk of being untrue. Conversely, with the surgeon who sketches or draws his operations, the result is apt to be intelligible only to him.

The training of a medical artist, like the training of a surgeon, is long and arduous. Alfred Feinberg is a recognized master in this field, as Dr. Madden is in his. Their joint venture in this book is a happy one. Each must have striven by long conferences and exchange of ideas to acquire some of the viewpoint and skill of the other. Brödel has written "A medical artist's eye should not work merely like a camera, it should digest the object and bring out the features which justify the task of picturing the case, without, of course, neglecting the realistic and truthful characteristics."

Severe limitations are imposed on the surgeon by this method. He must transmit to the reader highly focused technical methods which he knows full well are individualistic. Steps he takes are directed toward an objective which may be achieved by different instruments, by different exposure, and perhaps even by different attitudes. His depictions are then subject to minor and superficial criticisms which do not consider the objectives. Many of the illustrations of Dr. Madden's methods will almost certainly provoke the reaction "I do that differently." This is the price paid for completeness and definitiveness in the drawings. Such a reaction is on deeper thought a good lesson learned, particularly if both Dr. Madden and the reading student are referring to an operative maneuver as important as exposing the right hepatic artery in the early stages of a cholecystectomy. The point is that the artery is exposed.

The profit to a student reading this book is gained from what passes through his mind as he looks at the picture. The more profound the student, the greater the profit. Previous operative training, study of disease, experience, and intelligence contribute to the value of his thoughts. A number of factors combine to produce an idea which is only aroused by the picture.

The real test of the excellence of an illustration of operative technic is how such an illustration would stand without explanatory text. It would seem that the perfect drawing would require no text. Certainly an experienced surgeon, studying a good illustration, could compose an explanatory text of his own. Such a book as this, however, is for students at all levels of learning. For beginners to study the illustrated steps of an operation which they will subsequently be observing for the first time, an explanatory text is essential.

Another good feature of the book is that all the operations were performed by one surgeon in the presence of the artist making his sketches. Sketches drawn under such circumstances are the result not only of what the artist sees, but also of what he knows about the surgeon's plan and method for carrying out that plan. The final drawing is completed after a joint review of the sketches by both artist and surgeon. The book's unity of purpose precludes an encyclopedic presentation

1

of all surgical operations. The areas of specialization are not covered; only those procedures which one active general surgeon performs, and which therefore are the content of general surgery are shown.

In many drawings of operative technic the exposed structures are beautifully depicted as they appear at the completion of exposure. A student may see in such drawings how the field should look. What he ought to see is how to make the field look that way. For example, the mark of a skillful abdominal surgeon is his ability to reveal structures by accurate peritoneal incisions. The most important step in exposure of the biliary ducts and vessels is de-

lineation of peritoneum overlying them and a precise incision which unfolds the peritoneal layer. The drawings in this book carefully indicate these vital steps.

To paraphrase Abraham Flexner's statement about medicine—We should admit once and for all that surgery is difficult to learn and impossible to teach. There are no short cuts in time or method which will relieve a student of effort. He must develop himself. The stimulation of ideas through all his senses is as far as any aid can go. This book should serve well to promote thought by showing good drawings of good operations.

PRE- AND POSTOPERATIVE CARE WITH CONSIDERATION OF FLUID AND ELECTROLYTE BALANCE IN THE SURGICAL PATIENT

HENRY T. RANDALL

THE TASK of the surgeon is, by the training of his mind and the skill of his hands, to restore health to his fellow men who fall prey to a variety of diseases, accidents, and infections amenable to operative correction. Yet he who would be a surgeon, if he wishes to be more than merely a highly skilled mechanic of human tissue, must, in addition to developing skill and judgment in the operating room, learn the science and the art of patient care. In making the decision as to whether and when to operate, in the preparation of the patient for surgery, in the operation itself, and in the postoperative convalescence, the surgeon must take full responsibility for his acts and his judgment. Though the operation is the peak of the experience for both patient and surgeon, preparation and postoperative care often spell the difference between success and failure. Today's surgery involves increasing consideration of human physiology. The effect of the disease on normal function, the effect of trauma—including surgery—in producing a pattern of response, and the effect of the surgery in producing permanent alterations in normal function are all of great importance. The surgeon's responsibility is never finished, for if he is to evaluate critically what he has done and thus learn to do it better he must follow his patients carefully, keep accurate records, and compare his work with those of others, so that all may benefit.

The purpose of this chapter is to outline the high points of some major aspects of pre- and postoperative care, and to stimulate further interest in the how and the why of the patient's response to surgery.

PREOPERATIVE CARE AND EVALUATION

Surgical preoperative care begins the moment that a decision is reached that surgery should, or even might possibly, be used in the treatment of a patient. Its duration may vary from a few minutes of rapidly (though carefully) carried out preparation of the obvious surgical emergency while the operating room is being readied to many days of carefully thought out and systematic evaluation preceding an elective or semielective operation. The objective is to bring the patient into the operating room in the best possible physical and psychological state to withstand the procedure. Often great exercise of judgment in the patient's interest is involved to determine when he is ready for surgery.

Modified only by the degree of genuine emergency which exists, the beginning of preoperative care should consist of a careful and detailed history and physical examination of the surgical patient. The history should begin with the presenting complaint and with the diagnosis if established and should include in sufficient detail the patient's description of the onset and development of his illness together with the answers to certain guiding questions which occur to the examiner as he listens to the patient's story. All patients should be questioned with regard to their height, present weight, and whether or not they have lost weight. If he has lost weight, the patient should be asked how rapidly and over what period of time the loss has occurred. Those who have a positive history of weight loss should be interrogated concerning their dietary intake, particularly during the weeks immediately prior to admission. This will give a valuable clue with regard to nutritional status. All surgical patients should be questioned as to whether they have had previous surgery and if so of what type and when. They should be asked whether they had any particular untoward reactions to surgery or anesthesia, and these facts should be recorded. A history of severe injuries is also important, as is a history of drugs and medications which a patient is taking or has taken in the past. Clues to important other illnesses may be obtained in this fashion. A history of the use of alcohol and of tobacco is of considerable value in evaluating the surgical patient. So too is a sensitivity or allergy, particularly to any drug or medication, including antibiotics. This should be followed by a careful system review asking questions with regard to the central nervous system —including organs of special sense, respiratory tract, cardiovascular system, gastrointestinal tract system, genitourinary system—and a brief neuropsychiatric review. A menstrual history should be included for all adult female patients.

Physical examination, too often superficial on surgical services and confined to the immediate surgical lesion, should be sufficiently complete in detail to confirm the medical history and to evaluate the status of major systems. The anesthesiologist should never be the first individual to take the patient's blood pressure. A statement with regard to apparent age, sex, general appearance, and state of nutrition should be included. Do not forget that the ophthalmoscope gives ready access to the evaluation of the degree of arteriosclerosis which a patient has and that a rough approximation of the efficiency of the cardiovascular and respiratory systems can be obtained by the simple process of walking up a flight of stairs with the patient. It takes only a few minutes to check the Achilles, patellar tendon, and Babinski's reflexes of any patient; these should be recorded. A rectal examination should be made and recorded for all patients, and a pelvic examination should be made and recorded for all female patients except virginal ones.

The history taking and the examinations are time-consuming and in hospitals are usually assigned to the intern or to the junior assistant resident. The early development of a *systematic method* of taking a history and of doing a physical examination will not only greatly facilitate doing them but will also prevent overlooking occasional highly important findings.

BASIC LABORATORY DATA

No patient should go to the operating room for elective surgery without there being *recorded in the chart and observed by the responsible surgical team* at least:

1. A routine urinalysis, including microscopic analysis and determination of albumin and glucose. The specific gravity of the casually voided specimen is of doubtful significance. Remember that in female patients the microscopic examination of urine is of significant value only on a catheterized specimen.

2. A complete blood count which should include at least a hemoglobin determination, a total white cell count, and a statement concerning the apparent normality of distribution of platelets.

3. An x-ray or roentgenogram of the chest, or a documented chest film that was made within the previous six months without interval respiratory history.

In addition, elderly patients should have determinations of the fasting blood sugar and a BUN or NPN made; and if there is any suspicion of cardiac history, an electrocardiograph baseline should be taken. Debilitated patients with recent weight loss, many of whom are likely to have cancer, should also have the total serum protein determined and one or two basic liver function tests. In patients with emphysema, asthma, partial obstruction of the airway, pulmonary infection, or atelectasis, the baseline CO_2 and chloride of the plasma should be determined, and if possible a blood pH should be obtained, in order to assess the degree of compensation for the respiratory acidosis that exists in these conditions.

BLOOD TRANSFUSIONS AND BLOOD REPLACEMENT

While the hemoglobin and hematocrit are likely to be fairly good indices of the circulating blood volume and red cell mass in the otherwise healthy patient, certain types of surgical patients are likely to have a diminished blood volume which is *not necessarily reflected* in a change in hemoglobin and hematocrit. This is particularly true if the patient is simultaneously deficient in circulating blood and dehydrated. Notoriously likely to have diminished blood volumes are patients with cancer, particularly cancer of the gastrointestinal tract; patients who have had chronic bleeding, as seen with uterine fibroids and particularly with ulcerative colitis; and patients with chronic infection of any sort, particularly if it is sufficient to give them a low grade fever. This phenomenon, sometimes designated as "chronic shock," was first described by Clark and Lyons (1) and has since become generally recognized among surgeons. Patients whose blood volume is not restored before surgery are likely to become hypotensive under anesthesia and will tolerate any surgical procedure very poorly. Blood volume technics involving the use of either the Evan's blue dye or radioactive iodinated serum albumin are widely available and should be used when indicated (2, 3, 4). A rule of thumb method of assessment is to give the patient with a suspected deficit a 500 ml. blood transfusion, *wait 24 hours,* then determine the hematocrit and compare it with a baseline hematocrit. If the hematocrit is low initially and only a one or two percentage point rise occurs with a 500 ml. transfusion, give another 500 ml., wait 24 hours, and repeat the hematocrit evaluations. When a 500 ml. transfusion in a patient who is not dehydrated produces a rise of the hematocrit to a normal range with a jump of three to five percentage points 24 hours after the transfusion is given, one may assume that the cardiovascular system has its normal volume of blood.

In the patient who is acutely injured or who has just had a major hemorrhage, the red blood count and hematocrit will be deceptive. It takes one or two hours for the process of hemodilution to begin, and 24 hours for it to be complete following a loss of blood. Remember that patients with multiple fractures and crushing injuries, though they may not have lost blood externally, will lose large volumes of blood into the site of injury and thus effectively deplete their blood volume. The best replacement is, of course, whole blood. The next best is probably plasma. In emergencies, dextran or polyvinylpyrrolidone (P.V.P.) may be used. Remember to *take blood for cross matching before starting either dextran or P.V.P.* because both interfere seriously with crossmatching technics. A useful rule of thumb to remember in the patient acutely injured or suffering hemorrhage is that it takes approximately a 15 per cent loss of circulating blood volume to drop the systolic blood pressure to 100 in a normotensive patient. A 25 per cent loss of circulating blood volume will result in a systolic pressure of about 80. If the systolic blood pressure is 60 or less, one can assume that about *30 to 40 per cent* of the circulating volume has been lost. Since the blood volume averages about 8.5 per cent of the body weight of the normal adult, this means a loss of the order of 1,000 ml. to drop the systolic pressure to 100 mm., of 1,500 ml. to drop it to 80 mm., and of over 2,000 ml. to drop it below 60 mm. of mercury. Although in some cases 500 ml. of blood by transfusion may serve temporarily to raise the systolic blood pressure, this amount is inadequate to relieve the marked peripheral vasoconstriction and renal vasoconstriction which exist. Accordingly, 1,000 ml. or more of whole blood should be given initially when the adult patient is suffering from acute trauma or hemorrhage and has a systolic blood pressure of 80 mm. of mercury.

DEHYDRATION AND ELECTROLYTE LOSS OR IMBALANCE

Dehydration results when the patient is unable to take an adequate amount of water or when he loses an excessive amount through vomiting, diarrhea, and sweating, either alone or in combination. Almost invariably the dehydrated patient has some degree of electrolyte imbalance, for the dehydration is most often the result of malfunction of the gastrointestinal tract. Dehydration due to pure water loss is seen in surgical patients only in the event of obstruction of the esophagus and inability to swallow or in the rare event of a patient with obstruction of the gastrointestinal tract who is unable to vomit. Sometimes acute water loss dehydration is seen in the postoperative period in patients who receive an inadequate parenteral replacement of fluid. Usually, however, water is lost with electrolytes from the gastrointestinal tract in either vomitus or diarrhea or both. Relatively pure electrolyte loss with the development of the "low salt syndrome" is sometimes seen in patients with marked diarrhea who because of thirst take large amounts of water by mouth but who do not replace the lost electrolytes. The usual picture is a mixed dehydration consisting of both water loss and electrolyte loss, and this is the type which has been demonstrated to be the most dangerous (5, 6). In assessing dehydration, a history, if it can be obtained, is most important. How long has the patient failed to take in fluids by mouth? How long has the patient been vomiting or had diarrhea? What, if anything, has he been able to take in between episodes of vomiting? Remembering the total oral intake of water, including water in food, for the average patient in a day is of the order of 2,000 to 2,500 ml., a rough estimate of the deficit can be approximated.

Clinical symptoms of dehydration are dry tongue, dry mucous membranes, and loss of skin turgor; in severe cases, softness of the eyeballs, restlessness, and hypotension are also found. The urine is usually scanty and of high specific gravity. The hemoglobin and hematocrit are elevated unless the patient had a preexisting anemia, in which case they may be normal. The plasma protein is elevated during the first 24 hours of acute dehydration, and may give a clue to the extent of dehydration in a patient whose hemoglobin is unreliable because of possible preexisting anemia. An acute loss of 2 or 3 per cent of body weight as water is sufficient to produce symptoms, and an acute loss of 6 per cent of body weight by dehydration will produce peripheral vascular collapse. In the average 70 kg. adult, a rise in the hematocrit to 60 or in the serum protein to 9.4 gm. is indicative of a loss of extracellular fluid of the order of 4,000 to 5,000 ml. Acute dehydration is usually seen in the surgical patient with obstruction of the pylorus or of the small bowel and occasionally with obstruction of the esophagus. Volvulus, acute peritonitis due to rupture of a viscus, and acute pancreatitis present a similar picture, but in these instances the major fluid loss is by translocation within the patient rather than loss externally. In acute peritonitis and acute pancreatitis, the loss of plasma protein and plasma volume into the area of injury is sufficiently great so that the patient may present the picture of hemorrhagic shock; a full blown peritonitis or acute hemorrhagic pancreatitis is roughly equivalent to a 30 per cent third-degree body burn in the amount of fluid necessary for replacement.

A different picture entirely is presented by a chronic dehydration as seen, for example, in the patient with a slowly obstructing lesion of the sigmoid colon. Here, relatively enormous amounts of fluid may be lost, and the patient may lose 10 to 12 pounds in weight over a period of 10 days or so. The fluid losses are proportional to the total body water, being largely intracellular in type, and only a modest rise in hemoglobin and hematocrit and little or no rise in plasma protein are seen. The picture of dehydration is not nearly as acute as is seen with the loss of perhaps half as much fluid in a patient who has become dehydrated from small bowel obstruction in 24 hours.

Replacement depends upon the body compartment from which fluid is lost. In the case of hemorrhage, intravascular replacement of whole blood, plasma or plasma substitutes is indicated. In the case of acute dehydration due to excessive fluid loss from the gastrointestinal tract, in the first 48 hours the loss is almost entirely extracellular. If it is by vomitus, sodium chloride is the initial replacement fluid of choice. If the patient has been vomiting for more than 18 hours, it is wise to check the CO_2 and if this is below 18 mEq per liter (40 volumes per cent) a mixture of two thirds isotonic sodium chloride and one-third ⅙ molar sodium bicarbonate is a better initial replacement fluid since sodium chloride is initially *acid* in its effect on the extracellular fluid (the chloride content is 156 mEq per liter). Two or three liters may be run in rapidly during the period of time that the patient is getting abdominal x-rays and being prepared for the operating room. A good start in replacement of acute dehydration can be made within an hour, and *well indicated surgery for an acute intraabdominal emergency should not be delayed unduly by efforts at rehydration.* They can be continued through the operative period and into the postoperative period if necessary. On the other hand, it should be remembered that the dehydrated patient also has a dehydrated circulating blood volume, and shock is more likely to occur under anesthesia and surgery.

The chronically dehydrated patient presents a different picture entirely. Whereas 3 to 5 liters of saline or saline bicarbonate mixtures may be necessary to rehydrate the acutely dehydrated patient, an equivalent amount in a chronically dehydrated patient would result in overexpansion of the extracellular fluid space and might precipitate cardiac failure. The chronicaly dehydrated patient will take large amounts of glucose, water, and potassium salts *in a period of several days* to restore his intracellular compartments to relatively normal size. Only modest amounts of saline or saline and bicarbonate will be necessary to restore the extracellular fluid compartment to normal size. Patients who are dehydrated as a result of excessive diarrhea are very likely to have a metabolic acidosis as the result of the loss of excessive amounts of base in the stool. Such patients should be rehydrated by using a ratio of 2/3 volume of isotonic sodium chloride and 1/3 volume of 1/6 M sodium bicarbonate initially, and the amount of bicarbonate should be regulated by measurements of the CO_2 of the plasma.

It will be noted that no mention has been made of the administration of glucose. When patients require rapid rehydration the administration of a hypertonic solution such as glucose in saline should be avoided. Glucose cannot be administered to the average patient at a rate which exceeds about *0.5 gm. per kilogram of body weight per hour,* which sets the maximum speed of a 5 per cent glucose solution at an hour and a half per liter for the average patient. Administration at rates more rapid than this should be avoided as this is likely to result in an osmotic diuresis with the loss through the urine of as much as or more fluid than is administered. Glucose should of course be provided in parenteral fluids as soon as the rate of infusion can be slowed down sufficiently to permit its use. When starvation acidosis and ketonuria are present, a small amount of glucose should be administered from time to time during the rehydration process. In the presence of ketonuria, diabetic acidosis should be suspected. If the diagnosis is confirmed, solutions of glucose and insulin should be prescribed. Table 1 summarizes the types of dehydration and replacement therapy. The effectiveness of replacement of extracellular fluid may be judged by the rate of fall of the hematocrit, rising urine volume, and the improvement in the general clinical appearance of the patient.

PREPARATION OF THE GASTROINTESTINAL TRACT FOR SURGERY

Whenever abdominal, thoracoabdominal, or retroperitoneal surgery is to be undertaken, experience has taught that it is well to have the gastrointestinal tract at rest and at least moderately well cleaned out. The stomach should be empty before an anesthetic is administered, and if this is doubtful, gastric aspiration should be performed before the patient is anesthetized. This is of particular importance in patients who undergo emergency operations and who may well either have eaten food in the immediate past or have accumulated secretions in the stomach.

Many surgeons like to have a cleansing enema given the night before operation. Some like to add in addition a mild cathartic such as 15 to 20 ml. of 50 per cent magnesium sulfate given the afternoon before surgery, followed by a cleansing enema the night before surgery.

When more extensive bowel preparation is necessary, as for example in surgery of the large bowel, modern trends are toward the use of antibiotics either of the slowly hydrolyzed sulfa type or the broad spectrum mycin type, combined with cleansing enemas. It should be remembered that suppression of bacterial growth in the large bowel causes the body to be deprived of vitamin K which is formed by these organisms; therefore supplemental vitamin K, 5 to 10 mg. per day is necessary to prevent hypoprothrombinemia. Some surgeons still use extensive purgation in preparation of the large bowel. As a result of such purgation, the patient will become dehydrated and develop a metabolic acidosis as the result of loss of base with the diarrheal stools. Restitution of normal acid-base equilibrium and rehydration requires under these circumstances the administration of an average of 1,000 ml. of 0.9 per cent sodium chloride and 500 ml. of either 1/6 molar sodium lactate or sodium bi-

Table 1. Types of Dehydration and Replacement

	BLOOD PLASMA	EXTRACELLULAR FLUID, NaCl, HCO$_3$	INTRACELLULAR FLUID, K$^+$, HPO$_4$	GLUCOSE AND WATER
1. Hemorrhage	+ + + +	+	−	Baseline
2. Acute pancreatitis, diffuse peritonitis, burns, and crushing injury	+ + +	+ + +	−	Baseline
3. Acute dehydration < 48 hours with G.I. tract losses	+	+ + + +	Late potassium deficit likely	Baseline
4. Chronic dehydration > 48 hours to a week or more	±	+ +	+ + +	+ + +
5. Water deprivation	±	+ +	+	+ + + +

carbonate, usually the day before operation. Otherwise the patient will go into surgery both dehydrated and with a hyperchloremic acidosis (7).

The usual preoperative orders for patients include depriving them of all oral intake beginning at midnight the night before surgery. If the patient is an adult and the surgery is to be done the following morning, very little dehydration results. If, however, the operation is not scheduled until mid-afternoon, significant dehydration can result, and the patient should receive in the morning an infusion of approximately 1,000 to 1,500 ml. of 5 per cent glucose and water. With children the situation is more critical. Children should be scheduled with first priority on the operative schedule in the morning, and if for any reason their operation is delayed, they should be infused to prevent dehydration. Infants and young children are particularly susceptible to rapid dehydration on deprivation of fluid intake.

THE PSYCHOLOGIC PREPARATION OF THE PATIENT

Surgeons should never lose track of the fact that their patients are individual human beings. Brought into the strange environment of a hospital and subjected to a series of examinations and laboratory tests, they are often frightened and confused. A little time on the part of the surgeon devoted to sitting down and discussing with the patient what to expect will greatly ameliorate these fears. It is usually unwise to go into the details of a surgical operation; but it is certainly wise that the patient know the nature of the operation to be performed, approximately why it is to be performed, and what he can expect the day of operation and immediately postoperatively. Reassurance that anesthesia will be complete before the operation is performed helps allay the fear of pain. A simple description of the effect of preoperative medication is also helpful. Tell the patient where he will be on awakening from the anesthesia; forewarn him about tubes and the like if they are to be used; and reassure him about the ability to control postoperative pain. All this is exceedingly important. A little time spent in describing to a responsible member of the family the nature of the operation planned and your evaluation of the operative risk will give you a strong and loyal supporter instead of an uninformed,

often critical, and sometimes litigation-minded adversary.

THE PREPARATION OF THE SURGEON

Every surgeon should teach himself the discipline of personally checking all the aspects of the preoperative preparation of the patient before transportation to the operating room. A good rule, wise to cultivate early, is for the surgeon to examine the patient and review the work-up within 24 hours preceding the operation. A brief but complete summary note of the pertinent findings should be written in the chart; and the contemplated operative procedure, the reasons for choosing the particular procedure, and the evaluation of the patient as an operative risk should also be entered in the chart. The surgeon should never be too proud to review the technical aspects of an infrequently performed operation and the anatomic details of the operative area.

FURTHER FLUID AND ELECTROLYTE BALANCE CONSIDERATIONS IN SURGICAL PATIENTS

The term *balance* implies an equilibrium among two or more different things. Maintaining fluid and electrolyte balance in the surgical patient requires an understanding of the normal daily intake and output of water and the major electrolytes required for body economy. In addition, abnormal losses of water and electrolytes must be measured and replaced, and deficiencies or excesses acquired before treatment begins must be considered. The problem may be divided into three parts (8). The first of these, *baseline,* answers the question "What do I have to give the patient if he is wholly or partially deprived of oral intake but is otherwise in normal or relatively normal condition?" The second, which we have called *dynamic loss,* answers the question "What immediate losses does the patient have as the result of his disease or of the operative procedures, or of both, that are abnormal, and what is required to replace these losses?" The third category, *deficits* or *excesses,* answers the question "What preexisting deficiencies or excesses in water, electrolytes, and circulating blood volume does the patient have at the time I begin to treat him?" The total daily intake of water, electrolytes, and blood or blood replacements will be the sum of the baseline requirements plus the dynamic loss, plus a proportion of the deficiencies in water, electrolytes, and blood volume. Allowance is made for excesses if they exist.

When patients are dependent upon the surgeon for all or part of their intake requirements, at least a daily evaluation of the status of baseline, dynamic loss, and a critical evaluation of deficiencies should be made. When volumes of fluid and electrolyte turnover are large this evaluation may be required on a 12- or even an 8-hour basis.

One of the most important adjuncts to water and electrolyte balance is an accurate record of intake and output. All fluids administered to the patient, the type of fluids, and their electrolyte content should be recorded on the intake side of the ledger; and all measured losses and estimated insensible losses should be recorded on the output side. A daily recording of the patient's body weight is helpful in maintaining the fluid and electrolyte balance of the surgical patient. This can be done either with bed-type scales or improvised scales even with the sickest surgical patient, and it is for the sick patient that it is most needed. The average adult surgical patient should be expected to lose in body weight approximately 300 to 500 gm. per day, since it is not yet possible to maintain an adequate caloric intake parenterally. Larger amounts of weight loss are to be expected in patients with fever and of course in patients of larger body size.

1. Baseline. The average patient requires about 35 ml. of water per kilogram per day for baseline replacement. This amount is somewhat increased in the lean-bodied, young, athletic adult and approximates 45 to 50 ml. per day in the child 1 to 5 years old. In infants the daily requirement of water in proportion to body weight rises to remarkable levels and may reach as much as 150 ml. per kilogram per day. Fever increases the need for baseline water by increasing insensible loss through evaporation. An average of 500 ml. additional is required for each 3 degrees Fahrenheit increase in body temperature in the adult. The elderly patient, the obese patient, and the debilitated patient require less than the normal amount. A cardiac or nephrotic patient, who has an already overexpanded extracellular fluid space, benefits by the restriction of his baseline intake to approximately one half of average requirements. Thus, the average adult will require 2,000 to 2,500 ml. of water daily by parenteral route if he is deprived of all oral intake. To this is added water of oxidation within the body and preformed water obtained from destroyed cells to the amount of 300 to 500 ml. additional.

The electrolyte requirement for a baseline in surgical patients should not exceed a maximum of 4.5 gm. of sodium chloride per day (76 mEq of each ion), that contained in 500 ml. of 0.9 per cent sodium chloride. Only in the presence of excessive sweating should this baseline sodium chloride be increased, although much larger amounts of sodium chloride may be required to replace losses by abnormal routes or to replace deficits existing at the time of the onset of treatment. It is wise also to include in the baseline requirements, except in patients with renal failure, a daily intake of 40 to 60 mEq of potassium in the form of potassium chloride.

It has been shown that 100 gm. of glucose per day in the average adult will reduce nitrogen loss from starvation by 50 per cent. Therefore *100 gm. of glucose per day* is a minimum requirement in baseline parenteral fluid. This should preferably be given in two divided infusions, 8 to 12 hours apart. Loading the body with 100 gm. of glucose over a period of 2 or 3 hours, and allowing the patient to starve for the remaining 21, is expecting too much of the liver from the standpoint of glycogen storage. Additional calories should be given parenterally to the debilitated patient and to the patient who is to be on parenteral fluids for more than three or four days.

Parenteral amino acid administration replaces some of the nitrogen loss even though caloric intake may be inadequate. It is of doubtful value in the healthy adult who is to be on parenteral fluids for one to three or four days and who will then resume normal gastrointestinal tract intake of protein. It is of great value combined with glucose and, *when available,* intravenous fat in the debilitated patient and in the patient who must remain for long periods of time on parenteral fluids. However, from 35 to 60 calories per kilogram per day are required to maintain caloric balance in the postoperative patient, and this is as yet a relatively unachievable goal.

Table 2 illustrates in tabular form the basic requirements for baseline fluids and electrolytes in the normal adult, the debilitated patient, and the elderly or the obese patient. It may be observed that most of the require-

Table 2. Daily Baseline Requirements

	NORMAL ADULT	DEBILITATED PATIENT	ELDERLY OR OBESE
Water	35 ml./kg. Average 2,000 ml./day	30 ml./kg. Average 1,500 ml./day	25 ml./kg. (1,500)
Na+, Cl-	76 mEq/day maximum	less to 0	less to 0
K+	40 mEq	Usually > 40 mEq	40 mEq
Carbohydrate	100 gm. minimum	At least 150 gm. in divided doses	100 gm. minimum
*Parenteral vitamins	No demonstrable need except for vitamin C	B and C in therapeutic doses	Usually B and C in modest amounts
Protein (amino acids)	Some nitrogen-sparing action, but probably not needed	Essential	If on prolonged I.V. therapy

* Vitamin K in all patients with liver disease, jaundice, or on oral antibiotics.

ments can be met with solutions of 5 or 10 per cent glucose in water, and that relatively small amounts of electrolytes are required. A typical baseline order for a 70 kg. adult with 3 degrees of fever would be of 500 ml. of 5 per cent glucose in 0.9 per cent sodium chloride, and 2,500 ml. of 5 per cent glucose in water containing a total of 60 mEq of potassium chloride. *The potassium chloride solution should never exceed 40 mEq per liter in concentration.* The volume of replacement fluid prescribed should be given in divided doses, half in the morning and half in the evening.

2. Dynamic Loss. The surgical patient has two major routes for the abnormal loss of water and electrolytes: the gastrointestinal tract and wounds, particularly those that are exposed to the external environment. External abnormal losses should be replaced as nearly as possible volume for volume. The electrolyte content of these fluids varies with the type and site of their loss. Table 3 gives the average values.

Considering gastrointestinal tract losses, it may be noticed (Table 3) that with the exception of bile and pancreatic juice, gastrointestinal tract fluids are *hypotonic* to the plasma with respect to sodium and chloride ion concentration and therefore require somewhat less than isotonic electrolyte replacement. Most gastric juice is acid and contains chloride in excess of sodium. The excess of chloride loss is high in the patient with gastric or duodenal ulcer and low in the debilitated and elderly patient with achlorhydria. In most patients when chloride is lost by vomitus or gastric suction with gastric juice, sodium is excreted in the urine in the form of sodium bicarbonate, and the ultimate loss to the body is approximately equal in the two ions. For this reason, *sodium chloride is the replacement fluid of choice* for gastric juice loss.

Small intestinal fluid contains practically equal amounts of sodium and chloride ions although the amount of total base (sodium and potassium) lost increases progressively down the gastrointestinal tract. Because of the slightly increased base loss when compared with chloride, small bowel replacement when the volumes are large (1,000 ml. or more a day) requires the addition of small amounts of either sodium bicarbonate or sodium lactate to the replacement regime as shown in Table 3. Bile is in effect an ultrafiltrate of plasma containing no protein but sodium, potassium, and chloride in approximately the same concentrations as found in plasma. Pancreatic juice is exceptionally alkaline with a large content of sodium bicarbonate, and the loss of large volumes can cause a rapid and excessive loss of base and the occurrence of a metabolic acidosis. Losses from wounds are considered essentially the same as the loss of a plasma solution with electrolytes the same as in the plasma and the protein content only slightly less.

Table 3. Replacement of External Losses

APPROXIMATE VALUES MEQ. PER LITER LOSS*

	Na	K	Cl
1. Vomitus or Gastric Suction (acid)	60	20	100
2. Small Bowel Content (faintly alkaline)	100	10–30	96
3. Bile (quite alkaline)	140	5–10	100
4. Pancreatic Juice (very alkaline)	140	10	70
5. Diarrhea (above 500 ml.)	120–140	30	90
6. Wound Packing and Serous Drainage	140	10	100

(1) Replace gastric suction with ⅔ volume 0.9% NaCl and ⅓ as 5% glucose with 20 mEq KCl per liter.

(2) Replace small bowel and diarrheal losses with 70% volume 0.9% NaCl (with glucose), 20% volume glucose in water, and 10% volume with either M/6 sodium lactate or M/6 $NaHCO_3$. Potassium losses tend to increase, and ·chloride to decrease, the lower the point of change in small bowel. K^+ loss must be replaced.

(3) Replace bile loss as if it were a protein-free plasma filtrate. ⅔ volume as 0.9% NaCl (with glucose), ⅓ volume of M/6 $NaHCO_3$ or lactate (oral replacement for chronic fistulae 6 gm. enteric coated NaCl, 4 gm. $NaHCO_3$ per liter loss).

(4) Replace pancreatic juice with ½ volume 0.9% NaCl (with glucose) and ½ volume M/6 sodium lactate or $NaHCO_3$.

(5) Same as 2.

(6) Wound drainages are usually of the same electrolyte content as plasma, with variable amounts of protein up to 50 gm. per liter.

* When volumes of drainage are large (>1500 ml.), it is wise to determine the exact electrolyte content. The above values are averages, but considerable variability exists from patient to patient.

Internal fluid shifts are somewhat more difficult to assess but are not difficult to visualize when one considers the extensive edema of the burn, or the large volumes of fluid which can and do accumulate within the small bowel in adynamic ileus or intestinal obstruction. These volumes of fluid and their electrolytes *are effectively lost to the extracellular fluid during the period of their entrapment in a localized area.* Their losses must be replaced at least in part in order to maintain the extracellular fluid and the circulating blood volume. They differ from outright external losses only in that when the causative conditions are corrected, the fluid and electrolytes return to the general extracellular fluid volume. When this happens the patient receives in effect an auto-infusion which may seriously overload the extracellular fluid space *unless parenteral therapy is markedly curtailed.* Figure 1 illustrates this concept, which has been named the "third space" of injury and shows its formation, the effect of treatment and its resolution (8).

Major alterations in water and electrolyte balance result in two types of disability: *(a)* changes in the volume of extracellular fluid space, cell water, or circulating volume; and *(b)* changes in the relative electrolyte concentrations. Both phenomena usually exist together, although this is not necessarily the case. The surgeon should familiarize himself with the effect of relative changes of ion concentrations in the plasma and with the meanings of the terms *metabolic acidosis, metabolic alkalosis, respiratory acidosis,* and *respiratory alkalosis.* He should be familiar with the reasons why the CO_2 combining power of the plasma is *not* necessarily an indication of alkalosis when it is elevated or of acidosis when it is depressed. The CO_2 of the plasma is elevated

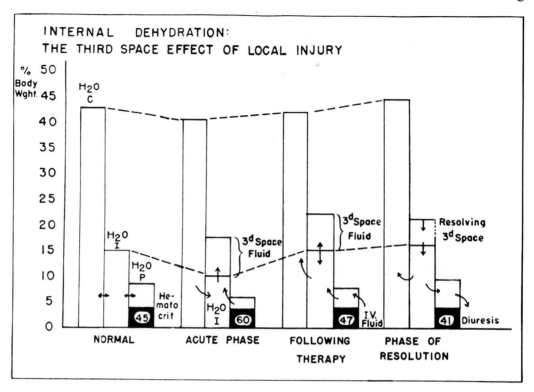

Fig. 1. Illustrating the effects of internal dehydration by injury or ileus with the creation of a third fluid space of unavailable fluid which dehydrates plasma and cells and diminishes available interstitial fluid. Replacement therapy restores normal volumes, and subsequent resolution of third space may overexpand available extracellular fluid. H_2O C is cell water, H_2O I is interstitial fluid, and H_2O P is plasma water.

both in metabolic alkalosis and in respiratory acidosis and is depressed in metabolic acidosis and respiratory alkalosis. Table 4 summarizes the major plasma changes found in these four states and indicates briefly the major causes of each (9).

3. Deficits or Excesses. As noted in the discussion of preoperative preparation, dehydration, loss of circulatory blood volume, and losses of electrolytes can occur in the postoperative period if adequate attention is not paid to the replacement of baseline and of dynamic losses. A rule of thumb to remember is this: *if deficits occur quickly, they may be replaced quickly, and if slow to occur, they must be replaced slowly.*

Excesses of water and extracellular fluid may exist in patients with chronic cardiac failure, in patients in the nephrotic stage of nephritis, and in patients with malnutrition and hypoproteinemia. Ascites and pleural effusions are special types of the same sort of problem. In general, baseline water should be reduced and sodium and chloride eliminated

in the parenteral replacement therapy of these patients. Large volumes of dynamic loss must, however, be replaced with appropriate electrolytes included.

Another special set of circumstances exists in the patient with acute renal failure from trauma, incompatible blood, hypotension, or renal poison. Baseline water is restricted to insensible loss (800 to 1,000 ml. per day). Ten per cent glucose is administered to reduce nitrogen breakdown, and small amounts of sodium bicarbonate are given to keep the CO_2 of the plasma at about 15 mEq. Articles on this subject should be consulted relative to the management of these cases (10, 11). *Certain iatrogenic problems* should be mentioned. Water intoxication, characterized by weakness, delirium, hypotension, and sometimes convulsions can be produced by injudicious administration of large volumes of glucose in water to patients who need electrolyte replacement. All serum electrolyte values are low in these cases. Small amounts (200 to 300 ml.) of 5 per cent sodium chloride solution should be

Table 4. Acidosis and Alkalosis

	Na	K	CO_2	Cl	CAUSES
1. Metabolic Acidosis pH ↓					
A. Renal	±↓	↑	↓	±↑	Acute or chronic renal failure, BUN ↑.
B. Metabolic	±	↑	↓	↓	Diabetes, hypoxia, adrenal insufficiency.
C. Hyperchloremia	±↓	±↑	↓	↑	NH₄Cl, Diamox, renal insufficiency, fistulas and diarrhea.
2. Metabolic Alkalosis pH ↑					
A. Alkali administration*	↑	↓	↑	±↓	NaHCO₃ excess.
B. 1° Cl⁻ loss*	±	↓	↑	↓	Vomiting, gastric suction.
C. Potassium deficiency**	±	↓	↑	↓	Prolonged alkalosis, surgical stress, no K intake.
D. Mixed K and Cl⁻ loss**	±	↓	↑↑	↓	Usual pattern of g.i. loss without K⁺ replacement.
3. Respiratory Acidosis					
A. Acute pH ↓	±	↑	±↑	±	Narcotics, anesthesia, atelectasis, obstruction.
B. Compensated pH ±	±	±	↑	↓	Asthma, emphysema, bronchiectasis.
4. Respiratory Alkalosis					
A. Early pH ↑*	±↓	↓	↓	↑	Hyperventilation due to
B. Compensated pH ±	↓	↓	↓↓	↑	fever, CNS lesions, NH₄ toxicity, salicylates, respirators.
C. Late pH↓**	↓	↓	↓↓	±↓	
(Marked dehydration)					

* Urine is alkaline.
** Urine is acid.

used discriminately to treat these cases.

Failure to administer potassium to patients with large losses will result in potassium deficiency, characterized by weakness, irritability, ileus, electrocardiographic changes, a plasma alkalosis, and an acid urine (8, 12).

Clysis of glucose in water will produce an active temporary drop in circulating blood volume and sometimes a shocklike state. This is an iatrogenic "third space" (13).

The requirements for fluid and electrolytes for a surgical patient equal *baseline, plus abnormal losses, and either plus an allocation for deficits or minus a deduction for excesses.* For example:

1. Male patient, 70 kg., with pyloric obstruction due to duodenal ulcer. Gastric aspirations, 2,000 ml.; urine volume, 1,100 ml.; infusion the previous day, 3,800 ml.

Think: Baseline	2,000 ml.	1,500 ml. 5% glucose in H₂O 500 ml. 5% glucose 0.9% NaCl 40 mEq KCl
Dynamic loss	2,000 ml.	1,500 ml. 0.9% NaCl 500 ml. 5% glucose in H₂O
Deficit or excess	none	40 mEq KCl 4,000 ml.

Order: A.M.—1,000 ml. 5% glucose 0.9 % NaCl + 20 mEq KCl
       1,000 ml. 5% glucose in H₂O + 20 mEq KCl
     P.M.—exactly the same as A.M.

2. Female patient, 60 kg., with ileus of small bowel, long tube in jejunum. Drainage previ-- ous 24 hours, 1,800 ml.; total infusion, 2,500 ml. Urine output, 400 ml.; specific gravity, 1.026. Patient is moderately dehydrated since previous day: CO_2 18 mEq, Cl 100 mEq, BUN 24, Na 136, K 5.3, hematocrit 52.

Think: Baseline
Dynamic loss
Deficit of extracellular fluid
Some acidosis, probably largely metabolic, dehydration basis, with some renal embarrassment
Potassium elevated slightly, probably due to dehydration

Prescribe: Baseline	2,000 ml.
Dynamic loss	1,800 ml.
To rehydrate (estimate)	1,500 ml.
	5,300 ml.
For baseline	1,500 ml. glucose in H_2O
	500 ml. glucose 0.9% NaCl
For tube drainage	1,000 ml. glucose saline
	500 ml. M/6 sodium lactate
	300 ml. glucose in H_2O
For rehydration	1,000 ml. glucose saline
	500 ml. M/6 sodium lactate
	5,300 ml.

Order: A.M.— 500 ml. M/6 sodium lactate
1,500 ml. 5% glucose 0.9% NaCl
1,000 ml. 5% glucose in H_2O
Check tube drainage for 8 hour volume; check urine volume.

P.M.— 1,000 ml. 5% glucose saline
500 ml. M/6 sodium lactate
800 ml. 5% glucose in H_2O
Order hematocrit and chemistries for A.M.

Think: She ought to be fairly well hydrated tomorrow, and probably her potassium will fall, as she has large losses. I will order some potassium chloride tomorrow morning if her urine volume is up, and I will check the report of the potassium serum level. When the ileus begins to resolve, some "third space" fluid will be absorbed. Accordingly, I will watch for this and reduce the volume of intravenous fluids as indicated.

OTHER ASPECTS OF POSTOPERATIVE CARE

1. Sedation. Children and elderly patients tolerate narcotics poorly. Narcotics tend to depress respiration in all patients and to produce respiratory acidosis. Use them sparingly. *Restlessness* in the postoperative patient is more likely to be due to *hypoxia* than to pain. Check! Remember that opiates depress G.I. tract function.

2. Antibiotics. Overuse of antibiotics results in resistance and may mask serious wound or intraperitoneal problems. The patient who has a clean wound with solid closure of viscus, good hemostasis, and no dead space, dead tissue, or retroperitoneal dissection does not need antibiotics. In the treatment of postoperative atelectasis, antibiotics are a poor substitute for coughing and intratracheal suction. Blind, routine ordering of antibiotics is bad treatment. Think before you prescribe.

3. Wounds. A surgical wound does not become infected unless bacteria are brought to it. Your wound dressing technics should be just as careful as your operating room technics. Use asepsis and avoid antisepsis.

4. Oral Intake. Patients with surgery of the extremities, including the head and neck, can usually tolerate fluids within 24 hours after operation and should have an adequate intake within 48 hours.

Abdominal surgery and retroperitoneal surgery *always* result in some degree of ileus. Also, many thoracic procedures do, but to a lesser degree. Do not rush oral intake; wait until peristalsis returns and *persists* for at least 12 hours. Then start slowly. Do not give a patient who is on gastric siphonage suction anything by mouth, because you only increase the loss of electrolytes from the stomach. If the security of the anastomosis is questionable, a delay in starting oral intake for an extra day or two longer is believed advisable. Also remember that there is no perfect substitute for oral intake either in nutrition or in water and electrolyte balance. Use nature's method as soon as it is safe to do so.

5. Remember that the normal response to surgery includes the following:

a. Antidiuresis for 12 to 24 hours
b. Fever of modest degree
c. Leukocytosis
d. Renal retention of Na+ and Cl−
e. Increased nitrogen and potassium loss
f. Some "third space" effect, from a little to a lot depending on wound size and how traumatic the surgery
g. A fall in serum sodium to levels of 135 mEq per liter or even 132 is *normal* following major operations and should not be treated per se.

6. Laboratory Tests. If a laboratory test does not fit the clinical picture, repeat the test. Don't treat numbers. Treat the patient!

Most patients will recover from surgery if they are not abused. It is only for the very sick patients that time and more time is required.

Avoid routine orders in fluid replacement therapy. Individualize each sick patient and treat that particular patient's problems. You can't substitute brine for brains!

REFERENCES

1. Clark, J. H., Nelson, W., Lyons, C., Mayerson, H. S., and DeCamp, P. Chronic shock: The problem of reduced blood volume in the chronically ill patient, Ann. Surg., 125:618, 1947.
2. Root, W. S., Roughton, F. I. W., and Gregersen, M. I. Simultaneous determination of blood volume by CO and dye (T-1824) under various conditions, Am. J. Physiol., 146:739, 1946.
3. Perry, F. A., Randall, H. T., Poppell, J. W., and Roberts, K. E. Blood volume replacement in surgical patients, S. Clin. North America, 36:301, April, 1956.
4. Aust, J. B., Chou, S. N., Marvin, J. F., Brackney, E. L., and Moore, G. E. The use of radioactive iodinated human serum albumin (RIHSA) for clinical total blood volume studies, Surgical Forum, Am. Coll. of Surg., p. 601, 1951.
5. Elkinton, J. R., Danowski, T. S., and Winkler, A. W. Hemodynamic changes in salt depletion and in dehydration, J. Clin. Investigation, 25:120, 1946.
6. ——— Winkler, A. W., and Danowski, T. S. The importance of volume and tonicity of body fluids in electrolyte shock, J. Clin. Investigation, 26:1002, 1947.
7. Roberts, K. E., Vanamee, P., Randall, H. T., and Walker, J. M. Common electrolyte abnormalities encountered in bowel surgery. Mechanism of hyperchloremic alkalosis, hypokalemic alkalosis and hyperchloremic acidosis, S. Clin. North America, 35:1189, 1955.
8. Randall, H. T. Water and electrolyte balance in surgery, S. Clin. North America, 32:445, April, 1952.
9. ——— and Roberts, K. E. The significance and treatment of acidosis and alkalosis in surgical patients, S. Clin. North America, 36:315, April, 1956.
10. Grollman, A. Acute Renal Failure, Springfield, Ill., Charles C Thomas, 1954.
11. Merrill, J. P. In Principles of Internal Medicine, Harrison, T. R., Editor, 2nd ed., New York, The Blakiston Company, 1954.
12. Randall, H. T. Habif, D. V., Lockwood, J. S., and Werner, S. C. Potassium deficiency in surgical patients, Surgery, 26:341, 1949.
13. Abbott, W. E., Levey, S., Foreman, R., Krieger, H., and Holden, W. E. The danger of administering parenteral fluids by hypodermoclysis, Surgery, 32:302, 1952.

ANESTHESIA

GEORGE A. KEATING

THE ACTIVITIES of an anesthesiologist can be divided into four phases. *First* is the preoperative visit to and evaluation of the patient. *Second* is the selection of the anesthetic agents and technic, with due regard to the safety of the patient, the nature of the surgical procedure, the abilities of the anesthesiologist, and the preferences of the patient and the surgeon. *Third* is the actual administration of the anesthetic and the management of the patient's condition during surgery. *Fourth* is the postoperative care and observation of the patient.

In the discussion that follows, the technics recommended in any particular instance do not attempt to set forth all the possible methods of solving an anesthesia problem. They are, however, practical opinions and technics, formulated mainly from close clinical observation of patients in the operating room and in the postoperative period.

THE PREOPERATIVE VISIT

The visit to the patient should be devoted first to obtaining as much information as possible concerning the patient's past history, the present illness, and the physical and laboratory findings. The results of this interview will help the anesthesiologist, working in cooperation with the surgeon, to determine how the patient may best be prepared for anesthesia and the operation. Ideally, this preoperative visit should take place not later than the day before surgery. However, in emergencies, a visit even 10 or 20 minutes before the operation is worthwhile. In addition to the usual medical and surgical history and a complete review of systems, a history of previous anesthesia experiences should be taken to avoid difficulties or a repetition of errors.

This personal contact with the patient is an important part of the preoperative preparation. There is no substitute for the calming effect of an unhurried visit, especially when the calmness is secured without the undesirable side effects accompanying opiates and barbiturates.

During the preoperative visit, the anesthetic technic planned for the operation should be discussed with the patient. A history of idiosyncrasies to drugs or a patient's mental aversion to some particular drug or technic may be elicited. Occasionally a patient has a morbid fear of being put to sleep. More often, he objects to some form of regional anesthesia, usually spinal, either because of hearsay or because of a previous personal experience. Unless there are specific contraindications, it is usually well to respect a patient's expressed desires, both from the standpoint of seeking a successful anesthesia and from the medicolegal aspect. Fairly often a careful but brief explanation of the anesthetic technic and an exposition of its particular value will be sufficient to sway the patient's feelings.

An important, and often little understood, part of this preoperative visit is the ordering of preanesthetic medication. This should not be allowed to become a mere routine but should be adjusted according to the particular requirements of the patient, the anesthesia, and the operation. Preanesthetic medication has four general purposes: (1) psychic sedation, or hypnosis; (2) elevation of the pain threshold; (3) reduction of metabolism; and (4) counteraction of undesirable side reactions from the anesthetic agent.

1. *Psychic depression* tends to place a protective cloak about the patient and spare him the unpleasant experience of anesthesia and surgery. While it may or may not provide actual amnesia, it should confer a state of indifference. A patient in such a state is more amenable to methods of regional anesthesia. Furthermore, the lack of excitement is an aid in the induction of general anesthesia.

2. *Elevation of the pain threshold* is particularly suited to regional anesthesia, because with this technic not all sensation is necessarily abolished. Pain perception may be blocked, but the deeper pathways conducting traction and pressure sensations remain active. These sensations are interpreted by many patients as pain.

3. *Reduction of tissue metabolism* causes a decrease in the amount and concentration of the various agents necessary to attain a satis-

factory plane of anesthesia or analgesia. This is closely allied to psychic depression, but it is concerned more with the patient's safety than with his comfort.

4. *Counteraction of undesirable side reactions* from the anesthetic agent is exemplified by the use of belladonna alkaloids to minimize the respiratory secretions caused by irritating inhalants and to decrease the incidence of laryngospasm, which is frequently associated with the administration of intravenous barbiturates. Another example is the effect of barbiturates in protecting against the convulsive effects of local anesthetic agents.

With the four purposes of preanesthetic medication in mind, a careful review of the drugs usually employed can be considered. All drugs have undesirable reactions as well as desirable ones, and they must be chosen as carefully as the anesthetic agent itself.

1. *Drugs used for psychic sedation* include the opiates, both natural and synthetic; the barbiturates and their related compounds; and the basal narcotic agents such as avertin. Of these, the opiates are the most commonly employed; they should be used with discretion, especially in the extremes of age. Caution is mandatory, first because of the effect of opiates in depressing respiration, and also because of their less recognizable effects in interfering with circulatory hemostasis. For this second reason opiates are avoided in all patients with any existing circulatory depression. This includes the patient who is either in shock or recently recovered from shock unless there is severe pain. Barbiturates in moderate amounts are useful in all age groups except in the occasional patient who experiences excitement rather than sedation. Patients in severe pain may also be excited by use of barbiturates. Basal narcotics are rarely used, since less potent and less depressing drugs may be more readily employed. Chlorpromazine and its related compounds have the disadvantage of frequently causing hypotension and a delay in the recovery period following general anesthesia.

2. *Principal drugs used for raising the pain threshold* are the opiates. Most patients about to undergo elective surgery do not have pain. Patients in shock usually do not have painful sensations until they attain a normotensive state. The use of opiates will only delay this recovery mechanism. Indeed, opiates given by the customary subcutaneous or intramuscular route may not be absorbed until the circulation returns to almost normal levels. It seems more logical to reserve the opiates for intra-

venous use during regional anesthesia either when the block is incomplete or when the patient misinterprets touch or pressure sensation as pain. In general, barbiturates are preferred to opiates for administration prior to anesthesia.

3. *Drugs for decreasing the metabolic rate* include opiates, barbiturates, and a variety of other sedatives. The preceding admonitions should govern their use.

4. *Agents used for counteraction of undesirable side reactions* include belladonna alkaloids and barbiturates. Atropine and scopolamine are prescribed for all patients, even when regional anesthesia is employed, in the event that general anesthesia may be required for supplementation. Because of its prolonged action, better drying of secretions, and additional hypnotic effect, scopolamine is preferred for all except the aged and those patients undergoing intrathoracic procedures. Atropine is probably more effective in blocking undesirable vagal reflexes, and it will not tend to disorient the aged patient.

The dosage of all these premedication drugs must be adjusted to the age and general physical condition of the patient. Patients less than one year of age generally receive no premedication with the exception of an occasional small dose of atropine (1/400 grain). Older children receive regular medication calculated according to age or, preferably, according to body weight. Doses of all types of drugs are markedly reduced in the elderly age groups.

Routinely, the preanesthetic medication is given either subcutaneously or intramuscularly one hour before the scheduled time of surgery. If less time is available, the intravenous route should be chosen with the dosage schedule unchanged. This routine has been adopted because morphine, a commonly used drug, reaches its peak effect approximately 90 minutes after subcutaneous administration, 45 minutes after intramuscular administration, and about 10 minutes after intravenous injection. Most other drugs reach their peak effect more rapidly.

After all the available information has been gathered concerning the patient, the premedication prescribed, and the confidence of the patient gained, the purpose of the preoperative visit has been achieved.

SELECTION OF ANESTHETIC TECHNIC AND AGENT

The second concern is the selection of the proper anesthetic technic and agents. The technic may be either regional or general. Regional anesthesia may be spinal, epidural, paravertebral block, regional nerve block, field block, or local infiltration. General anesthesia may be induced by inhalation and intravenous or rectal administration, each route permitting the use of a large number of technics. Various combinations of any of these methods may be used. For regional anesthesia the principal agents which we prefer are tetracaine, lidocaine, dibucaine, and chloroprocaine. Other available agents offer no particular advantages. Inhalation agents used include vinyl and ethyl ether, nitrous oxide, ethylene, and cyclopropane. The thiobarbiturates are employed intravenously, and either these drugs or avertin may be given rectally.

In choosing an agent and technic, the safety of the patient is the primary concern. This involves a thorough knowledge of the physical status of the patient, not only medically but also from the standpoint of age, sex, race, and psychic make-up. It also demands a complete understanding of the pharmacologic action of the anesthetics to be used, and how these anesthetics may affect the status of the patient as a whole. As an example, a patient with coronary artery disease should not be allowed to have a long, stormy induction with ether, even though ether might be considered the best anesthetic to use. Under such circumstances it is better to induce anesthesia with a small amount of a barbiturate administered intravenously and then subsequently maintain the anesthesia with ether. A barbiturate is not a good drug for prolonged anesthesia, but it serves an excellent purpose when its use is properly indicated.

As noted earlier, the next criterion governing the choice of anesthetic is the type, extent, and duration of the operation. Since this involves lengthy consideration, it will be discussed in detail in a separate section to follow. For the moment let us consider how the abilities of the anesthesiologist influence the choice of anesthetic. Most authorities think that the anesthesiologist should use the technic that best suits his abilities, regardless of whether it is the most generally favored method or not.

The anesthesia should be discussed with the patient during the preoperative visit and his fears or prejudices respected as far as possible. Many surgeons have their preferences, too. Those accustomed to the extreme relaxation afforded by spinal anesthesia may not be satisfied with inhalation anesthesia. Others may not care to operate on a patient who is conscious of all that transpires in the operating room.

The relationship of the anesthesia to the nature of the surgical procedure is best considered by grouping operative procedures according to their general anatomic localities.

OPERATIONS ABOUT THE NECK

These operations must all be considered to be major procedures from the viewpoint of anesthesia, whether the operation is for a sebaceous cyst or for a radical neck dissection. Once anesthesia is induced and the patient is prepared and draped for surgery, the anesthesiologist must work in a restricted area. Since there is always the possibility of interference with the airway by the surgical procedure and since there are many untoward reflexes encountered in this region, the use of an endotracheal tube is mandatory when general anesthesia is used. In a few unusually cooperative patients regional block may be employed.

If a patient has signs of respiratory obstruction preoperatively, or if there is a deep infection present, the endotracheal tube should be introduced under topical anesthesia while the patient is awake and in command of his own airway. If this is not feasible, an airway should be secured by performing a preliminary tracheostomy.

Probably the most common operation in the neck region is a thyroidectomy. While anesthesia for this procedure can satisfactorily be managed by performing both a superficial and a deep cervical plexus block, only rarely will a patient tolerate this method. The discomfort caused by unavoidable pressure and traction during the operation is not conducive to the patient's peace of mind.

Patients with toxic goiter almost universally require general anesthesia in order to avoid additional psychic stimulation. Premedication dosages in these patients are heavy. Frequently a basal anesthesia achieved by the intravenous or rectal route is used. Either light oxygen-ether or nitrous oxide–oxygen–ether is our anesthetic of choice. Ethylene is also an excellent agent. Cyclopropane is avoided in the toxic patient because of its effect on cardiac rhythmicity. Intubation may be facilitated by the use of a muscle relaxant. The thiobarbiturates have a cumulative effect and delay the time of reaction. Since these patients often have myocardial damage, careful observation of the cardiovascular status is important.

Fortunately the preoperative preparation of patients with hyperthyroidism, including the use of thiouracil and the iodides, has reduced the incidence of thyroid crises during anesthesia almost to the vanishing point. Anesthetic management of the nontoxic thyroid patient is essentially the same except that the cardiovascular status is usually better and basal anesthesia is not frequently employed.

In thyroid patients the airway problem is carried into the postoperative phase. Obstruction may occur as a result of vocal cord paralysis or paresis from edema caused by the endotracheal tube, or by surgical trauma and by tracheal collapse when there has been erosion of the cartilaginous rings by a tumor mass. For these reasons all thyroidectomy patients should have a tracheostomy set at the bedside for at least 24 hours postoperatively and be closely observed during that time for signs of airway obstruction.

Anesthesia for removal of thyroglossal or branchial cysts, parathyroid tumors, and hygromas is essentially the same as that required for thyroidectomy or nontoxic goiter. Anesthesia for radical neck dissection follows the same pattern. In this procedure the carotid sinus reflex may be markedly stimulated, with deleterious effects on the circulation. The surgeon may avoid this effect by careful dissection and retraction and by topical application of cocaine (4 per cent) or pontocaine (2 per cent) directly to the region of the carotid bifurcation.

In some procedures the surgeon may prefer to use the electrocautery. Then nonexplosive anesthetic agents must be used. Nitrous oxide combined with minimal amounts of thiobarbiturate administered intravenously or rectally, or avertin given rectally, is most commonly used.

OPERATIONS ON THE THORACIC WALL

These range from excision of simple cysts to removal of parts of the thoracic wall itself. With simple procedures, local or field block may be ideal. In more extensive operations, paravertebral blocks may be employed. Almost any inhalation or intravenous technic may be used since no relaxation is required. Furthermore, the anesthesiologist has access to the patient and can easily maintain a patent airway.

Mastectomy, simple or radical, involves only the soft tissues but can rarely be carried out under regional anesthesia because of the large area involved. General anesthesia with any of the inhalation agents is excellent. Because of the extensive tissue dissection required, a fairly large blood loss through constant oozing is common. Careful attention to the airway and to carbon dioxide elimination helps to keep the venous pressure from rising and increasing the blood loss. Often the use of an endotracheal tube to insure a good airway is advisable. Commonly, thiobarbiturate and nitrous oxide are used for preliminary excision of a lesion for examination by frozen section. If a radical operation is to follow, a volatile or gaseous agent is substituted.

INTRATHORACIC OPERATIONS

These involve surgery of the pleura, lungs, trachea, bronchi, mediastinum, and diaphragm. In general, the management of these procedures requires the highest degree of skill on the part of the anesthesiologist. Surgery of the thorax and its contained viscera has been until recently a last frontier.

Operations on the pleura may include the simpler procedures of removing collections of purulent material, blood, or fluid from the pleural space. These are performed under local or regional anesthesia. The operation may involve very extensive resections of tumors, necessitating the removal of a part of the thoracic wall or the decortication of fibrous tissue, either of which requires careful endotracheal technics. Cutaneous tracheobronchial fistulas often present a special problem which can best be solved by employing endobronchial intubation. This is most easily accomplished with the Carlens' double lumen tube.

Pneumonectomy may be partial or complete. Complete pneumonectomy is technically simpler. It requires the use of an endotracheal tube for anesthesia. Any of the inhalation agents may be used to attain the light plane of surgical anesthesia required. Because these patients commonly suffer from chronic pulmonary insufficiency, assisted or controlled respiration is necessary to maintain an adequate exchange. Controlled respirations are most easily attained by using cyclopropane, or by supplementary muscle relaxants. This technic gives a quiet operative field for the surgeon and is almost a necessity in some of the more delicate surgical procedures. The lung to be removed often contains large amounts of secretions, and the usual positioning of the patient places this side upward. Accordingly, frequent and vigorous tracheobronchial toilet is necessary in order to keep the normally functioning lower lung free and clear.

In lobectomy or in segmental lobectomy the problems are more complex because the surgery is more prolonged. In order to maintain assisted or controlled respirations, manual or mechanical inflation may be used. Each method has advantages and adherents. It is easier to interpret the patient's reactions with the manual method, but maintaining uniform and vigorous respirations for several hours without tiring is most difficult. The actual value of maintaining satisfactory respiratory exchange and aiding the circulation in the negative phase attributed to some mechanical respirators is open to question, but they are not believed harmful.

In our clinic the anesthesia of choice in most intrathoracic procedures involves a semiclosed system using nitrous oxide–oxygen–ether at a total flow rate of 3 to 6 liters per minute and with respirations either assisted or controlled. This is considered the best safeguard against carbon dioxide retention. Minute-to-minute control of the depth of anesthesia can be attained with the occasional supplementary use of cyclopropane. Except occasionally for induction, thiobarbiturate is not used because of its cumulative effect.

Other intrathoracic procedures involving the esophagus and mediastinal structures, or thoracic sympathectomy, are managed in the same manner as lung operations. A complicating factor may be the production of a bilateral pneumothorax. However, this requires mainly a slightly more vigorous effort at artificial support of the respiratory exchange.

Other intrathoracic operations becoming more common involve the aorta and great vessels and the heart itself. As a general rule, the anesthetic technics involve the same precautions and use the same agents as for all intrathoracic procedures. The plane of anesthesia is kept as light as possible while still allowing the patient to tolerate the endotracheal tube.

The pericardium is not very often the site of a surgical procedure. The most common operation is that for constrictive pericarditis. The most troublesome complication is an irritable myocardium. Otherwise, the same precautions relating to intrathoracic surgery in general are observed.

Because of the improvements in surgical technics, in anesthesiology, in diagnostic methods, and in the proper selection of patients, the correction of the various types of congenital anomalies of the heart is possible. One of the simpler procedures is closure of the patent ductus arteriosus. In general, the operation is done on children in whom the myocardium is in good condition. Except for a rise in diastolic pressure when the patent ductus is occluded, there are no special hazards to be expected. It is well for the surgeon to occlude this vessel temporarily while the anesthetist watches for changes in the circulatory dynamics before a permanent ligature is applied. Otherwise, the anesthetic management follows the course of any open thoracic procedure. The volume of blood replacement should equal the quantity that is lost. In these patients cyanosis is absent except in those who are either in congestive heart failure (cyanosis tardive) or in whom there is a reversal of flow with a right-to-left shunting of blood. Cyanosis due to reversal of flow is at present considered a contraindication to operation.

In operations to correct the tetralogy of Fallot, it must be remembered that these patients are cyanotic and have an increase both in the blood volume and in the hematocrit readings. Hence the volume of blood replacement should always be well below that which is lost. It is important in these and in other cyanotic cardiac patients to avoid an increase in the oxygen needs of the tissues by not allowing the patient's body temperature to rise. Such heat retention is common with closed "to-and-fro" anesthesia systems and, to a lesser degree, with closed-circle absorption systems. In such procedures it is well to employ a nonrebreathing or semiclosed absorption system for most of the time and to use the closed system only while it is necessary to maintain inflation of a collapsed lung.

When closely monitored, the body temperature of young patients under semiclosed anesthesia and in a cool operating room will usually fall three to four degrees below normal. Since this fall in body temperature reduces the oxygen demand of the tissues, it is a desirable state. Such a drop in temperature may be artificially obtained by the appropriate use of ice bags or a cooling blanket or mattress.

One of the most frequent operations performed on the heart valves is mitral valvotomy or commissurotomy. The cardiovascular status of these patients varies from reasonably good to poor. Auricular fibrillation, varying degrees of cardiac failure, and even unsuspected rheumatic activity may be present. The state of the myocardium depends on the severity and the duration of the lesion and also on the number and severity of the attacks of rheumatic fever. In patients with mitral stenosis, there is congestion of the pulmonary circulation, and since this blood is suddenly released into the systemic circulation after commissurotomy, the volume of the blood replacement should be less than the volume of the blood loss.

These procedures, like all cardiac procedures, are monitored on the cardioscope. Increase in the number of ventricular complexes or other changes in rhythm or conduction are indications to interrupt the operation, either temporarily or permanently, and to increase pulmonary ventilation. The amount of anesthetic agent required by these patients is remarkably little. It is our practice to induce anesthesia with a small amount (150 to 200 mg.) of thiobarbiturate and to maintain it with nitrous oxide–oxygen–ether using a semiclosed system. A very light plane of anesthesia is maintained, although not quite as light as that of so-called ether analgesia. Premedication is also very light. To prevent tachycardia, belladonna drugs are usually not used in patients who have a normal sinus rhythm. Opiates when prescribed are given in small doses. Frequently the use of intramuscular pentobarbital is preferred.

Aortic and pulmonic valvotomy may be accomplished by a blind technic, either inferiorly through the ventricular wall or superiorly through an artificially attached appendix made either of pericardium or of a combined cotton cloth and plastic material. Neither of these approaches involves any greater problem of anesthesia than any other cardiac procedure, except that patients with aortic lesions are more prone to disturbances in cardiac rhythm and have more changes in circulatory dynamics during and after the operation. There is a growing tendency to attempt the repair of these lesions as well as the repair of cardiac septal defects under direct vision. This necessitates either the temporary but complete interruption of the entire circulation in conjunction with hypothermia, or the use of the pump oxygenator to bypass the cardiopulmonary circulation.

Hypothermia has been used with some success. This allows complete occlusion of the circulation for short intervals of time and provides the advantage of operating on a relatively empty, though beating, heart. Total occlusion in our experience has not exceeded four and one-half minutes, and in the surviv-

ing patients no untoward effects have been observed.

The chief danger in hypothermia is the occurrence of ventricular fibrillation, a condition which is extremely difficult to correct in the cool heart. During cooling, close observation of the cardiac rhythm by electrocardiographic monitoring is essential. Any changes in rhythmicity at any point in the cooling are an indication for rewarming the patient and abandoning this technic.

Children and patients of small stature are more readily cooled, and their temperatures tend to drift to lower levels, almost uncontrollably at times. We have assumed a level of 85° to 86° F. to be a reasonably safe compromise between ventricular fibrillation at lower temperatures and cerebral damage during the period of circulatory occlusion at higher temperatures. The basic anesthetic agent is ether-oxygen, and induction is obtained with small amounts of either thiobarbiturate or cyclopropane. Controlled respirations are vigorously maintained throughout, using a semiclosed system. Every effort is made to avoid carbon dioxide retention. The anesthetic agent is given, in reduced amounts, even during the period of the lowest temperature. During circulatory occlusion, troublesome excursions of the diaphragm may be experienced, even though respirations were previously under complete control. Effective control may be obtained by administering *d*-tubocurarine about 10 minutes before occlusion.

Rewarming is started at the time of occlusion, but there is a lag of about 45 minutes before any temperature rise is detectable by observations of the rectal temperature. The rewarming blanket is never raised above a temperature of 120° F. in order to avoid burning the patient.

ABDOMINAL SURGERY

Like other types, abdominal surgery may be performed for conditions of either an acute or chronic nature. This strongly influences our choice of anesthesia. Anesthesia for upper abdominal surgery is more trying because of the difficulty in securing adequate muscle relaxation and because of the reflex effects of surgical manipulation on circulation and respiration.

Operations upon the biliary tract are the most common procedures in the upper portion of the abdomen. Because of the marked relaxation obtained and the lack of toxic effects on the liver, which may frequently be diseased, spinal anesthesia is preferred. It has three disadvantages, however: (1) hypotension may develop as a result of the sympathetic blockade, which produces analgesia to a level of the sixth thoracic dermatome or higher; (2) respiratory depression may occur because of intercostal paralysis; (3) the patient may complain of discomfort during traction on the abdominal viscera. These disadvantages are outweighed by the optimum operating conditions and by the usual lack of sequelae to the spinal anesthesia itself. Not only is there extreme muscle relaxation, but the intestines, constricted as a result of the spinal block, are easily retracted. This is believed to result in less trauma to the intestines and to lessen the incidence of postoperative ileus and vomiting.

The hypotension, if it occurs, can be corrected by the use of vasopressors, usually methoxamine or phenylephrine, administered intravenously either intermittently or in a continuous drip. Respiratory depression is controlled by manual compression of the rebreathing bag filled with oxygen. Discomfort from manipulation of the intraabdominal viscera is of short duration and may be controlled by nitrous oxide inhalation, demerol administered intravenously, or a combination of both. This combination of therapy can bring about the unwise use of a multiplicity of drugs, but this is the exception rather than the general practice. Often spinal anesthesia plus normal premedication is entirely adequate. Sometimes, in apprehensive patients, small amounts of one of the barbiturates given intravenously are used to allay fear and anxiety.

Arteriosclerotic heart disease, with or without hypertension, is considered a contraindication to spinal anesthesia. Instead, oxygen-ether or nitrous oxide–oxygen–ether is employed.

Spinal anesthesia is also used in most of the operations on the stomach, including subtotal gastrectomy, gastroenterostomy, and partial resection of the vagus nerves. The same variations of technics are employed as previously indicated to obtain the best type of anesthesia.

In gastric surgery for uncontrollable hemorrhage, the problem of hypovolemia is an important one. Under such circumstances cyclopropane anesthesia is preferred because of its tendency to interfere less with the circulatory homeostatic mechanisms than any other agent. Hypotension as a result of spinal anes-

thesia in a patient with a markedly reduced blood volume is a complication very difficult to control. It is because of this difficulty that spinal anesthesia is not used in cases of traumatic rupture of the spleen and hemoperitoneum. Cyclopropane is the first choice, light ether or nitrous oxide–ether the second. With either of these agents, muscle relaxants may also be employed as indicated.

In surgery of the spleen for hypersplenism and other forms of blood dyscrasia, spinal anesthesia is preferred. Theoretically, ether causes the normal spleen to contract, cyclopropane has no effect, and spinal anesthesia will cause dilatation. However, it is extremely doubtful that the pathologic spleen has the ability to contract or dilate according to the particular type of anesthesia that is administered.

Intestinal obstruction, if not severe, is managed best by spinal anesthesia. In any of these cases, spontaneous rupture of the bowel as a result of spinal anesthesia is a rarity. In cases of advanced intestinal obstruction with the patient acutely ill, dehydrated and in acid-base imbalance, and possibly in shock, spinal anesthesia is contraindicated. Despite the presence of a Levin tube in the stomach, there is a possibility that after the administration of a spinal anesthetic the patient may regurgitate and aspirate sufficient of the gastric contents to cause an immediate asphyxiation. Accordingly, the safest technic is to insert a cuffed endotracheal tube under topical anesthesia while the patient is conscious. Then the cuff is inflated to seal off the trachea and, using either cyclopropane or nitrous oxide–ether sequence, general anesthesia is induced.

Elective surgery of all types on the gastrointestinal tract is best accomplished with spinal anesthesia because of its excellent relaxation, constriction of the intestinal tract, minimal effect upon the acid-base and electrolyte balance, and less postoperative distention.

Spinal anesthesia should be given with caution to the patient with generalized peritonitis. The infection may well cause fixation of the abdominal wall muscles and the diaphragm. If the spinal anesthesia causes intercostal paralysis of any degree, respiratory exchange may be severely embarrassed.

Anesthesia for pelvic surgery is technically much simpler than that for other types of intraabdominal surgery. Gynecologic procedures are performed under spinal anesthesia with ease, and the problems of hypotension, respiratory insufficiency, and traction pain are minimal.

Prolonged spinal anesthesia may be obtained either by the addition of epinephrine in the amounts of 0.6 or 0.7 mg. to a single dose of the spinal anesthetic or by using the catheter spinal technic. The latter has become quite uncommon except in the replacement of the abdominal aorta by grafting after the excision of an aneurysm and in other time-consuming intraabdominal operations.

Intraabdominal surgery in children is performed under inhalation anesthesia—not because the value of spinal anesthesia is questioned, but because children in general seem to be temperamentally unsuited to any type of regional anesthesia. In the child, strange sights and sounds and the loss of sensation and motor power in a part of the body generally tend to cause a state of panic.

Herniorrhaphy of the abdominal wall is a very common surgical procedure which is performed most often in the younger, more vigorous age group. Chronic cough is frequently a contributing factor in the production of any hernia, congenital or acquired. Therefore, the anesthetic used should be designed to avoid irritation of the respiratory tract as much as possible.

Theoretically, local anesthesia would be ideal for inguinal hernia. However, local anesthesia for hernia repair requires considerable skill in its application and much gentleness in handling tissues to obtain the best results. In addition, the anatomy of the region is often distorted by the volume of anesthetic solution that is required. Last but not least, local anesthesia for hernia requires considerable fortitude on the part of the patient. Almost all hernia repairs in our clinic are completed under spinal anesthesia which may be complemented by intravenous barbiturate.

In emergency operations for strangulated or incarcerated hernias, spinal is again the anesthesia of choice. When a prolonged operation is anticipated, continuous spinal anesthesia is an excellent choice.

EXTRAPERITONEAL OPERATIONS

These involve many of the same problems as intraabdominal surgery. Operations on the kidney and ureter require maximum relaxation, which is satisfactorily obtained with spinal anesthesia, unless a rib resection is required. If this should prove necessary, the use of endotracheal anesthesia is mandatory.

The removal of either the normal adrenal glands in the treatment of certain forms of osseous metastases or the removal of a pheochromocytoma involves several complicating factors. *First,* the pleura may be torn in the manipulation. *Second,* there may be a period of a paroxysmal hypertension while the gland or tumor is being handled. *Third,* the blood pressure may descend to shock levels after the tumor or gland is removed. The first of these complicating factors is solved by the use of an endotracheal tube. The second is treated by adrenolytic or ganglionoplegic drugs. The third is corrected by the use of vasopressor drugs, notably phenylephrine and levo-arterenol. Because of the high titer of epinephrine in the circulating blood, the administration of cyclopropane is contraindicated. Ether or nitrous oxide-ether is the agent of choice.

SYMPATHECTOMIES

Thoracolumbar sympathectomy involves much the same considerations as operations upon the adrenals, particularly during the second stage of the operation. Endotracheal anesthesia is always employed because during the operation the pleura is regularly entered, either purposely or accidentally.

Lumbar sympathectomy, like ureteral surgery or inferior vena cava ligation, requires maximum muscle relaxation. Again, spinal anesthesia is the choice. The level must be carried relatively high on the side operated upon, reaching to at least the sixth thoracic dermatome.

SURGERY OF THE EXTREMITIES

Operations upon the extremities produce fewer anesthesia problems than most other procedures since this type of surgery usually has fewer systemic effects. Adequate anesthesia is obtainable with light planes of general anesthesia or by simple blocks of the more accessible nerves.

Minor procedures require only local infiltration or regional field block. For more extensive procedures in the lower extremities, it is well to employ spinal anesthesia. Nerve blocks about the elbow or knee and about the wrist or ankle also have a useful place, but they tend to be more time-consuming to perform and less positive in their results.

Major amputations for degenerative vascular disease are performed mostly on the lower extremities. These patients have circulatory insufficiency with or without an associated metabolic disease. Under such circumstances spinal anesthesia is preferred.

MANAGEMENT OF THE PATIENT DURING SURGERY

The choice of anesthesia and the method of administration are governed first by what is safest for the individual patient. During surgery the safety of the patient should continue to be the primary concern of the anesthesiologist. Most fatalities which occur during or immediately after anesthesia and which can be ascribed solely to the anesthesia are due to asphyxia. The term *asphyxia* indicates both oxygen lack and carbon dioxide excess. This may be caused by (1) failure to supply sufficient oxygen or failure to eliminate carbon dioxide properly because of defects in the anesthetic apparatus; (2) inadequate ventilation from respiratory obstruction, diminished intercostal and diaphragmatic activity, or failure to ventilate the patient artificially; (3) associated pulmonary disease that interferes with the gaseous exchange between the blood and the pulmonary alveoli; (4) the presence of anemia or diminished blood flow; (5) the inability of the tissue cells to utilize oxygen or eliminate carbon dioxide. These factors are under the control of the anesthesiologist, and he should observe them closely.

There have been instances where anesthetic gases have been accidentally attached to a machine in place of oxygen or where flowmeters or other parts have failed. Fortunately, these are extremely rare accidents. More commonly it is the insidious accumulation of carbon dioxide even in the presence of adequate oxygenation that results in respiratory acidosis and a train of unphysiologic effects. Respiratory obstruction, even of a minor nature, can produce both hypoxia and hypercarbia. Obstruction should be comparatively simple to recognize and correct, but it must be realized that even though an endotracheal tube is in situ, the airway may be inadequate. Decreased tidal exchange caused by the anesthetic or by some physical impairment of the patient must be carefully assessed. Its correction by rhythmic compression of the rebreathing bag should be simple. Inadequate efforts on the part of the anesthesiologist in maintaining assisted or controlled respirations are more difficult to assess. A good rule to remember is that it is almost impossible to overventilate a patient, but it is very easy to underventilate him. The presence of pulmonary disease interfering with gaseous exchange should be revealed by the preliminary clinical evaluation of the patient. Often little can be done to correct it, but vigorous ventilation or other efforts may help to compensate for it. The patient's blood volume and hemoglobin should be brought as nearly as possible to normal before any operation is performed. The anesthesiologist must carefully replace blood as it is lost during the operative procedure. In general, surgeons underestimate blood loss and anesthesiologists overestimate it.

The relation of asphyxia, usually partial, to the occurrence of cardiac arrest cannot be overemphasized. So-called vagovagal and other types of reflexes probably have little effect on the heart of a well oxygenated patient who is not suffering from respiratory acidosis. Careful and constant observation of the patient and reporting immediately to the surgeon the cessation of the pulse and the blood pressure are important, but even more important is the prevention of cardiac stoppage. In the event that cardiac arrest does occur, the well ventilated patient will be able to withstand the circulatory standstill with less rapid deterioration, since the tissues will have no oxygen debt or carbon dioxide excess. Not least important is the fact that in such instances the heart will respond more readily to resuscitative measures.

Cessation of the heartbeat usually has prodromal signs and frequently follows other significant events such as unreplaced blood loss or respiratory difficulty, active or passive. The actual interruption of the circulation must be recognized immediately, since normal brain tissues can withstand complete lack of blood flow for only about four minutes. It is in the early detection of the actual stoppage of the circulation that mechanical diagnostic aids may be of some benefit.

There must be no hesitation on the part of the surgeon or, if necessary, the anesthesiologist, to open the chest and institute effective manual massage of the heart as soon as the diagnosis of cardiac arrest is made. The massage must be sufficient to move enough blood through the vital centers to support life. Equally important is the necessity for the concomitant administration of a sufficient amount of oxygen to the lungs. This is usually done by rapid intubation of the trachea and artificial ventilation with 100 per cent oxygen. However, if equipment for endotracheal intubation is not immediately at hand, ventilation should be started with the conventional anesthesia mask. Once proper ventilation and circulation have been established, there should be no further deterioration of the vital brain centers. Then, other well recognized agents and methods for restoring efficient circulation may be employed in a comparatively leisurely manner.*

POSTOPERATIVE CARE AND OBSERVATION

Observation of the patient in the immediate postoperative period is a comparatively new aspect of the practice of anesthesiology. This aspect has always been implied, but it has been spelled out only in the past few years. The one person responsible for the care of the patient and the one who is able to make a proper and comprehensive assessment of the physiologic state of the patient is the anesthesiologist. He has seen the patient preoperatively; he has managed the patient during the anesthesia and the operation; and he should therefore possess the background of knowledge necessary to manage the patient properly during the immediate and precarious postoperative period. This control of the patient is effected best within the confines of a postoperative *recovery room*, where the patient has the benefits of all the concentrated talents available in the hospital and also of all the equipment necessary for the proper handling of any emergency that may occur. It is a fact that better service can be offered to the postoperative unconscious patients who are gathered in one area where all of the facilities necessary for their care are located than if these same patients were distributed throughout the various floors in the hospital.

In the immediate postoperative period the care of the surgical patient, whether in a special recovery area or in a private room or ward bed, is of great importance. The character of the respirations and the adequacy of the circulation should be carefully observed.

A most common and serious postoperative complication is interference with respiration. This may occur as a result of an obstruction of the upper respiratory passage by relaxed tissues which are no longer supported by an artificial airway. Obstruction also may be due to edema of the glottis secondary to endotracheal intubation. Tracheal collapse producing respiratory obstruction has occurred following the removal of an enlarged thyroid gland for

a benign or a malignant condition. More commonly, respiratory obstruction is due to retained viscid secretions and to aspirated vomitus. Whatever the cause of obstruction of the air passages may be, prompt recognition and correction are most important. Furthermore, the desirability of a tracheostomy should always be considered. All too frequently this operation is performed too late. Usually if one is in doubt as to the wisdom of doing a tracheostomy, it most likely should be done. It is much better to err by doing the tracheostomy too early than by waiting until it is too late.

In a patient who is restless and apprehensive postoperatively, particularly when there is an associated hypertension, one should assume hypoxia as the cause until it is proved otherwise. Too frequently opiates are administered to quiet the patient instead of investigating the causes of the restlessness. Sedation should be administered sparingly to the postoperative patient and preferably by the intravenous route to observe more closely its effect. Even then it should be given only after all efforts have been made to insure the adequacy of the respiratory exchange and the absence of a distended urinary bladder.

The pulse and blood pressure should be recorded at stated intervals and carefully observed for any untoward fluctuations. If hypotension should occur, the patient should be examined to determine the cause. This may be secondary to an inadequate replacement of blood or to cardiac failure, vasomotor instability, a sudden decrease in a previously elevated carbon dioxide level in the blood, or to rough handling in moving or changing the position of the patient. The factor or factors which are responsible should be promptly recognized and corrective treatment prescribed.

Finally, the postoperative care of the patient includes strict attention to other details such as infusions and transfusions, observations for allergic reaction to drugs or to blood, and the care of the nasogastric tube and suction siphonage apparatus as well as of water-seal drainage systems employed following intrathoracic procedures. Furthermore, inspection of the wound dressing for hemorrhage should also be made. Most of this type of care is the responsibility of the members of the surgical staff rather than the anesthesiologist. The importance of attention to details in the satisfactory postoperative recovery of the patient cannot be too strongly emphasized.

---

* For a scientific and practical discussion of the subject of cardiac arrest, see the monograph on Cardiac Resuscitation by Robert Hosler.

RIGHT PARAMEDIAN INCISION

A. The location of the incision in the lower part of the abdomen is depicted by the dotted line.

B. The incision is deepened through the subcutaneous fatty tissue layer, and the wound margins are retracted to expose the line of incision in the anterior sheath of the rectus fascia.

C. The medial cut margin of the anterior rectus sheath is grasped by clamps and upward traction is maintained. The mobilized portion of the rectus muscle is displaced laterally by manual retraction overlying a moist gauze pad, and the medial border of the lower portion of the rectus muscle is separated from its midline attachments by scalpel dissection.

D. The right rectus muscle is retracted laterally to expose the underlying related structures as labeled.

E. The surgeon and the first assistant "pinch up" small segments of the posterior rectus sheath and peritoneum preparatory to severance with a scalpel.

F. The incision into the peritoneal cavity is made, and the cut margins of the posterior rectus sheath and peritoneum are grasped in clamps. A segment of a moist gauze sponge is inserted beneath the peritoneum for protection of the underlying bowel, and the incision is extended upward by scissor dissection.

Plate 1

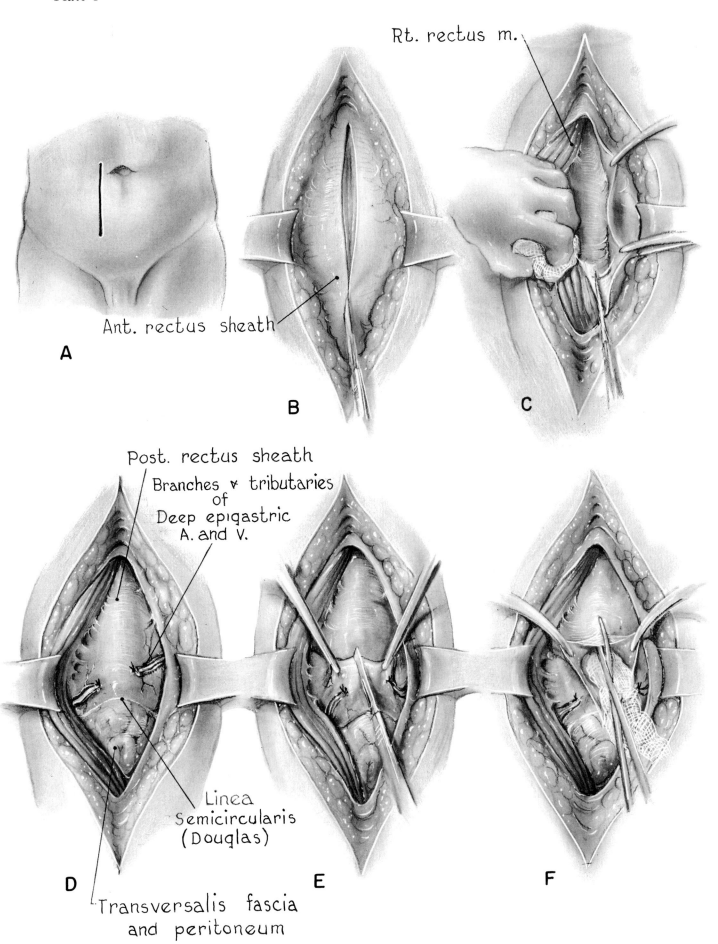

Rt. rectus m.

Ant. rectus sheath

A

B

C

Post. rectus sheath
Branches & tributaries
of
Deep epigastric
A. and V.

Linea
Semicircularis
(Douglas)

D

E

F

Transversalis fascia
and peritoneum

RIGHT PARAMEDIAN
INCISION

G. The upward extension of the incision is completed and its downward extension is commenced by scalpel dissection. Here a scalpel is preferred because it does not require the surgeon to assume an awkward position of the arm and hand as is required when scissors are employed.

H. The opening into the peritoneal cavity is completed, and the related underlying intra-peritoneal viscera are visible.

I, I′. The posterior rectus sheath and peritoneum are sutured with either a continuous interlocking double strand suture of 00 chromic catgut (I) or a series of interrupted everting mattress sutures alternating with simple interrupted sutures of 00 silk (I′).

J. The rectus muscle is returned to its normal position, and the closure of the anterior rectus sheath is partially completed using interrupted sutures of silk (00). Thus the muscle acts as a buttress interposed between the lines of closure of the peritoneal and fascial layers.

K. The closure of the skin with interrupted sutures of 000 silk completes the operation.

The proclaimed advantage of this incision is that it does not predispose to nerve injury and resulting muscle atrophy. Furthermore, interposition of the muscle layer between the lines of closure of the anterior and posterior rectus sheaths is considered an additive support to the security of the wound closure. This incision is used almost routinely for operations in both the upper and lower portions of the abdomen, and it is highly recommended.

Plate 2

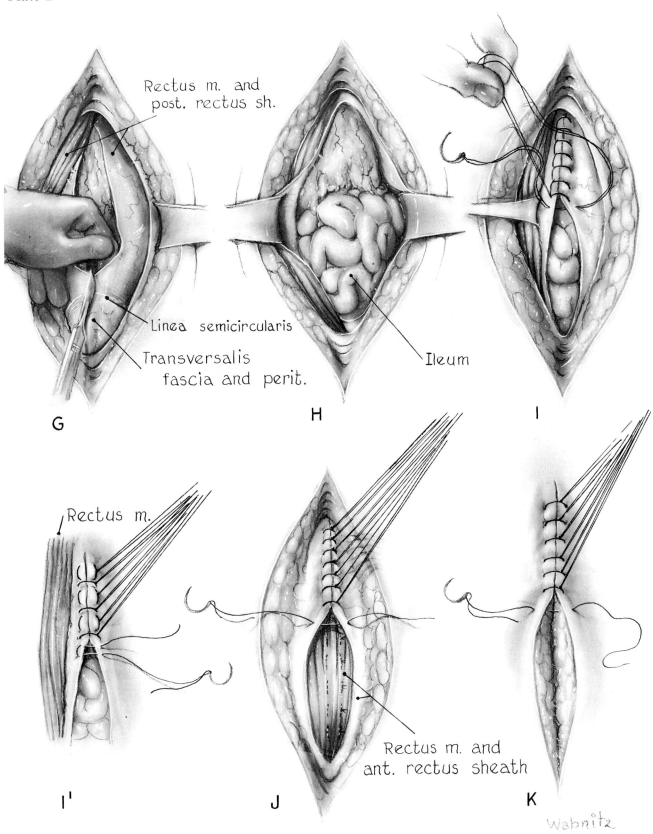

Rectus m. and
post. rectus sh.

Linea semicircularis

Transversalis
fascia and perit.

G

Ileum

H

I

Rectus m.

I'

Rectus m. and
ant. rectus sheath

J

K

Wabnitz

BATTLE–JALAGUIER–KAMMERER–LENNANDER INCISION

A. The incision overlying the outer third of the infraumbilical portion of the right rectus muscle is shown by the solid line.

B, C. The incision is deepened through the anterior rectus sheath, and the lateral border of the rectus muscle is manually displaced medially as the mobilization of its lower portion is completed by scalpel dissection.

D. The lateral border of the right rectus muscle is retracted medially to show the intercostal nerves, the linea semicircularis, and, in the lower portion of the wound, the deep epigastric vessels and a branch and tributaries from the same to the posterior belly of the right rectus muscle.

E. The opening in the peritoneal cavity is completed, and the wound margins are retracted to expose the underlying intraperitoneal viscera.

F. Closure of the incision is commenced by suture of the fascia-peritoneal layer by everting mattress sutures of silk (00).

G, H. To complete the wound closure, the rectus sheath (G) and the skin (H) are approximated with interrupted sutures of 00 and 000 silk respectively.

Although frequently used, the objection to this incision is the necessity for interrupting the nerve supply to the segment of the rectus muscle that is exposed in the field of operation. This causes an atrophy of the muscle, and the resulting weakness of the abdominal wall theoretically predisposes to the occurrence of a postoperative ventral hernia.

Plate 3   31

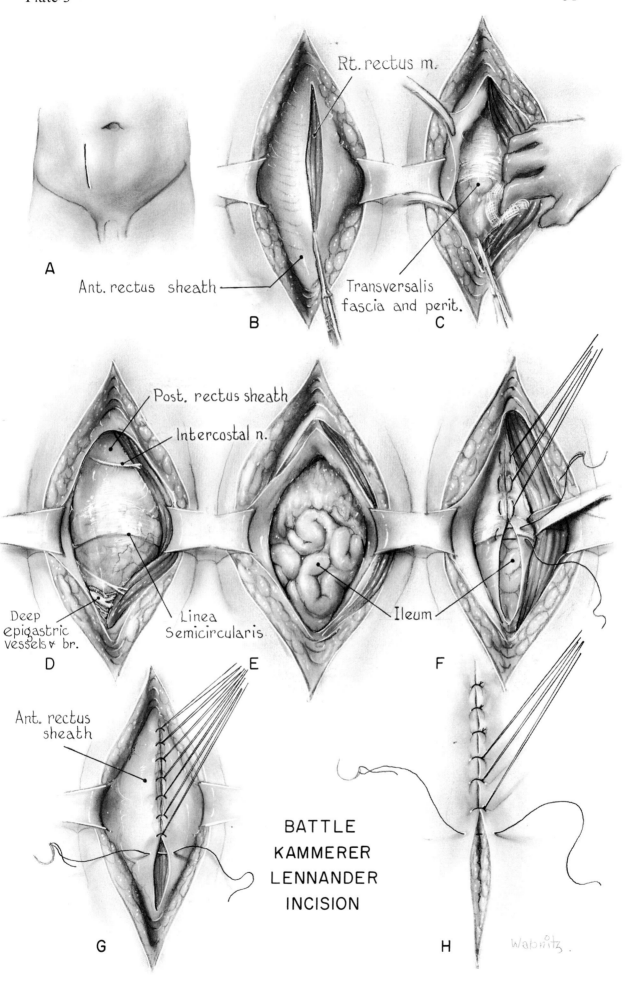

A

Ant. rectus sheath

B

Rt. rectus m.

Transversalis fascia and perit.

C

Post. rectus sheath

Intercostal n.

Deep epigastric vessels & br.

Linea Semicircularis

Ileum

D   E   F

Ant. rectus sheath

G

BATTLE
KAMMERER
LENNANDER
INCISION

H

Wabritz.

McBURNEY INCISION

A. The outline of the incision and McBurney's point are indicated. McBurney's point is located 4 cm. from the anterior superior iliac spine on an imaginary line drawn from the umbilicus to the anterior superior iliac spine. The incision, traversing McBurney's point, extends in an oblique direction one third above and two thirds below the plane of this line.

B, C, D. The incision is deepened through the fibers of the external oblique muscle and its aponeurosis and the internal oblique and transversus abdominis muscles. In the separation of the fibers in the plane between the internal oblique and transversus abdominis muscles, caution must be observed to avoid an avulsion injury of the intercostal nerves which are depicted in D.

E. Small segments of the transversalis fascia and peritoneum are tented by tissue forceps preparatory to being incised transversely with a scalpel.

F. The peritoneal cavity is entered, and the wound margins are retracted to expose the ileocecal region and the appendix.

G. The fascia-peritoneal layer is closed using interrupted everting matress sutures of silk (000).

H, I. The separated margins of the transversus abdominis, internal oblique, and external oblique muscles are approximated loosely with interrupted sutures of 000 silk.

J. The closure of the skin with interrupted sutures of silk (000) completes the operation.

This incision is considered most anatomic and conducive to less trauma because exposure is obtained by separation of the muscles in the direction of their fibers. There is also less likelihood of injury to the nerve supply of the muscles. It is believed that this incision, though widely used and recommended by many, is employed too routinely and, as a consequence, operative exposure may frequently prove inadequate. It is particularly useful for the performance of appendectomies in young children and adult males. In women, even though the diagnosis of acute appendicitis is the most likely one, a right paramedian incision is preferred. In fact, this type of incision is used rather than the McBurney regardless of the age and sex of the patient. Although the McBurney incision has been advocated, particularly for the drainage of intraperitoneal abscesses, no difficulty has occurred when similar drainage was required through a paramedian incision.

Plate 4

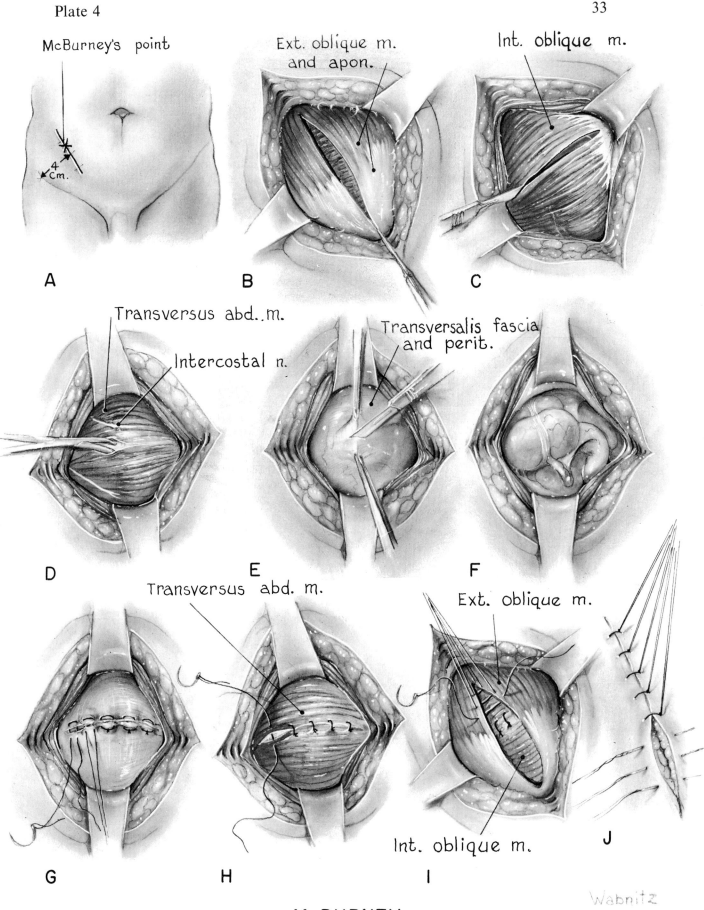

McBurney's point

A

Ext. oblique m. and apon.

B

Int. oblique m.

C

Transversus abd..m.

Intercostal n.

D

Transversalis fascia and perit.

E

F

Transversus abd. m.

G

H

Ext. oblique m.

Int. oblique m.

I

J

Wabnitz

McBURNEY
INCISION

PFANNENSTIEL INCISION

A. The location of the curvilinear transverse incision, with its convex border down and within the hair line of the pubes, is shown.

B. The rectus fascia is severed transversely in the same plane as the skin incision to expose portions of the rectus muscles.

C. Curved clamps (Kelly) are applied to the cut margin of the upper leaflet of the rectus fascia, and, with traction maintained, this fascia is mobilized from the surface of the rectus muscles by scalpel dissection.

D. The lower leaflet is similarly dissected downward, and the separated medial borders of the rectus muscles are retracted laterally, and the fascia-peritoneal layer is opened longitudinally with a scalpel to enter the peritoneal cavity.

E. The opening into the peritoneal cavity is completed, and the wound margins are retracted to expose the pelvic and related viscera.

F. The closure of the fascia-peritoneal layer is almost completed using continuous interlocking double strand suture of 00 chromic catgut.

G. The medial margins of the rectus muscles and the rectus fascia are sutured with interrupted sutures of 00 silk.

H. The operation is completed by closure of the skin incision with interrupted sutures of 000 silk. Sutures are not inserted in the subcutaneous fatty tissue layer regardless of the depth of this particular layer.

Plate 5

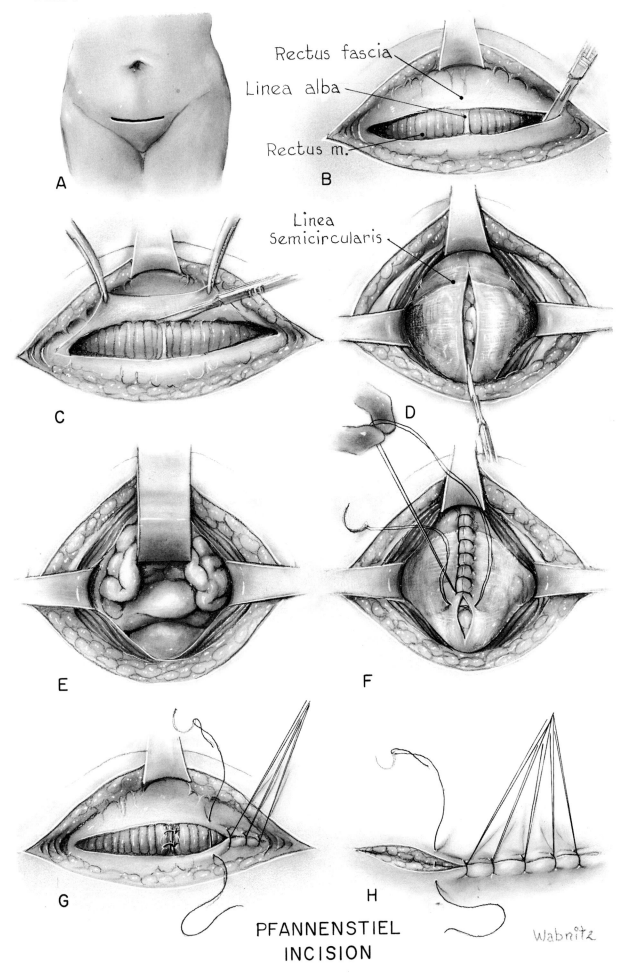

Rectus fascia

Linea alba

Rectus m.

Linea
Semicircularis

A

B

C

D

E

F

G

H

PFANNENSTIEL
INCISION

Wabnitz

SUBCOSTAL (KOCHER) INCISION

A. The extent and location of the incision in relation to the right costal margin is demonstrated.

B. The incision is deepened through the subcutaneous fatty tissue layer, and the underlying structures are depicted.

C. The anterior rectus sheath is incised, and the incision is continued laterally through the aponeurosis and fibers of the external oblique muscle.

D. The rectus muscle is transected, and the internal oblique muscle and its aponeurosis are exposed.

E. The aponeurosis and the fibers of the internal oblique muscle are severed, and the relation of the posterior lamella of the aponeurosis of the internal oblique muscle and the fascia of the transversus abdominis in the formation of the posterior rectus sheath may be seen.

Plate 6   37

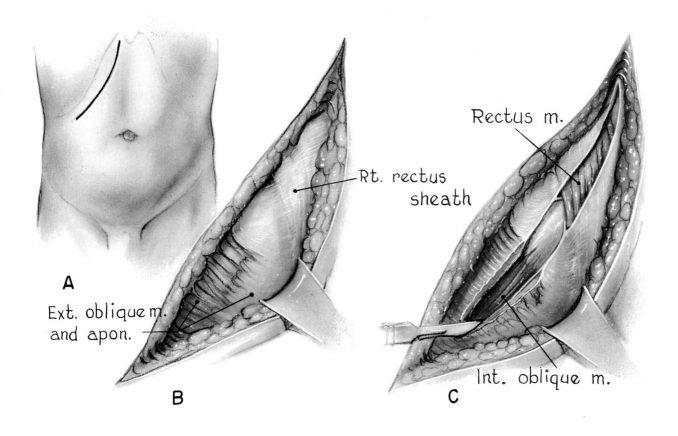

A

Rt. rectus
sheath

Ext. oblique m.
and apon.

B

Rectus m.

Int. oblique m.

C

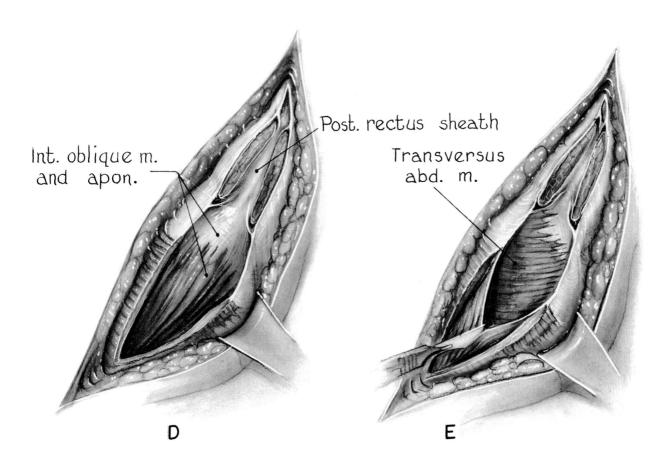

Int. oblique m.
and apon.

Post. rectus sheath

Transversus
abd. m.

D

E

SUBCOSTAL (KOCHER)
INCISION

F. The incision is extended through the posterior rectus sheath, the transversus abdominis muscle, and the peritoneum to expose the underlying intraperitoneal viscera.

G. Closure of the incision is commenced by the suturing of the transversus abdominis muscle and the underlying peritoneum laterally and the posterior rectus sheath and underlying peritoneum medially with interrupted sutures of silk (00). If desired, closure with the use of a continuous suture of chromic catgut, or interrupted figure of 8 or everting mattress sutures of silk (00), may be employed.

H. The internal oblique muscle and its aponeurosis and the anterior rectus sheath are approximated with interrupted sutures of 00 silk.

I. The closure of the external oblique muscle and its aponeurosis and the anterior rectus sheath is completed using interrupted sutures of 00 silk.

J. In the closure of the skin, a series of small straight (Cambric) needles are all first inserted, then withdrawn individually and the sutures tied. These sutures may be cut either individually after they are tied or after they have all been first inserted and tied.

This incision is one of the most popular in use for operations upon the biliary tract. Nevertheless, the preference of the author is a longitudinal oblique paramedian muscle-retracting (lateral) incision as depicted in the illustrations of the technic for cholecystectomy.

Plate 7   39

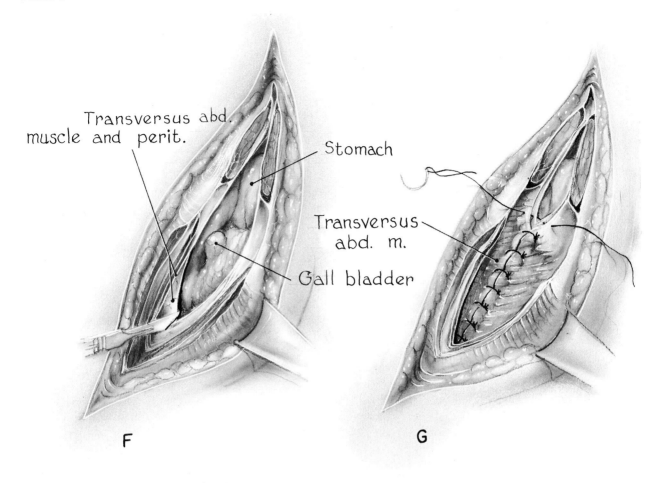

Transversus abd.
muscle and perit.

Stomach

Transversus
abd. m.

Gall bladder

F

G

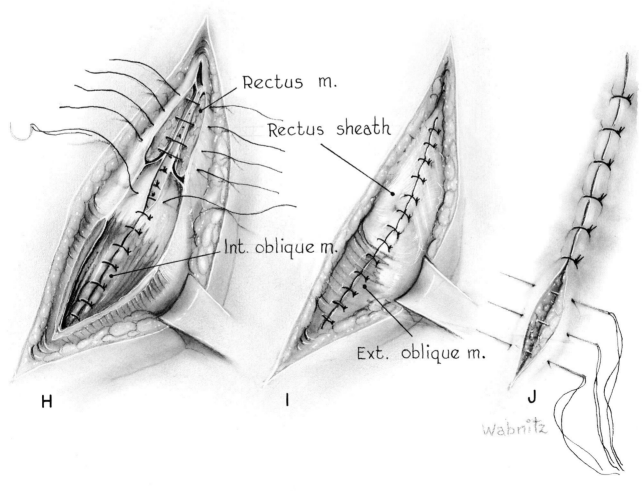

Rectus m.

Rectus sheath

Int. oblique m.

Ext. oblique m.

H

I

J

Wabnitz

KEHR INCISION

A. The skin incision is commenced in the midline at the level of the tip of the xiphoid process and extends vertically downward to a point approximately midway between the xiphoid and umbilicus. It is then directed obliquely lateralward to terminate just beyond the outer border of the right rectus muscle.

B. The incision is deepened through the subcutaneous fatty tissue plane, and the line of fascia fusion of the rectus sheaths (linea alba) is incised.

C. The underlying properitoneal fatty areolar tissue layer and peritoneum are incised, and the peritoneal cavity is entered. Usually one or two vessels in the areolar tissue layer are clamped, severed, and ligated, using ligatures of fine (0000) silk. The direction of the incision for transection of the anterior rectus sheath and the underlying rectus muscle is indicated by the dotted line.

D. The transection of the rectus muscle is completed, and the line of incision in the posterior rectus sheath is demonstrated (dotted line).

E. The incision is completed into the peritoneal cavity, and it is extended laterally by partial severance of the fibers of the transversus abdominis muscle. The falciform ligament is doubly clamped and severed at the site indicated by the dotted line.

Plate 8   41

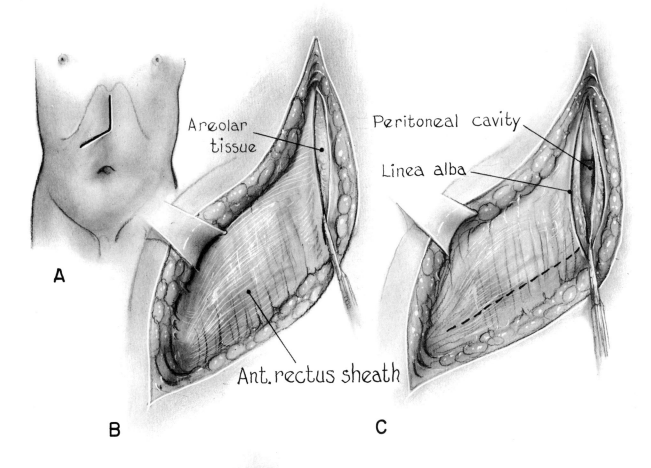

A

Areolar tissue

Peritoneal cavity

Linea alba

Ant. rectus sheath

B   C

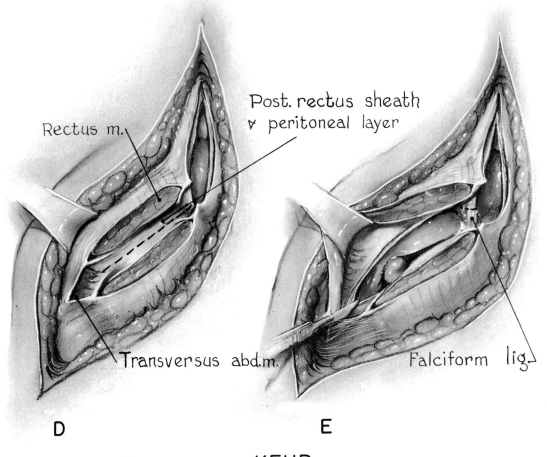

Rectus m.

Post. rectus sheath
& peritoneal layer

Transversus abd.m.

Falciform lig.

D   E

KEHR
INCISION

F. The incision is completed, and the adequacy of the exposure obtained is demonstrated.

G. Closure of the incision is commenced by suturing the peritoneal and fatty areolar tissue layers in the midline and continuing the closure in an obliquely transverse direction to approximate the posterior rectus sheath and peritoneum. A continuous interlocking double strand suture of 00 chromic catgut is used. However, if preferred, interrupted everting mattress sutures of silk (00) may be employed.

H, I. The fascia and skin layers are approximated using interrupted sutures of 00 and 000 silk respectively.

The particular advantage of this type of incision in operations upon the gallbladder and bile ducts has been recently emphasized by Holman.

Plate 9   43

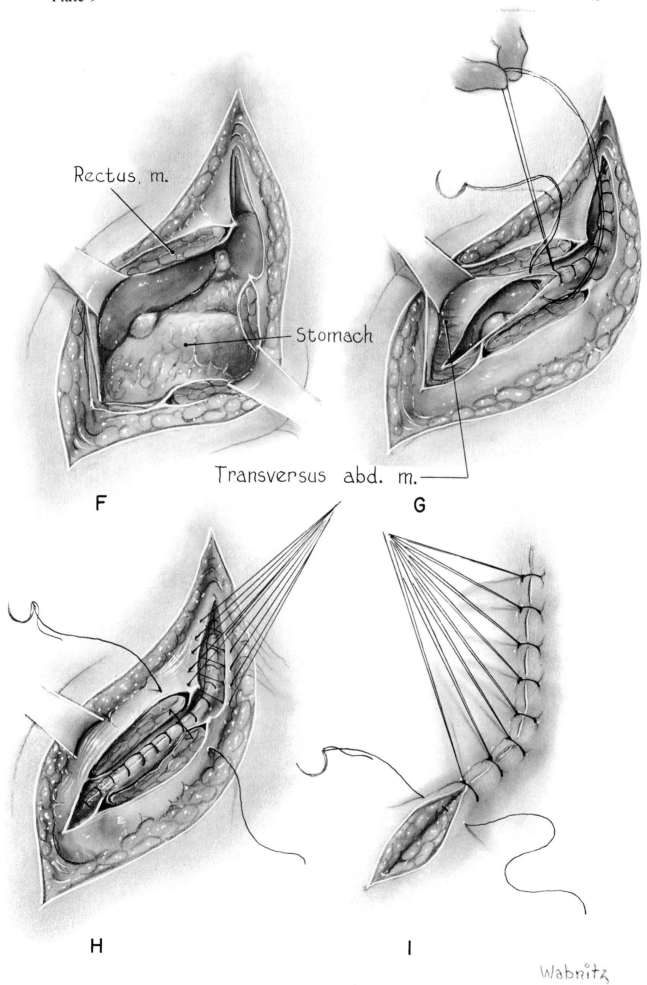

Rectus. m.

Stomach

Transversus abd. m.

F

G

H

I

Wabnitz

MARWEDEL INCISION

A. The incision commences in the costoxiphoid angle and extends downward to a level approximately 1 inch below and lateral to the umbilicus. Just above the umbilicus, a transverse extension of the incision is made which is directed lateralward to form a modified T-shaped pattern. In the original article in which this incision is described, it is shown on the right rather than on the left side as illustrated.

B. The incisions through the subcutaneous fatty tissue layer are completed, and the anterior sheath of the rectus is incised longitudinally in the left paramedian plane.

C. The transection of the left rectus muscle is completed, and the musculofascial flap is retracted upward to expose the costal arch and a portion of the transversus abdominis muscle. The opening into the peritoneal cavity is visible.

D. The main portion of the costal arch and its related costal cartilages are severed with a scalpel preliminary to retraction of the costal arch.

E. The fascia, peritoneum, and the transversus abdominis muscle are severed in a horizontal plane, and the musculochondral flap is retracted upward to complete the operative exposure.

This incision is used only rarely in modern surgery. An advantage proclaimed for this type of incision was that one could obtain maximum exposure for surgery within the upper portion of the abdomen without entering into the pleural cavity. However, in present-day surgery there is not the same fear of entrance into the pleural cavity. Accordingly, abdominal incisions may be extended into the thoracic cavity when this is required to obtain more adequate exposure. Therefore, the use of the compromise type of incision described by Marwedel would be rarely required.

DISCUSSION—DR. EDMUND HORGAN. To properly carry out a surgical procedure on the abdominal wall or within the abdomen, it is desirable and necessary that the placement and size of the incision be such that the site of the surgical operative field will be adequately exposed. Furthermore, the incision should be large enough to allow complete exploration of all the structures within the abdomen and the retroperitoneal structures, such as the kidneys, adrenals, abdominal aorta and iliac arteries, unless it is contraindicated on account of perforation or abscess.

In making an abdominal incision, consideration should be given to its closure, and preparation for the closure in anatomical layers should be made. When multiple surgical procedures, such as total cystectomy and construction of an ileal conduit bladder, are necessary, multiple surgical incisions are needed. When combined surgical procedures, such as total colectomy for chronic ulcerative colitis and construction of an ileostomy by the method of Turnbull, are performed, multiple incisions are required. Multiple incisions are also required in the Duhamel method for Hirschsprung's Disease.

In the excellent work of Rodney Maingot on abdominal operations four T-incisions for use in abdominal surgery are illustrated. By using the T-incision that is indicated, the upper abdomen, the lower abdomen, the right side of the abdomen, or the left side of the abdomen can be well approached to do an extensive surgical procedure. For most conditions in the upper abdomen requiring treatment, a diagonal incision in either the right or the left upper quadrant, whichever is indicated, can be used. The incision begins high, starting between the xiphoid and the border of the ribs and extending diagonally downward, lower than the umbilicus, toward the lateral border of the rectus muscle. If adequate exposure cannot be obtained, a transverse lateral incision can be made from its midportion to convert it to a T-incision. Generally, the long diagonal incision is adequate, especially with the anesthetic agents and muscle relaxants that are now used. May I say that with the careful administration of these substances and the controlled and coordinated use of them by our anesthetists, there is little risk in their use. Therefore, complicated incisions are not necessary today when available anesthetic substances and muscle relaxants are supplemented by controlled respiration and respiratory ventilation. But incisions large enough and properly placed must be used.

For an acute or subacute abscess within the abdomen, if it can be located, the planned approach should be direct. The incision should be sufficient only for aspiration and drainage. Exploration should not be done. Definitive surgery should be deferred until clinical studies can determine the cause of the abscess and that the surgical procedure indicated can be carried out.

Abdominothoracic incisions, right and left, have a well-established place. On the right side, an abdominothoracic incision may be used for excision of a chronic ecchinococcus cyst of the liver, an adenoma or hemangionendothelioma of the liver, and the right lobe of the liver; reconstructive surgical operations of the biliary tract and portacaval

Plate 10   45

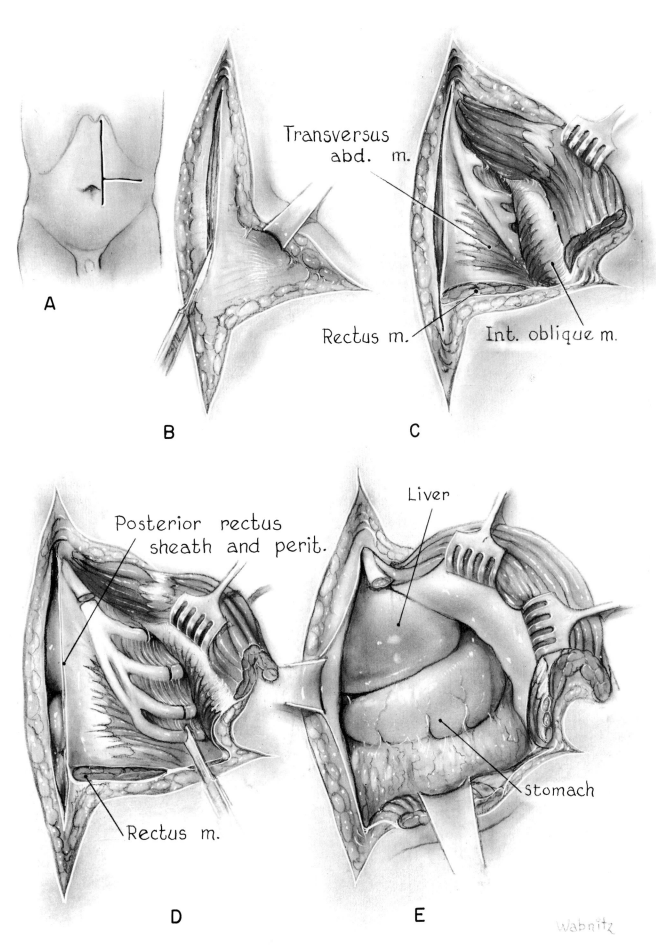

Transversus
abd. m.

Rectus m.   Int. oblique m.

A

B   C

Posterior rectus
sheath and perit.

Liver

Rectus m.

stomach

D   E

Wabnitz

MARWEDEL
INCISION

shunts. On the left side, an abdominothoracic incision may be used for the performance of total gastrectomy, splenectomy, when the perisplenitis (aque cake) is severe and of long standing with marked adhesion to the diaphragm, and splenorenal shunts. Pheochromocytomas and lesions (benignant and malignant) of the cardiac portion of the stomach and lower esophagus may similarly be excised. It may also be used for the Longmire procedure of re-establishing the continuity of the biliary tract with the gastrointestinal tract by anastomosing the left intrahepatic bile duct with the jejunum.

A transverse right rectus incision, a transverse left rectus incision, or a transverse right and left rectus incision may have a useful place as an abdominal approach. I have described the use of a high right transverse incision as an approach for doing the Fredet-Rammstedt pyloromyotomy in infantile hypertrophic pyloric stenosis. A high transverse incision is made over the right rectus abdominis muscle through the skin and subcutaneous connective issue. The anterior sheath of the right rectus muscle is incised transversely and dissected upwards and downwards. The right rectus muscle is retracted mesially or incised transversely, exposing the posterior sheath of the muscle. The posterior sheath and peritoneum are incised transversely, exposing the edge of the liver and the stomach. The hypertrophied pylorus can easily be delivered into the incision and the pyloromyotomy procedure performed. The posterior and anterior rectus sheaths can be approximated by using a few interrupted sutures in each and the skin can be sutured. There is little strain on the incision, and there is little likelihood of dehiscence of the wound. A transverse incision usually does not cause as much discomfort and pain as a longitudinal incision, since there is not as much tension or voluntary splinting of the sutured wound.

For the newer surgical procedures, where extensive and meticulous surgery is carried out, there are newer surgical approaches and maneuvers to obtain and maintain adequate exposure of the surgical operative site. This is accomplished by shifting the position of anatomical structures and immobilization of transposed anatomical structures by the use of gauze packs, the use of the plastic bag of Lahey for the intestines, and the use of self-retaining and manual retractors.

With the great interest in adrenalism, adrenal tumors, pheochromocytoma, occlusion of the renal arteries, and excision of the adrenals in certain forms of malignancy where both renal and adrenal areas have to be explored and exposed, an anterior approach has to be made. It is mandatory that these bilateral areas be carefully explored before a surgical procedure is carried out on either one. In order to accomplish this, a wide tranverse curvilinear incision is made across the upper abdomen. Beginning on one side, just below the twelfth rib, the incision is curved upward and passes across the upper abdomen below the xiphoid cartilage and is continued across the opposite side in the reverse manner. When the incision has been made through the skin and subcutaneous tissues, the concavoconvex edges stand open opposed to one another.

The fascia and muscles of the upper abdomen on each side can be divided in their anatomic layers. The peritoneal cavity can be entered, and, after doing so, the round ligament and falciform ligament of the liver can be sectioned. With these structures transected, the upper part of the abdomen is easily brought into view. By dividing and ligating the splenocolic omentum and mobilizing and retracting the splenic flexure of the colon, the left renal and adrenal areas can be exposed to view. On the right side, the posterior peritoneum can be incised lateral to the duodenum, the hepoduodenal ligament, and the head of the pancreas so that the maneuver of Kocher can be carried out to retract all of the inclusive structures mesially and the right renal and adrenal areas exposed to view. The advantage of this anterior approach is so apparent to those who use it that the posterior approach is no longer considered. The remarkable fact about the anterior approach is that it facilitates the excision of tumors, the control of the arterial and venous blood flow, and the surgical correction of arterial occlusions of the renal vessels and makes possible aortorenal by-pass by the use of a synthetic dacron graft. Through the incision, an adrenal tumor can be excised and the opposite side can be explored to determine if an adrenal tumor is or is not present. Bilateral adrenalectomy may be done and, in doing so, the venous and arterial circulation are under control because the adrenal vein can be so well exposed that it can be easily ligated and divided; and, the several adrenal arteries can be clamped and ligated. The exposure on the left side is ideal for the performance of a splenorenal shunt. Through this incision a choledochojejunostomy (Roux "en-y") may be done for obstructive conditions of the external biliary tract or in combination with other procedures. This incision may be used for vagotomy in conjunction with resection of the duodenum and stomach, pyloroplasty, or gastrojejunostomy for duodenal ulcer. It may also be used for total gastrectomy or resection of the lower esophagus followed by esophagogastrostomy. Hernias of the esophageal hiatus can be corrected through this approach by doing an infradiaphragmatic abdominal hernioplasty consisting of excision of the hernial sac and suturing of the esophogeal hiatal crus of the diaphragm. Dr. Madden has described his precise and meticulous method of doing pancreaticoduodenectomy with pancreaticojejunostomy and choledochojejunostomy for carcinoma of the head of the pancreas through a longitudinal right rectus incision. Apparently, with proper preparation of the patient, proper surgical facilities, and proper anesthesia with muscle relaxants, the longitudinal incision is excellent. The same operative technic might be utilized if the upper abdominal transverse curvilinear incision were used, but his surgical procedure within the abdomen could not be improved upon by this incision.

A condition that has recently been prominently presented by Doubilet, Puestow, Goldman, and others is the surgical excision of a stone or stones within the pancreatic duct, followed by pancreaticojejunostomy. To facilitate this procedure, it is necessary to have a wide transverse incision or the high curvilinear incision described above.

For total cystectomy combined with transplantation of the ureters into an ileal conduit bladder and pelvic exenteration combined with a similar reconstructive procedure, the lower abdomen and pelvis must be fully exposed. To make such an approach and give such an exposure, an abdominal incision was devised by Cherney. This incision transects the recti abdominis muscles above the symphysis pubis. Then the incision is extended diagonally upwards in the direction of the fibers of the aponeurosis of the external oblique muscle, the internal oblique, and the transversus abdominis muscles, together with the transversalis fascia on each side. With these structures incised, the peritoneum may be incised, and, in doing so, the urachus and the obliterated hypogastric vessels may be transected. The value of this incision in such procedures was noted in a series of patients in whom it was used at the Mayo Clinic. In using the Cherney incision, I have found it most helpful in gaining access to the structures of the lower abdomen and pelvis because of the splendid exposure of these structures and because it allows an ample operative field to carry out extensive exenteration, particularly if spinal anesthesia is used in combination with sodium pentothal.

In the surgical treatment of chronic ulcerative colitis, Turnbull has pointed out the need for a total colectomy to eradicate the diseased condition and remove a pathologic condition that has a high incidence of cancer. When total colectomy is done, it becomes necessary to do an ileostomy by using the sectioned end of the terminal ileum. For this complete procedure two incisions are used. A long left paramedian incision is made for the total colectomy. The incision begins at the spine of the pubis and extends upwards well above the umbilicus. A circular disk of skin is excised at the site selected for the single-barrelled ileostomy. The subcutaneous fatty connective tissue is entered to expose the fascia. A circular disk of fascia is excised exposing the underlying muscle. With a Kelly forcep, a stab wound is made through the abdominal wall into the peritoneum. Turnbull has stressed the fact that the stab wound must be dilated large enough to admit two fingers, in order not to interfere with the blood supply to the terminal ileum when it is brought through the wound. With preservation of the blood supply, a sufficient length of ileum can be brought through to make a mucous membrane covered projecting functional ileostomy that can be utilized to drain into a Rutzen bag. The end of the ileum of an ileal conduit bladder of Bricker may be brought out by the method of Turnbull so that the urine can drain directly into a bag.

There are various forms of colostomies. Most of them are done to decompress the proximal side of the colonic lesion and to defunctionalize the distal. Some are temporary and some are permanent colostomies. When a temporary colostomy is being contemplated, consideration should be given to its final closure and re-establishment of colonic continuity. Therefore, the placement should be one that will allow excision of the colostomy, re-establishment of colonic continu-

ity, and secure closure of the wound. Some colostomies are made through the primary surgical wound, and some are made through a separate wound. I do not like to place a colostomy in the primary surgical wound because of the contamination that might result in infection, suppuration, and sloughing, which might bring about weakness of the incision with dehiscence. If dehiscence does not occur, the weakness of the wound might be great enough to result in an incisional hernia. I prefer to make the colostomy in an additional wound, so that when the time arrives for closure, the colostomy can be excised by using two curvilinear incisions, with the ends meeting. The colostomy with its stomata and scar tissues can be excised and colonic continuity can be re-established by "open" end-on-end anastomosis. The colon can be returned to the abdomen and the colostomy wound of the abdomen sutured in anatomical layers. I do this because I do not think that the use of crushing clamps to crush spurs is a sound surgical procedure. Left lower quadrant colostomies and transverse colostomies can be closed in the same manner.

A cecostomy can be made through a relatively small incision in the lower right quadrant of the abdominal wall. The peritoneum can be sutured to the taenia of the cecum. The wound can be allowed to remain open, without the use of sutures, but packed with vaseline sulfathiozole, penicillin gauze. From 12 to 48 hours later, the cecum can be opened by the use of the electrosurgical knife along the exposed taenia. A tube or catheter is not used. Decompression can be facilitated by the use of castor oil or magnesium sulphate. After definitive surgery, the cecostomy usually closes spontaneously. If it does not, the cecostomy can be excised, the stoma closed, and the wound sutured.

Many intra-abdominal surgical procedures have to be done where previous first-stage or emergency measures have been employed in the management of traumatic, pathologic, or concomitant pathologic conditions. In some of these, an approach has to be made through another surgical incision. But the approach may have to be made by excising the scar of the former surgical wound; or, by excising the scar of the former surgical wound where a gastrostomy, ileostomy, cecostomy, or colostomy is present. In any one of these conditions there may be an old incisional defect, which must be considered in making the surgical incision so that a secure closure can be made that will leave an intact abdominal wall. The anatomic layers must be prepared in making the surgical approach. If the anatomic layers cannot be separated, the coalesced fascia must be prepared so that it can be imbricated in making the closure.

Since the surgeon is responsible for the surgical wound, he should plan for its closure and healing. Good judgement must be used in the placement of the incision, the handling of the tissues of the wound, the prevention of contamination of the wound, and the accomplishment of hemostasis so that with careful suturing of the anatomical layers favorable conditions will exist for healing.

DISCUSSION—DR. RAYMOND P. SULLIVAN. Abdominal incisions require careful consideration by the surgeon for adequate exposure and in anticipation of a safe and satisfactory closure. Improper incisions contribute to additional time consumption and may add to the surgical risk. An adequate incision permitting free access to the abdominal contents will always prove not only safer but conducive to less trauma and more efficient teamwork. The choice of abdominal incision is primarily a matter for the surgeon's consideration of the physiologico-anatomic factors in such a way as to avoid mutilation of the abdominal wall. It should always be borne in mind that any incision is safest when anchored to the fundamental rules of asepsis, hemostasis, adequate exposure, and team work. These are the important factors of safety which contributed so much in the development of surgery after the introduction of anesthesia and the transition from antiseptic to aseptic technic.

In the upper portion of the abdomen the Kocher subcostal incision as illustrated is used for lesions of the gallbladder, bile ducts, pancreas, duodenum, and on occasions for resection of the colon. It is not a physiologic incision because it cuts obliquely the underlying musculature of the anterolateral abdominal wall and consequently injuries two or three of the intercostal nerves. However, it is believed less harmful than other forms of nonphysiologic incisions. In place of this type of incision, especially in the obese patient, the incision described by James Masson (Plate 11, A2) is believed more satisfactory, especially if lower abdominal exploration is necessary. This incision extends obliquely downward from the tip of the xiphoid to a point immediately below and 2 to 3 cm. lateral to the umbilicus. The anterior rectus sheath is severed and the fibers of the rectus muscle are split longitudinally at the junction of its inner and middle thirds. The posterior rectus sheath and peritoneum are then incised longitudinally, and the peritoneal cavity is entered.

The longitudinal paramedian incision which is shown may also be used in the upper abdomen. However, when it is used and drainage is deemed necessary, this should be done through a lateral stab wound opening as suggested by Fred Lund. This enables the surgeon to obtain a complete closure of the original wound and lessens the predisposition to the occurrence of a postoperative incisional hernia. This type of incision is always preferred to one of the midline type.

Still another incision, available in place of the Kocher incision, would be the one described by Mayo-Robson (Plate 11, B1) which is frequently referred to as the hockey stick incision. The Bevan (Plate 11, A1, B2) modifications of this incision may prove equally useful. Furthermore, a transverse incision including the skin, fascia, muscle, and peritoneum gives excellent exposure and easy access to all of the upper abdominal contents. It may be employed in operations upon the stomach, pancreas, liver, bile ducts, and spleen. It is an incision which is the least likely to injure nerves and blood vessels and, accordingly, it is less apt to be asociated with the occurrence of an incisional hernia.

The Marwedel incision as depicted provides an excellent exposure for operations upon the liver, stomach, spleen, hepatic flexure, transverse colon, and splenic flexure. This incision gives ready access to the subdiaphragmatic space and may be particularly useful in the performance of total excision of the stomach.

The Kehr incision as demonstrated was designed particularly for operations on the gallbladder and bile ducts. It gives excellent exposure but is not believed as physiologic as some of the others previously described. It is a type of incision which requires minute attention to detail in the closure of the wound in order to obtain satisfactory union.

In the lower abdomen, the incision that is probably the most frequently used is the one described by McBurney. This incision is most physiologic because it does not cause injury to nerves, muscles, or blood vessels, and, therefore, theoretically it is less likely to result in the occurrence of a postoperative incisional hernia. It is primarily indicated for appendectomy, cecostomy, and drainage of lower quadrant abscesses. However, this type of incision limits the opportunity for really adequate exploration, and, furthermore, if the appendix is fixed either in the pelvis or high in the retrocecal position, the necessity for enlargement of the incision may make the operation more difficult technically. To obtain better exposure the incision may be extended by the method described by Weir—the transection of the rectus sheath and either retraction or severance of the underlying rectus muscle.

The Battle-Kammerer-Lennander incision as shown in the drawings is preferred to the gridiron type, especially in adults or in the obese patient. This type of incision may be extended readily when necessary for more adequate exposure in the performance of a general exploration or to do a bowel resection. However, in children when there is little doubt of the diagnosis of appendicitis, the McBurney type of incision is routinely employed.

The Pfannenstiel lower abdominal incision is used principally in gynecologic surgery. This incision is not strictly a physiologic one because at this level the fusion of the aponeuroses of the internal oblique and transversus abdominis muscle enters into the formation of the anterior sheath only. Hence the longitudinal part of the incision posterior to the rectus muscles is confined chiefly to the transversalis fascia and the peritoneum.

Regardless of the type of incision that the surgeon may employ either in the upper or lower portion of the abdomen, attention to detail relative to hemostasis and prevention of tissue trauma should always be of prime consideration. Tissues should be handled with the utmost gentleness and minimal amounts of tissue should be grasped in the hemostatic forceps. Ligatures and suture ligatures of fine silk or fine catgut are preferred. The peritoneal cavity should not be entered until hemostasis in the wound layers is complete. Sterile towels are fixed to the skin margins, and the application of moist laparotomy pads to the sides of the wound will not only protect against trauma but will aid in the control of capillary oozing. If the surgeon is diligent about these necessary details and accordingly is "kind to the tissues," the tissues will be in turn "kind to the surgeon" and healing of the wound per primam will be the expected outcome.

Plate 11   49

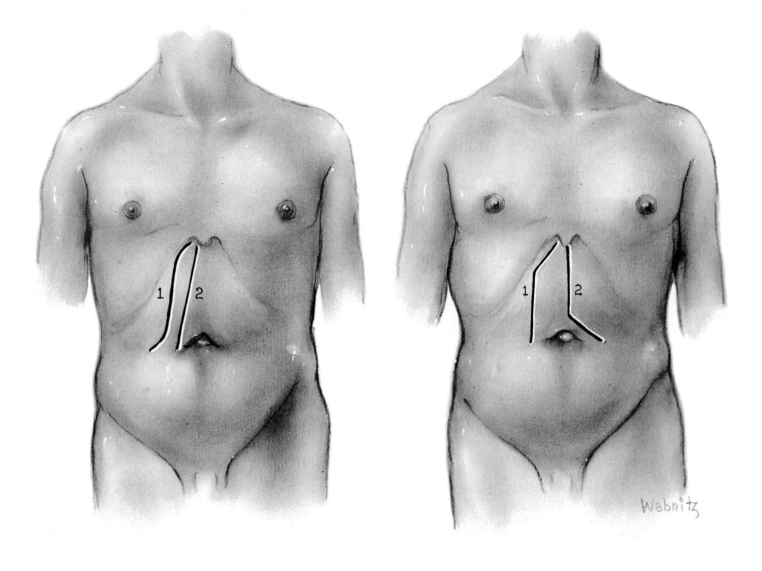

A

B

I. BEVAN   INCISION "OLD"   I. MAYO-ROBSON INCISION

2. MASSON   INCISION   2. BEVAN   INCISION "NEW"

THE THORACOABDOMINAL INCISION

The thoracoabdominal incision, either right or left, is of distinct value if used when properly indicated. It converts the pleural and the peritoneal cavities into one main cavity and thereby gives excellent exposure of the operative area. However, closure of the wound is time-consuming and there is a predisposition to more frequent postoperative complications. Furthermore, it is believed that this type of incision is employed too frequently as a routine when either an abdominal or a thoracic incision alone would suffice for the operation that is planned.

The right thoracoabdominal incision, as depicted in the artist's illustrations, may be particularly useful in reconstructive operations upon the common duct, total excision of the right lobe of the liver, and shunt operations between the portal vein and the inferior vena cava. The left thoracoabdominal incision may be used effectively in resections of the lower end of the esophagus, total gastrectomy, the removal of large and adherent spleens, and in the performance of shunt operations between the splenic and the left renal veins.

A. The incision overlying the eighth interspace and extending across the right costal margin onto the anterior abdominal wall is shown.

B. The incision is deepened through the skin and the subcutaneous fatty tissue layers to expose the underlying musculature of the anterolateral thoracic and the anterior abdominal walls.

C. The exposed muscles—the latissimus dorsi, the serratus magnus, and the external oblique muscle and its aponeurosis—are severed with a scalpel to expose the eighth and ninth ribs and the intervening external intercostal muscle.

D. The incision is continued through the external intercostal muscle layer, and the fibers of the internal intercostal muscle which course in a different plane are depicted.

Plate 12

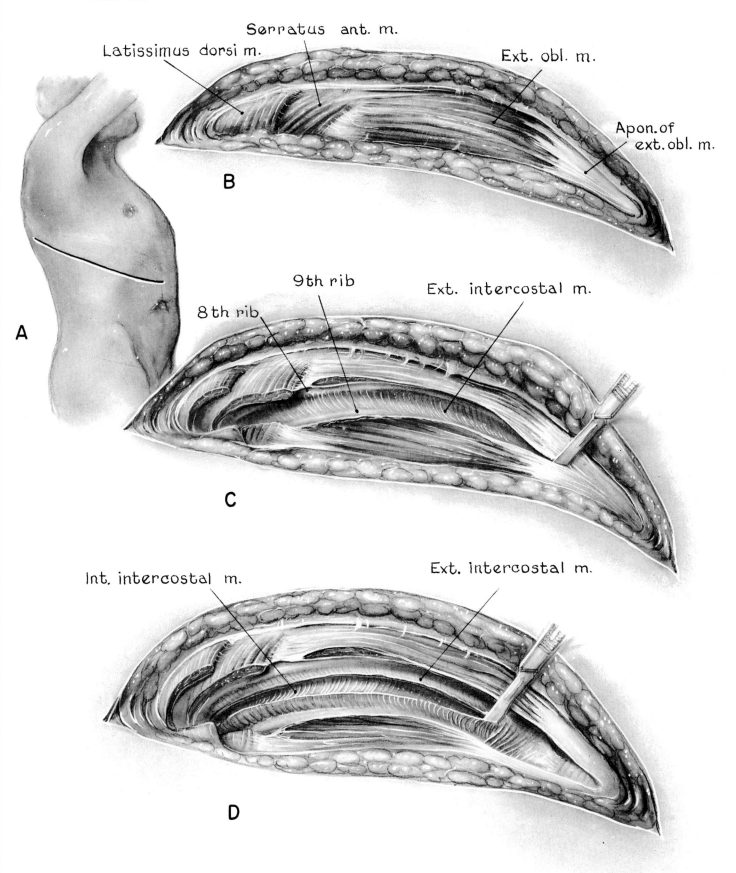

Serratus ant. m.

Latissimus dorsi m.

Ext. obl. m.

Apon. of
ext. obl. m.

B

A

9th rib

Ext. intercostal m.

8th rib

C

Int. intercostal m.

Ext. intercostal m.

D

E. The incision is deepened posteriorly through the internal intercostal muscle, the endothoracic fascia, and the parietal pleura to enter the right pleural cavity. This incision is then extended anteriorly to the costal arch severing the fibers of the internal intercostal muscle and the underlying fibers of the right leaflet of the diaphragm.

F. The incision is continued across the costal arch and through the musculature of the anterior abdominal wall to enter the peritoneal cavity.

G. The incision is completed, and the adequacy of the exposure of the operative field obtained by the conversion of the pleural and peritoneal cavities into a common cavity is shown.

Plate 13   53

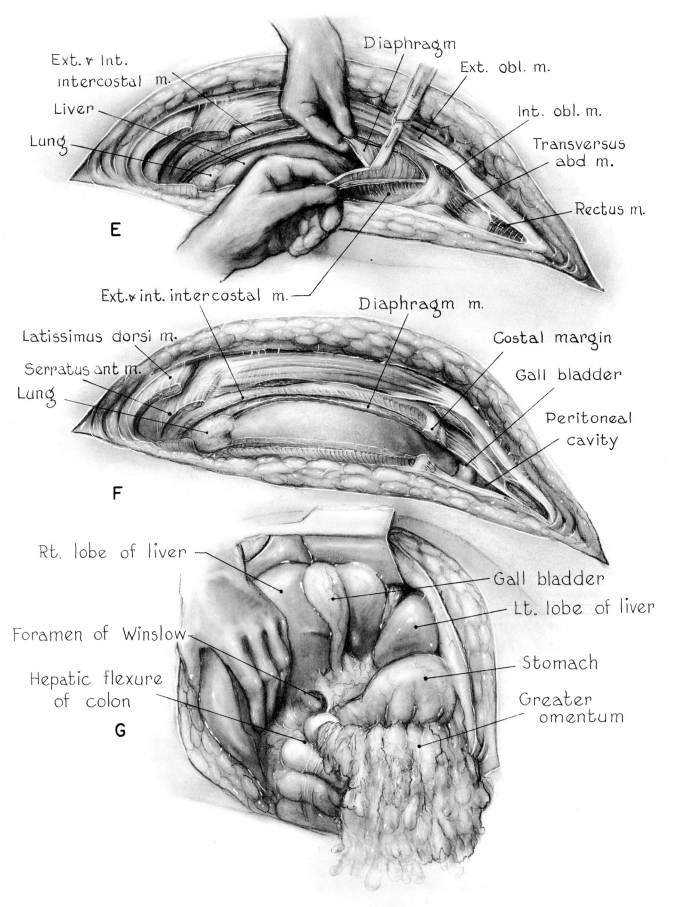

E

Ext. ᵥ Int. intercostal m.

Liver

Lung

Diaphragm

Ext. obl. m.

Int. obl. m.

Transversus abd m.

Rectus m.

F

Ext. ᵥ int. intercostal m.

Latissimus dorsi m.

Serratus ant m.

Lung

Diaphragm m.

Costal margin

Gall bladder

Peritoneal cavity

G

Rt. lobe of liver

Foramen of Winslow

Hepatic flexure of colon

Gall bladder

Lt. lobe of liver

Stomach

Greater omentum

H. The closure of the incision is begun by the approximation of the cut margins of the diaphragm with interrupted sutures of silk (00). The surrounding related structures are indicated.

I. Two pericostal sutures of double strands of No. 2 chromic catgut are inserted preliminary to the approximation of the eighth and ninth ribs. Prior to the insertion of these sutures periosteal "windows" are made along the inferior border of the lower or ninth rib. This is done to prevent the impingement of the sutures upon the periosteum and thereby possibly lessen both the incidence and/or the severity of post-thoracotomy pain.

J. The rib cage is approximated with a self-retaining Bailey–Gibbons rib approximator, and the pericostal sutures are tied and cut. The sutures of silk (000) in the intercostal muscle layers are first inserted and, after approximation of the ribs, they are then tied and cut. A figure of 8 mattress suture of No. 1 braided silk is inserted to unite the cut margins of the costal arch.

Plate 14

55

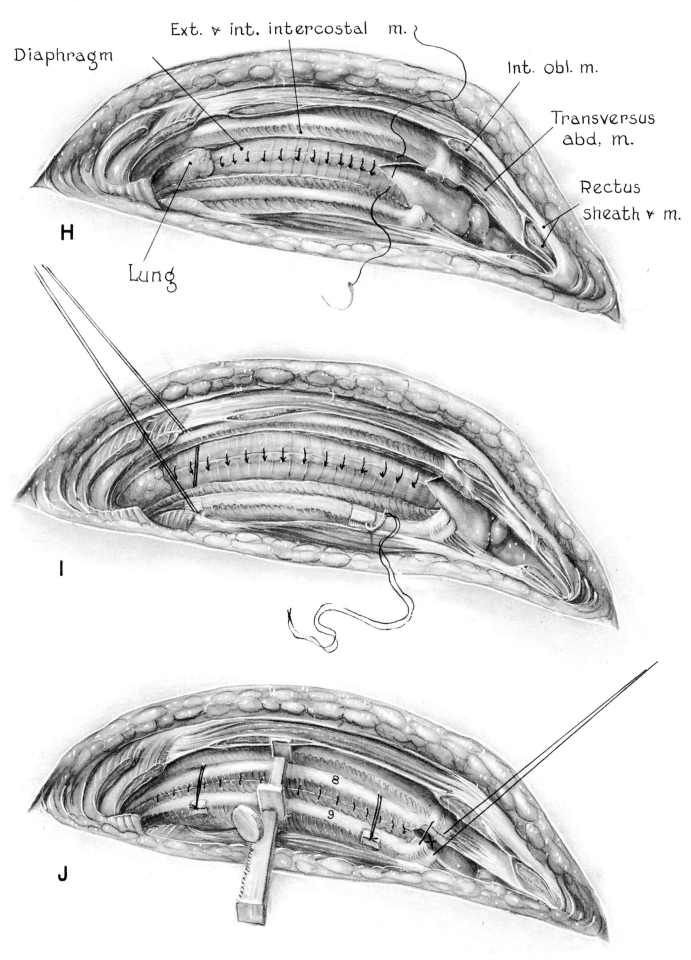

Diaphragm

Ext. & int. intercostal m.

Int. obl. m.

Transversus
abd, m.

Rectus
sheath & m.

H

Lung

I

J

K. The closure of the rib cage is completed, and the cut margins of the serratus anterior and the external oblique muscles are sutured with interrupted sutures of silk (00).

L. Close-up showing the approximation of the severed fibers of the latissimus dorsi muscle with interrupted silk (00) sutures.

M. The transversus abdominis muscle layer is approximated with a series of interrupted sutures of silk (000), which are shown inserted but not tied.

N. The closure of the transversus abdominis muscle is completed, and the suturing of the internal oblique muscle is begun using sutures of silk (000).

O. The closure of the muscle layers is completed by suturing the aponeurosis of the external oblique muscle and the anterior rectus sheath. Although not illustrated in the drawings, water-seal drainage of the pleural cavity is routinely employed.

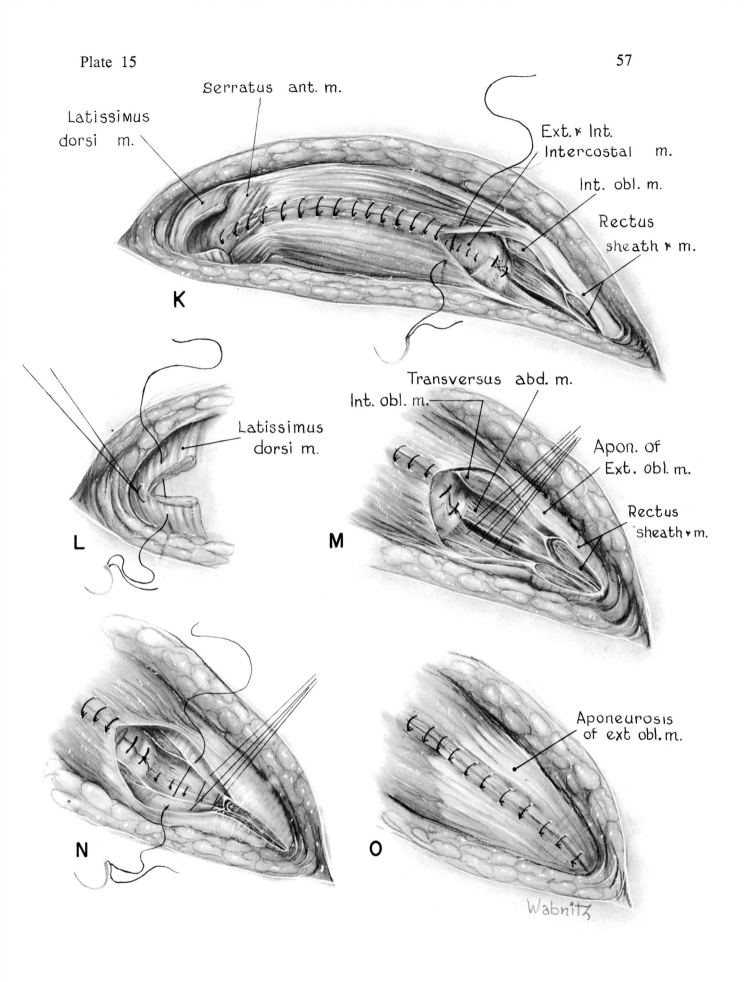

Plate 15

57

Latissimus
dorsi m.

Serratus ant. m.

Ext. × Int.
Intercostal m.

Int. obl. m.

Rectus
sheath × m.

K

L

Latissimus
dorsi m.

Transversus abd. m.

Int. obl. m.

Apon. of
Ext. obl. m.

Rectus
sheath × m.

M

N

O

Aponeurosis
of ext obl. m.

Wabnitz

HERNIORRHAPHY—INDIRECT INGUINAL HERNIA
MODIFIED FERGUSON-ANDREWS REPAIR

A. An oblique inguinal incision approximately 6 cm. in length and about 3 cm. medial and parallel to the inguinal ligament is outlined and crosshatched to facilitate later closure. The proximal end of this incision extends to a point midway between the pubic tubercle and the anterior iliac spine. The extension of the incision to the level of the anterior iliac spine, so frequently depicted, is not necessary.

B. The skin incision is deepened through the superficial layer (Camper) of the subcutaneous fascia to expose the vessels between this layer and the underlying deep layer (Scarpa) of the subcutaneous fascia. The external superficial epigastric vessels have been doubly clamped, severed, and occluded with ligatures of fine (0000) silk. The external superficial pudendal vessels are being severed between clamps with a

scalpel. The incision to be made through Scarpa's fascia is in dotted outline.

C. An incision is made through the fatty areolar tissue layer beneath Scarpa's fascia to expose the underlying aponeurosis of the external oblique muscle.

D. The fatty areolar tissue layer is most easily separated from the aponeurosis of the external oblique muscle by blunt digital dissection with a piece of dry gauze over the index finger.

E, F. A small incision is made with a scalpel through the external oblique aponeurosis, and the incision is extended downward by scissor dissection through the external ring.

G. The medial and lateral leaflets of the aponeurosis are mobilized and retracted to expose the structures as depicted.

DISCUSSION—DR. S. W. MOORE. When incisions are crosshatched (Plate 16, A) to facilitate closure, usually the cross marks are not accurately approximated and at times leave an unsightly scar. The incision may be accurately approximated by insertion of the middle suture first, one bite of which it may be necessary to place lower on one side than on the other. In general incisions for hernias are placed too far laterally. It is believed that the incision should extend well over the pubic spine as this is the location where the repair is to

be performed.

It is the practice of some surgeons not to remove the fatty areolar tissue from the fascia (Plate 18, O) since it is believed that this is an important source of blood supply. Personally, however, I prefer to have the fascia as clean as possible. In the illustration, Plate 16, G, the ilioinguinal nerve is clearly shown. Normally it is best to leave this nerve intact, but if it should interfere with the repair, it may be severed without any ill effect.

Plate 16   59

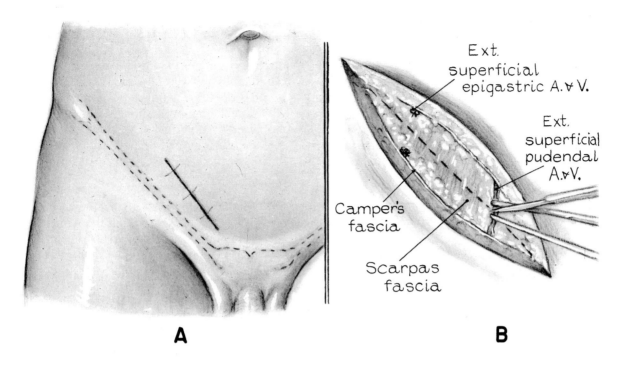

A

Ext. superficial epigastric A. & V.

Ext. superficial pudendal A. & V.

Camper's fascia

Scarpas fascia

B

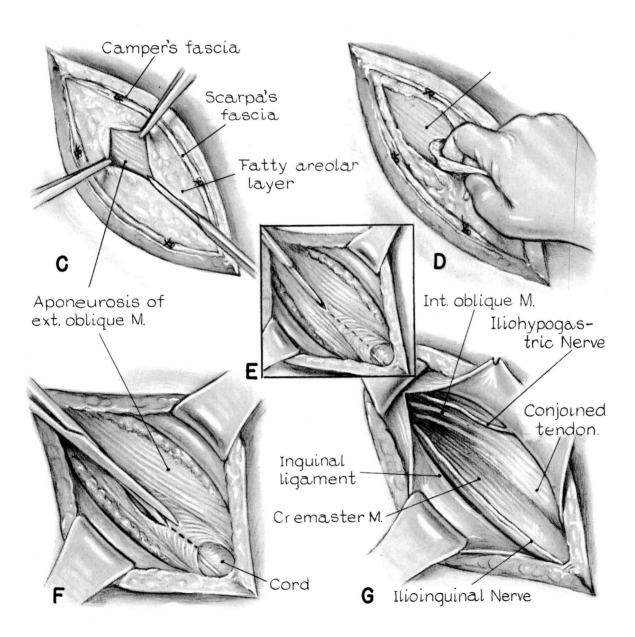

Camper's fascia

Scarpa's fascia

Fatty areolar layer

C

Aponeurosis of ext. oblique M.

D

E

Int. oblique M.

Iliohypogastric Nerve

Conjoined tendon.

Inguinal ligament

Cremaster M.

F

Cord

G   Ilioinguinal Nerve

H. The cord structures and the overlying "veil" of cremaster muscle fibers are displaced medially to expose the external spermatic and pubic vessels which are faintly visible beneath the cremaster muscle.

I. The cremaster muscle "veil" is incised, and mobilization of the cord is commenced.

J. The mobilization of the cord is continued, and its relation to the surrounding structures is indicated. The dotted line depicts the site of the incision in the areolar tissue plane between the vas deferens and the external spermatic and pubic vessels that is required to mobilize completely the cord structures.

K. The mobilized cord, encircled by a gauze strip, is retracted laterally, and scissor dissection of the hernial sac is commenced. In indirect inguinal hernias, excluding those of the sliding type, the hernial sac is anteromedial to the cord. The V-shaped defect uniformly present in the transversalis fascia may be seen.

L. The sac is completely mobilized, and the relation of the neck of the sac to the internal spermatic vessels, the vas deferens, the deep epigastric vessels, and the V-shaped defect in the transversalis fascia is shown.

The dotted line indicates the site of the opening to be made in the sac. A technic for mobilizing the sac, preferred by many, is to make an incision into the lumen of the sac immediately upon its identification. A finger is then inserted into the lumen, and, with digital traction maintained, the sac is mobilized by blunt gauze dissection. However, mobilization by sharp dissection as indicated is preferred.

M, N. A high transfixion suture ligation of the neck of the sac, using 00 silk, is performed, and the redundant sac tissue is subsequently removed. In large hernias a preliminary resection of a portion of the redundant sac is done as indicated in dotted outline (M). If the neck of the sac is unduly large, closure by interrupted mattress sutures of silk to avoid tissue tension is preferred. The divergence of the internal spermatic vessels and the vas deferens and their relation to the posterior surface of the neck of the sac are visible. Rethreading of the long ends of the transfixion suture for anchorage to the internal oblique muscle is neither practiced nor recommended. The use of such a method is believed an expression of inadequate mobilization of the sac because the ligated stump of a sac that has been completely mobilized will automatically retract beneath the internal oblique muscle.

DISCUSSION—DR. MOORE (cont.)

I prefer to open the sac as quickly as possible and consider this a technical aid in its further mobilization by a combination of blunt gauze and sharp scalpel dissection. In long sacs, portions of the sac are excised as the dissection proceeds toward the neck. If, in the course of this dissection, an opening is accidentally made in the lower part of the sac, it is immediately continued into the main opening. Following the completion of the mobilization of the sac, the neck may be occluded by a high transfixion suture ligation as demonstrated (Plate 17, M, N). However, in some instances, particularly in sacs in which the neck is of a wide diameter, closure of the neck of the sac from the inside using either a circular or a series of interrupted sutures is preferred.

Plate 17   61

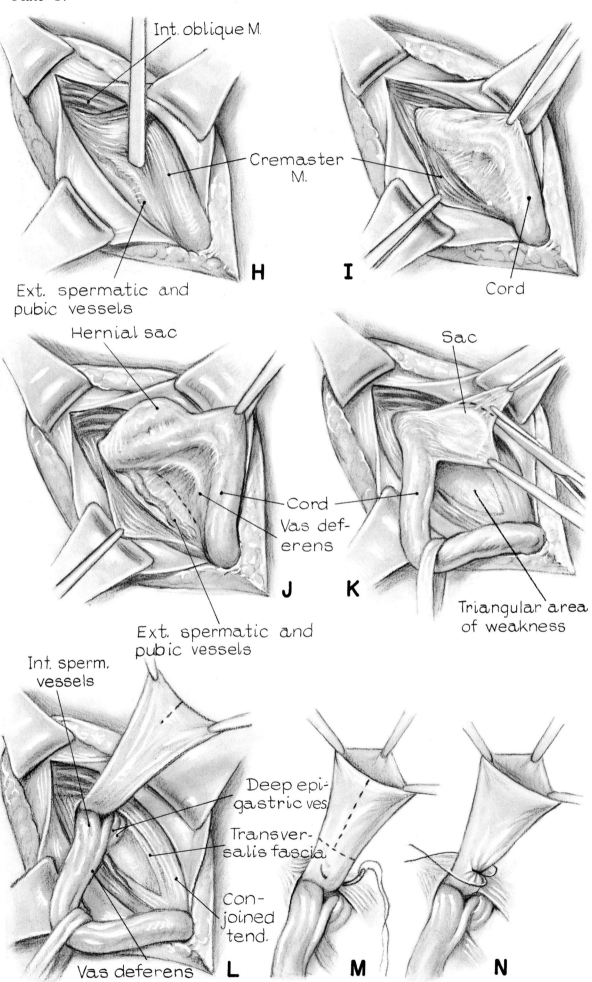

Int. oblique M.

Cremaster M.

Ext. spermatic and pubic vessels

H

Cord

I

Hernial sac

Sac

Cord

Vas def-erens

J

Triangular area of weakness

K

Ext. spermatic and pubic vessels

Int. sperm. vessels

Deep epi-gastric ves.

Transver-salis fascia

Con-joined tend.

Vas deferens   **L**

M

N

O. The ligated stump of the hernial sac, retracted beneath the internal oblique muscle, is shown in dotted outline. The external spermatic and pubic vessels and their parent trunk, the deep epigastric vessels, are clearly shown. In the closure of the V-shaped defect in the transversalis fascia, the two uppermost silk (000) sutures are anterior and the remaining sutures posterior to the external spermatic and pubic vessels.

P. The closure of the defect in the transversalis fascia with interrupted sutures of silk (000) is completed. The external spermatic and pubic vessels have their exit below the two uppermost sutures. If desired, a segmental resection of these vessels may be performed prior to the closure of the transversalis fascia.

Q. The cremaster muscle "veil" may be loosely approximated as shown, and the medial leaflet of the external oblique aponeurosis is enfolded and sutured to the shelving edge of the inguinal ligament using interrupted sutures of silk (000). In this technic a fascia-to-fascia approximation without tension is obtained. The Bassini type of repair in which the conjoined "tendon" is sutured to the inguinal ligament is not practiced. The objection to this type of repair is twofold: (1) it is believed anatomi-

cally unsound and places undue tension upon the structures that are approximated; (2) the conjoined tendon is most frequently not tendinous but generally a frayed musculofascial structure of limited holding power.

R. The approximation of the medial leaflet of the external oblique aponeurosis to the shelving edge of the inguinal ligament is completed, and the imbrication of the lateral leaflet about the cord, using sutures of fine silk (0000), is commenced.

R′. Inset to demonstrate the Stetten maneuver of cutting the lateral leaflet to prevent constriction of the cord at its exit from the internal ring. Although this method is in common usage, the technic shown in R is preferred.

S. The imbrication of the lateral and medial leaflets of the external oblique is being completed. The sutures which approximated the medial leaflet of the external oblique aponeurosis to the shelving edge of the inguinal ligament may be seen as faintly visible black dots.

T, U. The superficial fascia and skin layers are approximated using interrupted sutures of 0000 and 000 silk respectively.

DISCUSSION—DR. MOORE (cont.)

In repairing the defect as illustrated in Plate 18 (O) I like to get rid of as much excess tissue in the cord structures as possible in order to diminish its diameter and thereby have a small opening at its site of exit in the fascia repair. Therefore, all of the fat and usually the cremaster muscle is excised frequently, leaving only the vas deferens and the cord vessels. At times the vas deferens and the cord vessels are separated completely and brought out through different openings in the fascial repair.

In the Halsted I type of repair, where the exter-

nal ring is placed over the internal, I no longer incise the lateral leaf of the external oblique aponeurosis as depicted in Plate 18 (R′), but actually make a very short inguinal canal, measuring approximately 1.5 cm. in length, between the two openings placing the external opening cephalad. When the tissues are thinned out and weakened and in instances where there have been two or more attempts at the repair of a hernia, the cord may be severed and/or the testicle removed to effect a better chance for cure.

Plate 18

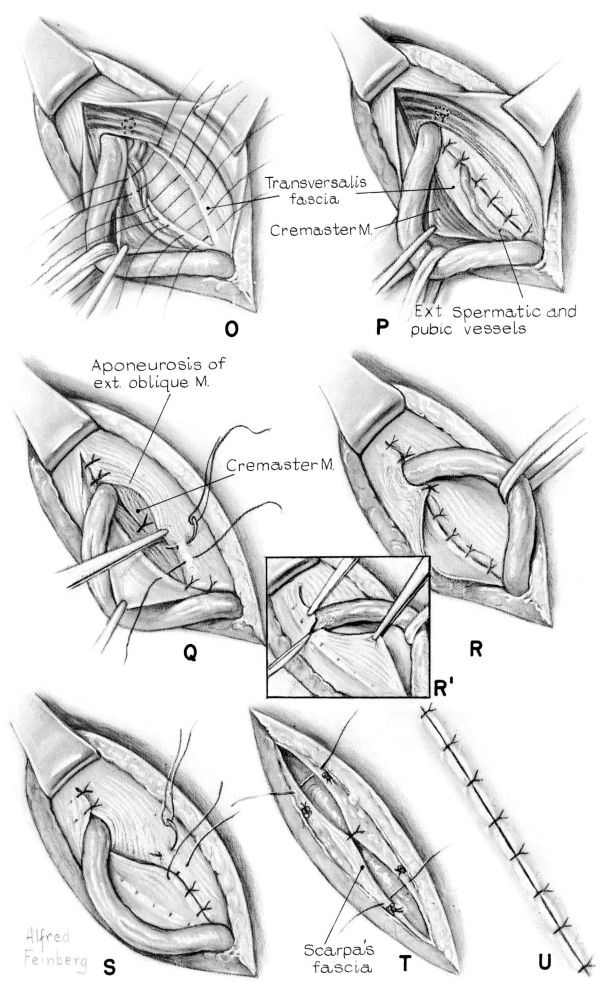

Transversalis fascia

Cremaster M.

Ext. Spermatic and pubic vessels

O

P

Aponeurosis of ext. oblique M.

Cremaster M.

Q

R

R'

Alfred Feinberg

S

Scarpa's fascia

T

U

DISCUSSION—MR. W. J. LYTLE. The skin incision illustrated is a satisfactory one and could with advantage be extended farther outward if the internal ring were to be repaired. It is important to expose cleanly the shining fibers of the external oblique aponeurosis (E) in order to avoid the intervention of fatty and areolar tissues in the subsequent line of suture, which would prevent firm union of this aponeurosis. In G, the ilioinguinal nerve can be removed without ill effect if it gets in the way.

Regarding H, the external spermatic artery and veins, which enter the inguinal canal through its posterior wall, medial to and below the internal ring, and the genital branch of the genitofemoral nerve are rarely depicted in hernia illustrations; if roughly handled, they can cause troublesome bleeding. The cremaster "veil" (I) should be divided widely and well below the external ring to give good exposure to the deeper dissection.

At the stage shown in L, I recommend that the internal (deep) ring be identified and repaired. In my view the repair of the ring when it is strong is of major importance, because the ring stands as a guardian at the exit of the spermatic cord and provides at this opening an active closure mechanism that can be demonstrated at hernia operations under local anesthesia. In oblique hernia the internal ring is gradually enlarged as the hernia increases in size, and it is important to reduce this opening to normal size in order to allow the closure mechanism to function properly. When, as in L, the sac has been mobilized and opened, the ring edges can be clearly demonstrated by passing the index finger through the neck of the sac. The finger draws forward and exposes to view the white shining fibers of the ring. This is the most important step in the operation, and opportunity should be taken to assess the strength of the posterior wall of the inguinal canal by pressing forward with the finger inside the peritoneal cavity. With the finger behind the ring, a few touches of the knife will free and define its margin, which is then picked up in artery forceps. The ring, held forward in forceps, is separated from the neck of the sac, to which it is often closely adherent, and from the spermatic cord. This step must be carried out before the sac is tied off; otherwise, the stump of the sac retracts and carries the ring backward out of view. After removal of the sac, the edges or pillars of the ring, when strong, are sutured together with fine silk, starting medially and working laterally until the ring fits snugly around the cord.

The lower or outer pillar of the ring is often found to be weak. If defective in this way, the upper or inner pillar, which is usually strong, is stitched to the inguinal ligament to close the ring opening around the cord. If both pillars of the ring are unsatisfactory or if the posterior inguinal wall has been found defective by the exploring finger within the peritoneal cavity, a posterior wall repair like that for direct hernia (O) is carried out; otherwise, with a good ring and good posterior wall, this step seems to be unnecessary or even damaging.

To digress briefly, I should like to describe the anatomy and function of the internal (deep) inguinal ring. The U-shaped ring is a sling composed of thickened transversalis fascia with two pillars that are firmly attached above to the posterior aspect of the aponeurosis of the transversus abdominis muscle, whose fibers lie obliquely in the inguinal region.

The protective action of the internal ring is explained as follows. During acts of coughing and straining, the muscles of the anterior abdominal wall contract. If during contraction there is any attempt at protrusion of the abdominal contents through the ring, its pillars are pulled upon. This pull is transmitted to the fibers of the transversus muscle, and, as a result, the contraction of the transversus muscle is greatly increased. Because the fibers of the muscle lie obliquely in the inguinal region, the ring is drawn in an upward and outward direction to close around the emerging spermatic cord. This action, which I described in 1945, is an example of the stretch reflex of Liddell and Sherrington, who showed that when a muscle is caused to contract, a stretch applied to it enhances its contraction to a considerable degree.

Surgeons have overlooked the internal ring if they have not known how to expose it at operations. Anatomists have also failed to find it, because the ring can only be seen when the posterior aspect of the anterior abdominal wall is examined with the bony pelvis preserved intact around it. Hesselbach described the internal ring with the bony pelvis in situ in 1816, and Henry O. Marcy, the pioneer surgeon of Boston, Massachusetts, described the operation for repair of the ring in 1871.

Over many years I have found that repair of the internal ring, as described above, has led to a considerable decrease in the number of recurrences.

To explain further the action of the internal ring, it may be of interest to relate how by chance I found that it possessed mobility and was not merely an inert opening in the transversalis fascia. On February 13, 1943, I was operating on a man with oblique inguinal hernia and had isolated the internal ring and tied and removed the sac when the patient, who was under light anesthesia, began to cough. The ring, which was held by forceps under tension and ready for suture, was suddenly pulled out of my hand. With each cough the ring moved upward and outward under cover of the internal oblique muscle. Movement of the ring was observed only when it was held under tension. This observation, confirmed by operations under local anesthesia, encouraged me to turn to the older anatomists and surgeons, and I found that Hesselbach had described the ring with beautiful illustrations in 1816 and that Marcy had first repaired it in 1871. Marcy wrote several articles on repair of the ring and published his large and well-illustrated book in 1892.

Plate 34 97

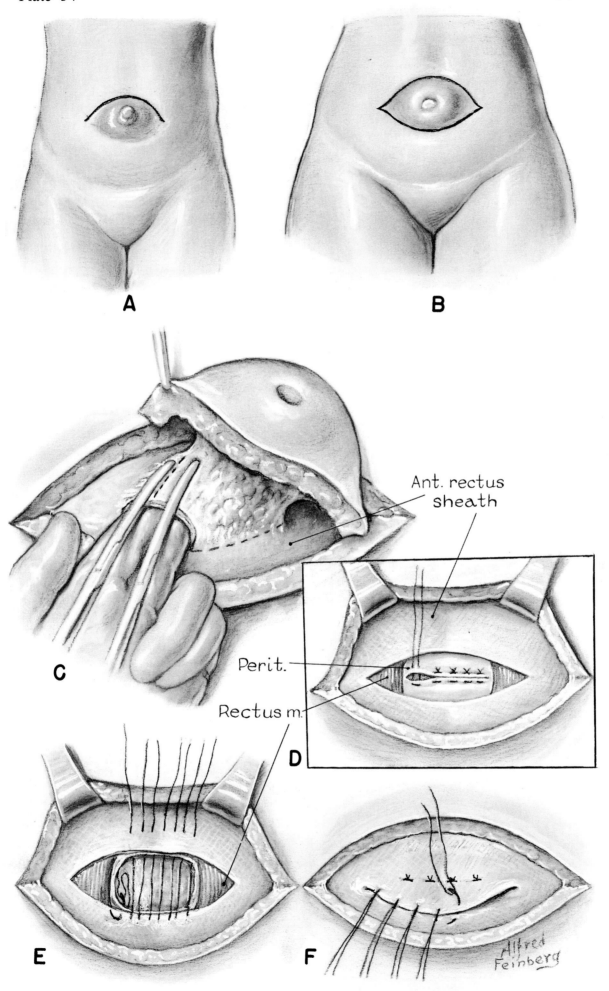

A

B

Ant. rectus
sheath

C

Perit.

Rectus m.

D

E

F

Alfred
Feinberg

DISCUSSION—MR. W. J. LYTLE. The illustrations show clearly the Mayo method of repair for umbilical hernia.

Preservation of the umbilicus in children for cosmetic reasons is recommended; its removal may subject children to ridicule at school.

The great advantage of the Mayo operation is its transverse closure, for the repair is not pulled apart by contraction of the lateral abdominal muscles.

The operation is also greatly favored because of the increased strength given by the overlap of the rectus sheath, but there are some obvious weaknesses in this view. The repair is weak at the lateral angles, where the degree of overlap is slight or absent. In E both peritoneum and extraperitoneal fat are sandwiched between the layers of the overlap and tend to act as buffers against firm fibrous union. When the peritoneum is repaired separately, as in D, extraperitoneal fat, unless carefully removed, also intervenes between the two flaps.

I venture to put forward a plea for approximation of the cut edges of the rectus sheath without overlap, after suturing the peritoneum separately. This should give, and in my experience does give, good union at the line of suture, where there is free release of fibroblasts.

DISCUSSION—DR. CHESTER B. McVAY. The management of the umbilical hernia as presented follows my concepts exactly. In the small umbilical hernioplasty I frequently do not imbricate or close in a "vest over pants" fashion but simply approximate the thickened edges in a linear fashion with closely placed sutures. In the infant umbilical hernia I use fine silk sutures, as depicted. In the larger umbilical hernias in the adult I use wire sutures of stainless steel. The concept of closure of the umbilical defect in the transverse plane is a very sound concept. The direction of muscle pull is entirely lateral, and if the defect is closed in a vertical plane, every abdominal wall strain tends to disrupt the suture line.

A. The incisional scar overlying the hernial protrusion is excised in an elliptical manner as indicated in the dotted outline.

B. The elliptical excision of the operative scar is completed, and the thinned out fibrous tissue (false hernial sac) which encases the hernial contents is shown.

C. Sterile towels are fixed to the skin edges with towel clips through which upward and outward traction is maintained as scalpel dissection is commenced beneath the subcutaneous fatty tissue plane. This dissection is extended widely on either side to the margins of the lateral abdominal wall. This is considered an essential basic step in the operative repair of incisional hernias. Following the completion of the dissection on one side several warm moist gauze pads are placed beneath the mobilized flap and a similar dissection is performed on the opposite side.

D. The mobilization of the flaps is completed, and the relation of the hernial protrusion to the surrounding fascia and muscles of the anterolateral abdominal wall is depicted.

E. An incision is made parallel to the lateral margin of the hernia through the line of junction of the true and false fascia, and a portion of the underlying rectus muscle is exposed. Clamps are applied to the cut edge of the true fascia, and with lateral traction maintained, the incision is continued distally to join the lower portion of a similar incision completed on the opposite side.

F. Scalpel dissection is continued and the medial border of the rectus muscle is separated from the side of the false hernial sac exposing the underlying layer of transversalis fascia and peritoneum.

DISCUSSION—DR. DANIEL F. CASTEN. The occurrence of incisional hernias is dependent upon many factors: location of incision, type of suture material, infection, postoperative stress upon the incision, and poor technic of abdominal wall closure. Some of these factors are definitely amenable to correction, and with properly placed incisions, careful attention to every detail of closure, and avoidance of postoperative distention, the incidence of incomplete wound dehiscense should be materially decreased. The work of Dunphy and others has increased our knowledge considerably in the field of hormonal and metabolic factors concerned in the healing of incised wounds, and clinical application of these data should prove rewarding.

These illustrations define the ideal repair for abdominal incisional hernias. The layers of the abdominal wall are cleanly dissected and delineated. They appear to be of satisfactory strength and texture, and the defect is small enough to permit a layer closure with an anterior rectus sheath overlap. This is the goal for our surgical repair: reapproximation of anatomic layers in normal sequence and without tension. The use of nonabsorbable sutures, as illustrated, is essential for the maintenance of the repair until fibroplasia is complete.

Unfortunately, however, one is frequently unable to approach this ideal. The layers of the abdominal wall at the site of herniation may be scarred and fused. The false hernial sac, as demonstrated (Plate 35, B) represents fusion of remnants of fascial elements with peritoneum. The tissues adjacent to the sac may also be involved in this process of fusion and scarification and, therefore, are frequently unsatisfactory for use as a buttress. Furthermore, the sac may be so ad-

herent to the underlying viscera that separation is virtually impossible. Finally, the defect may be so large or so located that approximation of the edges cannot be accomplished. The rectus muscles in these larger hernias become attenuated and are useless for purposes of repair; the fascial layers, having been replaced by scar tissue, may appear strong, but, because of loss of elasticity, are unable to resist the forces of intraabdominal pressure.

Many alternative procedures have been recommended to meet these situations. The treatment of the sac, for example, varies considerably. I believe, with Dr. Madden, that excision is desirable if possible, but it has been my practice to leave portions of the sac behind if the visceral adhesions render separation hazardous. Methods of inversion of the sac by serial rows of sutures without opening into the peritoneal cavity are dangerous since one does not expose the underlying viscera. Furthermore, this method may predispose to postoperative intestinal obstruction.

If the fascial and peritoneal layers are fused, individual closure, as depicted in Plate 36 (I, J, and K), is impossible. In these individuals an overlap procedure of the fused layers in a vertical or transverse axis similar in principle to the Mayo technic for closure of umbilical hernias is adequate and satisfactory. Relaxing fascial incisions may be employed when necessary, and many seemingly impossible repairs can be effected. In small defects, I prefer a transverse closure since the lines of force exerted upon the abdominal wall during stress tend to approximate rather than separate the edges. Large defects, of necessity, require a vertical closure.

Plate 35   101

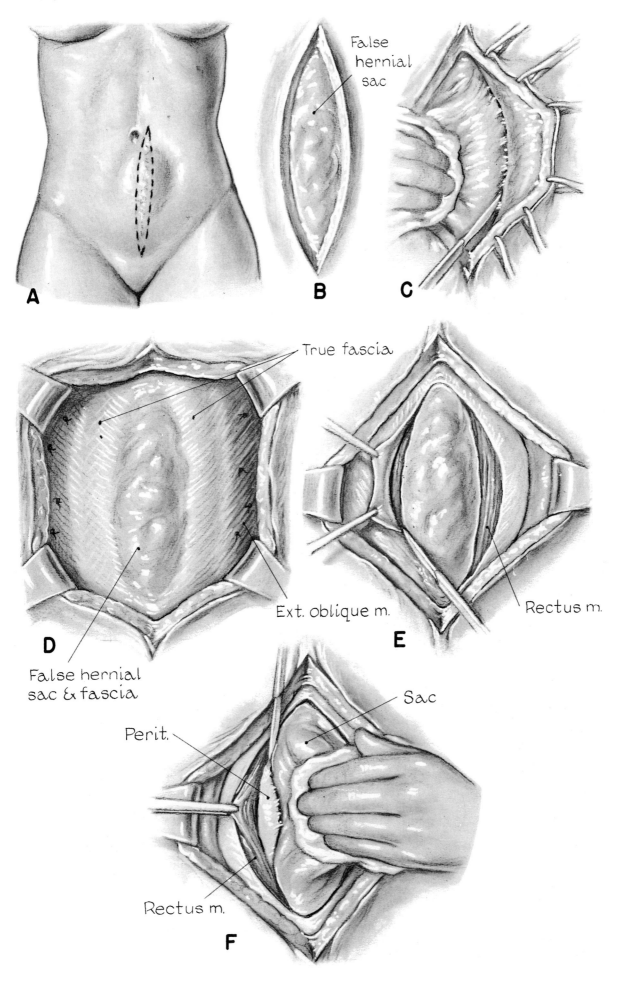

False
hernial
sac

A

B

C

True fascia

Ext. oblique m.

Rectus m.

D

E

False hernial
sac & fascia

Sac

Perit.

Rectus m.

F

G. The mobilized musculofascial layers are retracted, and, using a scalpel, the dissection of the false hernial sac is completed.

H. An elliptical excision of the false hernial sac (dotted lines) along the line of junction with the normal fascia-peritoneal layer is commenced.

I. The excision of the false hernial sac is completed, and the closure of the fascia-peritoneal layer, using interrupted mattress sutures of silk (00), is begun.

J. The fascia-peritoneal closure is completed, and the muscle layer is loosely approximated with simple interrupted sutures of silk (00). In many instances the closure of this layer is omitted because of either the atrophy of the muscles or the excessive tension on the suture line.

K. An imbrication type closure of the anterior fascial layer is performed using both horizontal mattress and simple interrupted sutures of 00 silk. If undue tension on the suture line is present, linear relaxing incisions in the fascia laterally on either side are made.

L. The closure of the skin incision with interrupted sutures of silk completes the operation. Because of the extensive undermining of the flaps of skin and subcutaneous fatty tissue, drains are frequently used and have their exit through stab wounds lateral to and on either side of the skin closure.

DISCUSSION—DR. CASTEN (cont.)

Herniations in the subcostal areas or in the upper midline offer certain difficulties. In the former, the unyielding upper costal edge presents a barrier to closure, and in the latter, the relatively fixed fascial layers present a challenge to adequate mobilization and sufficient relaxation for secure repair. In these hernias and in all large hernias through the abdominal wall my preference is the use of tantalum mesh for the repair as advocated by Koontz. The peritoneal and fascial layers are defined and approximated as carefully as possible without tension, and the residual defect is covered with a sheet of tantalum mesh. Considerable experience with this method has demonstrated its value and prolonged follow-up observations have confirmed this impression. A firm, unyielding proliferation of fascia occurs through the interstices of the mesh, and even though this frequently becomes fragmented, the closure remains firm. The use of tantalum or surgical steel mesh is preferred to fascial flap or graft procedures.

As a final note, a recent experience with preoperative pneumoperitoneum, as advocated by Russo and Mazzini in the preparation for operation of a patient with a huge incisional hernia which had lost its "right of domicile," and some past unfortunate experiences in the forceful reduction of these hernias has suggested the more frequent employment of this method.

DISCUSSION—MR. W. J. LYTLE. The operation so clearly illustrated is the well-tried and satisfactory repair for incisional hernia. The anatomic layers are clearly defined in the drawings, as they should be at operation, and each layer is united in its normal plane. It would be a great advance if this principle could be followed in the repair of groin hernia.

An alternative operation is closure of the layers of the abdominal wall over unopened peritoneum. This method is valuable for "poor risk" patients. It has the advantage of not disturbing the peritoneal cavity and avoiding tedious dissection of intestinal adhesions that are usually present. There is, in consequence, less risk of chest complications and postoperative abdominal distention. If the hernial protrusion does not reduce easily and completely, the operation may be followed by intestinal obstruction. The obstruction may be caused, for example, by a loop of small intestine imprisoned in a loculus that has been pushed back into the abdomen.

In huge hernias of long duration, especially in fat patients, the abdominal cavity cannot accommodate the hernial contents. A suitable belt and diet restrictions may enable the operation to be carried out at a later date.

DISCUSSION—DR. CHESTER B. MCVAY. The incisional hernia problem has so many facets that it is impossible to cover it in a brief discussion. The incisional hernia that is presented and figured is repaired by sound surgical principles and offers no room for disagreement. I use stainless steel wire instead of silk and in recent years have tended to simply approximate the scarred and fused margins of the aponeurotic defect without making any attempt to dissect out the separate layers. I have not evaluated long-term results in this simplified method of closure, but, as an anatomist, I cannot resist the opportunity to point out that if all abdominal incisions were transverse the incisional hernia problem would not be so complex.

Incisional hernias do occur in transverse incisions, but their repair is usually quite simple. The all-important transversus abdominus layer can be approximated without tension, because the fibers have been separated by the hernial mass and not transected by the surgeon's knife. The wide retraction of the margins of the aponeurotic defect in an incisional hernia in a vertical incision, on the other hand, coupled with the fixed contracture of the corresponding muscle fibers, frequently makes the problem of incisional hernioplasty a formidable one.

Plate 36

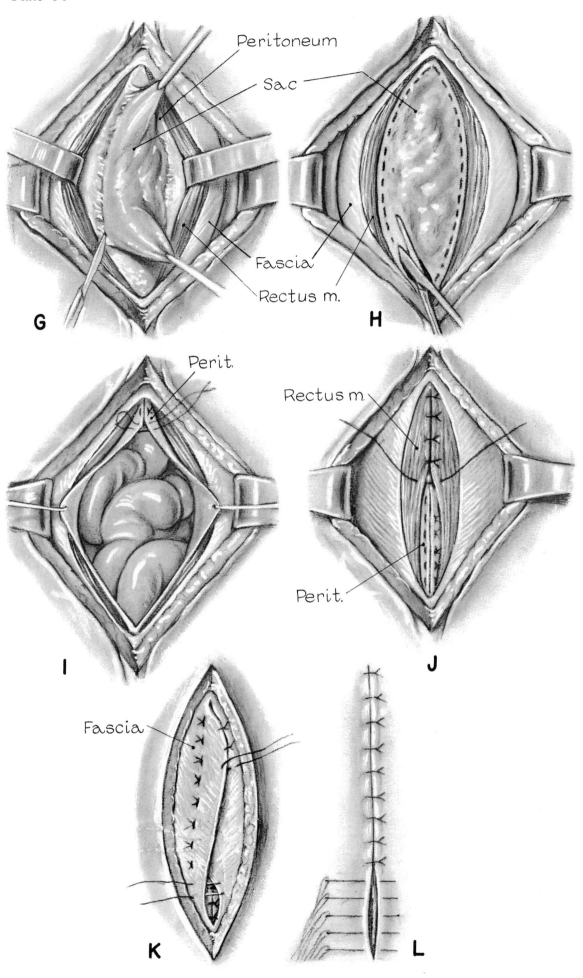

Peritoneum

Sac

Fascia

Rectus m.

G

H

Perit.

Rectus m.

Perit.

I

J

Fascia

K

L

COMBINED OPERATION FOR CONGENITAL INGUINAL HERNIA AND UNDESCENDED TESTICLE

A. The incision, which partly overlies the protuberance caused by the undescended testicle, is indicated by the solid black line. The empty scrotum on the left side is visible.

B. The skin incision is deepened through Camper's fascia, and the external superficial epigastric vein, doubly clamped, is being transected with scissors. The ligated stumps of the external superficial pudendal vein are visible caudad. These vessels are located between the fascia of Camper (superficial) and that of Scarpa (deep).

C, D. Scarpa's fascia is incised (C), and the underlying fatty areolar tissue is removed from the surface of the aponeurosis of the external oblique muscle by blunt digital dissection using a piece of dry gauze (D).

DISCUSSION—DR. GEORGE A. FIEDLER. Surgical treatment of cryptorchism has as its main purpose the placing of the testis in its normal position in the bottom of the scrotum and at the same time preserving its blood supply and the vas deferens. Whether even after this all the functions of the testis reach a normal physiologic level is never certain. Consequently there is a wide difference of opinion as to what is the appropriate age for the success of this procedure.

The decision to operate having been made, it is most important to choose the surgical procedure most likely to preserve the blood supply (or the least likely to impair it) and lengthen the spermatic cord. One sees at once the need for meticulous care in teasing out the vessels from the tissues in which they always seem to be enmeshed. The skill and patience of the surgeon, his respect for delicate structures, and a thorough knowledge of the anatomy of the region will insure, more than anything else, the success of the operation.

The anatomic relations so clearly shown in the drawings will be lost unless great care is taken after the skin incision is made. The operation chosen by Dr. Madden and illustrated shows clearly the various tissue layers encountered in surgery of the cryptorchid that is most commonly seen—namely, the one which lies somewhere in the inguinal canal, and accessible through the incision over the canal. In the case of a testis within

Plate 37   105

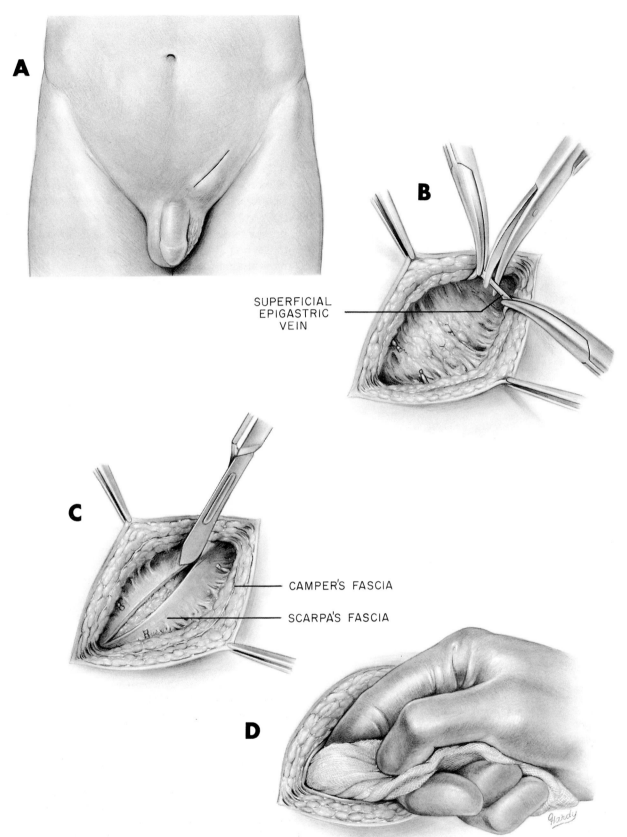

A

B

SUPERFICIAL
EPIGASTRIC
VEIN

C

CAMPER'S FASCIA

SCARPA'S FASCIA

D

E, F. The wound margins are retracted, and a short incision is made cephalad in the external oblique aponeurosis (E) and then extended caudad (broken line) through the external ring by a pushing motion with the tips of the partially open blades of the scissors (F). The undescended testicle is protruded through the external ring (E, F).

G. The leaflets of the external oblique aponeurosis are retracted, and the underlying structures are exposed. An opening made in the cremaster muscle "veil" is being extended caudad to unroof the dislocated testis, which is held taut by clamp (Babcock) traction through the gubernaculum.

H. The cremaster fibers are transected distally, which permits the elevation of the cord structures encased by the sac of the accompanying congenital hernia. The sac, mobilized in forceps, is being severed (broken line) with scissors. The proximal cut ends of the cremaster muscle are visible in the caudad angle of the incision.

I. The hernial sac is severed anteriorly, and saline is being injected between the posterior wall of the sac and the cord structures to facilitate their separation. The broken line indicates the incision to be made preparatory to the completion of the mobilization of the posterior wall of the hernial sac. A portion of omental fat is seen protruded from the peritoneal cavity.

DISCUSSION—DR. FIEDLER (cont.)

the abdomen or in an ectopic position, however, the same incision would very likely be employed.

It has been my practice to employ, when possible, the well-known method of Torek. In this operation the exposure and dissection of the restricting fibrous tissue is performed to give as much length to the cord as possible, or at least sufficient to place the testis as low as possible in the scrotum. Then the testis is carried through an incision in the skin of the scrotum and attached to the deep fascia of the anteromedial aspect of the thigh of the same side. The type of sutures seems to be of little consequence, but silk is more dependable than catgut for attachment of the testis to the fascia. The silk can be either removed or left behind for three to six months, when the testis is detached at the second stage of the operation.

Observation of the results of many operations by many surgeons for cryptorchism have convinced me of the advantages of this procedure. Whether the testis, which appears to be a more normal one when seen at the second stage, is due to its low position or to additional temporary blood supply has always been controversial. For some reason, which cannot be logically explained, it appears larger. But the addition of fat removed from the thigh and carried with the testis back into the scrotum will often make the organ appear larger.

Plate 38   107

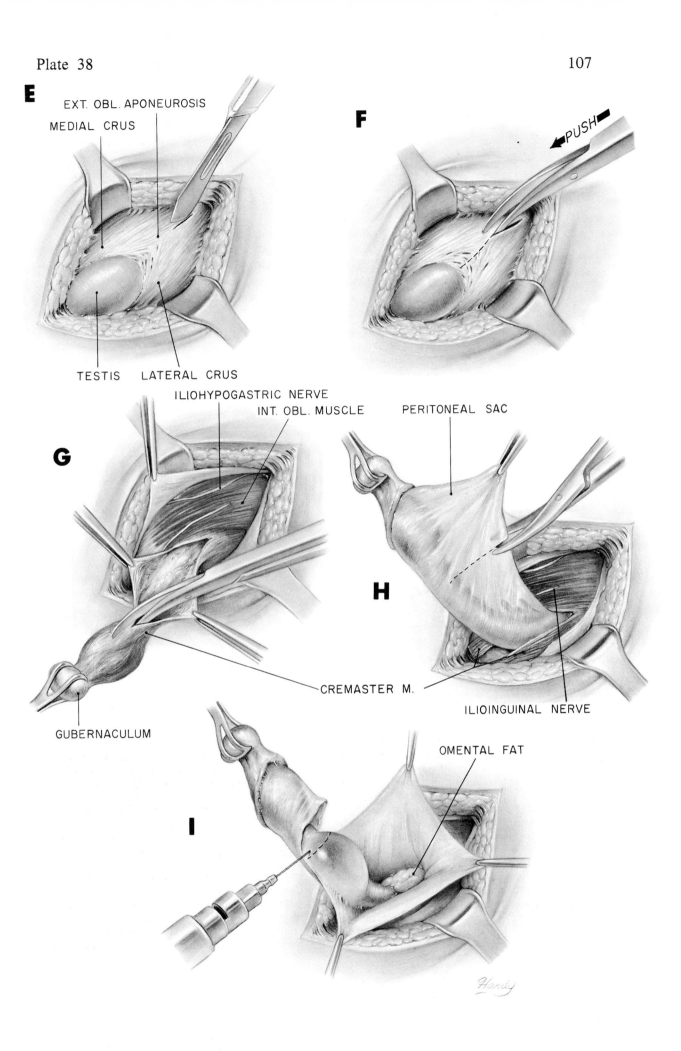

E

EXT. OBL. APONEUROSIS

MEDIAL CRUS

TESTIS   LATERAL CRUS

F

PUSH

ILIOHYPOGASTRIC NERVE

INT. OBL. MUSCLE

G

PERITONEAL SAC

H

GUBERNACULUM

CREMASTER M.

ILIOINGUINAL NERVE

OMENTAL FAT

I

J. The partially mobilized posterior wall of the hernial sac is held up in forceps for traction as its separation from the cord structures is being completed (broken line) by scalpel dissection.

K, L, M. The neck of the mobilized hernial sac is occluded with a suture ligature of 000 silk (K, L) and the redundant sac tissue excised (M).

N, O, P. The anterior wall of the patent tunica vaginalis is severed with scissors in a longitudinal plane (N), and its everted cut margins are sutured (000 silk) together posterior to the testicle (O, P).

DISCUSSION—DR. FIEDLER (cont.)

As stated before, it is my feeling that the most important part of any type of operation for cryptorchism is the very careful dissection of the fibrous tissue from the internal spermatic vessels in order to give the greatest possible length to these vessels in order to elongate the cord. The success of the operation hinges on this feature of the procedure more than on any other. Of lesser importance is lack of tension on the cord, and this is the advantage of the use of the rubber band. The closure of the various layers over and around the cord in a normal anatomic manner, to avoid constriction of this structure, is also important.

Both functions of the testis—sperm production and androgen secretion—must be kept in mind. In successful operations for cryptorchism (especially bilateral) the vas frequently is not sufficiently patent to transport the sperm to the seminal vesicles. This is the best argument for early operative intervention, preferably before the age of six; many surgeons suggest operation as early as one to two years of age. Whether or not spermatogenesis is more likely to be preserved or accomplished in the earlier age of one or two is controversial. It is generally agreed that surgery before the age of six gives the best results.

The administration of intramuscular injections of gonadotrophin to encourage the descent of the cryptorchid is again controversial. Whether this hormone may permanently injure the undescended

Plate 39   109

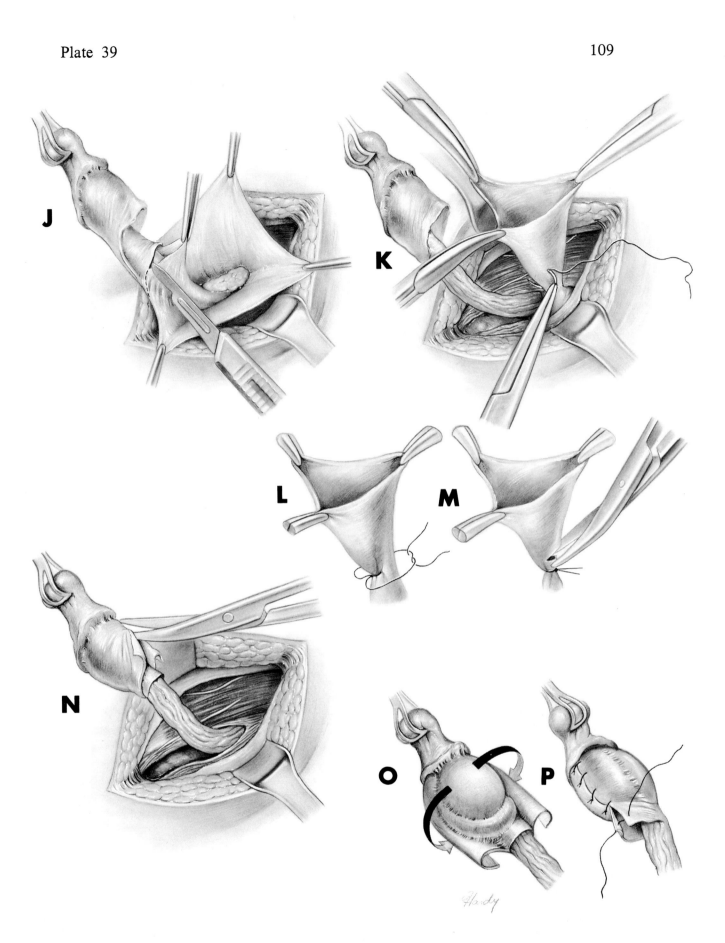

Q. The vas deferens and the blood vessels that comprise the cord structures are "skeletonized" by scissor dissection to obtain the maximum length of the cord.

R. The cord structures are completely mobilized, and the commonly present defect in the transversalis fascia is repaired, using interrupted sutures of 000 silk. The ligated stump of the hernial sac is visible between the blood vessels laterally and the vas deferens medially. The deep epigastric vessels and their relation to the cord structures, and the defect in the transversalis fascia are also visible.

S. The closure of the defect in the transversalis fascia is completed, and the strands of a silk (00) suture inserted in the gubernaculum have their exit through separate sites in the base of the scrotum. Immediately preceding this step, a scrotal "bed" is made for the testicle by forceful digital dissection from within the incision.

T. The cut margins of the congenitally foreshortened cremaster muscle are approximated anterior to the cord structures. This is usually done after the testicle is placed in the scrotum. The distal segment of the cremaster is visible as a rim of tissue between the lower pole of the testicle and the gubernaculum.

DISCUSSION—DR. FIEDLER (cont.)

testis is sometimes questioned. However, it is thought by most observers to be safe when no more than 20,000 I.U. are employed. The hope, of course, is that these injections, given in one or two courses of 500 to 3,000 I.U. per dose, with a total of 10,000 to 20,000 I.U., will result in the normal descent of the testis.

When to employ gonadotrophin varies according to the success observed by those who have employed it. Unfortunately, these results very likely include many patients in whom normal descent would have taken place anyhow, or in patients with retractile (pseudo-cryptorchism) testes. Many patients referred to me for cryptorchism have simply retractile testes. Overly anxious parents too often insist on something being done. It is in the patient with retractile testes that injections of gonadotrophin, or surgery, have proved equally satisfactory.

My personal experience with gonadotrophin has been disappointing, but I have not seen evidence of injury in any patient to whom it was given. Injury to the undescended testis by gonadotrophin has, however, been advanced as a reason for avoiding its use. Temporary changes in the opposite scrotal testis have been observed. Therefore, when the injections fail, most surgeons suggest operation as soon as possible.

The high incidence of malignancy of the undescended testis is considered by many physicians to be sufficient reason for orchiopexy. In the scrotum, changes in the size of the testis produced

Plate 40   111

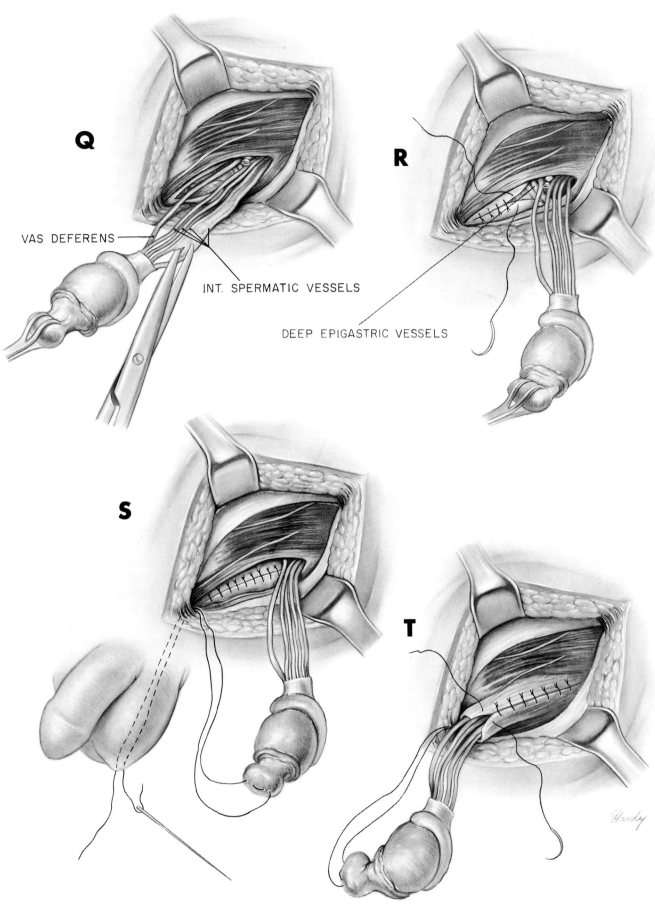

VAS DEFERENS

INT. SPERMATIC VESSELS

DEEP EPIGASTRIC VESSELS

U. The suture strands are tied to form a loop, which is encircled by a rubber band for traction. When the proper amount of traction is obtained, the rubber band is fixed to the thigh with one or two strips of adhesive. This traction is maintained for five to seven days.

V. The cut margins of the aponeurosis of the external oblique muscle are approximated with interrupted sutures of 000 silk. The relation of the closure of the cremaster

muscle and the ilioinguinal nerve to the external inguinal ring may be seen.

W. The subcutaneous fascia layers (Camper and Scarpa) are sutured as a single unit with interrupted sutures of 0000 silk.

X. Skin hooks are inserted into each angle of the incision and the margins approximated with straight (cambric) needles. The needles are all first inserted, withdrawn individually and the suture strands tied and then cut to complete the operation.

DISCUSSION—DR. FIEDLER (cont.)

by malignancy are more likely to be observed at an early stage. This is important when one considers statistics that indicate malignancy occurs 50 times more frequently in the undescended testis than in the scrotal one. The abdominal testis is four times more likely to become malignant than the undescended inguinal testis. In spite of successful surgery or descent by use of gonadotrophin for cryptorchism, it is generally agreed, that the incidence of malignancy remains the same. This has led some to suggest orchiectomy in all cases of true cryptorchism.

A final reason for orchiopexy is the psychic effect on the individual. In my own experience this has been much overemphasized. In most cases it

has appeared to be due to the attention drawn to the condition by the anxiety of the parents.

In conclusion, the operation for cryptorchism in my opinion should be performed before the age of six if possible, and if gonadotrophin is employed and fails, surgery should follow immediately. After the age of six, even in spite of arguments to the contrary, gonadotrophin and surgery should be employed before puberty, and surgery alone after puberty.

Since I have not seen malignancy develop in a case of cryptorchism before or after orchiopexy, I do not take the view that orchiectomy should be advised to prevent malignancy of the testis.

Plate 41   113

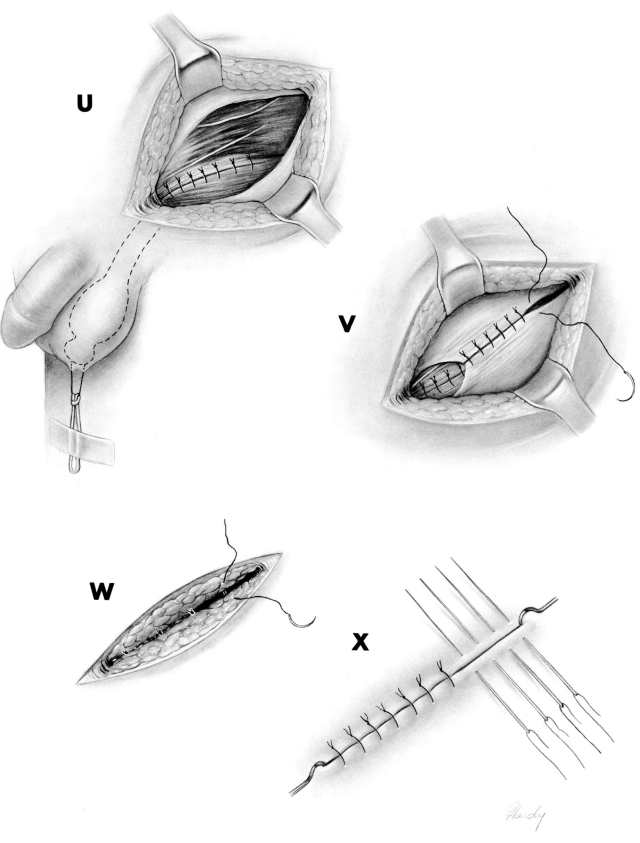

HYDROCELECTOMY

A. The patient is in the supine position, and the oblique inguinal incision is indicated by the broken line. This incision, 2 cm. medial to and paralleling the inguinal ligament, extends obliquely cephalad from the level of the pubic tubercle for a distance of approximately 7 cm. A scrotal incision may be used, but, because of the increased incidence of infection and hematoma formation and the greater discomfort to the patient, the inguinal incision is preferred.

B, C. The incision is deepened through the superficial (Camper) and deep (Scarpa) layers of the subcutaneous fascia (B) to expose the aponeurosis of the external oblique muscle and the external inguinal ring (C). The incision in the cremaster muscle is indicated by the broken line medial to the ilioinguinal nerve (C).

D. The wall of the hydrocele is exposed, and the incision in the overlying cremaster muscle is being extended cephalad by scissor dissection.

E. The hydrocele and its relation to the spermatic cord structures and an accompanying properitoneal lipoma are depicted.

F. The cord structures are secured in a vascular type of Babcock clamp * and elevated to show the external spermatic and pubic vessels as they course in the base of the "mesentery" of the cord. These vessels are branches and tributaries of the deep epigastric artery and veins, respectively.

DISCUSSION—DR. THOMAS H. JOHNSON. The technic illustrated implies a principle that is primary to any technic: *If a hydrocele is to be treated at all, the treatment should be open surgery.* This statement appears less dogmatic after even a brief consideration of the pros and cons of open surgery versus the alternatives of (1) needle or trocar puncture and evacuation and (2) puncture and evacuation plus introduction of sclerosing material.

Though tapping a hydrocele may appear conservative and safe to the patient because it is an office procedure, this is purely an illusion. It is more dangerous *because* it is an office procedure and lacks the aseptic disciplines of the operation room. Whereas open surgery is definitive and final, tapping is but the first of a sequence of repetitions and entails each time the same hazards intrinsic to the procedure. The frequency of treatment is determined by the period of refilling. The possibility of introducing infection into the residual hydrocele fluid is always a risk. The fact that the medium is a space-filling liquid removed from the immunologic responses of the blood stream adds to the danger. Furthermore, there is always the potential complication of hemorrhage secondary to blood vessel trauma induced by the tip of the needle. Added to all these objections is the inability of the operator to observe any associated pathologic conditions.

Every one of the contraindications to simple aspiration of a hydrocele applies to aspiration and injection of a sclerosing agent, plus such strong and obvious additional objections that the procedure may be discounted with no further comment.

---

* Manufactured by Edward Weck & Co., Long Island City, N.Y.

Plate 42   115

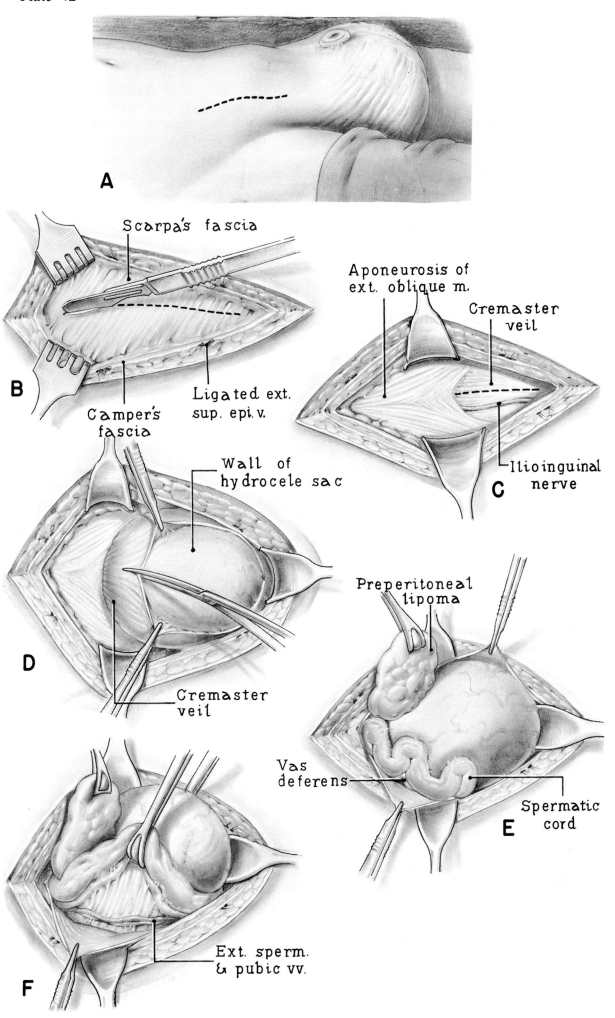

A

Scarpa's fascia

B

Camper's
fascia

Ligated ext.
sup. epi. v.

Aponeurosis of
ext. oblique m.

Cremaster
veil

Ilioinguinal
nerve

C

Wall of
hydrocele sac

Cremaster
veil

D

Preperitoneal
lipoma

Vas
deferens

Spermatic
cord

E

Ext. sperm.
& pubic vv.

F

G, H, I. The hydrocele is decompressed by suction siphonage, using a trocar and cannula (G). Clamp traction is maintained upward on the wall of the decompressed sac, and its relation to the tunica dartos of the scrotum is visible (H). By scissor dissection the sac is separated from the tunica dartos (I). The cord structures and the testis in relation to the sac are now seen (I).

J, K, L. The decompressed sac is incised, as indicated by the broken line (J). After the lumen is widely entered (K), the redundant sac tissue about the testicle is excised (K, L).

DISCUSSION—DR. JOHNSON (cont.)

The statement that treatment of hydrocele should be open surgery suggests a pointed question: Why should operation be performed? There are two basic reasons: (1) Hydroceles undergo a predictable increase in size with time, and this is associated with increasing intensity of symptoms. (2) Operation permits inspection of the testicle to rule out an associated malignancy or other lesion more significant than the hydrocele itself.

The choice of technic, whether through a scrotal or an inguinal approach as illustrated, should be determined by the experience and preference of the surgeon. Specialty traditions, area familiarity, and procedural habit play a role with both the general surgeon and the urologist. Specific indications exist for each approach. The natural conclusion is that both the urologist and the general surgeon should be equally adept to use either approach. However, it is generally observed that the urologist employs a scrotal incision and the general surgeon elects the inguinal approach. In the absence of specific indications for the use of a particular approach, either may be used with satisfaction, provided the accepted and basic surgical principles are followed.

The inguinal technic is illustrated clearly and well and requires elaboration on only one point. I suggest drainage for a short period (48 hours) of the most dependent aspect of the scrotal bed. The drain should not extend to the inguinal incision; it is, in fact, contrary to principle if it does. The reason for suggesting drainage lies in the nature of the scrotal tissue itself. The scrotum is dependent and capable of stretching more than any other cutaneous structure in the body. Unfortunately, it can do so rapidly and attain immense

Plate 43

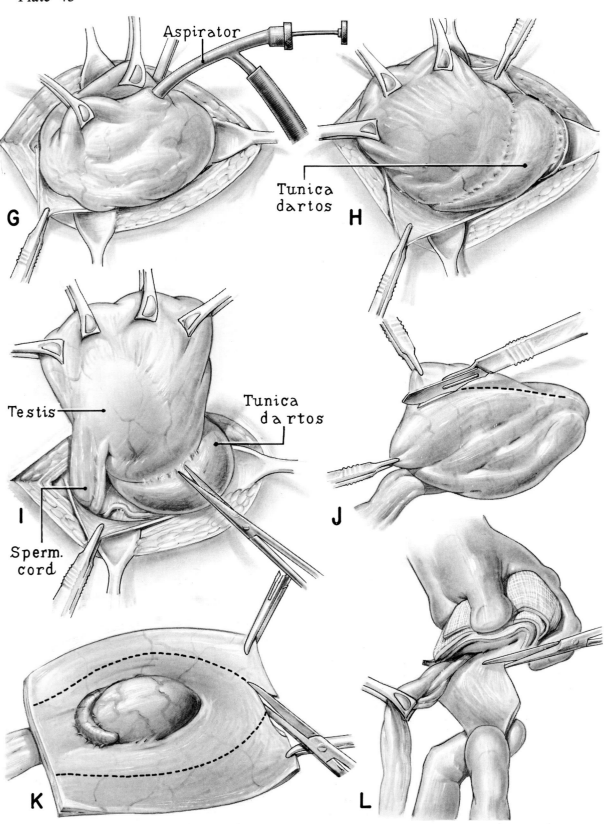

G

Aspirator

H

Tunica
dartos

Testis

Tunica
dartos

I

Sperm.
cord

J

K

L

M, N. The cut margins of the sac remaining are everted and approximated posterior to the testicle, using a continuous suture of 00 chromic catgut.

O. The excision of the hydrocele is completed and the testis is replaced into the scrotal "bed." Although on occasions the hydrocele has been resected in toto, the technic illustrated is simple and practical.

In this patient there was an accompanying properitoneal lipoma, which was excised. The broken line indicates the incision in the aponeurosis of the external oblique muscle, which is extended through the external ring.

Its relation to the surrounding structures is depicted.

P. The properitoneal lipoma is mobilized and a high transfixion ligation (00 silk) of its "neck" is performed. The lipoma is then transected with scissors distal to the ligature. There was no accompanying hernial sac.

Q. The associated defect in the transversalis fascia and its relation to the external spermatic and pubic vessels (cremasteric) and their parent trunks, the inferior (deep) epigastric vessels is visible.

DISCUSSION—DR. JOHNSON (cont.)

proportions. Since there is no absolute control over the postoperative seepage of blood, drainage of the scrotum is the best prophylaxis for the complication of a scrotal hematoma. The easiest method for the insertion of a drain is to pass a clamp down to the most dependent aspect of the scrotum and tent the scrotal wall. A small skin incision is then made over the tip of the clamp, and a narrow Penrose plain rubber tissue drain is withdrawn by the clamp into the scrotal "bed."

The use of counterpressure dressings is not practiced. In fact, there is good logic in dependent drainage only and not forcing fluid in other directions by pressure. Furthermore, the application of counterpressure may result in postoperative urinary retention by urethral compression and distortion. The few hours of pressure are of doubtful value and have been abandoned by me for the

better. One final caution in the matter of hematoma prevention: beware the dry field after the use of a local anesthetic that contains a vasoconstrictor; this may be followed by the rapid occurrence of a huge hematoma.

Dr. Madden mentions some general reasons for preferring the inguinal approach. It is believed that this approach should be used when there is a question of communication with the peritoneal cavity, a concomitant hernia, or associated cord findings similar to the example illustrated. In the event of a suspected testicular tumor the inguinal approach permits a more proximal or higher transection of the cord.

K and L show the resection of the redundant sac tissue and the eversion and approximation of the cut margins by a continuous suture of 00 chromic catgut (M, N). This is the procedure of

Plate 44

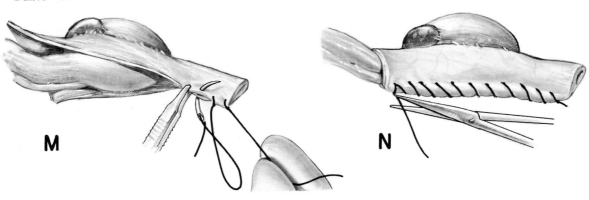

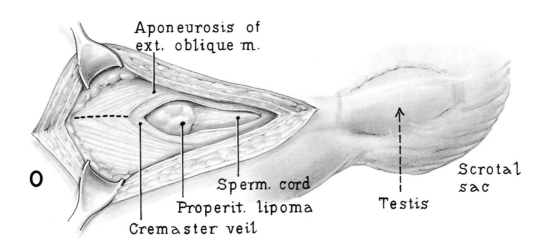

Aponeurosis of
ext. oblique m.

O

Sperm. cord

Properit. lipoma

Cremaster veil

Testis

Scrotal
sac

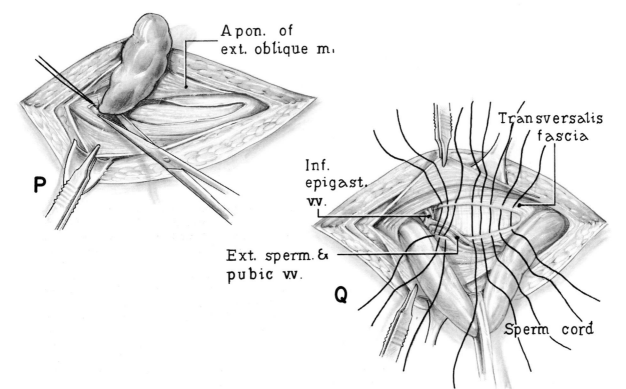

Apon. of
ext. oblique m.

P

Transversalis
fascia

Inf.
epigast.
v.v.

Ext. sperm. &
pubic v.v.

Q

Sperm cord

R. The fascial defect is closed (Q, R), both cephalad and caudad, to the external spermatic and pubic vessels, using interrupted sutures of 000 silk.

S. The cord is placed on the reconstructed fascial "floor," and the cremaster muscle layer is sutured over the cord, using interrupted sutures of 000 silk.

T. The cut margins of the aponeurosis of the external oblique muscle are approximated using interrupted sutures of 000 silk.

U, V, W. The closure of the subcutaneous fascia layer with interrupted sutures of 0000 silk (U) and the skin with interrupted sutures of 000 silk (V) completes the operation (W).

DISCUSSION—DR. JOHNSON (cont.)

choice. To attempt total resection of the hydrocele intact is meaningless and time-consuming and adds to the bleeding hazard. At the other extreme, merely everting the entire sac without its excision may result in a postoperative scrotal mass of a size that equals the original hydrocele.

The scrotal approach has the general advantages of ease and directness. It is specifically indicated for bilateral hydrocele repair using a single incision in the scrotal raphe, and also when the hydrocele is unusually large, when plastic work on the scrotum is anticipated, and when previous inguinal operations have been performed. The same precautions relative to drainage apply. In the case of small hydroceles the elastic tissue of the scrotal wall may reduce the "bed" to such an extent that the repaired testicle and residual sac cannot be replaced. Stretching of the scrotal "bed" with the index fingers permits the ready replacement of the testicle.

In the wound closure, the use of deep vertical mattress sutures, which include all layers, is preferred. Such sutures are excellent for hemostasis. Minimum difficulty has been experienced with the use of chromic catgut (00) sutures which are absorbed and do not require removal. If nonabsorbable sutures are used, they should be cut long, since the scrotum has proved an effective hiding place for sutures that have short ends.

Plate 45   121

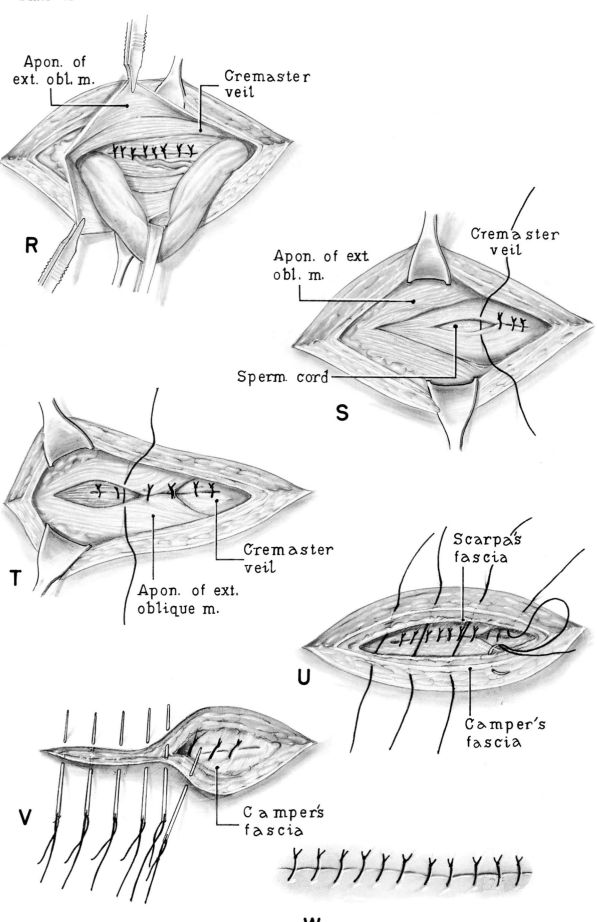

Apon. of
ext. obl. m.

Cremaster
veil

R

Apon. of ext
obl. m.

Cremaster
veil

Sperm. cord

S

Cremaster
veil

Apon. of ext.
oblique m.

T

Scarpa's
fascia

Camper's
fascia

U

Camper's
fascia

V

W

EXCISION OF PILONIDAL CYST

A. The patient is placed in the prone and modified "jackknife" position, and the buttocks are separated by strips of adhesive tape which are fixed to the sides of the operation table. The sites of attachment of these strips to the skin of the buttocks is reinforced by short lengths of adhesive tape applied at right angles to the underlying layer, forming a T-shaped pattern. The elliptical incision about the orifices of the pilonidal sinus is outlined. The injection of methylene blue into the orifices of the sinuses is neither practiced nor recommended. The technic of excision depicted in the subsequent illustrations is essentially a modification of the method previously described by Dunphy and Matson.

B, C. The incision is deepened through the thick subcutaneous fatty tissue layer, first on one side and then the other, to expose the sacral fascia in the depths of the wound. In this dissection it is most important that all of the diseased tissue is excised. Accordingly as the dissection proceeds, the lateral walls of the wound are carefully inspected for small islands of grayish gelatinous tissue which resemble tapioca pudding in appearance. If such islands of diseased tissue are seen, the area of excision should be extended laterally as far as necessary to assure their complete removal.

D. Traction, with the aid of Kocher clamps, is maintained on the cut margins of the elliptical skin segment to be excised, and the tissue attachments to the sacral fascia are severed as indicated (dotted line) by scalpel dissection.

Plate 46

123

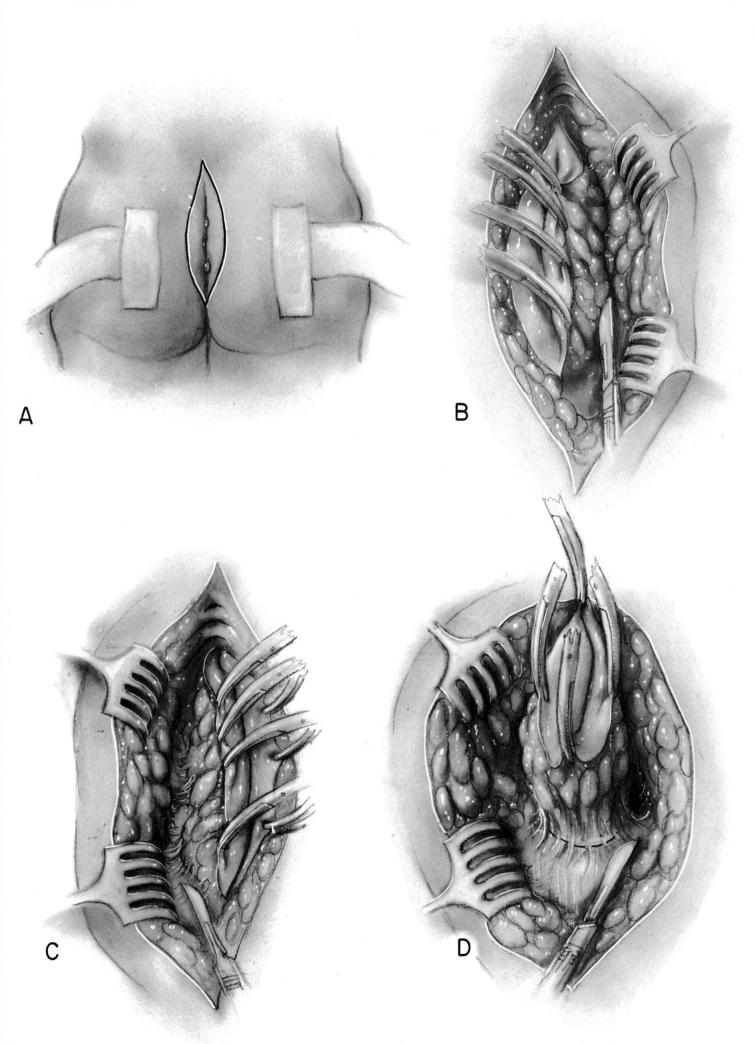

E. The severance of the tissues in the depths of the wound from the sacral fascia is continued cephalad, and the excision of the pilonidal cyst is completed (F).

F. After completion of the excision of the cyst, rake retraction is maintained on the wound margin, and the attachment of the fibrofatty tissue layer to the surface of the gluteus maximus muscle is separated by sharp scalpel dissection. During this dissection active bleeding from the cut vessels in the gluteus maximus muscle always occurs and requires the application of clamps for the control of hemorrhage.

G. The dissection of the fibrofatty tissue layer on each side of the wound is completed, and hemostasis within the gluteus maximus muscle is obtained with suture ligatures of silk (000).

H. A series of four interrupted skin retention sutures of silk (No. 1) are inserted, each of which incorporates a "bite" of the sacral fascia.

DISCUSSION—DR. WILLIAM F. MACFEE. Pilonidal cysts and sinuses have been treated by a variety of methods, but most surgeons rely upon wide excision which is intended to encompass the possible ramifications of the sinus tract. The usual procedure begins with an elliptical incision which includes the openings of the sinuses with a narrow zone of surrounding skin. The excision comprises a considerably wider area of subcutaneous fat extending down to the sacrococcygeal fascia in the center and to the gluteal fascia at the margins.

With respect to the actual technic of excision, the injection of methylene blue or other dye into the sinus serves no useful purpose. The dye not only obscures the operative field but may actually be misleading through its failure to reach all parts of the sinus tract and its possible ramifications. After the skin incision has been made, the surgeon proceeds according to the plan of excision he considers best. As the first step, the drawings B, C, and D, Plate 46, show the lateral incisions carried to their full extent. Following this, the tissues in the depth of the wound are severed from the sacral fascia in a cephalad direction (Plate 47, E).

An objection which may be offered to the early completion of the lateral incisions is the fact that the slight ooze of blood from these incisions tends to run down and obscure the field during the dissection of the tissue mass from the sacrum. If, instead, the incisions are carried to the required depth only at the inferior angle of the ellipse and then progressively deepened as the tissues are dissected from the sacral fascia, a much clearer operative field is obtained with less effort.

On the management of the wound created by the excision, opinions differ. Some favor primary closure while others prefer to leave the wound open, or at least partially open, and pack it with gauze. Another method of closure designed to obliterate dead space and reduce raw surface is the suturing of the skin edges to the sacral fascia along, or near, the midline.

Closure of the wound by primary suture is the ideal method, provided primary healing follows. However, virtually all such wounds are contaminated in some degree, and the combination of a small residual dead space with the presence of a few bacteria is sufficient to cause failure. The tissues beneath the skin become separated by a hematoma or an abscess, and the wound then must heal by granulation.

Packing of the open wound is, in effect, an acceptance of a type of healing that is slow but assumed to be sure. Unfortunately, healing is by no means sure. Regardless of frequent changes of packing, the process of granulation tends to proceed more rapidly along the surfaces of the subcutaneous fat than in the depth of the wound, over the sacrum, where granulations apparently form more slowly and grow less luxuriantly. The result is a constant tendency of the wound to close superficially, leaving a deep zone of incomplete healing over the sacral fascia. Low grade infection may persist at this level and become active after healing appears to be complete. It may be regarded as a recurrence of the original condition and the patient subjected to a second excision. The tissue removed at the second operation frequently discloses a sinus tract leading down through scar tissue, but without epithelial lining.

Closure by suture of the skin edges to the sacral fascia obliterates dead space by bringing the relatively vascular walls of the wound down into a position of direct contact with the sacral fascia. An uncovered area of fascia, usually not more than one cm. wide, is left between the skin edges, either to epithelialize naturally or to be grafted. If this type of closure is selected, the residual raw surface must receive the surgical attention normally required by any superficial granulating wound. Whatever the type of operation, a common cause of failure is inadequate treatment of the residual wound.

Plate 47

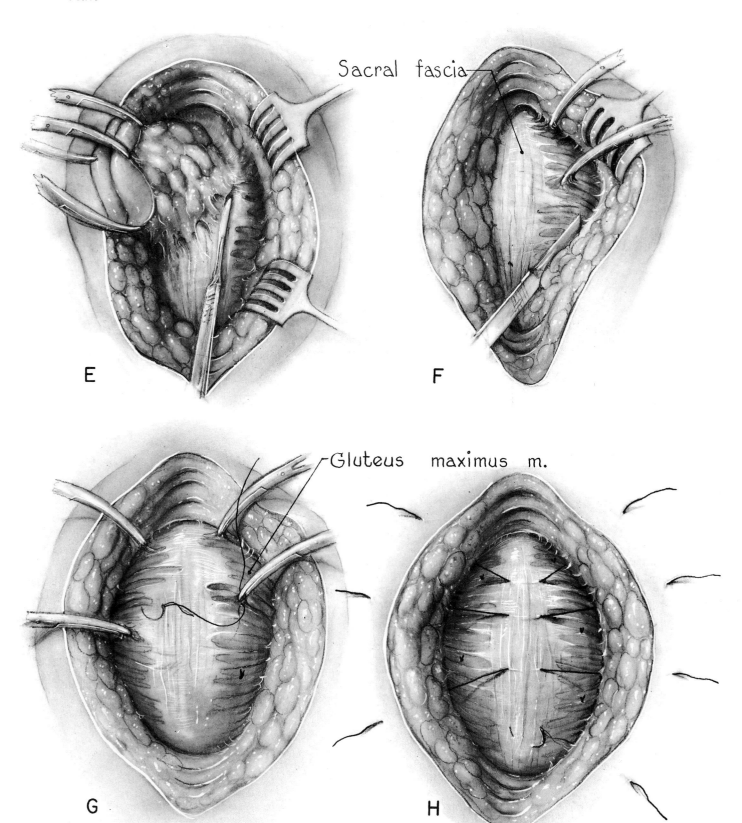

Sacral fascia

Gluteus maximus m.

E

F

G

H

I. Drains (two) are inserted in the upper and lower angles of the wound down to the sacral fascia, and the suture of the fibrofatty tissue layer is commenced. This layer, which was previously separated from the surface of the gluteus maximus muscle, possesses good holding power and its approximation effects a strong layer of closure in the depths of the wound. Immediately prior to this closure, the traction tapes of adhesive separating the buttocks are released to prevent tension on the suture line.

J. The closure of the deep fibrofatty tissue layer about the drains is completed, and the closure of the skin margins of the wound is partially completed, using interrupted sutures of silk (000). If preferred, vertical on-end mattress sutures (MacMillan) may be used for the skin closure.

K, L. Following completion of the skin closure, the drains are incorporated in a gauze dressing over which a gauze roll is applied. The retention sutures are then tied firmly over the gauze roll and dressing to effect an obliteration of the underlying dead space. The application of two additional layers of gauze and a firm adhesive dressing completes the operation.

Postoperatively a regular diet as tolerated is prescribed and no attempt is made to inhibit bowel motions by the use of various medications. The retention sutures and the drains are removed routinely on the fourth day and the skin sutures on the eighth day postoperatively. The day after the skin sutures are removed tub baths are prescribed and continued daily thereafter for a period of five to seven days.

DISCUSSION—DR. MARTIN J. HEALY. The primary closure technic illustrated (I, J, K, L) is only one of several acceptable methods of surgical management of pilonidal cyst or sinus. These are excision with open packing, excision with primary closure, and excision with partial closure. All these methods have the common objective of complete en bloc excision of all pilonidal tissue without unnecessary sacrifice of surrounding normal soft tissues, particularly the overlying skin. Conservative enucleation, marsupialization, or unroofing of pilonidal cysts or sinuses is not recommended.

Excision with open packing of the resulting wound is a time-honored procedure, and the long-term end results are good. However, the morbidity is great, months being required for scar epithelium to gradually cover the large granulating surface. The final stages of this process are frequently very prolonged, and the resultant scar, adherent to the underlying sacrum, is subject to trauma, infection, and "recurrence." I use this procedure infrequently, preferring methods with less morbidity. However, the technical requirements are less exacting, and it probably represents the procedure of choice for the occasional operator.

Excision with primary closure, such as that illustrated, gives the least morbidity with excellent functional results. However, I feel that this technic should be restricted to the midline, noninfected cyst or sinus. Attempts to perform primary closure after excision of large infected cysts or those with multiple or eccentric sinuses too frequently result in a residual "dead space," which fills with blood and serum. Since this area is nearly always contaminated, low-grade infection may follow, resulting in a closed space lined with granulations.

Subsequent persistent drainage completes the picture of the so called "recurrence." Perhaps nowhere else in the body are the technical niceties of surgery more essential for wound healing than in attempting primary closure in this area. Gentle handling of tissues, use of fine ligature material, absolute hemostasis, and obliteration of all "dead space" without undue tension are "musts" if this technic is to succeed.

With reference to the specific steps illustrated, I would emphasize preoperative preparation of the area by the patient with pHisohex or a similar detergent, daily for three to five days prior to surgery. The anus should be draped out of the operative field with a towel clipped to the midline skin. I agree wholeheartedly with the injunction against the use of methylene blue or other dye materials, which cannot be trusted to reach all ramifications. Failure to encounter the dye may give false reassurance that excision is complete. If the dye escapes from the cyst, the flooding and staining of the operative field makes the remaining dissection obscure.

I would prefer the sacrifice of less skin than is illustrated in A, preferring to take the narrowest ellipse consistent with removal of involved skin and the sinus openings. Likewise, in deepening the incision (B, C), the dissection should be kept as close as possible to the pilonidal disease process in order to diminish the size of the ultimate "dead space." I prefer to ignore all but the most vigorous bleeding points until excision is completed; otherwise, the field is rapidly obscured by clamps.

In E, when upward traction is made and the cleavage plane is found in the inferior angle of

Plate 48   127

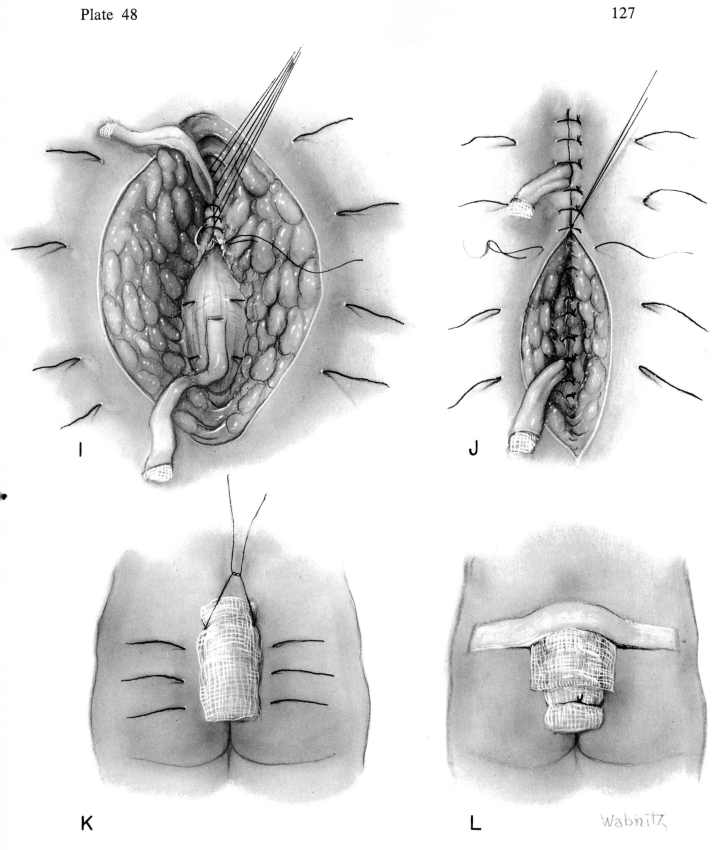

I

J

K

L

Wabnitz

the wound, care must be taken not to cut through the anococcygeus muscle or rectal wall, which is easily drawn upwards into the operative field. The raising of musculofascial flaps, as shown in F, is nearly always essential to overcome the "dead space" but can occasionally be eliminated if the excised tissue bloc is small.

I prefer not to use drains (I) for fear of introducing infection into the depths of the wound. If hemostasis is complete, the wound is thoroughly irrigated with saline prior to closure, and a firm elastoplast pressure dressing applied. This minimizes serum accumulations. If drainage is felt desirable, I would prefer the use of a centrally perforated polyethylene tubing, the ends of which should be brought out at a distance from the cephalad end of the main incision and attached to a portable suction device, such as the Hemovac.*

Postoperatively, I prefer to limit early ambulation until the fourth or fifth day, because walking places tension on the muscle flaps. Since the operation is usually performed in the younger age group, systemic postoperative complications are infrequent. However, I have seen wound separations and fluid collections that I believe have been brought about by premature walking, squatting, and sitting. Such activities are restricted for two to three weeks until wound healing is sound and complete. For up to three months or longer, my patients are advised to avoid prolonged automobile rides or sitting on hard surfaces.

In a comparative analysis of various closure methods in 229 unselected consecutive cases of pilonidal cyst, Dr. Paul Hoffert and I (1) found that "recurrences" are equally common regardless of the technic used. I have been able to diminish the frequency of recurrences by using a special technic of partial closure in all cases with large cysts, with infection, or with eccentric skin openings. In this procedure, the "dead space" is obliterated by developing undermined flaps which are sutured to the sacral fascia, as originally described by MacFee.

The incision outlines all sinus openings with a minimum sacrifice of skin. The skin edges are then sharply beveled outward and the subcutaneous fat undercut at a 45 degree angle until the fascia overlying the gluteus maximus muscles is reached. En bloc dissection is then completed just superficial to the gluteus and sacral fascia. After removing the adhesive straps, used for skin traction, the wound edges are brought into apposition with the sacral fascia, usually meeting in the midline without tension. Effective obliteration of the "dead space" and accurate maintenance of the skin edges against the sacral fascia are accomplished by a series of loop or Sturmdorf sutures of 00 silk or dermalon threaded on a large cutting edge needle. The suture begins 3 to 4 cm. from the skin edge,

* Manufactured by Zimmer Co., St. Louis, Missouri.

traversing the thickness of the flap, picks up a bite of sacral fascia near the midline, and then bites back through the skin 3 to 4 mm. from its edge. The loop is completed by reversing the three steps, taking in turn skin edge, fascia, and skin flap, each several millimeters from its counterpart. Pulling up on the two free ends of the suture engages the skin edge within the loop, holds it snugly against the fascia, and at the same time obliterates the "dead space" beneath the flap. Sutures are first placed at close intervals around the periphery, and after final irrigation of the wound, all sutures are pulled up at once. Each is then tied over a short piece of soft rubber tubing to prevent cutting through the skin. The sutures are left long and tied over a fluffed gauze tampon, and a pressure dressing is applied. Details of this technic and its modifications for eccentric sinuses or for unusually heavy buttocks have been described in detail elsewhere (1). The end result is complete obliteration of the operative wound, leaving at most a narrow central strip of fascia to granulate in. Postoperative care is essentially the same as for primary closure, sutures being removed on the sixth to eighth postoperative day.

The partial closure technic preserves the internatal cleft by placing the scar deep, where it is protected by the buttocks. The scar usually becomes mobile, rarely breaks down, and provides an excellent anatomic and functional result. Morbidity and postoperative care are comparable to primary closure. Its adaptability to complicated cases, its lesser technical requirements, and its low "recurrence" rate recommend it as an adjunct to the technic described in the text.

Finally, in choosing between open packing and primary or partial closure, the surgeon should consider all factors, including the size, type and extent of the disease process, length of hospital stay, morbidity, and the occupational and functional requirements of the patient. After critically appraising his own technical capabilities, he should choose that method which will, in his hands, most probably achieve the result intended.

REFERENCES

1. Healy, M. J., Jr., and Hoffert, P. W. Pilonidal sinus and cyst: A comparative evaluation of various surgical methods in 229 consecutive cases, Am. J. Surg. 87:578, 1954.
2. ——— and Hoffert, P. W. Pilonidal sinus and cyst, S. Clin. North America, 35:1497–1502, Oct., 1955.
3. ——— and Hoffert, P. W. Pilonidal disease, in Robert Turell. Diseases of the Colon and Anorectum, Philadelphia, W. B. Saunders & Company, 1959, chapter 57, volume 2, pp. 1169–1194.

Plate 47   125

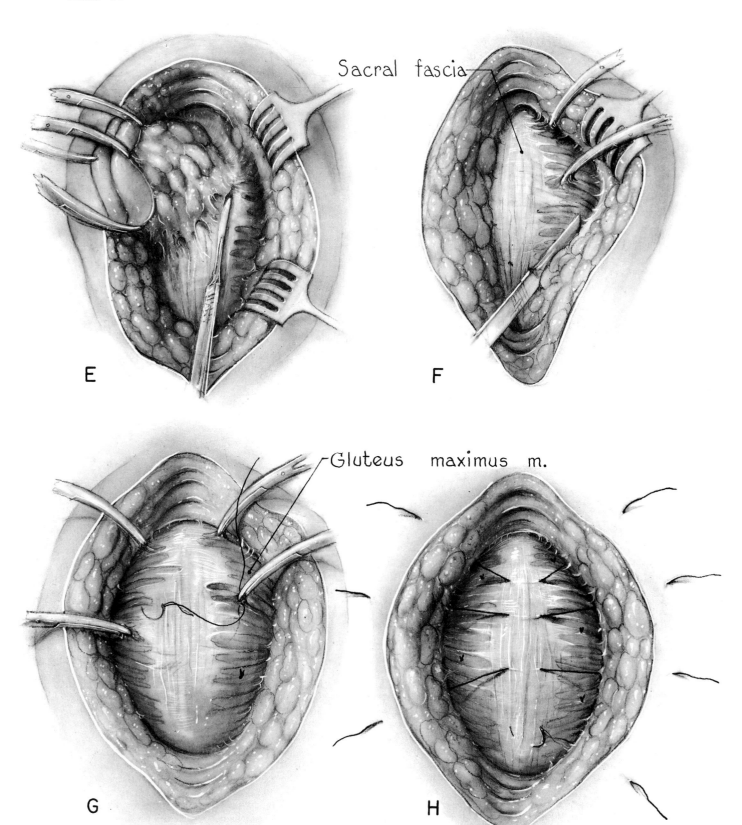

Sacral fascia

E

F

Gluteus maximus m.

G

H

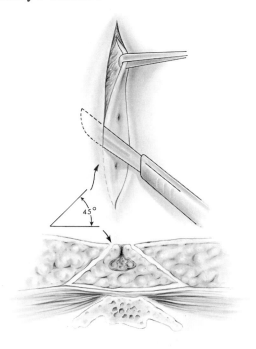

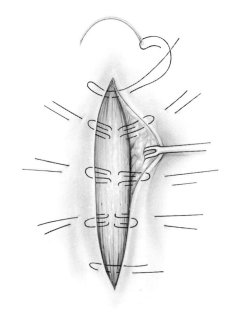

1. An elliptical incision, with minimal sacrifice of skin, is made and undercut at a 45° angle until the fascia overlying the gluteus maximus muscle is encountered. Cross section demonstrates general configuration of en bloc tissue excised by sharp dissection just superficial to the sacral and gluteal fascia.

2. A series of loop or Sturmdorf sutures are first placed at 2 cm. intervals, using 00 silk or dermalon on a cutting edge needle. Bites in the sacral fascia are taken near the midline so that, when drawn taut, the opposing flaps meet. The upper and lower angles of the wound are closed with end-on mattress sutures, which also take a bite of the sacral fascia.

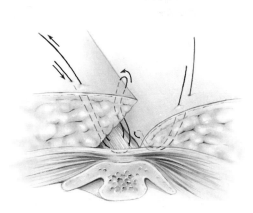

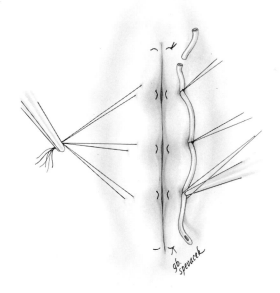

3. This illustration shows in detail the loop suture. Using a needle with a medium to large cutting edge, the suture is started about 3 cm. from the edge and takes a liberal bite of the sacral fascia and then a 2 mm. bite of the skin edge. The steps are now reversed, emerging a short distance medial to the starting point.

4. When hemostasis is complete, the wound is irrigated, and all of the sutures are drawn up simultaneously. A soft catheter or rubber tubing is placed on either side between the free ends of each loop suture. Each suture is then individually tied, as the assistant depresses the catheter to permit setting the knot with just enough tension to hold the skin edge against the sacral fascià. Occasionally an interrupted silk suture (000) may be required between the loop sutures to provide snug approximation of the skin to the fascia. The sutures are left long, and each is tied to its opposite fellow over a fluffed gauze or absorbent cotton tampon. A large elastic adhesive pressure dressing is applied.

EXCISION OF MAMMARY DUCT PAPILLOMA

The patient, a 51-year-old white married woman, was admitted to the hospital because of painless bleeding from the nipple of the right breast. Two days before admission, bleeding occurred for the first time and was accidentally discovered when blood stains on her nightgown were observed. On examination of the breast, a small mass was palpable in the supra-areolar region of the breast at about "11 o'clock." Digital compression overlying the mass caused a discharge of bloody fluid from the nipple. The affected breast segment was excised, and the histopathologic diagnosis was benign intraductal papilloma.

A. Circumferential digital pressure is made in a serial manner about the areola of the breast, and the site of compression that is associated with the discharge of blood from the nipple is observed. In this patient it was located at "11 o'clock."

B, C. The duct orifice in the nipple through which the blood exuded is first canalized and then dilated, using graduate sized lacrimal duct dilators. A curvilinear incision is made in the areolocutaneous margin overlying the affected duct and breast seg-

ment (B) and deepened into the underlying fatty areolar tissue (C).

D. The wound margins are retracted, and the breast segment, held taut in a clamp (Babcock), is mobilized by scalpel dissection.

E. The remaining tissue attachments of the breast segment are severed by scissor dissection. Forceful retraction of the lower skin margin has caused an inversion of the nipple into the operative field. Accordingly, caution must be observed to avoid nipple injury.

Plate 49

131

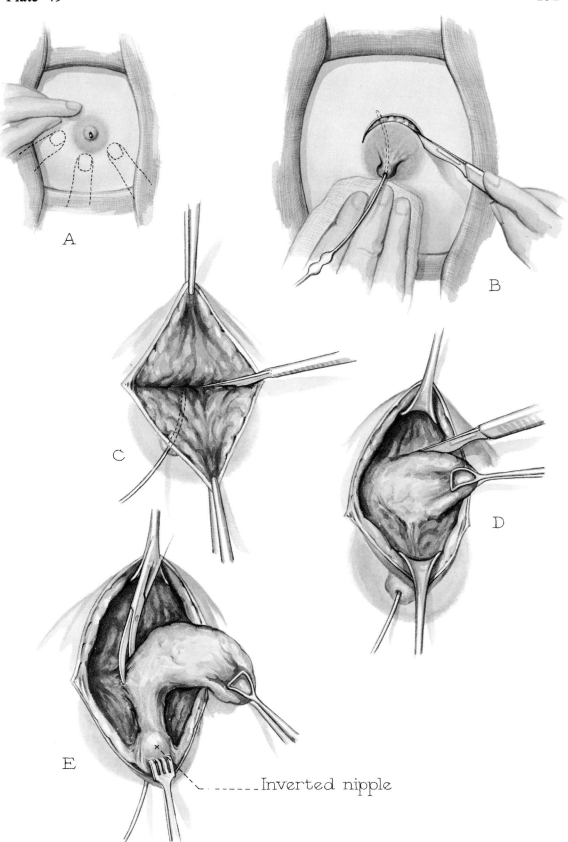

Inverted nipple

F. The mobilized breast segment and contained duct are transected with a scalpel at the base of the nipple.

G. The filling defect in the mammary gland is obliterated by approximation of the cut margins with interrupted sutures of 00 chromic catgut. Because of the firmness and thickness of the mammary tissue, the use of a cutting-edge needle is required for the insertion of the sutures.

H. The appearance of the operative field on completion of the skin closure is shown.

Plate 50

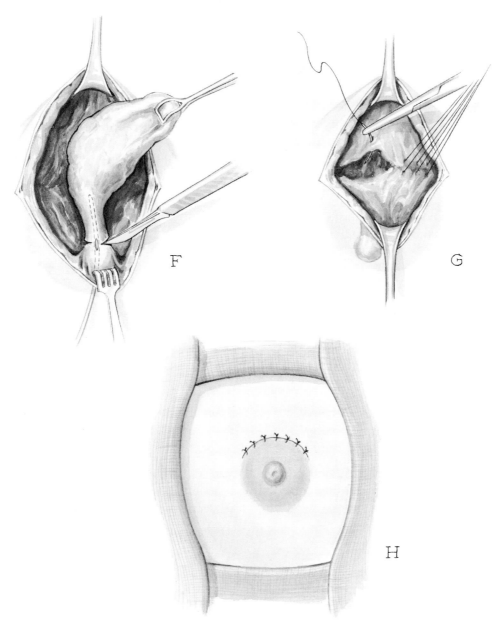

F

G

H

RADICAL MASTECTOMY

A. The patient is placed in the supine position and the left side of the thorax is elevated on a pillow support. The location of the tumor in the lower medial quadrant of the left breast is visible and the outline of the skin incision is depicted. The incision used, a slight modification of the Willy Meyer (1894) and John B. Deaver (1917) incisions, is one that has proved the most universally applicable. Extension of the incision onto the upper third of the arm is neither necessary nor desirable. Alternate types of incision which are in general use are depicted in Plates 55, 56, and 57.

B, C. A sterile moist towel folded once longitudinally is attached to the cut margin of the lateral skin flap with towel clips. Traction is maintained upward on the lateral skin flap, and scalpel dissection is continued both laterally and posteriorly until the anterior border of the latissimus dorsi muscle is exposed.

D. In like manner, a folded sterile moist towel and towel clips are applied to the cut edge of the medial flap, and with traction maintained, the scalpel dissection is continued in the superficial subcutaneous plane until the mobilization of the flap is completed to the right border of the sternum. In the elevation of the skin flaps, a wide dissection in the superficial subcutaneous tissue plane is routinely performed and a thin layer of subcutaneous fat is permitted to remain on the undersurface of either flap.

E. Upon completion of the mobilization of the medial and lateral skin flaps, the island of skin overlying the breast tumor and the surrounding breast tissue is covered with a small dry sterile towel, the edges of which are anchored to the skin margins with a series of Kocher clamps.

Plate 51   135

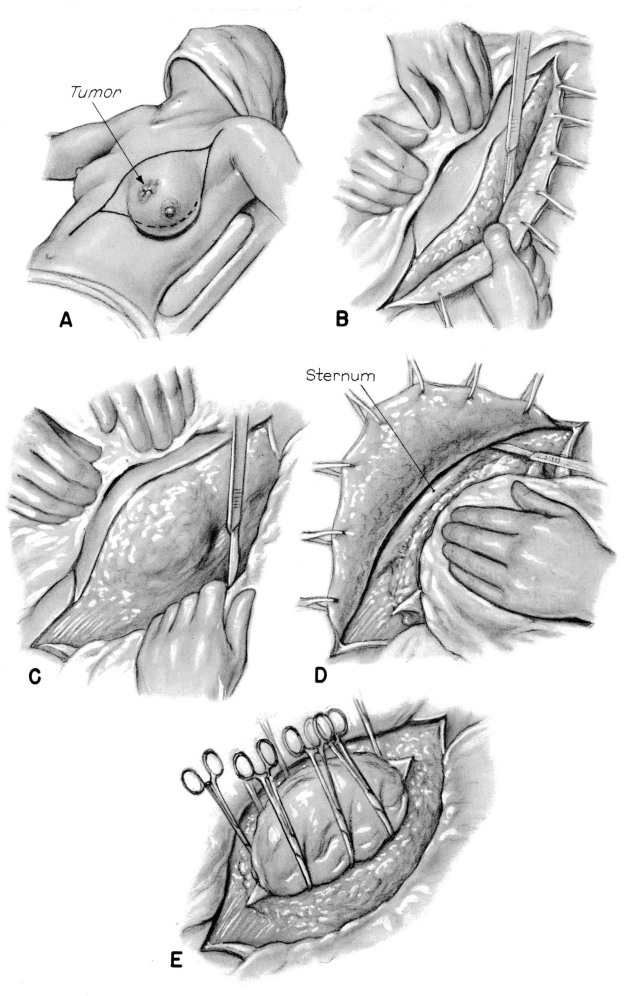

Tumor

Sternum

A

B

C

D

E

F. To facilitate manipulation of the breast by the assistant, the handles of the Kocher clamps are secured together about a crumpled sterile towel with a piece of gauze tape.

G. The cephalic vein, an anatomic landmark for the deltopectoral groove, is first identified, and then a cleavage plane between the fibers of the pectoralis major and deltoid muscles is obtained. The tendon of insertion of the pectoralis major is encircled by the left index finger of the surgeon, and the characteristic twisting of its fibers prior to insertion into the humerus along the lateral crest of the bicipital groove is shown. This tendon of insertion and the origin of the clavicular portion of the pectoralis major are severed as indicated by the dotted lines. The clavicular portion of the pectoralis major is resected routinely in the performance of a radical mastectomy.

H. The mobilized portion of the pectoralis major muscle is turned downward and medially to expose the line of incision in the costocoracoid membrane (coracoclavicular or clavipectoral fascia) which forms a thin and somewhat transparent covering over the tendon of insertion of the pectoralis minor muscle into the coracoid process of the scapula. The coracoid process is also the site of origin of the coracobrachialis muscle and the short head of the biceps brachii muscle. Scissor dissection of the costocoracoid membrane is commenced preliminary to the mobilization of the tendon of insertion of the pectoralis minor muscle.

I. The scissor dissection of the costocoracoid membrane is completed, and the tendon of insertion of the pectoralis minor muscle is elevated upon the left index finger preparatory to its severance from the coracoid process as indicated by the dotted line.

J. The mobilized tendons of insertion of both the pectoralis major and minor muscles are turned downward and the line of the axillary dissection is shown. This dissection commences medially in an area cephalad to the brachial plexus and axillary vessels. The outlines of the axillary vein and its tributaries are faintly visible.

Plate 52   137

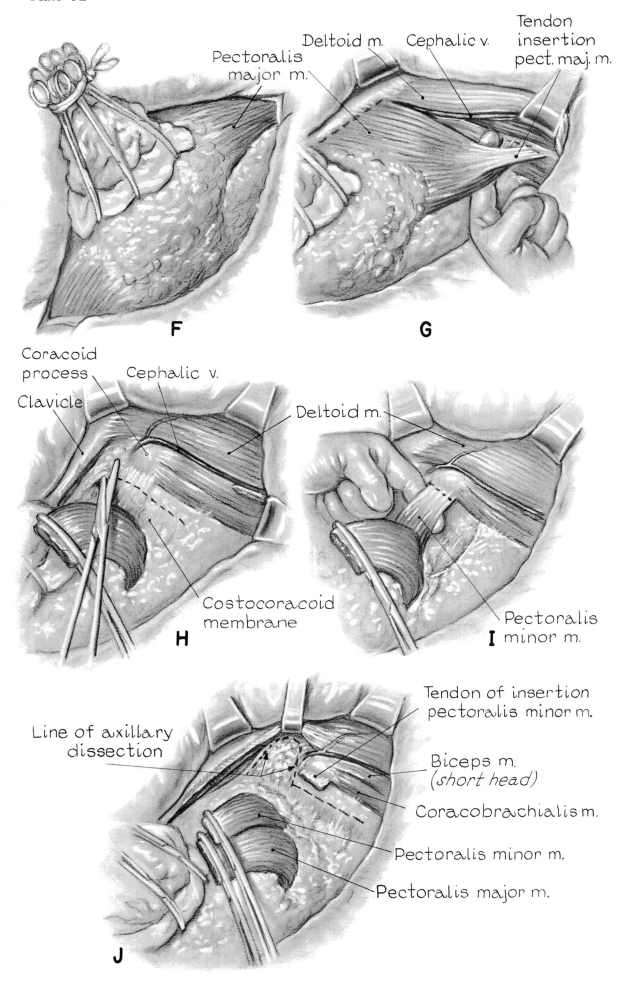

F

Pectoralis major m.

Deltoid m. Cephalic v. Tendon insertion pect. maj. m.

G

Coracoid process Cephalic v.

Clavicle

Deltoid m.

Costocoracoid membrane

H

Pectoralis minor m.

I

Line of axillary dissection

Tendon of insertion pectoralis minor m.

Biceps m. (short head)

Coracobrachialis m.

Pectoralis minor m.

Pectoralis major m.

J

K. The axillary dissection cephalad to the brachial plexus is completed, and the fatty areolar tissue is turned downward over the brachial plexus and its encased axillary artery to expose the axillary vein. The skeletonization of this vein is begun by incising the overlying adventitia layer as shown.

L, M. The mobilization of the breast mass is continued and the tributaries of the axillary vein and the branches of the axillary artery are doubly clamped, severed, and ligated (0000 silk) as they are exposed and isolated.

N, O. Upon completion of the skeletonization of the axillary vein, the fatty lymphoareolar tissue is cleared from the apex of the axilla, and scalpel dissection of the breast mass is continued onto the upper portion of the rectus abdominis muscle. Bleeding points in the muscle are occluded with suture ligatures of silk (000), and the scalpel dissection is continued upward onto the anterior chest wall (O).

Plate 53   139

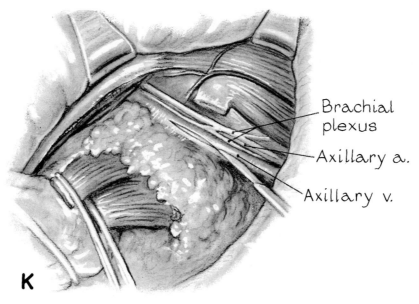

Brachial
plexus

Axillary a.

Axillary v.

K

Subclavius m.

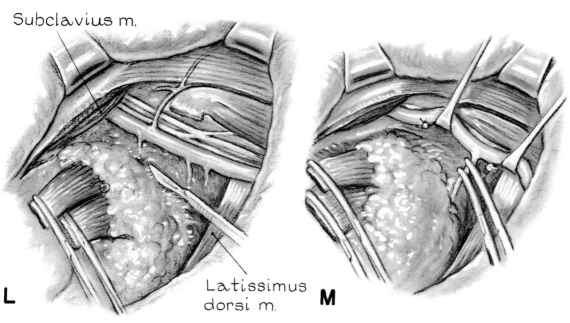

Latissimus
dorsi m. **M**

L

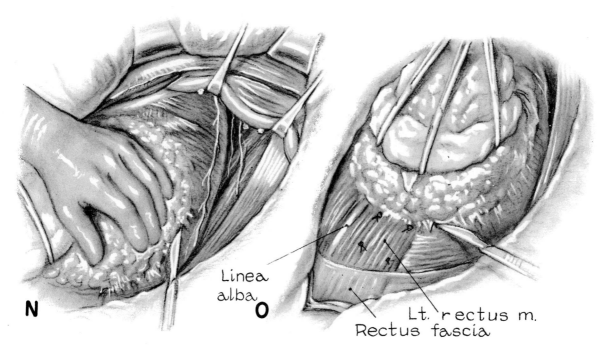

N

Linea
alba **O**

Lt. rectus m.
Rectus fascia

P. The breast mass is displaced downward and laterally, and the sternal origin of the fibers of the pectoralis major muscle and the costal origin of the pectoralis minor muscle are severed by sharp dissection with a scalpel. During this dissection, the perforating branches of the internal mammary artery are first identified in continuity and then doubly clamped and severed. In the event of bleeding from an accidentally severed perforating branch the immediate control of hemorrhage is best obtained by digital compression. Subsequently the severed vessel may be secured with a clamp, the points of which are applied in a horizontal rather than a vertical plane to avoid a puncture wound into the subjacent pleural cavity.

Q. The remaining tissue attachments of the breast are severed from a lateral to a medial direction because of the better visualization of the cleavage plane between the breast mass and the fibers of the serratus anterior muscle.

R. The operative field following the completion of the left radical mastectomy is shown. Although in this particular patient all of the nerves were spared, they are sacrificed with impunity if this is necessary to avoid leaving diseased tissue behind. Despite the location of the tumor in the medial quad-

rant of the breast, dissection of the internal mammary chain of nodes was not performed.

S. The primary closure of the skin flaps is completed, and the sites for the insertion of the catheters (18 F) are shown. The catheters are joined by a Y-tube connection through which constant suction (Stedman pump) is applied for 72 to 96 hours. This method obviates the need of pressure dressings and has proved much more comfortable for the patient. Primary closure of the incision is usually obtained. However, it must be emphasized that one should never condone an inadequate removal of skin in order to obtain primary closure of the incision. To obviate such a tendency, Follis suggested that the surgeon who performs the radical mastectomy should not be the one to close the incision. In this regard, the teaching of W. Sampson Handley of England (the removal of an adequate area of the skin surrounding the tumor and the resection of a much wider area of the underlying fascia) is followed. This teaching differs from Halsted who advised the wide removal of a circular area of skin surrounding the tumor and the routine use of primary split thickness skin grafts of the Ollier-Thiersch variety for the immediate closure of the skin defect.

Plate 54   141

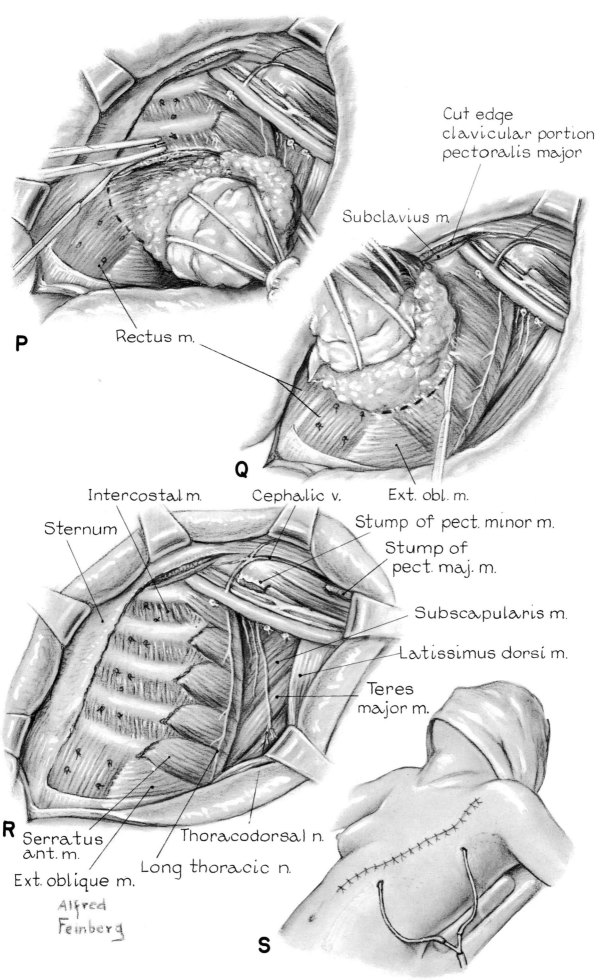

Cut edge
clavicular portion
pectoralis major

Subclavius m.

P   Rectus m.

Q

Intercostal m.   Cephalic v.   Ext. obl. m.

Sternum   Stump of pect. minor m.

Stump of
pect. maj. m.

Subscapularis m.

Latissimus dorsi m.

Teres
major m.

R Serratus
ant. m.   Thoracodorsal n.

Ext. oblique m.   Long thoracic n.

Alfred
Feinberg

S

DISCUSSION—DR. WILLIAM CRAWFORD WHITE. Before entering into a discussion of the operative technic as shown by the drawings, it would be well to consider the problem of diagnosis of cancer of the breast. In early cases, this is often impossible without the aid of a biopsy. Tissue for diagnosis may be obtained either by a needle biopsy or an incisional biopsy. The advocates of the needle biopsy speak of its simplicity and convenience. Although admittedly this is true, they neglect to say that a competent pathologist, who is completely familiar with this technic, is very necessary and furthermore that a negative report does not exclude the diagnosis of cancer.

The incisional biopsy, which is the preferred method, is done at the time that the patient is in the hospital operating room and prepared for major surgery. The technic consists of skin incision, excision of the tumor, ligation of the bleeding vessels, followed by the closure of the wound which is done while the frozen section is under study by the pathologist. If the report is a benign tumor, the operation is over. If the pathologist is unable to make a diagnosis until the preparation of the paraffin sections is completed, the operation is also over, at least temporarily. However, if the pathologist reports that the tumor is a cancer, then it is indicated to proceed immediately with a radical mastectomy. Prior to this, a rubber dam is placed over the incisional wound and glued to the skin. The whole area is then resterilized, the gowns and gloves are changed, and a new set of sterilized instruments are used. We have demonstrated cancer cells on both the instruments and gloves after a biopsy of a malignant tumor. Accordingly, all this "fuss" is indicated to prevent the transplantation of cancer cells to the raw wound that is to be made.

The outline of the incision illustrated in Plate 51 (A) is excellent. It is wide of the tumor with a radius of at least two-and-one-half inches from the tumor as suggested by Sampson Handley. Even after vigorous and widespread deep undercutting of the flaps, this means that in many cases the incision may not be closed primarily without the necessity for skin grafting. In my own experience, about 30 per cent of my patients have required skin grafting. The advantage of this widespread removal of the skin is that one thereby reduces the percentage of local recurrences (or persistence) as we have demonstrated in a control series.

Drawings F and G, Plate 52, indicate well the method of isolating and separating the pectoralis major muscle from its neighbors. Many feel strongly that the whole of this muscle should be removed. Contrariwise, others have elected to leave in its clavicular portion in order to avoid the marked depression which occurs caudad to the clavicle when complete removal is practiced. It is believed that saving the clavicular portion does help the postoperative appearance of the chest and in my opinion it has not affected adversely the success of the operation.

Illustrations H, I, and J, Plate 52, demonstrate well the steps in cleaning out the axilla after the severance of the insertion of the pectoralis major. Perhaps it looks easier than it is. Certainly, if one goes anterior to the axillary vein and then cephalad to it in order to clean out the area anterior to the brachial plexus, there will be more difficulty than usual, and furthermore the need for it has not been proved. The metastatic nodes ascend into the axilla and into the neck, both posterior and mesial to the brachial plexus. However, when the growth is extensive and inoperable, there is a generalized involvement of the nodes in this region.

I personally like the technic illustrated in K, L, M, N, and O, Plate 53, but it is doubtful if the removal of the rectus sheath is either indicated or necessary. In illustration N the nerves are shown intact. However, if there is any doubt as to the complete removal of cells in the surrounding area because the nerves and vessels are left intact, one must not hesitate to sacrifice both the long thoracic and the thoracodorsal nerves as suggested by the author.

It will also be observed that the author has not excised the internal mammary nodes despite the fact that the tumor was located in the medial aspect of the breast. This procedure has been advocated by some competent surgeons, especially when the cancer is located in the mesial half or the central portion of the breast. The value of this additional step to the procedure of radical mastectomy, which is illustrated, is not yet established. It is still in the experimental stage and the proof of its value remains to be demonstrated. Instead, roentgen therapy could be administered to the mediastinum and the surgeon spared the increased mortality and morbidity that would result if the whole surgical community routinely undertook this procedure. It is also to be observed that those surgeons who do the mediastinal extension of the operation never do a skin graft and, therefore, I do not believe that they do a sufficiently radical procedure relative to the breast itself.

Another additional procedure in the performance of a radical mastectomy—the routine dissection of the neck on the same side when the axillary nodes are involved—was advocated by Halsted in 1894 and subsequently abandoned. Now it has been recently revived by Wangensteen and Dahl-Iversen. Time will be needed to check on their efforts. It is my present attitude that Halsted's belief, that metastasis to the supraclavicular nodes was an index of incurability, was correct.

At times, it may be possible to close primarily a large wound by first undercutting widely and deeply in all directions. Rodman used to undercut so far on the other side that after he had closed the wound, the remaining breast appeared to be in front of the sternum. He referred to it as the "Cyclops" operation. Later he claimed the breast would return to its normal position. Nevertheless, this method has some merit in avoiding the necessity for skin grafting. The addition of suction to the rubber tube drains, as suggested by the author, is believed an important contribution to the surgical technic for radical mastectomy.

Plate 55   143

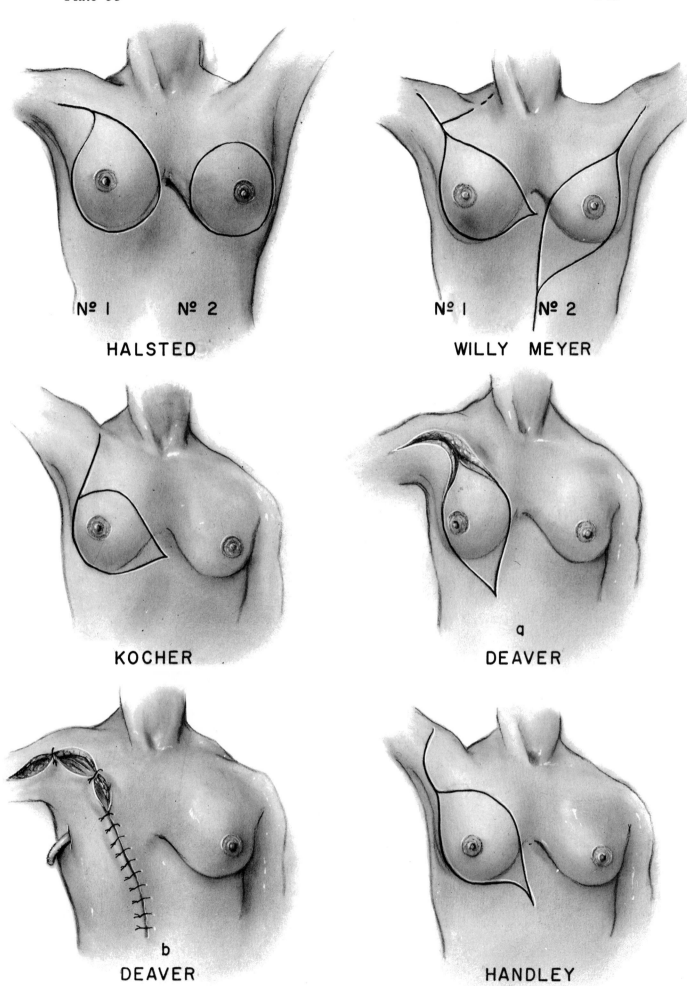

N° 1   N° 2

HALSTED

N° 1   N° 2

WILLY   MEYER

KOCHER

DEAVER

DEAVER

HANDLEY

DISCUSSION—DR. CHARLES ECKERT. Not shown in the illustrations is the incision used for biopsy of the primary tumor. The need to establish histologic proof of diagnosis prior to radical mastectomy is to be emphasized even in those cases in which clinical evidence of cancer seems incontrovertible. When biopsy is not done routinely, a small but definite frequency of erroneous diagnoses will be made, with resulting overtreatment. It has been said, "You can always remove a breast, but you cannot replace one." The recommended technic of biopsy consists of incisional biopsy of large tumors (over 3 cm. in diameter) and excisional biopsy of small tumors. In either case representative tissue from the tumor must be obtained for the pathologist's examination. Immediate frozen section technic leads to exact diagnosis in 90 to 95 per cent of cases; the remaining cases require permanent sections. After closure of the biopsy incision, the field is reprepared and the biopsy incision is excluded from the field of radical mastectomy with a plastic dressing that is cemented to the skin. All instruments, drapes, gowns, and gloves used for the biopsy are discarded in order to minimize risk of contamination.

Preliminary biopsy using the Vim-Silverman needle is preferred by some. When done 24 to 48 hours prior to definitive treatment, this technic reduces the operative time, further minimizes risk of contamination, and—provided a positive diagnosis is established—has no serious disadvantages. Of course, the pathologist must be willing and able to work with the small pieces of tissue provided him.

The incision illustrated in A is a good one, but it is my belief that the surgeon should be prepared to vary the incision, depending upon the position of the tumor within the breast. The considerations involved in the choice of incision are as follows: a viable flap for coverage of the axillary structures must be assured; a sufficient amount of skin (four fingerbreadths) must be included around all margins of the tumor; the incision should not cross the anterior axillary fold in the axilla, for resultant postoperative scarring may interfere with abduction of the arm; and, finally, the scar should permit the wearing of a moderately low-necked gown without being seen. A primary desire to close the wound should not influence the surgeon. It should also be noted that the incision illustrated removes all of the skin overlying the breast. Since mammary tissue is in close relation to the skin, incomplete mastectomy may result from attempts to preserve a part of the skin overlying the breast itself.

In elevating the skin flaps, firm, steady traction on the skin edges with countertraction on the underlying subcutaneous tissue will help to maintain an even plane of dissection. The proper plane is just beneath the nutrient blood vessel running parallel to the dermis in the subcutaneous layer. As the limits of the flap are approached, the plane should be gradually deepened to the deep fascia. This will give a smooth flap that, in the absence of excessive trauma and excessive length, should heal satisfactorily. If tenacula are used on the edges of the flap, as shown in B and D, they should be placed close to the edge; this thin zone can subsequently be excised. In the axilla the flap must be very thin because the axillary tail of the breast lies just beneath the dermis.

Except in cases in which the primary tumor occupies the extreme superior portion of the breast, I believe the clavicular fibers of the pectoralis major muscle need not be removed (G). There is no evidence that this will adversely affect the results of the operation; neither does it interfere with exposure of the axillary structures. The saving of this portion of the pectoralis major will provide some protection for these structures and also avoid an infraclavicular depression, which is cosmetically superior to the result following complete removal of the muscle. The point of separation between the sternal and clavicular fibers is in most cases clearly visible, and bleeding from the few small blood vessels crossing the line of demarcation is easily controlled.

After cutting the tendon of insertion of the pectoralis major (G), division of the upper fibers of origin from the sternum and costal cartilages 2 and 3 will improve exposure for dissection of the axilla. Downward traction on the clamps on the tendons of insertion of the pectoral muscles also aids in the subsequent dissection of the axilla.

Although most surgeons do not carry the axillary dissection above the axillary vein, I agree that the areolar tissue, lymphatics, and lymph nodes overlying the cords of the brachial plexus and axillary artery should be included in the dissection (J, K). In my experience this has not materially increased the difficulty of the operation.

It has been suggested by Mustard that the adventitial sheath of the axillary vein be preserved in an effort to reduce the frequency and severity of postoperative lymphedema chirurgica of the arm. This concept may or may not be correct and awaits substantiation. In ligating branches of the axillary vein and artery, care should be taken to avoid leaving a stump of the vessels, for this may lead to propagating thrombus formation.

Seldom is it necessary to sacrifice the long thoracic nerve, for it lies beneath a fascial covering invasion of which by tumor would be tantamount to inoperability. The thoracodorsal nerve, however, is in close relation to potentially involved lymph nodes; accordingly, it should be sacrificed. Relatively little disability attends the loss of latissimus dorsi function.

The maneuver of dissecting the breast from a lateral to medial dissection over the serratus anterior muscle shown in Q is an excellent one, for it is far easier to stay in the proper plane of dissection by so doing, thereby avoiding injury to the muscle as well as troublesome bleeding.

Plate 56

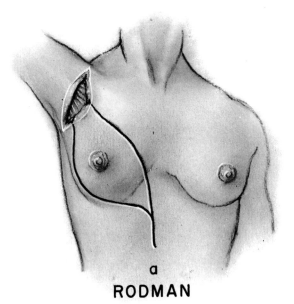

a
RODMAN

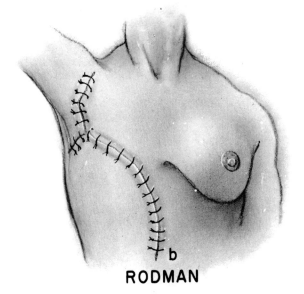

b
RODMAN

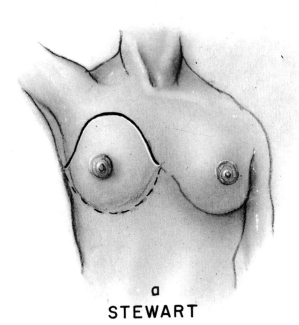

a
STEWART

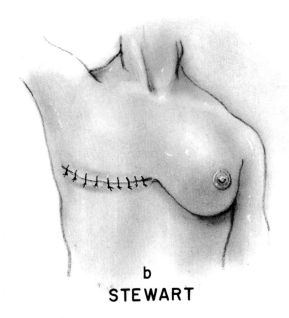

b
STEWART

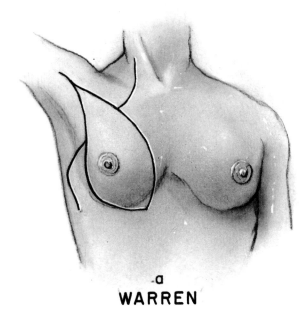

a
WARREN

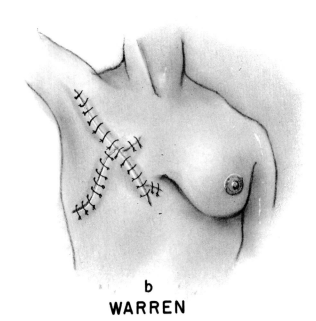

b
WARREN

DISCUSSION—DR. ECKERT (cont.)

Although the tumor illustrated in A occupies the medial hemisphere of the breast, the author has not recommended en bloc resection of the internal mammary lymph nodes (Urban). Routine performance of this addition to the standard procedure can be expected to materially increase morbidity and possibly mortality as well. Until further data are forthcoming on follow-up of a significant series in which the Urban operation has been done and in which the internal mammary lymph nodes are involved, this procedure should be considered experimental. Similarly, the value of extending the operation to remove supraclavicular lymph nodes, which was first tried by Halsted and more recently by Wangensteen and Dahl-Iversen and Anderson, is unproved.

Following removal of the breast and control of bleeding, the wound should be thoroughly irrigated to remove small blood clots, loose fat, and the like. Examination of the irrigating fluid has shown healthy-appearing cancer cells in a surprising proportion of cases. For this reason, the final irrigation should be done with a solution which will destroy these cells. I use a 5 mg. per cent solution of nitrogen mustard for this purpose. In this concentration I have not observed problems in wound healing that could be attributed to this agent. The skin flaps should then be carefully examined; if viability along the margins is questionable, questionably viable tissue should be debrided. Through this practice prolonged treatment of sloughing wound edges can be avoided.

Seldom do I find it possible to perform a primary closure without tension, and I greatly prefer to apply a split thickness skin graft to the midportion of the wound. I emphasize this point not because I believe the wider removal of skin will increase curability, but because primary healing reduces postoperative morbidity. An important factor in the genesis of necrosis of the flaps in addition to the above is the collection of blood or serum beneath the flaps. This is best avoided by use of catheter suction drainage, as illustrated in S. If a skin graft is used, one catheter is inserted beneath the medial flap and another beneath the lateral flap. A pressure dressing over the catheters is not only unnecessary but may result in pressure necrosis of the skin overlying the catheters. Therefore, the skin flaps at the margins of the defect to be grafted are sutured to the chest wall. Pressure on the graft is achieved through use of a "tie-over" or "stent" dressing.

In conclusion, despite the many questions raised over the effectiveness of radical mastectomy in curing mammary cancer, the fact remains that for patients truly operable according to the modified criteria of Haagensen and Stout, it continues to be the operation that gives the best chance for control of the disease. There are data to refute the therapeutic nihilists, the advocates of simple mastectomy and proponents of the "Edinburgh experiment." This statement should not be construed as complacency over the present situation, for in only approximately 25 per cent of patients with mammary cancer will the type of treatment used alter the eventual outcome.

Plate 57   147

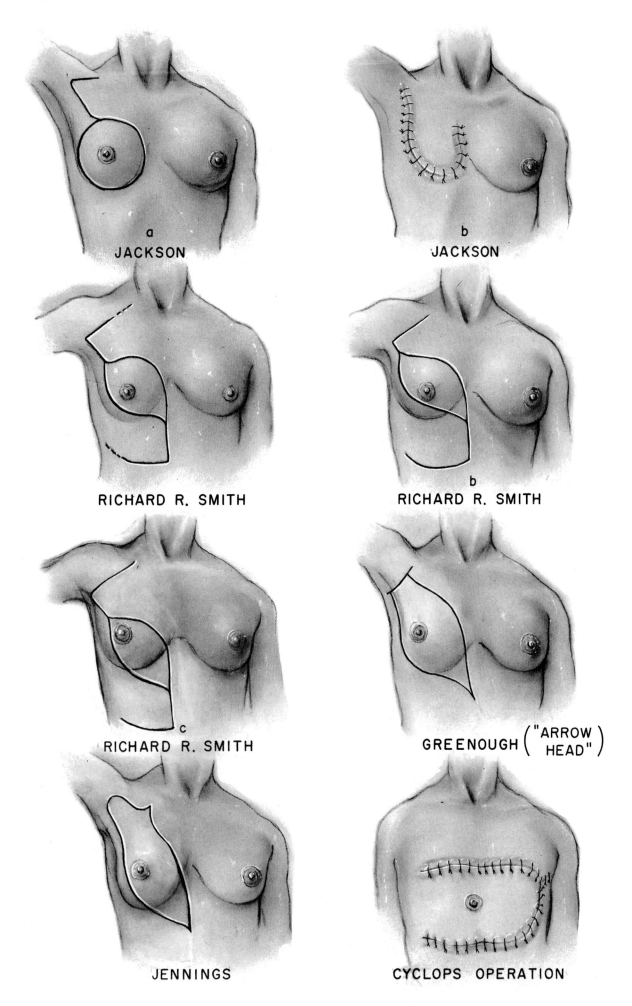

a
JACKSON

b
JACKSON

RICHARD R. SMITH

b
RICHARD R. SMITH

c
RICHARD R. SMITH

GREENOUGH ("ARROW HEAD")

JENNINGS

CYCLOPS OPERATION

TRACHEOSTOMY

A tracheostomy may be performed either electively or as an emergency operation. Frequently it is done as an emergency procedure and, unfortunately, it is oftentimes performed too late. A good dictum to follow is that if the necessity for the performance of a tracheostomy is seriously questioned, it is usually a good indication for the operation. The technic for an elective tracheostomy is illustrated.

A. The two types of incision employed, the transverse and longitudinal, are indicated. The transverse incision is preferred.

B. The incision is deepened through the subcutaneous tissue plane, and its continuation through the fibers of the underlying platysma muscle is shown.

C. The upper and lower flaps of skin, subcutaneous fat, and platysma muscle are retracted and, with a scalpel, the anterior or investing layer of the deep cervical fascia is incised in the midline.

D. The sternohyoid muscles are retracted, and the underlying anterior borders of the sternothyroid muscles may be seen. An incision is made through the middle or pretracheal fascia layer of the deep cervical fascia to expose the isthmus of the thyroid gland.

E. The left finger of the surgeon is inserted downward beneath the pretracheal fascia, and the incision in this fascia is extended caudad by scissor dissection.

DISCUSSION—DR. EDGAR L. FRAZELL. The choice of the skin incision for tracheostomy is usually dictated by the circumstances of the individual case. When performed electively it is usually done as an integral part of some other operative procedure about the head and neck region.

The type of incision must then conform to the necessities of the primary operation. As an emergency measure, tracheostomy is both dramatic and life-saving. Rapid exposure of the trachea with minimal dissection of skin flaps is imperative in such cases. I find this is facilitated by the use of the vertical midline incision as it minimizes blood loss from the distended veins in the area. Furthermore, the incision through subcutaneous tissue and fascia corresponds to the natural cleavage plane between the pretracheal

muscles. Additional exposure is obtained by extension of the incision in either direction to allow for variations in the position of the thyroid isthmus. The latter structure may be retracted superiorly or inferiorly or rapidly divided between clamps to expose the second or third tracheal ring.

The important objective in an emergency tracheostomy is to establish an artificial airway in the shortest possible time. Simple incision of two or more tracheal cartilages is usually sufficient for introduction of the canula, though some surgeons prefer excision of a window. The latter technic tends to delay spontaneous closure of the fistula after the emergency is past. Suture of the wound about the tracheostomy may lead to troublesome subcutaneous emphysema in some cases and cellulitis in others.

Plate 58

149

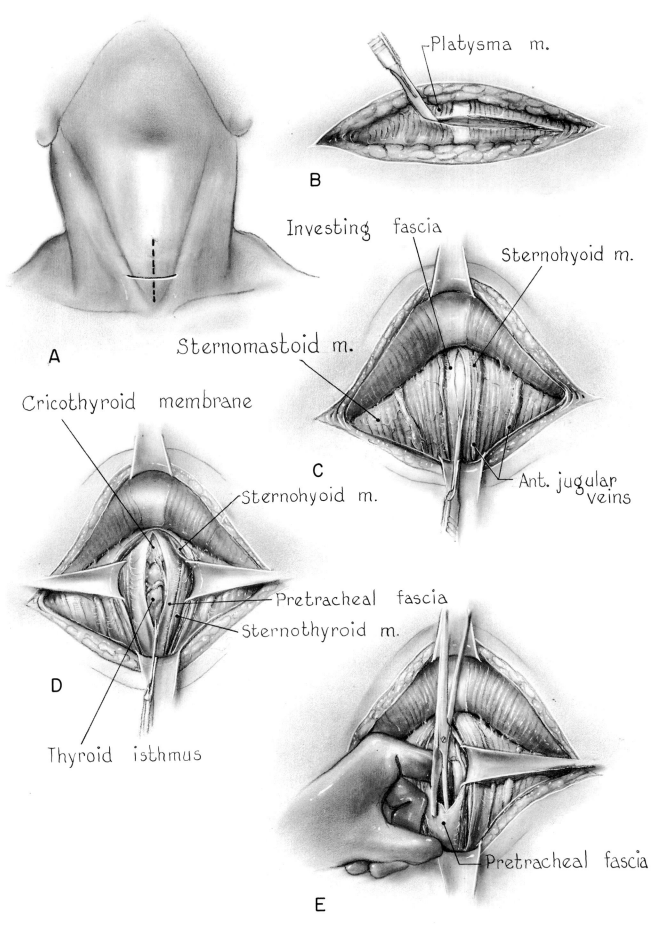

A

B

Platysma m.

Investing fascia

Sternohyoid m.

Sternomastoid m.

C

Ant. jugular veins

Cricothyroid membrane

Sternohyoid m.

Pretracheal fascia

Sternothyroid m.

D

Thyroid isthmus

E

Pretracheal fascia

F. The incision in the pretracheal fascia layer is completed, and a portion of the trachea is exposed. The inferior border of the isthmus of the thyroid gland is grasped in anatomic forceps, and its attachment to the anterior surface of the proximal portion of the trachea is freed by scissor dissection.

G. The isthmus of the thyroid gland is retracted upward, and the oval segment of the trachea to be incised is indicated in dotted outline. A segment of the third and frequently the fourth tracheal rings is included in this excision. Entrance into the trachea above this level is avoided to prevent the subsequent occurrence of laryngeal stenosis. Immediately prior to opening into the trachea, 8 to 10 minims of cocaine (10 per cent) is injected into its lumen as depicted. This maneuver, originally suggested by Sir St. Clair Thomson, lessens the cough as the tracheal lumen is entered.

H, I. The severance of the remaining attachment of the oval segment of the anterior portion of the trachea is being completed (H) prior to the insertion of the tracheostomy tube (I). In the adult, the No. 5 and No. 6 tubes are the two sizes most commonly employed. In the infant child and adolescent, tubes ranging in size from No. 0 to No. 4 may be used.

J. The tracheostomy tube is inserted and the obturator removed to complete the operation. One or two skin sutures to approximate loosely the skin margins may be inserted. This type of wound is always potentially infected and accordingly a layer or tight closure of the incision is avoided. In some instances no sutures are used, the wound being covered by a moistened sterile split piece of gauze.

Plate 59

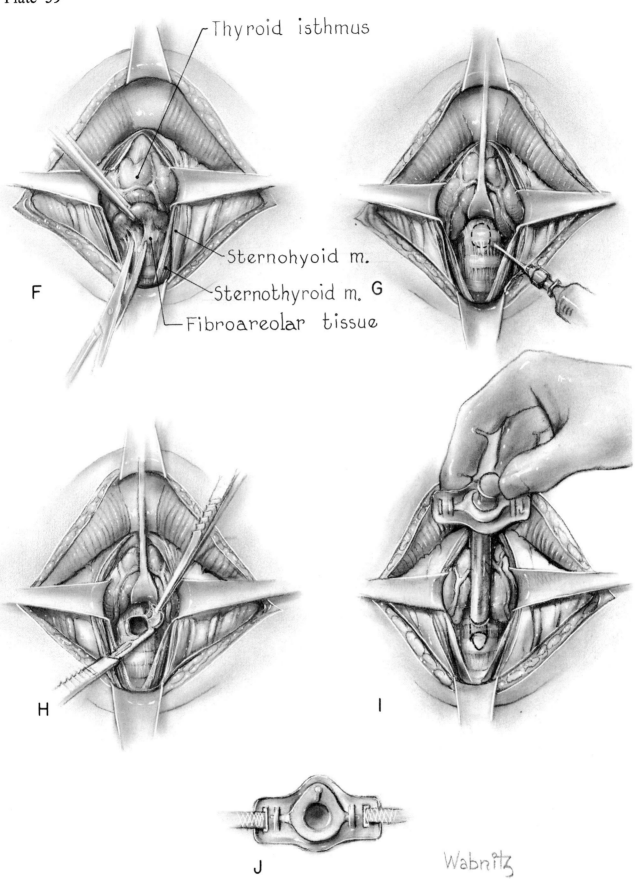

Thyroid isthmus

Sternohyoid m.

Sternothyroid m.

Fibroareolar tissue

F

G

H

I

J

Wabnitz

SCALENOTOMY

A. The site of the incision overlying the subclavian triangle of the neck is represented by a dotted line. This incision, located approximately 4 cm. cephalad to the clavicle, is bound anteriorly by the posterior border of the sternomastoid muscle and posteriorly by the external jugular vein.

B. The skin incision is deepened through the subcutaneous fatty tissue plane to expose the platysma muscle.

C. The fibers of the platysma muscle are severed transversely, and the incision in the anterior layer of the deep cervical fascia (investing layer) is visible.

D. The clavicular belly of the sternomastoid muscle is retracted anteriorly, and the incision in the middle layer of the deep cervical fascia between this muscle and the in-ferior belly of the omohyoid muscle is indicated by the dotted line.

E. The middle layer of the deep cervical fascia (omohyoid "fascial carpet") is incised, and the underlying fat pad, a characteristic anatomic landmark, is protruded into the incision.

F. A portion of the fat pad is held in tissue forceps and displaced posteriorly to expose portions of the scalenus anterior muscle and the phrenic nerve. A blood vessel accompanying the nerve may also be seen.

G. The lowermost portion of the scalenus anterior muscle is elevated on a clamp, and the transection of its fibers in layers is begun. The internal jugular vein, the transverse scapular vessels, and the phrenic nerve with its accompanying vessel are demonstrable.

DISCUSSION—DR. JAMES T. DANIELS. The apparently simple procedure of dividing a muscle such as the scalenus anticus can be appreciated as complex when the important structures lying in proximity to it are visualized. The illustrated technic of approach through the subclavian triangle to the scalenus anticus muscle demonstrates graphically the intricate relationship of these structures to the muscle. It is essential to recall that the entire nerve and blood supply to the upper extremity and one-half the nerve supply to the diaphragm are contained within this small area, lying much deeper than it is possible to indicate in a two dimensional illustration. The maneuvering within this confined space is conducted with care in order to avoid injuring the adjacent structures.

From the viewpoint of operative surgery alone, relief of disturbing neurovascular symptoms due to compression by scalenotomy is achieved by knowledge of the anatomic relationship of the local and adjacent structures, proper exposure, and careful technic. Illustrations designed to serve as a guide for this purpose can be expected to fulfill these requirements. A knowledge of the normal anatomic arrangement of the elements present in the vicinity of the scalenus anticus muscle is presumed. The need for this knowledge is obvious when consideration is given the fact that lying nearby the scalenus anticus muscle and the structures contained within the precise boundaries of the subclavian triangle are the pleura, the carotid sheath and its contents, and the subclavian and jugular veins. For the careless operator there are many opportunities for disaster.

Individual preferences based on experience suggest various considerations for slight alterations of technic. These variations present themselves by anticipating certain anomalies or abnormalities the surgeon may encounter in this region. For example, the anterior approach as illustrated is preferable to the lateral, particularly when a cervical rib of significant proportion is to be resected. In this instance a "collar" incision passing 5 to 6 cm. upward and backward from a point slightly above the sternoclavicular articulation is advantageous. This affords exposure of the tendinous clavicular attachment of the sternocleidomastoid muscle. Division of the clavicular attachment provides considerable space and exposure of the proximal portion of the subclavian artery and obviates difficult retraction. It is readily sutured with mattress sutures. The incision repre-

Plate 60   153

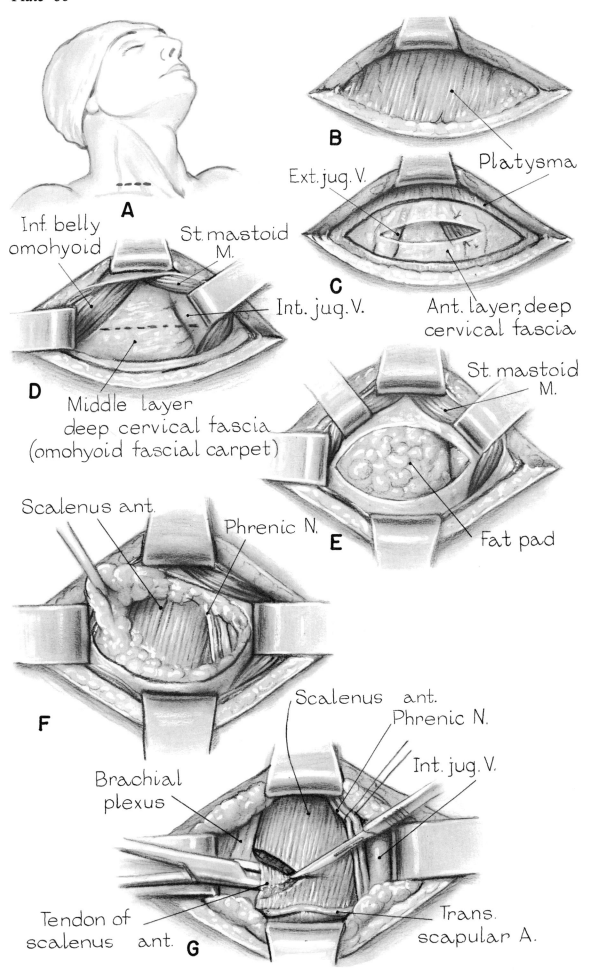

A

B

Platysma

Ext. jug. V.

C

Ant. layer, deep
cervical fascia

Inf. belly
omohyoid

St. mastoid
M.

Int. jug. V.

D

Middle layer
deep cervical fascia
(omohyoid fascial carpet)

St. mastoid
M.

E

Fat pad

Scalenus ant.

Phrenic N.

F

Brachial
plexus

Scalenus ant.
Phrenic N.

Int. jug. V.

Tendon of
scalenus ant.   G

Trans.
scapular A.

H. The transection of the remaining tendinous portion of the scalenus anterior muscle is about to be completed. In this regard, it is most important to sever completely all of the muscle and tendinous fibers to obtain complete release of the compression effect upon the subjacent subclavian artery.

I. The scalenotomy is finished, and the relation of the ends of the completely tran-

sected muscle to the surrounding structures is visible.

J, K. The fat pad is replaced, and the middle (J) and the anterior (K) layers of the deep cervical fascia are approximated with interrupted sutures of fine (0000) silk.

L. The skin is being closed with interrupted sutures of 000 silk. Each suture is threaded on a straight cambric or milliner's needle.

DISCUSSION—DR. DANIELS (cont.)

sented in A, Plate 60, is well suited to this purpose by slight extension anteriorly. The sternocleidomastoid are omohyoid muscles are retracted together as shown in Plate 60 (D). Only occasionally is it necessary to sever the omohyoid.

It may be suggested that, when the incision is made closer to the clavicle, the transverse cervical and suprascapular arteries will cross horizontally along the line of approach to the scalenus anticus muscle, particularly its tendinous insertion. These are readily isolated, clamped, severed, and ligated or electrocoagulated. At this low level, the phrenic nerve has, in coursing downward, obliquely crossed the scalenus anticus from its lateral to its medial border. The nerve lies medial and may be difficult to find beneath the sternocleidomastoid muscle. It is readily found higher up, and it should be identified, liberated, and displaced medialward where it can be protected for some distance.

In the lateral aspect of the exposure, the brachial plexus is found emerging from behind the scalenus anticus muscle at its lateral border. The surgeon must be aware that the distal portion of the subclavian artery lies inferior to the plexus, after arching posterior to the scalenus anticus muscle. This is illustrated in Plate 61 (I). Therefore it is signally important to anticipate possible injury to the subclavian artery. Occasionally, atheromatous plaques form on the vessel as the result of prolonged compression and irritation. Such plaques have been dislodged and fatal hemorrhage reported. If forceps are to be passed posterior to the muscle, it must be done with great care. My own preference is to free the plexus from the lateral border of the scalenus anticus muscle, to place a cotton strip upon the plexus, and to move it gently medialward as the muscle is divided in the same direction. Direct visualization is thus achieved and injury to the artery avoided. It is considered safer to sever the muscle in a piecemeal manner by grasping a few fibers in tissue forceps and carefully inspecting each group before sectioning with scissors.

Plate 61 (I) demonstrates the presence of a few fibrous adhesions attached to the inferior border of the arching subclavian artery. These are occasionally situated about the vasa vasorum. If they are injured, troublesome extravasation of blood will occur between the muscular and adventitial layers of the subclavian artery. This is best avoided by severing the fibrous adhesions some distance from the vessel.

The layers of the deep cervical fascia—the socalled "fat pad," which, incidentally, harbors Virchow's lymph node on the right side—contain many fine blood vessels. These are disrupted in this procedure, and care must be taken to avoid oozing which will stain the surrounding structures, making identification difficult. They can readily be electrocoagulated, or, if such a unit is not available, ligation may be necessary.

Irrigation of the operative area with warm saline, gentle suctioning, and the use of wet cotton strips or "paddies" used for sponging, quite satisfactorily serve the purpose of maintaining the normal appearance of tissues. When sectioning the scalenus anticus muscle, the oozing encountered can be minimized in this fashion, thus enabling the surgeon to identify precisely the structure he is about to divide.

In closing the wound, in addition to the readily recognized necessity for closing the deep cervical fascia over the "fat pad" to avoid a troublesome postoperative "lump" beneath the incision, two considerations are noteworthy. They are, first, that a deeply placed suture near the clavicle can perforate the subclavian vein, and second, that an attempt should be made to avoid a resultant ugly scar, especially in a female patient. The wound should, of course, be closed in layers, preferably with interrupted 0000 silk sutures as Doctor Madden suggests. This should include a subcuticular layer placed deeply enough to be well covered by the thin skin in this area.

A very careful skin closure with 000000 "arterial silk" and an "atraumatic needle" will afford accurate approximation of the wound edges and prevent an unsightly scar.

Plate 61   155

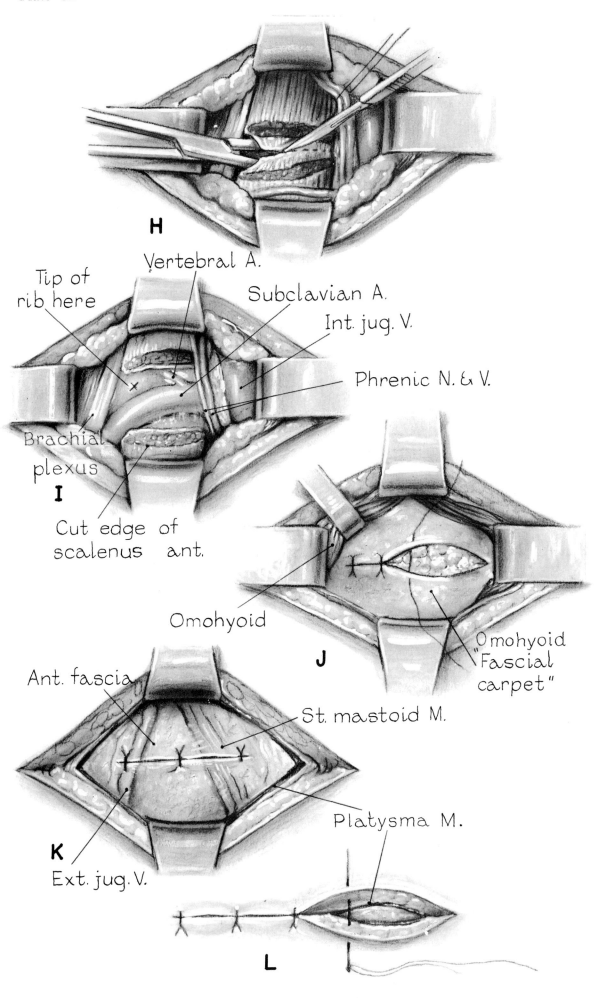

H

Tip of
rib here

Vertebral A.

Subclavian A.

Int. jug. V.

Phrenic N. & V.

Brachial
plexus

I

Cut edge of
scalenus ant.

Omohyoid

J

Omohyoid
"Fascial
carpet"

Ant. fascia

St. mastoid M.

K

Ext. jug. V.

Platysma M.

L

EXCISION OF THYROGLOSSAL DUCT CYST

A. A pillow support is placed in the midline posteriorly between the shoulders, and the head is hyperextended on the neck. The site of the transverse incision between the hyoid bone and the thyroid cartilage is indicated by the solid black line.

B. Sagittal view to show the relation of the cyst and sinus to the surrounding structures, particularly the hyoid bone and the base of the tongue. The passage of the sinus through the hyoid bone and its opening on the base of the tongue at the foramen caecum are visible.

C. The incision is deepened through the subcutaneous fatty tissue and the platysma muscle layers and the previously mobilized wound margins are retracted to expose the underlying structures.

D. The incised margins of the anterior or investing layer of the deep cervical fascia are grasped in clamps, and the extensions of the longitudinal incision in this fascia are indicated by the dotted lines and arrows.

E. The sternohyoid muscles are retracted to show both the prominence of the thyroglossal cyst in the midline and the subjacent thyrohyoid muscles laterally.

F, G, H, I, J. The cyst is alternately displaced in various directions as the scissor dissection in the surrounding tissues is continued to mobilize completely the cyst down to its attachment to the hyoid bone.

Plate 62

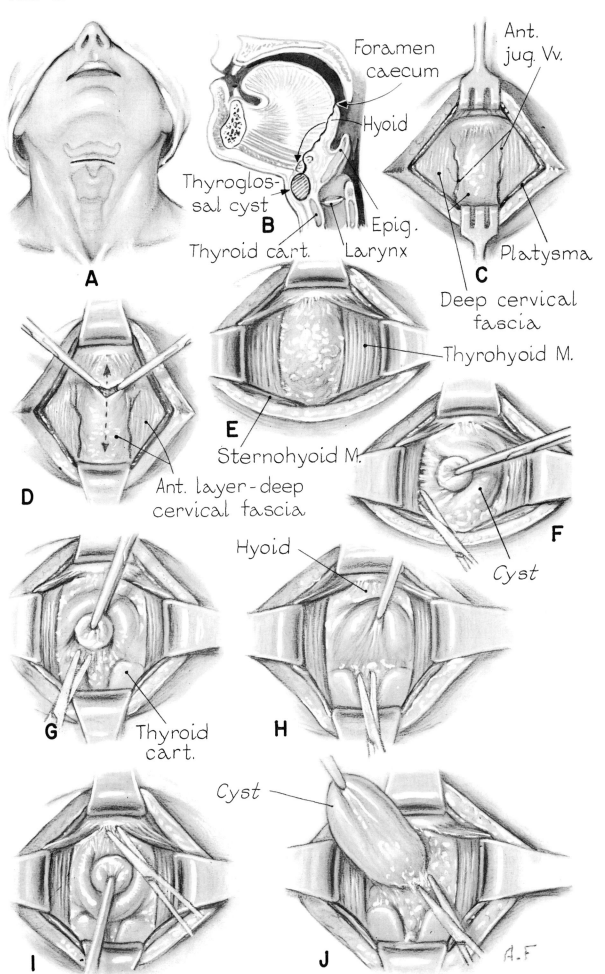

A

Foramen
caecum

Hyoid

Thyroglos-
sal cyst

Thyroid cart.

Epig.

Larynx

B

Ant.
jug. Vv.

Platysma

C

Deep cervical
fascia

Thyrohyoid M.

D

E

Sternohyoid M.

Ant. layer-deep
cervical fascia

F

Cyst

Hyoid

G

Thyroid
cart.

H

I

Cyst

J

A.F.

K. A portion of the wall of the summit of the cyst is grasped in a clamp, and with downward traction on the cyst maintained, the transection of the hyoid bone with scissors is begun. In some instances the use of bone-cutting forceps for this transection may be required. The length of the segment of hyoid bone to be removed is indicated by the dotted lines.

L. The excision of a segment of the hyoid bone is completed, and the line of severance of the fibers of the mylohyoid muscles is shown by the dotted line.

M. The dissection of the thyroglossal duct within the fibers of the geniohyoid and the genioglossal muscles is completed, and a transfixion suture of silk (000) is being in-serted through the cephalad part of the duct which will be transected immediately caudad when the ligature is tied.

N. The excision is completed, and a drain is inserted prior to closure of the thyrohyoid muscles. Neither the mylohyoid muscles nor the cut ends of the hyoid bone are approximated.

O, O′. A drain is inserted through the line of closure of the muscles (O), or preferably through a lateral stab wound drain in the sternohyoid muscle (O′).

P. The skin incision is closed about the drain, using interrupted sutures of silk (000). The exit of the drain laterally, rather than in the midline of the incision as depicted, is preferred.

DISCUSSION—DR. EDGAR L. FRAZELL. Since the technic of excision of a thyroglossal duct cyst is so standardized, one wonders at the frequency of recurrence of these lesions. It is probable that prior infection may hinder complete excision of all portions of the sac. Failure to excise a portion of the hyoid and any portion of the tract leading toward the foramen caecum are likely sources of error. Injection of a few ml. of methylene blue into the sac preoperatively may be of value in some cases.

Plate 63   159

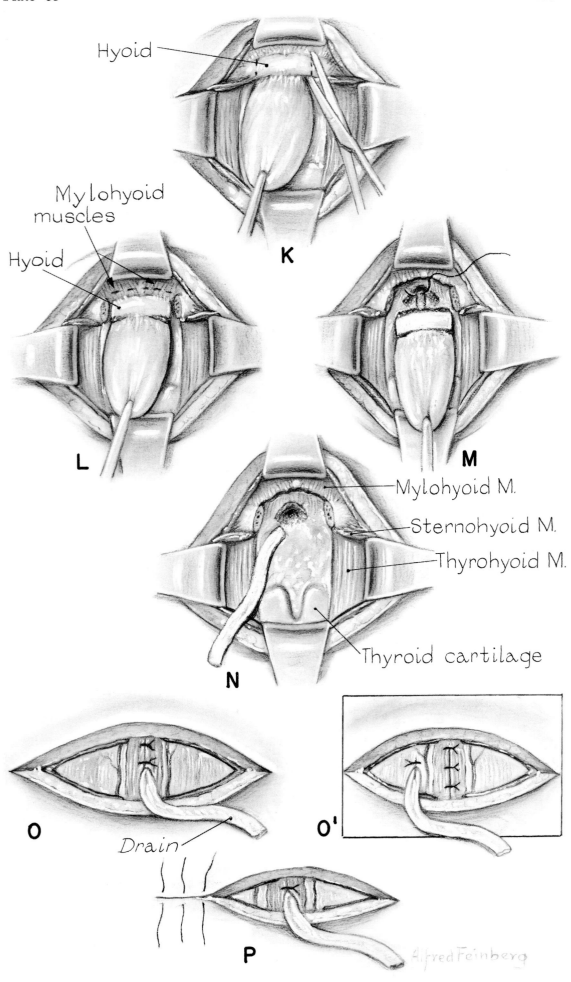

Hyoid

K

Mylohyoid
muscles

Hyoid

L

M

Mylohyoid M.

Sternohyoid M.

Thyrohyoid M.

Thyroid cartilage

N

O

Drain

O'

P

AlfredFeinberg

THYROIDECTOMY

A. The incision is outlined by pressure with a fine silk (0000) thread approximately 4 cm. above the suprasternal notch. Previous to this three small cross hatch marks are made: one in the midline anteriorly and each of the other two overlying the anterior border of either sternomastoid muscle. The larger the gland the higher and the more transverse the incision.

B, C, D. The incision is deepened through the underlying platysma muscle and the upper flap is mobilized by a combination of first sharp and then blunt dissection to a level slightly above the superior notch of the thyroid cartilage. During this dissection of the upper flap, one or two perforating vessels generally require clamping and ligation. The importance of an adequate elevation of the skin and platysma flaps cannot be overemphasized. Dissection of the flaps beneath the platysma muscle, rather than in the subcutaneous tissue plane superficial to the muscle, is preferred.

E. The lower flap is mobilized both by sharp and blunt dissection downward to the level of the suprasternal notch. In the mobilization of the flaps, the main and most extensive part of the dissection is in the midportion rather than in the lateral aspects of the incision. If desired, either routine or selective transection of the prethyroid ("strap" or "ribbon") muscles may be employed as shown by the dotted lines (F). In this event, a preliminary dissection and retraction of the corresponding anterior border of the sternomastoid muscle is performed. A high transection (upper third) of the muscles is performed to avoid injury to their nerve supply through the hypoglossal nerve.

Clamps are not placed across the muscles prior to their severance as it is believed that they cause unnecessary tissue trauma. The anterior jugular and communicating veins are first ligated with suture ligatures of silk on either side of the proposed line of transection, and the muscles are then severed by scalpel dissection.

F. The mobilization of the flaps is completed, and the incision in the anterior (investing) layer of the deep cervical fascia between the anterior jugular veins and overlying the line of junction of the sternohyoid muscles is shown in dotted outline.

G. The sternohyoid muscle, the superficial of the prethyroid or ribbon muscles, is retracted to expose the underlying deep ribbon muscle, the sternothyroid, and the line of incision in the middle layer of the deep cervical (pretracheal) fascia. This layer of fascia is frequently referred to as the "false" or "surgical" capsule of the thyroid gland.

H. Digital dissection is commenced in the plane beneath the pretracheal fascia or "surgical" capsule preparatory to the mobilization of the right lobe of the thyroid gland. This is believed a most important technical step in the operation because, if the proper plane of dissection is not entered, troublesome bleeding is most likely to ensue. The fibers of the sternothyroid muscle are intimately adherent to the thyroid gland, and their complete separation is required to facilitate its mobilization. In the dissection laterally and posteriorly beneath the "false" capsule, particular care should be taken to avoid injury to the middle thyroid vein, a tributary of the internal jugular vein.

DISCUSSION—DR. LAWRENCE W. SLOAN. The routine thyroidectomy may be expeditiously carried out in steps essentially as illustrated. Recalling the fact, however, that nothing in surgery is really routine and that, in the surgery of nodular goiter in particular, one is usually operating because the suspicion exists that the goiter is malignant, the procedure must frequently be modified by the gross findings at operation and the knowledge one has about the likelihood of malignancy. Today, lobectomy is performed much more frequently than in the past. The reason for this is the greater awareness of the likelihood of cancer and the possibility of producing implants or spread of the cancer by needle or incisional biopsy.

The routine type of thyroidectomy is adapted especially for toxic diffuse goiter which is seldom malignant.

In dealing with any nodular goiter, the surgeon should be aware of the possibility of malignancy. In fact, except for actual or threatened compromise of the airway, or because of clinical manifestations of toxicity, the primary indication for operation is the belief that the nodular tumor is either malignant or potentially malignant.

It must be remembered that if cancer is present in the gland, the field has been entered upon making the incision. After raising the flaps, the surgeon should be alert to the presence of lymph nodes which may

Plate 64   161

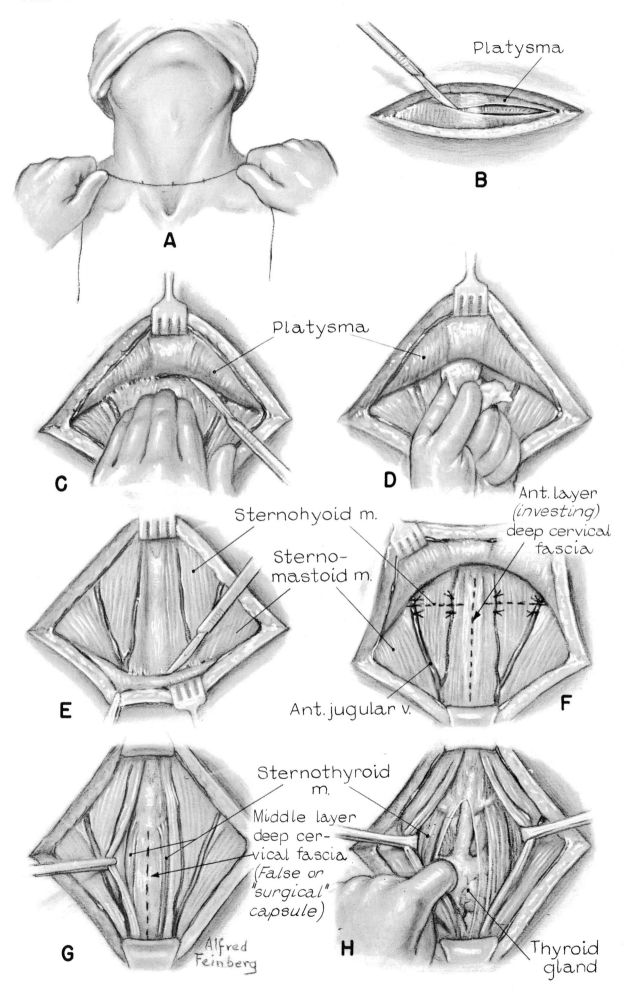

Platysma

B

Platysma

A

Platysma

C   **D**

Sternohyoid m.

Sterno-
mastoid m.

Ant. layer
(investing)
deep cervical
fascia

Ant. jugular v.

E   **F**

Sternothyroid
m.

Middle layer
deep cer-
vical fascia
(False or
"surgical"
capsule)

Alfred
Feinberg

G   **H**

Thyroid
gland

I. By digital retraction, the right lobe of the thyroid is displaced toward the midline and the middle thyroid vein is doubly clamped prior to its division. If desired, ligatures rather than clamps may be used. This is done before attempts are made to mobilize the gland. Otherwise an avulsion tear of the vein and troublesome hemorrhage may occur. In some instances a second venous tributary may require ligation and division.

J. The gland is displaced downward and to the left, and the ribbon muscles are retracted upward and to the right to expose the superior pole of the right lobe of the gland. Displacement of the gland by digital manipulation is generally preferred to the use of clamps which may tear the tissues and cause annoying hemorrhage. Mobilization of the vascular pedicle of the superior pole is commenced by blunt dissection medially with a clamp inserted through an opening previously made in the fibroareolar tissue layer. Subsequently, the relatively dense layer of tissue posteriorly, which binds down the superior pole, is incised as depicted by the dotted line. After incising this tissue, the left index finger is inserted into the space behind the superior pole. This space is bound posteriorly by the cervical vertebrae and laterally by the carotid artery. By digital dissection in this space the superior pole of the lobe and its vascular pedicle may be completely mobilized.

J', J''. These insets depict the findings at operation in two successive patients and show the intimate relation of the external branch of the superior laryngeal nerve to the vascular pedicle of the superior pole of the thyroid lobe. It is believed that this relation has not been sufficiently stressed. This nerve accompanies the superior thyroid vessels in their descent toward the superior pole of the lobe. At a variable distance above this pole the nerve passes medialward in relation to the inferior constrictor and cricothyroid muscles. It lies on the surface of the cricothyroid muscle immediately subjacent to the line of insertion of the sternothyroid muscle into the thyroid cartilage and may be seen on elevation of the upper portion of this muscle. In the application of clamps to the isolated vascular pedicle of the superior pole, it is believed that this nerve should always be demonstrated to prevent injury to it. In fact, in one instance (J'), selective clamping, ligation, and division of the superior thyroid vessels was necessary to avoid injury to the nerve. Several "blind" methods have been proposed for the avoidance of injury to this nerve during the dissection, isolation, and division of the superior thyroid vessels. However, none of these methods is absolutely safe because there may be anatomic variations in the distribution of the nerve which may be determined only by direct vision. In the performance of a thyroidectomy the importance of the proper identification and prevention of injury to the recurrent laryngeal nerve is repeatedly stressed. It is believed that the same should apply also to the external branch of the superior laryngeal nerve. Injury to this nerve, which innervates the cricothyroid muscle, causes a roughness, weakness, and early fatigue of the voice. Confirmation of the nerve injury is obtained by indirect laryngoscopy. The affected cord will be lax and have an oblique, wavy concavity. This is in contradistinction to the straight midline position of the affected cord, the so-called "cadaveric" position, in paralysis of the recurrent laryngeal nerve.

K, L. The vascular pedicle of the superior pole is isolated, and after proper identification of the external branch of the superior laryngeal nerve, the pedicle is triply clamped and severed between the two most distal clamps.

M, M'. The proximal stump of the vascular pedicle is occluded with a proximal ligature and a distal transfixion suture ligature (M') of 00 silk. The relation of the external branch of the superior laryngeal nerve to the inferior constrictor and cricothyroid muscles and to the ligated stump of the superior thyroid vessels may be clearly seen.

N. Dissection is commenced in the avascular areolar tissue space between the thyroid gland medially and the carotid artery laterally to expose the inferior thyroid artery. The related surrounding structures are appropriately labeled.

N'. Inset to show the inferior thyroid artery encircled by an untied silk (00) ligature and the commencement of the isolation of the vascular pedicle of the inferior pole by clamp dissection.

O. The isolated vascular pedicle is triply clamped, and the site of severance between the two proximal clamps is indicated by the dotted line.

Plate 65   163

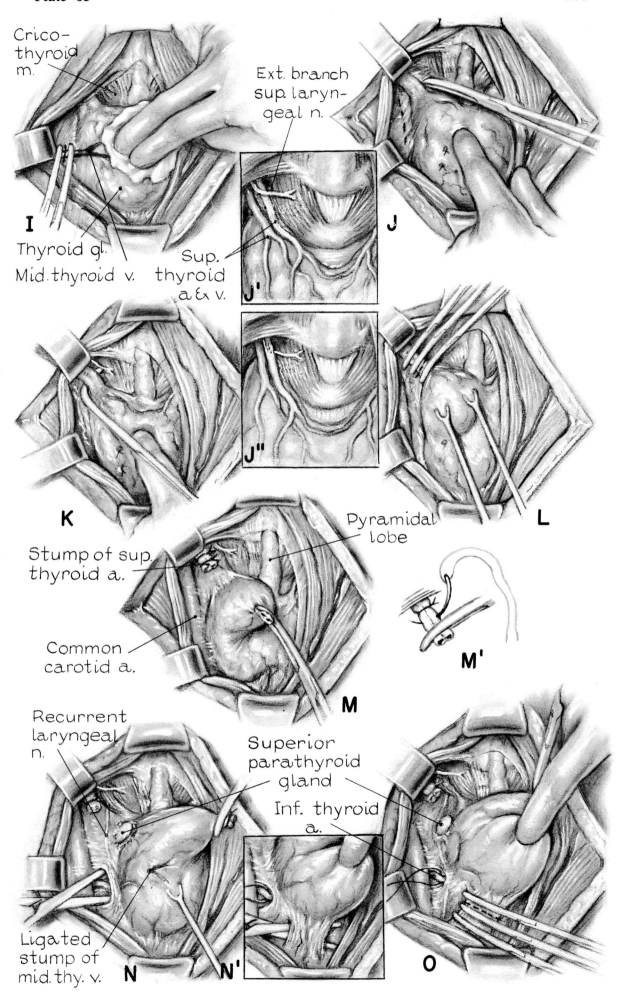

Crico-
thyroid
m.

Ext. branch
sup. laryn-
geal n.

I

Thyroid gl.
Mid. thyroid v.

Sup.
thyroid
a & v.

J'

J

J"

K

Pyramidal
lobe

L

Stump of sup.
thyroid a.

Common
carotid a.

M

M'

Recurrent
laryngeal
n.

Superior
parathyroid
gland

Inf. thyroid
a.

Ligated
stump of
mid. thy. v.

N

N'

O

P. The mobilized superior and inferior poles of the right lobe of the thyroid gland are approximated, and the gland is retracted toward the midline. The inferior thyroid artery is ligated in continuity and its two branches have been doubly clamped, severed, and ligated in preparation for the total removal of the right lobe. In this patient the recurrent laryngeal nerve was located anterior to the inferior thyroid artery at the site of its bifurcation. The relation of this nerve to the superior parathyroid gland and its entrance into the larynx beneath the lower border of the inferior constrictor muscle is shown. This is immediately posterior to the site of articulation of the inferior horn of the thyroid cartilage with the cricoid cartilage.

P′, P″. These insets depict the alternate positions commonly observed in the relation of the recurrent laryngeal nerve to the inferior thyroid artery and its branches. The nerve may pass either between the branches (P′) or behind (P″).

Q. The vascular fibroareolar tissue attaching the gland to the cricothyroid ligament and commonly called the suspensory ligament is doubly clamped prior to its severance as indicated by the dotted line.

[The operative technic illustrated up to and including this step is the same regardless of whether a total or subtotal lobotomy of the thyroid gland is performed.]

R, R′, R″. These illustrations show the sub-

sequent steps in technic for bilateral subtotal thyroidectomy (R′) and unilateral subtotal lobectomy (R″). In the partial resection of a lobe (R), clamps are applied to the gland superiorly, inferiorly, and posterolaterally. The clamps posterolaterally are inserted into the gland substance immediately proximal to the entrance of the branches of the inferior thyroid artery. Only five or six clamps are required. Ligation in continuity of the main trunk of the inferior thyroid artery is routinely performed. The site of the incision for the subtotal resection of the right lobe is indicated by the dotted line. Following the completion of the resection, hemostasis in the remaining segment of the lobe is obtained by suture ligatures of silk (000). Similarly hemostasis in the clamped and severed isthmus (R″) will be obtained with suture ligatures of silk (000). Following the completion of either a unilateral or a bilateral subtotal thyroidectomy, the remnant of the lobe is anchored to the pretracheal fascia with sutures of silk (000) as shown in R′. This particular step in technic is an aid in the control of bleeding from the cut surface of the gland.

S, S′. The operation for total removal of the right lobe of the thyroid gland is now continued. A cleavage plane between the isthmus and the anterior surface of the trachea is obtained by blunt dissection, and the isthmus is serially clamped and severed as demonstrated (S′).

DISCUSSION—DR. SLOAN (cont.)

first be found in the midline as the median raphe is incised and the sternohyoid muscles separated. It is good practice in dissecting these muscles free to keep close to the under surface, leaving the thin fibroareolar tissue and nodes attached to the anterior surface of the gland (or to the "surgical capsule") to be removed with the specimen should the goiter actually turn out to be malignant. If in separating these muscles one of them should be found to be adherent to the gland, especially over a nodule, it would be important to excise the muscle. This will usually be the sternothyroid muscle, but, of course, both muscles may be removed without producing either undue deformity or disability. Under such circumstances lobectomy should probably be performed and begun by transection of the isthmic part of the lobe which is thought not to be involved. In such cases it is my practice to reflect the fragment of the uninvolved lobe together with the prelaryngeal and pretracheal fatty tissues (which contain lymph nodes) toward the side of the involved lobe (Figs. 1 and 2). The superior ves-

sels are divided high, clearly identifying and often ligating them individually with fine silk. If nodes are present alongside the vessels, they are included in the resected specimen.

The sternomastoid muscle is freed, and the carotid sheath is entered. The dissection is kept close to the deep surface of the muscle so that any nodes within the sheath may be reflected toward the gland with the fascia. The nodes, if present, and the sheath over the internal jugular vein, vagus nerve, and common carotid artery are reflected toward the gland. Approaching the lateral posterior margin of the gland, the inferior thyroid artery is isolated, divided, and ligated, and the recurrent laryngeal nerve is identified. If the gland is malignant, the most common site of involved nodes will be the small lymph glands in close proximity to the primary tumor. These nodes will be frequently found in the fatty paratracheal and paraesophageal tissues, paralleling and medial to the recurrent laryngeal nerve, and follow the descent of this nerve into the mediastinum encircling sometimes

Plate 66   165

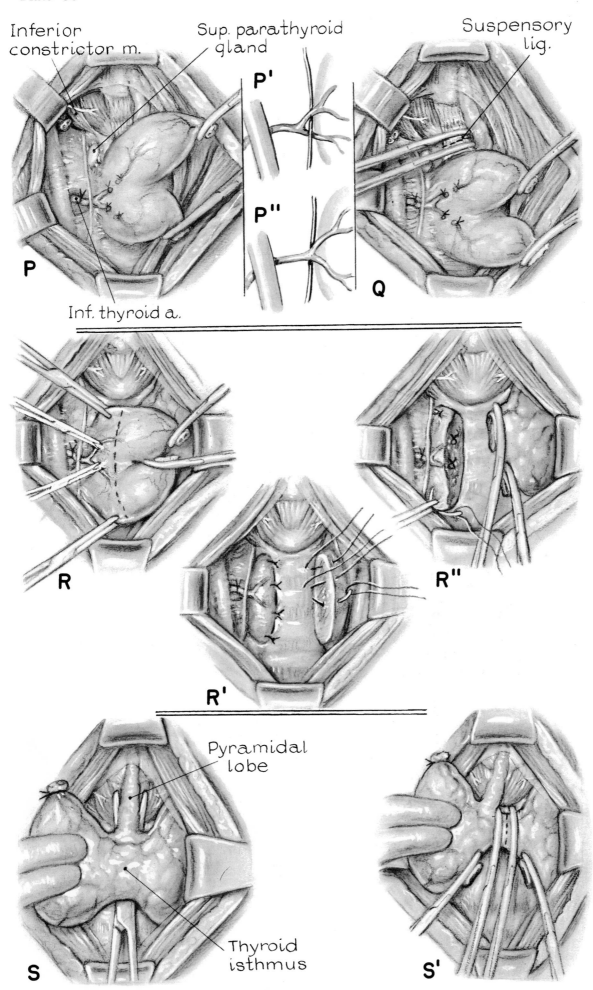

Inferior
constrictor m.

Sup. parathyroid
gland

Suspensory
lig.

P'

P"

P

Q

Inf. thyroid a.

R

R"

R'

Pyramidal
lobe

Thyroid
isthmus

S

S'

T, U. The severance of the isthmus is completed, and the clamps are replaced with hemostatic suture ligatures (00 silk). The previously mobilized pyramidal lobe is clamped, and the severance of its site of attachment is shown by the dotted line (U). This tissue attachment of the pyramidal lobe is clamped before it is severed because of the contained blood vessel normally present. For clarity the clamp is not shown.

V. The right lobe of the thyroid gland is again retracted toward the midline, and the remaining attachment of the right lobe to the pretracheal fascia is severed by scalpel dissection.

W. The operative field and the related struc-

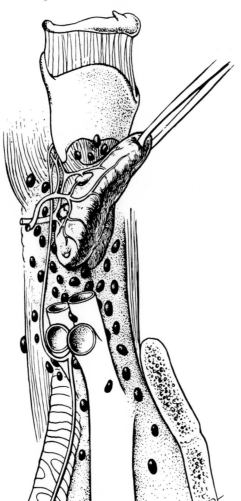

Fig. 1. "Corner" of the gland and paraglandular spaces: paratracheal, paraesophageal, paralaryngeal, anterior and superior mediastinal. Note intimate relationships between recurrent laryngeal nerve and vessels especially at point of entrance of dividing nerve to intrinsic laryngeal muscles. The fascialike structure "suspending" the gland at this point is often quite tough and dense. Lymph nodes in the paraglandular areas are small but frequently involved in papillary or mixed cancer of the thyroid. These are clustered about the gland and extend toward or into the superior and anterior mediastina not infrequently just beyond the level which can be reached through the usual cervical incision.

tures following the completion of the total right lobectomy are depicted.

X, Y. The sandbags are removed from between the scapulae and the sternothyroid (X), and the sternohyoid (Y) muscles are approximated with interrupted sutures of 000 silk.

Z, Z'. The skin and platysma muscles are closed together as one layer (Z), and the application of a sterile dressing (Z') completes the operation. In general, drains are not employed regardless of the size of the gland removed. However, if the use of a drain is considered indicated, it is brought out between the fibers of the sternomastoid muscle as recommended by Lahey.

DISCUSSION—DR. SLOAN (cont.)

the trachea and the esophagus. These tissues are carefully dissected from the recurrent laryngeal nerve and the superior parathyroid gland, being careful to avoid compromise of the blood supply to this gland. The superior parathyroid gland is usually located anterior to the recurrent laryngeal nerve near its entrance into the larynx and accordingly it may be easily identified and preserved. However, the inferior parathyroid gland is located among the nodes which should be removed with the specimen and cannot be as easily preserved without compromising the completeness of the dissection. The removal of the involved tissues is carried down as low as possible along the nerve and, occasionally, on the right side, to its point of origin. Here, not infrequently, involved nodes are found either during the neck dissection or during the mediastinal dissection performed subsequently if nodes along this route of spread have been found to contain cancer at the primary operation. The lobe, together with the paraglandular tissues described, is freed from the trachea and submitted to the pathologist. The diagnosis is usually established by gross and frozen section examination of the resected specimen. If the disease is benign, the neck incision is closed, usually without drainage. If it is malignant, the other lobe is removed together with the paraglandular tissue on the opposite side. The rationale for this step is twofold: (1) Thyroid cancer is frequently multifocal and may be present even in microscopic foci in the grossly uninvolved lobe. (2) The likelihood that the nodes in the paraglandular areas closest to the primary focus will be involved is so great that a thorough dissection of these areas at a time when it can be done without undue risk of injury to the nerves and the parathyroid glands is most desirable.

The conventional neck dissection that is frequently performed for cancer of the thyroid gland metastatic to the cervical lymph nodes, does not take into consideration the important areas described above, because the operation was devised for metastatic cancer from primary lesions of the face, mouth, or pharynx. Malignant tumors originating in these sites do not spread along the routes which are most frequently followed in the dissemination of thyroid cancer from its primary site. The knowledge we now have about the spread of thyroid cancer must of necessity revise our ideas about the surgical procedures in dealing with this type of neoplasm. If cancer is found in the

Plate 67   167

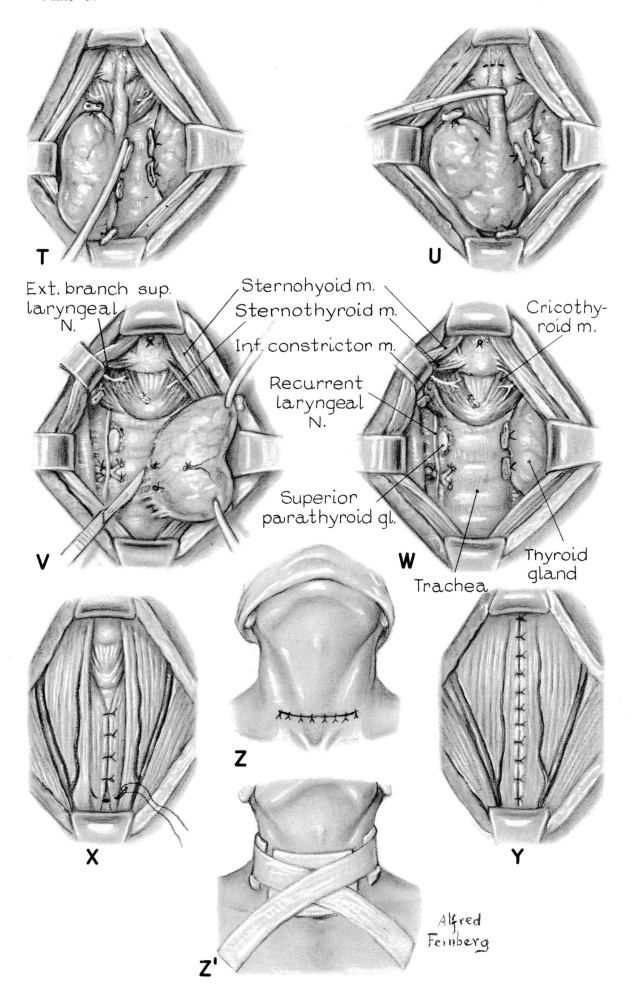

T

U

Ext. branch sup.
laryngeal
N.

Sternohyoid m.

Sternothyroid m.

Inf. constrictor m.

Recurrent
laryngeal
N.

Superior
parathyroid gl.

Cricothy-
roid m.

Thyroid
gland

Trachea

V

W

X

Z

Y

Z'

Alfred
Feinberg

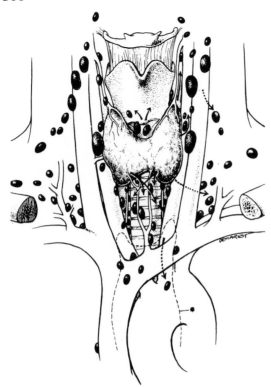

Fig. 2. Routes of local and regional lymphatic spread of thyroid cancer. There is little spread from the anterior aspect of the gland. The drainage appears to be along major vessels and nerves. Distribution therefore occurs chiefly from the poles, along the posterolateral borders of the gland, and along the recurrent laryngeal nerves. Mediastinal involvement when present is most dense near the lower border of the gland but often just out of reach through a cervical incision. Lymphatics encircle the trachea and esophagus particularly below the gland level so that occasionally para and retrotracheal and esophageal nodes will be found involved contralateral to the primary focus.

DISCUSSION—DR. SLOAN (cont.)

surgical specimen, and these paraglandular tissues have not been removed, their subsequent removal will be a most important step in extirpating the disease. However, such secondary operations will be fraught with the danger of injury to the parathyroids and the recurrent laryngeal nerve. The removal of the paraglandular tissues is referred to as "clearing the gland area," which is most opportune to do at the time of the first procedure.

Other modifications of the large variety of routine procedures which may be used in doing a thyroidectomy are dependent upon the circumstances relative to a particular type of goiter. In some instances division of the anterior thyroid muscles (Plate 64, E) is used, and in others, for example a large posterior mediastinal goiter, a drastic modification of the operative technic may be required (Fig. 4). Knowledge of the anatomy involved is of particular importance in these somewhat exceptional situations because of the anatomic distortions or variations that are frequently present.

SUBSTERNAL, INTRATHORACIC, AND POSTERIOR MEDIASTINAL GOITER

Intrathoracic goiter is usually acquired. Substernal goiters are common and congenital aberrant goiters are rare.

The usual intrathoracic goiter is anterior; that is, it lies within the anterior mediastinum in front of the trachea and the great vessels. It may produce compression of the trachea, the esophagus, and the vessels from either before, backward, or obliquely, at the level of the thoracic inlet (Fig. 3).

In the usual operation for intrathoracic goiter, division of the "strap" muscles is generally desirable to provide good exposure. A good light is absolutely essential. Partial lobectomy of the smaller lobe is carried out first unless there is unilateral enlargement only of the gland. In that event, regardless of its size and consistency, benignancy of the enlarged lobe should be questioned, and a total lobectomy should be performed. In any event, it is most important to free the superior part of the intrathoracic portion of the goiter before attempting its removal from the chest. This includes securing the superior thyroid vessels, division of the so-called suspensory ligament, transection of the isthmus of the gland, and, of equal importance, freeing the lobe to be resected from alongside of the trachea (Fig. 3). After accurately establishing the lateral plane of dissection on the surgical capsule of the gland, the lateral veins are ligated in this plane as they are encountered. Following this the intrathoracic portion of the gland can usually be eased upward and forward out of the chest. During this procedure, and especially before incising the surgical capsule laterally or inferiorly, careful search should be made in a dry, well illuminated field for an attenuated, displaced nerve. If found, it should be carefully freed and the lobe displaced toward the midline before resection. If this is done, the parathyroids also will usually be identified and protected from injury.

Frequently, a substernal goiter, which is far more common than a truly intrathoracic goiter, will be called intrathoracic, including the *goitre plongeant*. However, the operative technic is essentially the same as in a routine thyroidectomy. A word about this technic should be said in relation to the large, "solid" variety of substernal goiter which, in a patient with a short, thick neck, may produce severe pressure on the trachea. Over a long period of time, this can produce softening of the tracheal cartilages to such a degree that tracheal collapse may occur either at operation or subsequently because the supporting effect of the thyroid is removed. A tracheotomy may be required and should be done if there is any question whatsoever about a competent airway. An alternative procedure is occasionally available if the area of softening is detected at operation and if it lies close to the origins of the sternohyoid and sternothyroid muscles. Sutures from the origins of these muscles to the adjacent tracheal fascia may be employed to keep the softened wall from collapsing until the scarring and fixation of healing provide sufficient support for the trachea. If the area of compression is not in proximity to the muscle origins, collapse of the trachea will not

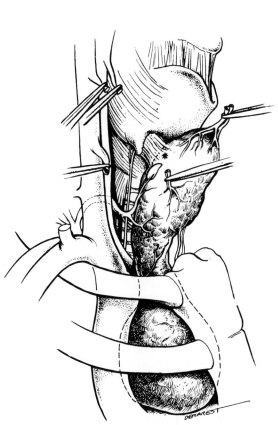

Fig. 3. The usual (anterior type) of intrathoracic goiter. Freeing the superior pole, dividing the "suspensory ligament," the isthmus of the gland, and the tracheal attachments of the lobe to be removed are preliminary to delivering the intrathoracic part of the goiter. The intrathoracic portion of the goiter lies anterior to the great vessels. Part of its vascular attachments may be in the mediastinum.

* "Corner" of the gland.

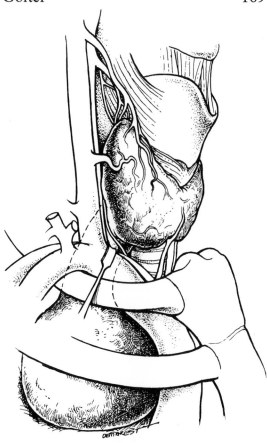

Fig. 4. Posterior mediastinal goiter. The cervical portion of the gland is often lower than shown. The mediastinal portion of the goiter is shown springing from the posterior aspect of the gland close to the trachea, thus displacing the recurrent nerve laterally into a vulnerable position. The goiter lies posterior to the major vessels, displacing them forward. The trachea and esophagus are usually displaced forward and to the left. All of these structures may also be compressed. The internal and external branches of the superior laryngeal nerve are shown exaggerated to remind the surgeon of the proximity to the superior thyroid vessels.

DISCUSSION—DR. SLOAN (cont.)

be prevented by suturing the tracheal wall to the muscles or to their aponeuroses and accordingly should not be done. The zone of compression in an intrathoracic goiter is usually at the thoracic inlet and in such instances the discusser has found the above described procedure of distinct value. In determining whether there is softening and whether the expedient described is effectual, the cooperation of the anesthetist is essential. The endotracheal tube should be withdrawn slowly to a point just above the tracheal cartilages involved but not above the glottis. The area of softening may be easily detected by the surgeon feeling the trachea as the tube is moved.

In dealing with large goiters, especially if the enlargement is unilateral and associated with rotation of the trachea and larynx as well as displacement, one must always be aware of the possibility that the recurrent nerve may be stretched over the gradually expanding mass and lie in a vulnerable position. Under such circumstances, inadvertent injury to the nerve is not uncommon, especially if it lies in front of (or

external to) the inferior thyroid artery and its branches rather than in its usual positions posterior (or medial) to the artery or between its branches.

In large goiters (and sometimes in small ones) the capsular veins are large and so fragile that they are easily torn, causing annoying and, at times, serious bleeding, which may be a threat to the successful outcome of the operation. Securing the major vessels, particularly the inferior thyroid vessels, before resection is a recommended procedure, but at times in the attempt to expose these vessels, the bleeding from the large capsular veins may predispose to injury of the recurrent laryngeal nerve, the parathyroid glands, and the internal jugular vein. A maneuver which has been found helpful in such instances is to pass mass suture ligatures of fairly heavy material through the gland substance. These are tied snugly and the ends cut long to use as retractors. The use of hooks and small shallow ligatures in these glands usually causes excessive bleeding because of the abundant network of superficial and friable veins.

Rarely, in removing a large and adherent intrathoracic goiter, the sternum may have to be split. However, the maneuver described by Lahey many years ago may be employed in dealing with the usual type of nontoxic nodular intrathoracic goiter which is composed largely of colloid and degenerating thyroid tissue. The finger is inserted into the top of such a mass, breaking it up and removing enough of its contents so that the intrathoracic component can be compressed and delivered into the neck through the thoracic inlet. In this type of gland the risk of hemorrhage from this procedure is minimal.

Posterior mediastinal goiter, a type of intrathoracic goiter which is not common, arises from the posterior aspect of the gland and extends as it enlarges downward into the chest *behind* the carotid sheath. In about 75 per cent of the cases, the downward extension is on the right side between the sheath and the trachea (Fig. 4). In those instances in which the gland lies low in the neck, the goiter may be entirely intrathoracic although usually there is a sizeable cervical component. The intrathoracic extension, connected to the cervical goiter by a small and inconspicuous isthmus, may not be recognized at operation and only be discovered later by roentgenographic studies either incidental to or because of symptoms of tracheal or esophageal compression. The differential diagnosis of these goiters is sometimes puzzling. Radioactive iodine studies have proved helpful. Expansion downward produces deviation of the trachea and esophagus forward and to the side opposite the goiter, with or without compression. They sometimes attain a large size and may encroach significantly upon the upper lobe of the lung. The recurrent laryngeal nerve usually is in its normal location, but the extension of the goiter downward may begin low in the gland between the trachea and the nerve where it deviates from the trachea, especially on the right side. This position exposes the nerve to an added risk of injury, a fact the surgeon should always remember.

When small, a posterior mediastinal goiter can usually be removed through a cervical approach. In any event, if this type of goiter is suspected, even when large, the initial approach should be made by the cervical route because of the location of the major blood supply which is in the neck. Exploration of the gland, determination of the position of the recurrent nerve, control of the major vessels of the gland, and possibly even removal of the goiter through the neck wound may be accomplished by retraction of the carotid artery, internal jugular vein, and vagus nerve in one direction and the trachea and the esophagus in the other. One should recall, however, that the intrathoracic component may have acquired or already possesses good sized vascular channels. Accordingly, the surgeon should not persist unrelentingly in the attempt to remove the mass by this route but should remove it through a thoracotomy incision suitably placed. It is obvious that splitting the sternum for removal of this type of goiter has not the same rationale as in dealing with the unusually large anteriorly placed intrathoracic goiters.

DISCUSSION—DR. GEORGE CRILE, JR. Although I am in full agreement with the general principles expressed by Dr. Madden, the technic that I prefer differs from his in a few respects. For approximately 10 years, I have eliminated completely the raising of skin flaps. When a thyroidectomy incision is made high, as it should be to obtain the best cosmetic results, there is no need to raise flaps at all. The dissection can be carried straight on down through the platysma and through the strap muscles, separating the strap muscles only on the affected side in the case of a unilateral goiter, until it reaches the thyroid gland. The sternomastoid muscle can be set back by a little dissection, so that it will not be injured. The incision can then be spread by digital traction up and down on the sides of the incision, so that adequate exposure is obtained.

I have never seen a goiter too big to be removed in this way, nor one in which raising a flap would give better exposure. The raising of flaps leaves a place for serum to accumulate or hematomas to form. There is no cosmetic advantage to raising flaps. It is time-consuming and I believe unnecessary.

I prefer No. 60 cotton to silk because, in the years when I used silk, I saw more extrusion of sutures than I have since I switched to cotton. The superficial vessels are electrocoagulated.

Dr. Madden mentions the necessity of removing all of the muscular capsule of the thyroid before attempting to mobilize the gland (H). This in my opinion is the most commonly disregarded technical aspect of thyroidectomy. Young surgeons in training do not seem to be able to distinguish readily between the exposed true capsule of the thyroid and the adherent muscular capsule. They try to rotate the gland before it has been released from the muscles which bind it down.

Dr. Madden speaks of routine ligation of the lateral thyroid vein (I). This is doubtless feasible, but it is often unnecessary. Although I believe the course of the vein should be identified, I do not think that it always has to be ligated extracapsularly. In many cases, the vein hugs the posterior capsule of the thyroid and does not go straight across from the anterior surface of the thyroid to the jugular. In such cases rotation can be accomplished without separate ligation of the vein.

In describing the dissection of the superior pole (J), Dr. Madden emphasizes the medial part of the dissection separating the pole vessels from the larynx, but he says nothing of the necessity of doing a similar dissection on the lateral side isolating completely the superior pole from the carotid sheath. I find it much easier if I have completely separated the superior pole from the carotid sheath before starting the medial portion of the dissection.

I would find it difficult to identify the external branch of the superior laryngeal nerve in all cases (J', J"), because it is quite small and irregular in its distribution. This, I presume, is because I have not been trained to recognize this nerve. I think some surgeons could waste a great deal of time searching for it, and I am sure that it can be avoided in the vast majority of cases by staying very close to the thyroid vessels on the medial side and not ligating them too high. I have never noted any untoward effects from a unilateral injury of the nerve but agree that a bilateral injury causes definite morbidity.

RADICAL NECK DISSECTION: LEFT

A. The double-Y incision used is outlined. The four insets show other types of incisions that may be chosen in the performance of a radical neck dissection.

B. The mobilized skin flaps to which the platysma muscle is attached are retracted to show the underlying anatomic structures.

C. The external jugular vein is doubly ligated in continuity and severed between the ligatures. The anterior or investing layer of the deep cervical fascia overlying the fatty tissue layer posteriorly is being incised. This incision, which severs branches of the cervical cutaneous nerves, will be continued medially to transect the sternomastoid muscle just proximal to its clavicular and sternal insertions.

DISCUSSION—DR. ARTHUR G. JAMES. The neck lends itself to block dissection more readily than any other region of the body. It is indicated for many primary tumors of the neck as well as for metastatic carcinoma originating in oral-pharyngeal primaries. I employ the double-Y incision as shown in A. The upper arm of this incision is made in the upper cervical crease. Although the diagram does not show this accurately, it is possible with this incision to have equal angles—each 120°—thus lessening the possibility of skin necrosis due to impaired circulation. The incision diagramed in A_4 is more cosmetic, but it should be pointed out that it does not afford the exposure to the entire side of the neck that the double-Y incision does. When one is dealing with a malignant process, it is more important that adequate exposure be obtained for complete resection rather than a good cosmetic scar that possibly covers incomplete excision of tumor.

The platysma muscle may or may not be left with the skin flaps (B). If one is dealing with a malignant melanoma, which very often spreads by the superficial lymphatics, it is better to take the platysma muscle. The skin flaps will survive whether or not the platysma muscle is left.

After the deep vein is doubly ligated and transected (D), it is helpful to ligate the transverse cervical vessels prior to proceeding with the posterior neck dissection. The blood supply to this part is reduced, and the posterior dissection is less vascular. The posterior belly of the digastric muscle is a good landmark. Until one reaches this muscle in the posterior triangle, he may be assured that nothing of consequence will be severed and that the brachial places will be protected. I do not believe that a lower neck dissection can be complete without sacrificing the spinal accessory nerve, which is shown transected in D. There is some morbidity associated with transecting this

Plate 68

173

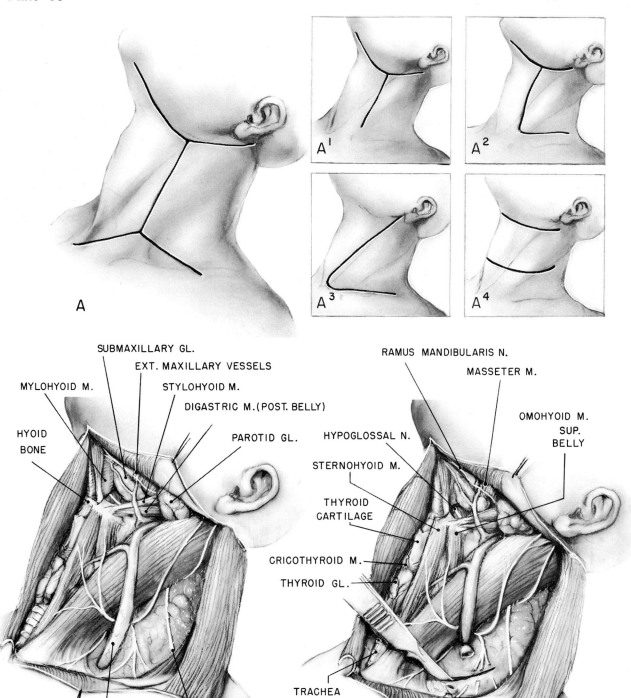

A

A¹ A² A³ A⁴

B

SUBMAXILLARY GL.

EXT. MAXILLARY VESSELS

MYLOHYOID M. STYLOHYOID M.

DIGASTRIC M.(POST. BELLY)

HYOID BONE PAROTID GL.

EXT. JUGULAR V.

ACCESSORY N.

C

RAMUS MANDIBULARIS N.

MASSETER M.

HYPOGLOSSAL N. OMOHYOID M. SUP. BELLY

STERNOHYOID M.

THYROID CARTILAGE

CRICOTHYROID M.

THYROID GL.

TRACHEA

PLATYSMA M.

STERNOMASTOID M.

D. The proximal transected portion of the sternomastoid muscle is held in clamps and retracted upward. The partially mobilized internal jugular vein is being encircled by a ligature of 00 silk preliminary to its ligation. The broken line indicates the incision to be made in the middle layer of the deep cervical fascia, the omohyoid fascial "carpet." This incision will transect the "pulley" tendon of the omohyoid muscle.

D'. The internal jugular vein is doubly ligated (00 silk) in continuity, and a transfixion suture ligature (000 silk) is inserted in juxtaposition to the caudad ligature.

D". The ligated vein is severed between the two proximal ligatures.

E. The omohyoid fascial "carpet" is incised, and the omohyoid muscle is transected to expose the fat pad that overlies the scalenus anticus muscle.

E', F. The tissue "bloc" is mobilized cephalad by sharp dissection, and the underlying muscle and neurovascular components are exposed. The superior belly of the omohyoid muscle is being severed at its insertion into the hyoid bone (F). In this patient the superior thyroid artery arose from the common carotid artery rather than from the usual site, the external carotid.

DISCUSSION—DR. JAMES (cont.)

nerve; with proper exercise and physiotherapy, however, these objections can usually be overcome.

When the carotid bifurcation is approached, it is well to inject the carotid body with a local anesthetic agent. This very simple procedure does prevent shock from an overactive carotid sinus, which occurs in a definite number of patients.

When dissecting medially to the carotid in the region of the superior thyroid artery, it is important to avoid damaging the superior laryngeal nerve. This nerve may be endangered if the carotid bifurcation is overly rotated during the course of the dissection. It originates from the vagus nerve and proceeds medially deep to the carotid vessels to enter the larynx just above the greater cornu of the thyroid cartilage. If it is transected, partial anesthesia of the glottis results, and the

patient may have serious difficulty because of aspiration of food and water.

As shown in I, the submaxillary space is beautifully exposed by retracting the mylohyoid muscle superiorly and medially. The duct of the submaxillary gland runs between the hypoglossal nerve below and the lingual nerve above, and these two structures should be identified before the duct is transected. The illustration indicates a transection of the lower end of the parotid gland, which may be performed without fear of salivary fistula as long as the salivary duct system is patent.

I utilize the same type of closure as that shown in L, and I have been much impressed with the suction drainage rather than the bulky compression dressings. I employ two catheters, one medially and one posteriorly in the wound, and usually attach them to a portable suction apparatus.

Plate 69   175

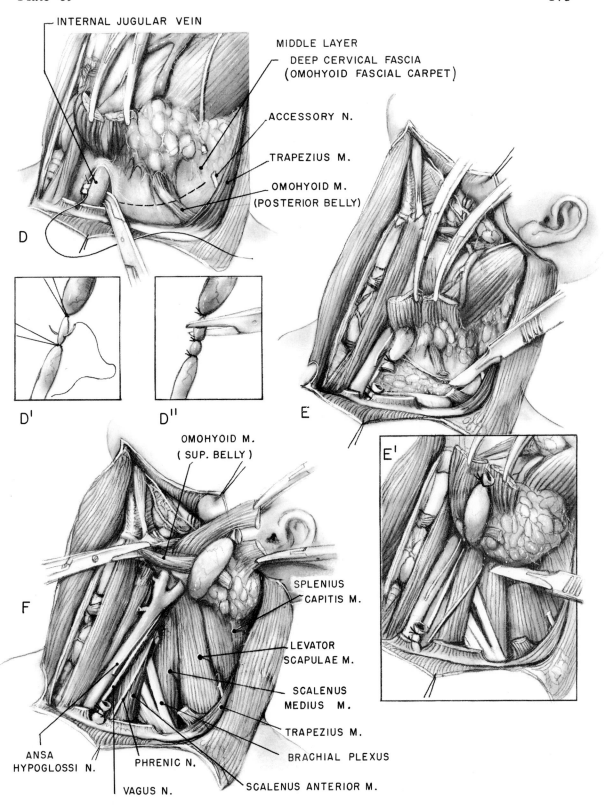

INTERNAL JUGULAR VEIN

MIDDLE LAYER
DEEP CERVICAL FASCIA
(OMOHYOID FASCIAL CARPET)

ACCESSORY N.

TRAPEZIUS M.

OMOHYOID M.
(POSTERIOR BELLY)

D

D'

D''

E

E'

OMOHYOID M.
(SUP. BELLY)

F

SPLENIUS
CAPITIS M.

LEVATOR
SCAPULAE M.

SCALENUS
MEDIUS M.

TRAPEZIUS M.

BRACHIAL PLEXUS

ANSA
HYPOGLOSSI N.

PHRENIC N.

SCALENUS ANTERIOR M.

VAGUS N.

G. The mobilized tissue "bloc" is covered with a moist gauze pad and depressed downward and medially as the sternomastoid muscle is transected just proximal to its insertion into the mastoid bone.

H. The lower pole of the parotid gland is next transected, caution being taken to isolate the enclosed posterior facial vein, which is shown being severed between ligatures of 000 silk.

H'. The facial (external maxillary) artery, which courses in a groove on the posterior surface of the submaxillary gland, and the anterior facial (external maxillary) vein, which lies on the anterior surface of the gland, are doubly clamped and severed (broken line). Care should be taken to avoid injury to the mandibular branch of the facial nerve. This nerve, unusually wavy in appearance, is narrow in diameter and located anterior to the facial vessels. Its severance results in an immediate flattening of the ipsilateral side of the lower lip, which is accentuated on motion of the lips.

I. The submaxillary gland, grasped in a clamp, is displaced downward, and the mylohyoid muscle is retracted to show the submaxillary (Wharton's) duct on the surface of the hyoglossus and its relation to the lingual nerve above and the hypoglossal nerve below. The internal jugular vein, between and deep to the transected parotid gland and sternomastoid muscle, is first doubly ligated (00 silk) in continuity. Then a transfixion suture ligature of 000 silk is inserted in close proximity to the cephalad ligature preliminary to the severance of the vein between the two caudad ligatures.

J. The mobilization of the tissue "bloc" is continued cephalad by scalpel dissection. Shown clearly are the carotid bulb and the ligated stumps of the superior thyroid (caudad) and lingual (cephalad) arteries, which are branches of the external carotid artery.

DISCUSSION—DR. OLIVER H. BEAHRS. The diagrams are well done, adequately demonstrating the important anatomic structures and their relationships as seen in the course of a radical neck dissection. If the reader is well acquainted with the anatomy of the neck (which he should be if he is to operate on this region), the legends are a satisfactory outline of Dr. Madden's surgical approach and technic.

The kind of incision (A) probably is not too important, but it provides adequate exposure of all portions of the operative site. Dr. Madden prefers the double-Y incision, while we at the Mayo Clinic prefer the T incision, primarily because, with adequate retraction, exposure is just as good and difficulty with the blood supply to the skin flaps, which results in slough of tissue, occurs less often. This is true also of incisions shown in A² and A³. The transverse incision (A⁴) should give the best cosmetic result, but, unfortunately, edema develops in the upper skin flap and remains after neck dissection, thus offsetting the benefit of an incision along normal skin lines.

The neck dissection should be carried out in an orderly fashion, and that proposed by Dr. Madden is like that used at this clinic except for a few minor details. After first exposing the entire operative site (B), we detach the structures from the lower margin of the mandible, preserving the marginalis branch of the facial nerve, and divide through the parotid gland to remove its lower pole and the subparotid and infraparotid lymph nodes, as is done later in the illustrated procedure.

Rather than transect fascia in the lower posterior cervical triangle at this time (C), we first detach the origin of the sternocleidomastoid muscle, elevating it medially and upward. Tension in this manner facilitates removal of the contents of the posterior cervical triangle inferiorly and posteriorly along the clavicle and the border of the trapezius muscle.

At the time of isolating and transecting the lower end of the jugular vein, care must be taken to protect the thoracic duct, which projects upward from the mediastinum into the neck for 1 to 3 cm. and then downward, usually to enter the

Plate 70   177

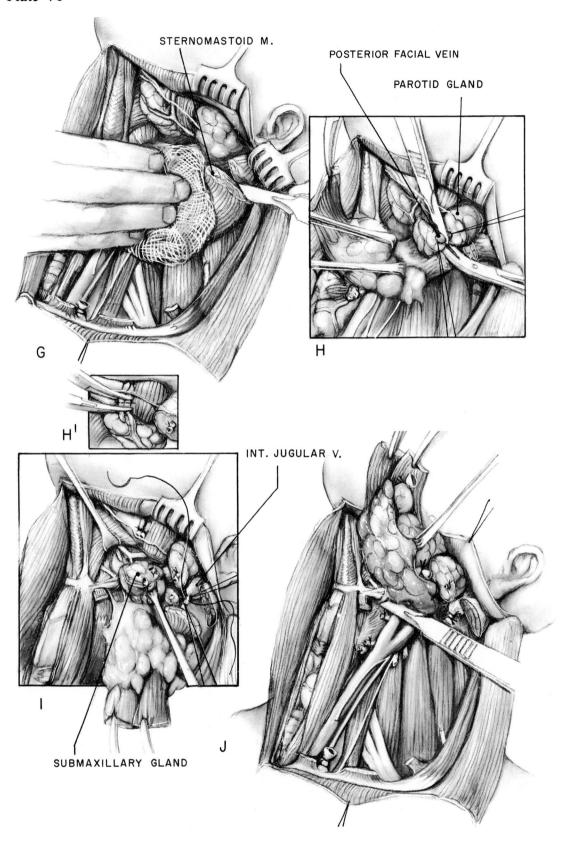

STERNOMASTOID M.

POSTERIOR FACIAL VEIN

PAROTID GLAND

G

H

H'

INT. JUGULAR V.

I

J

SUBMAXILLARY GLAND

K. The classical left radical neck dissection is completed, and the component structures of the operative field are depicted.

L. The skin flaps are approximated with interrupted sutures of 000 silk, and a catheter (16-18 F) for continuous suction siphonage drainage has its exit through a stab wound in the posterior flap. This is preferred to the use of a large compressive gauze dressing.

DISCUSSION—DR. BEAHRS (cont.)

subclavian vein near the internal jugular vein. If the duct is intentionally or accidentally sacrificed, the proximal end should be ligated to prevent chylous drainage from the neck or the development of a chylous fistula.

D shows the spinal accessory nerve transected; later it is sacrificed. For many years we did this routinely, but recently, since approximately 30 per cent of our patients showed a significant morbidity associated with loss of function of the trapezius muscle, we have been preserving this nerve whenever clinical evidence of metastasis is not present in the upper part of the neck and gross metastasis is not encountered in the course of dissecting the nerve free of other tissues sacrificed during the operation. Our impression at the time of this writing is that the prognosis in cases in which the nerve has been preserved has not been less favorable.

Although it is not of great importance, it might be better to sacrifice the ansa hypoglossi to the level of its origin because of its close proximity to the middle deep jugular nodes, rather than to transect it at the strap muscles and then leave it in situ, as illustrated in F.

Care in preserving the marginalis branch of the facial nerve is mentioned (H'). It should be pointed out, however, that, although the nerve is usually at the lower border of the mandible, it might be 1 cm. or more below it on occasions. If submaxillary lymph nodes are grossly involved by metastasis, the nerve often should be sacrificed.

There is no objection to preserving the digastric and stylohyoid muscles (K); however, their function is not missed by the patient, and sacrifice of these muscles does permit better and easier en-bloc removal of the submental and upper deep jugular nodes. Suction drainage, as illustrated in L, is much preferred to the use of soft Penrose-type drains only. However, the catheter might function better if, rather than merely inserting its tip of the catheter into the lower posterior portion of the operative site, several perforations were made in it and it was then inserted upward for a greater distance into the center of the operative site.

Plate 71   179

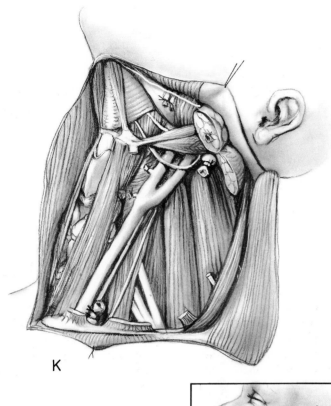

K

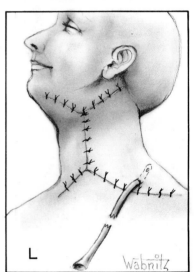

L

COMBINED RADICAL NECK DISSECTION (RIGHT), HEMITHYROIDECTOMY, AND TOTAL LARYNGECTOMY

A. A tracheotomy is first performed, and an endotracheal tube is inserted for the continued administration of a general anesthesia. The double-Y incision used is outlined.

B. The respective skin flaps are elevated, and the external jugular vein is doubly ligated and transected. When the severance of the clavicular and sternal heads of the sternomastoid muscle is completed, the investing layer of the deep cervical fascia overlying the fat layer posteriorly will be incised as indicated by the broken line.

C. The transected ends of the sternomastoid muscle proximally are retracted upward, and the internal jugular vein is elevated on a clamp preparatory to being encircled by a ligature.

D, D'. The internal jugular vein is doubly ligated and doubly clamped in continuity and transected between the two clamps (broken line). Each clamp is replaced by a suture ligature of 000 silk (D'). The middle layer of the deep cervical fascia the omohyoid fascial "carpet," the omohyoid muscle, and the vagus nerve are incised as indicated.

Plate 72   181

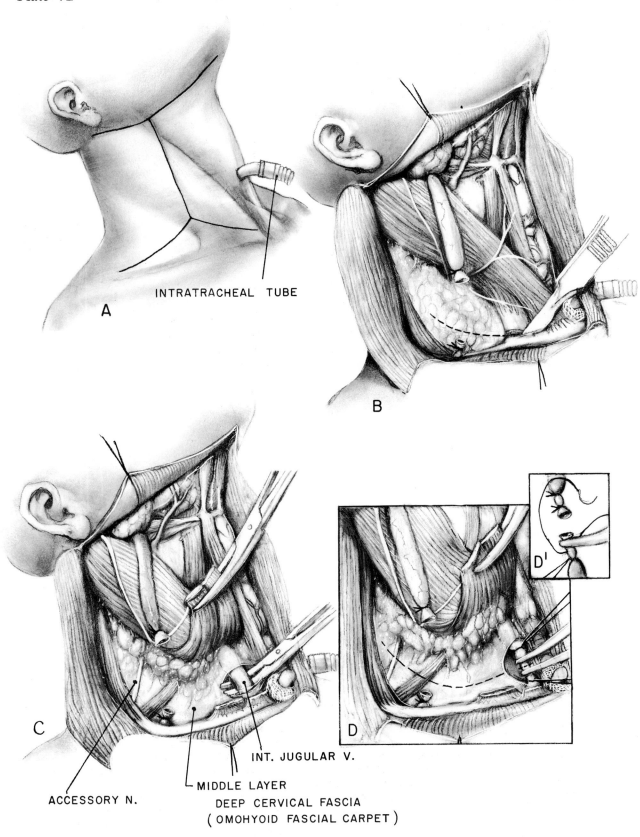

INTRATRACHEAL TUBE

A

B

C

D

D'

ACCESSORY N.

MIDDLE LAYER
DEEP CERVICAL FASCIA
(OMOHYOID FASCIAL CARPET)

INT. JUGULAR V.

E. The partially mobilized tissue block is elevated, including the strap muscles (sternohyoid and sternothyroid) on the right side. The middle thyroid vein tributary of the internal jugular vein is being encircled by a ligature of 000 silk.

F. The middle thyroid vein, doubly ligated in continuity, is cut between the ligatures (000 silk) with scissors.

G. The superior belly of the omohyoid muscle is transected, and the carotid "bulb" is exposed. The mobilization of the tissue block posteriorly is being continued cephalad by scalpel dissection. The characteristic anatomic relation of the external branch of the superior laryngeal nerve to the superior thyroid vessels, the cricothyroid muscle (which it innervates), and the undersurface of the sternothyroid muscle just proximal to

its site of insertion on the thyroid cartilage is visible.

H. The superior thyroid vessels are triply clamped and severed between the two clamps caudad. During the application of the clamps to the superior thyroid vessels, care must be taken to prevent injury to the external branch of the superior laryngeal nerve. Injury to this nerve causes weakness of the voice, huskiness (often mistakenly called postoperative tracheitis), and early fatigue on talking. On indirect laryngoscopy a concave "bowing" of the affected cord is observed, in contradistinction to its midline appearance (cadaveric) when the recurrent laryngeal nerve is injured.

I. The severed ends of the superior thyroid vessels are doubly ligated (000 silk) cephalad, and the isthmus of the thyroid gland is being serially clamped and severed.

DISCUSSION—DR. ARTHUR G. JAMES. One may begin with a tracheostomy as indicated in A, or one may complete the entire operation and establish anesthesia connection with a tracheal stoma when the trachea is severed from the larynx. In some cases in which the patient presents laryngeal obstruction, it is essential that the tracheostomy be performed and the endotracheal tube be inserted at the beginning of the operation. In the patient in whom obstruction is not a problem, however, there is a definite advantage in not performing the tracheostomy first. One must contend with the endotracheal tube as he is mobilizing the larynx, and it is definitely in the way.

This operation is indicated for the primary carcinoma of the larynx with neck node metastases. Some also believe that the neck dissection should be done with a definite extrinsic type of carcinoma of the larynx even though nodes cannot be palpated. This adequate surgical procedure has increased the cure rate of extrinsic cancer of the larynx about three- to fourfold. The five-year salvage rate with radiation therapy was approximately 7 to 12 per cent, but since this type of surgery has been instituted, the cure rate for similar lesions has increased to between 35 and 40 per cent.

In general, I agree with all the technics diagramed. However, I prefer to proceed as follows, in order that the larynx, thyroid lobe, and the neck dissection tissues are removed in continuity and as one surgical specimen. The neck dissection is begun inferiorly and extended posteriorly to the mastoid region. The submental and submaxillary

Plate 73   183

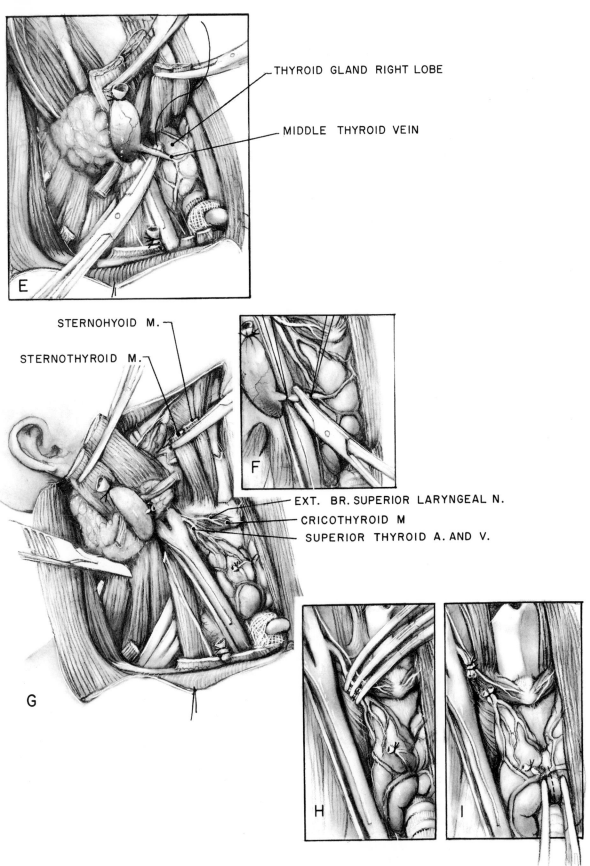

THYROID GLAND RIGHT LOBE

MIDDLE THYROID VEIN

E

STERNOHYOID M.

STERNOTHYROID M.

F

EXT. BR. SUPERIOR LARYNGEAL N.
CRICOTHYROID M
SUPERIOR THYROID A. AND V.

G

H   I

J. The total lobectomy of the right lobe of the thyroid gland is completed. The lingual artery, arching above the greater cornu of the thyroid cartilage and the superior laryngeal nerve, is doubly ligated in continuity and severed.

K. This inset shows the submaxillary gland almost completely mobilized. Its duct (Wharton's), located on the surface of the hyoglossus muscle between the lingual (above) and hyoglossal (below) nerves, is doubly ligated in continuity and severed (broken line).

L. The right radical neck dissection is completed, and the total laryngectomy is commenced. The trachea is severed between the third and fourth tracheal rings, and the endotracheal tube is inserted into the open end of the distal segment. An incision is made through the thyrohyoid membrane to enter the pharyngeal cavity. If desired, the incision may be made above the hyoid bone, which would then be included in the resected specimen.

DISCUSSION—DR. JAMES (cont.)

spaces are dissected free, and, finally, the neck dissection specimen is held only by its attachments to the larynx. The larynx is then freed on the left side of the neck, and as the laryngectomy procedure is completed, it is removed in conjunction with the neck dissection specimen.

E does not indicate the fact that a feeding tube is inserted into the esophagus prior to the completed closure of the pharynx. This may be introduced either through the nose and advanced into the esophagus and stomach or through a pharyngostomy opening in the side of the neck.

I prefer to remove the hyoid bone in each case where a laryngectomy is performed. This adds an additional margin of safety in the resection, especially of the extrinsic carcinoma of the larynx, and also facilitates closure of the pharyngeal stoma. This is all the more important when it is necessary to remove much of the pharyngeal wall because of tumor involvement.

If one chooses not to perform a tracheostomy at the beginning of the procedure, the lower medial end of the double-Y incision should be extended in a transverse collar fashion approximately 2 cm. above the sternoclavicular junction. The tracheal stoma can then be brought out through this incision, which avoids another incision in the medial flap.

Plate 74   185

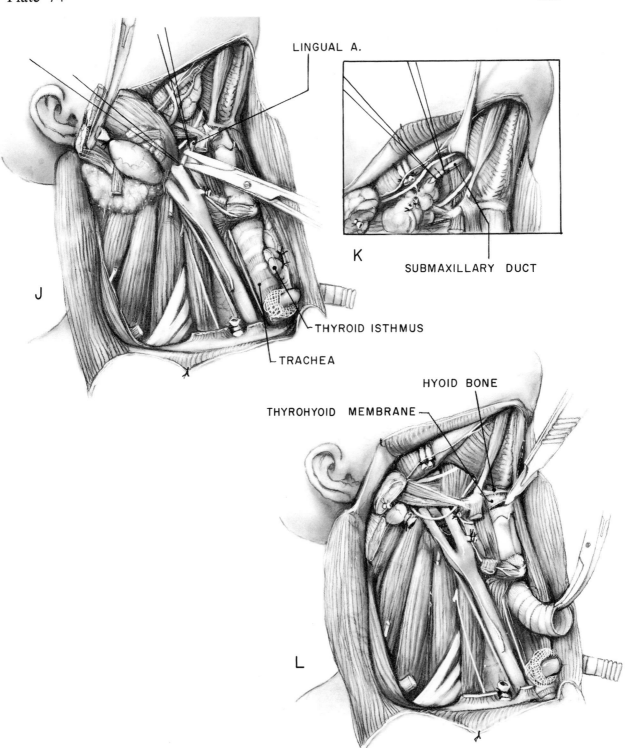

LINGUAL A.

SUBMAXILLARY DUCT

K

J

THYROID ISTHMUS

TRACHEA

HYOID BONE

THYROHYOID MEMBRANE

L

M. The epiglottis and proximal cut end of the trachea are grasped in clamps, and as outward traction is maintained, the lateral wall of the pharynx is severed by scissor dissection. The tumor mass in relation to the glottic chink is visible.

N. This is a close-up view of the preceding (M).

O, P, Q. The closure of the opening in the pharynx using continuous sutures of 00 chromic catgut is depicted.

R. Formation of the tracheostomy stoma (tracheostome) by suture of the distal transected end of the trachea to the margins of the tracheotomy incision, using interrupted sutures of 00 silk, is shown.

S. This is the operative field on completion of the wound closure. A catheter (18 F), used for continuous-suction drainage, has its exit through a stab wound opening in the posterior skin flap.

DISCUSSION—DR. OLIVER H. BEAHRS. General comments regarding dissection of the neck have been made previously. Further comments relate to the extended operation.

A preliminary tracheotomy is essential in many cases of cancer of the larynx. If obstruction to the airway is not present, however, an intratracheal tube might serve satisfactorily until a later stage in the laryngectomy. If this is possible, time is saved and the operative site is kept more orderly during the first part of the operation.

Although the hemithyroid can be removed separately, as shown in J, it might be better to remove it with the neck structures if jugular nodes are involved. If those nodes are not involved, it would be better to remove it en bloc with the larynx, so that the tracheoesophageal nodes, which might be involved by metastatic cancer, can be more skillfully and more adequately excised.

Rather than transecting the trachea straight across, as illustrated in L, cutting it in an oblique direction offers a distinct advantage in that the posterior wall of the distal trachea is longer than the anterior wall. This makes possible a larger stoma and one that is less likely to contract or become stenosed.

The hyoid bone need not always be removed, as shown in L and M, but sacrifice of it does permit a wider field laryngectomy. For this reason, I usually include the hyoid bone with the tissues removed.

Plate 75   187

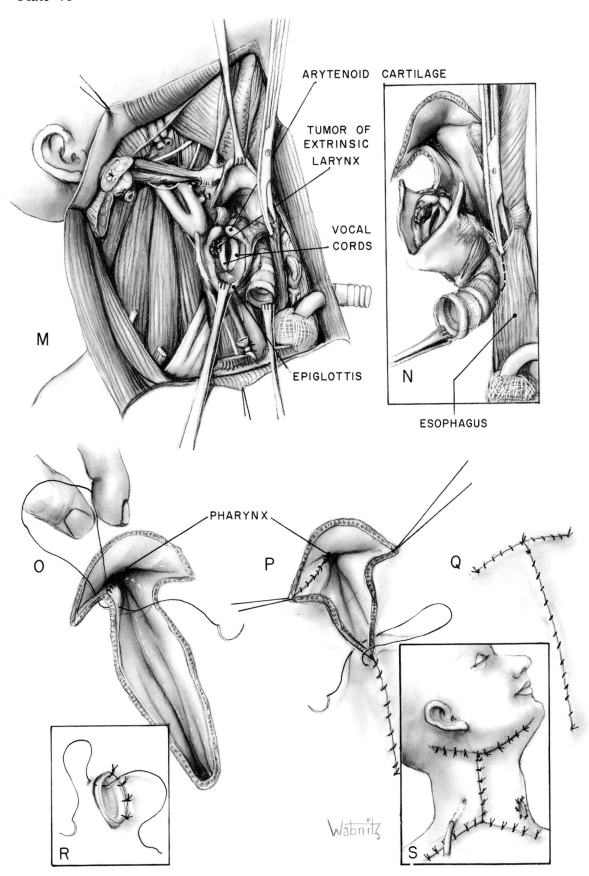

ARYTENOID CARTILAGE

TUMOR OF
EXTRINSIC
LARYNX

VOCAL
CORDS

EPIGLOTTIS

M

N

ESOPHAGUS

PHARYNX

O

P

Q

R

S

Wabnitz

RESECTION OF PHARYNGOESOPHAGEAL DIVERTICULUM

Diverticula of the esophagus are classified into two types: traction and pulsion. Traction diverticula most commonly occur on the anterior wall of the midportion of the thoracic esophagus in the region of the tracheal bifurcation. These diverticula are secondary manifestations of a surrounding inflammatory reaction and are true diverticula in that they contain all of the coats of the esophagus. However, this type of esophageal diverticulum is of little surgical significance.

The pulsion types of diverticula are most commonly found in the cervical region at the pharyngoesophageal level. They most commonly protrude on the left side, but they may be bilateral or protrude in the midline posteriorly. They may occur infrequently in the lower third of the esophagus just above the diaphragm, the so-called epiphrenic diverticula, and protrude either toward the right or the left side in the posterior mediastinum. The pulsion type of diverticulum is classified as false in that the mucosa of the esophagus herniates through the layers of overlying muscle fibers, and, accordingly, the diverticulum does not consist of the whole thickness of the wall of the esophagus. In the cervical region this protrusion usually occurs in the space between the lowermost fibers of the inferior constrictor muscle of the pharynx and the fibers of the cricopharyngeus muscle. Occasionally the protrusion may occur through the uppermost fibers of the cricopharyngeus muscle.

Pulsion diverticula are more commonly found in males (4:1) and occur most frequently in the sixth and seventh decades. However, in the illustrated technic the drawings were from sketches made by the artist while observing the operation performed in a 30-year-old man who had symptoms of progressive dysphagia of 14 months duration.

A. The patient is anesthetized, using intratracheal anesthesia. The oblique linear incision employed, paralleling the anterior border of the sternomastoid muscle, is depicted in dotted outline. Rarely, a right-side approach may be indicated for the exposure and the removal of a pharyngoesophageal diverticulum.

B. The incision is deepened through the platysma muscle and the anterior or investing layer of the deep cervical fascia to expose the fibers of the left sternomastoid muscle.

C. The anterior border of the sternomastoid muscle is mobilized and retracted laterally to expose the middle or pretracheal layer of the deep cervical fascia and its contained carotid sheath. The adjacent muscle structures are depicted.

D. The tendinous pulley, uniting the superior and inferior bellies of the omohyoid muscle, is elevated by a guy suture of silk (0) and retracted downward and medially. Severance of this tendon may be performed but this is generally not necessary. The retraction of the superior belly of the omohyoid muscle medially exposes the posterolateral portion of the left lobe of the thyroid gland and its overlying fascial (pretracheal) covering.

E. The middle or pretracheal fascial layer of the deep cervical fascia is incised to expose clearly the thyroid gland and the contents of the carotid sheath: the internal jugular vein, the vagus nerve, and the common carotid artery. In this patient there was an unusually large tributary vein as depicted which entered the internal jugular vein in the region conforming with the site of drainage of the common facial vein. Although it was in close approximation to the operative area, ligation and severance of this vein was not required.

F. The superior belly of the omohyoid muscle and the underlying sternothyroid muscle are retracted anteriorly and medially, and the sternomastoid muscle and the structures contained in the carotid sheath are retracted posteriorly and laterally to expose more clearly the posterolateral aspect of the left lobe of the thyroid gland. The inferior thyroid artery, a branch of the thyrocervical trunk of the subclavian artery, crosses horizontally beneath the carotid artery and divides into ascending and descending branches prior to its entrance into the gland structure. The inferior thyroid artery is a useful landmark for the identification of a pharyngoesophageal diverticulum which is usually located immediately subjacent to this vessel.

Plate 76

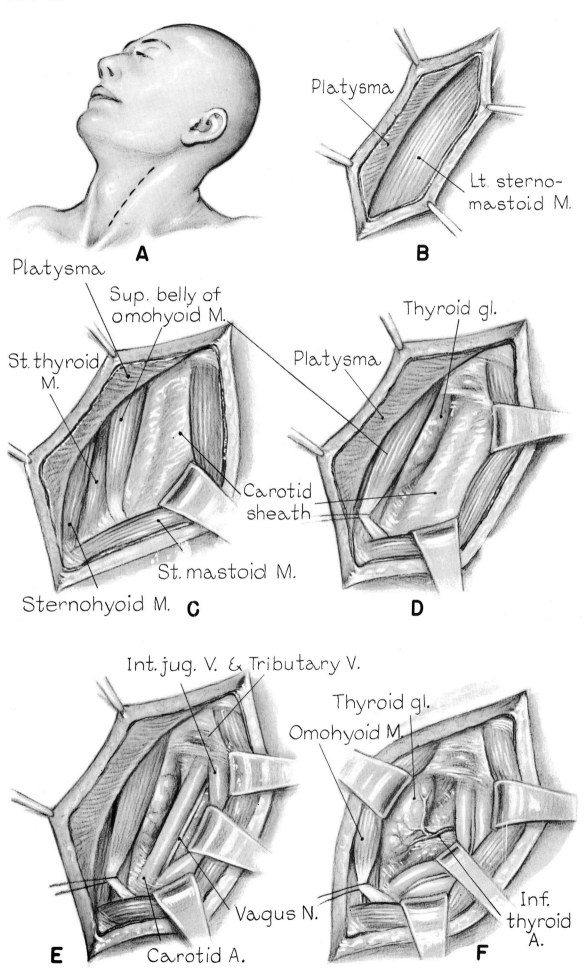

A

Platysma

Lt. sterno-
mastoid M.

B

Platysma

Sup. belly of
omohyoid M.

St. thyroid
M.

Platysma

Thyroid gl.

Carotid
sheath

Sternohyoid M. **C**

St. mastoid M.

D

Int. jug. V. & Tributary V.

Thyroid gl.

Omohyoid M.

Vagus N.

Inf.
thyroid
A.

E Carotid A.

F

G, H. The inferior thyroid artery is doubly ligated and severed (G) and the thyroid gland is retracted medially to expose the esophagus, the diverticulum, and the recurrent laryngeal nerve (H).

I. The recurrent laryngeal nerve, encircled by a guy suture of silk (000), bifurcated just prior to its passage beneath the lowermost fibers of the inferior constrictor muscle and its entrance into the larynx. The identification and isolation of this nerve is important in the prevention of injury to it during the operative procedure. The diverticulum, covered by fibroareolar tissue, may be seen to protrude through the space between the lower border of the inferior constrictor muscle of the pharynx above and the fibers of the cricopharyngeus muscle below. In some instances the protrusion may occur through the uppermost fibers of the cricopharyngeus muscle.

J, K. A Babcock clamp is applied to the fundus of the partially mobilized diverticulum (J), and, with traction maintained through the clamp, the mobilization of the diverticulum from the surrounding structures is completed by scissor dissection (K).

L. Inset showing a magnified view of the completely mobilized diverticulum and the demonstration of a technic for the determination of the level of the true neck of the diverticulum. In this particular patient the neck of the diverticulum appeared unduly wide in diameter. Accordingly, a catheter (16 F) was inserted through an opening in the fundus of the diverticulum and into the lumen of the distal portion of the esophagus where its tip could be readily palpated by the left index finger impinged against the outer wall of the esophagus. In this manner the true neck of the diverticulum was defined and the line for the resection indicated.

DISCUSSION—DR. KENNETH W. WARREN. It has been an almost invariable practice at the Lahey Clinic to employ a long, oblique incision along the anterior border of the left sternomastoid muscle in approaching pharyngoesophageal diverticula. The choice of this type of incision is based upon the observation that one cannot prophesy preoperatively which diverticulum will be easily exposed, delivered, and dissected and which—because of its size, its adherence to the esophagus or related cervical structures—will prove to be difficult to manage. Until recently the majority of pharyngoesophageal diverticula treated at the Lahey Clinic were removed by the two stage operation. The long, oblique incision placed along the sternomastoid muscle afforded ample opportunity in this two stage procedure to permit fixation of the fundus of the diverticulum high in the cervical region so that the most dependent portion of the diverticulum would be at the junction of the sac with the longitudinal esophagus. Over 90 per cent of esophageal diverticula currently treated at the clinic are excised in a one stage maneuver. We still prefer this incision.

The skin and platysma are incised, and the anterior edge of the sternomastoid muscle on the left is reflected laterally, thus exposing the anterior belly of the omohyoid muscle. We have preferred to remove the anterior segment of this muscle completely rather than to retract it as is demonstrated in Plate 76 (D). The advantages of re-

moving this segment of the omohyoid (while it is not necessary in every instance) are very great. This maneuver exposes the internal jugular vein with its branches running to the thyroid gland. After division of these lateral thyroid veins, the left lobe of the thyroid is elevated and rotated anteriorly and medially, thus exposing the common carotid artery which is then retracted laterally. Retraction of the carotid artery affords access to the inferior thyroid artery which is then divided between clamps and ligated. This division permits a greater degree of mobility of the left lobe of the thyroid. The left recurrent laryngeal nerve is then identified and its entire cervical course is exposed, but manipulation of this structure is avoided insofar as possible.

The preceding maneuvers expose the region of the pharyngoesophageal diverticulum which can now be identified. The fundus of the sac is grasped with Babcock forceps and the junction between the inner edge of the sac and the longitudinal esophagus is demonstrated. In some instances, the sac will be enveloped by a considerable thickness of fibers of the cricopharyngei which may make its identification difficult. In other instances, the sac may be extremely large and extend well down into the mediastinum. The delivery of such a large diverticulum from the mediastinum must be done with great care lest the diverticulum be perforated during this maneuver.

It should be borne in mind that the pharyngoesophageal diverticulum prior to its dissection lies

Plate 77   191

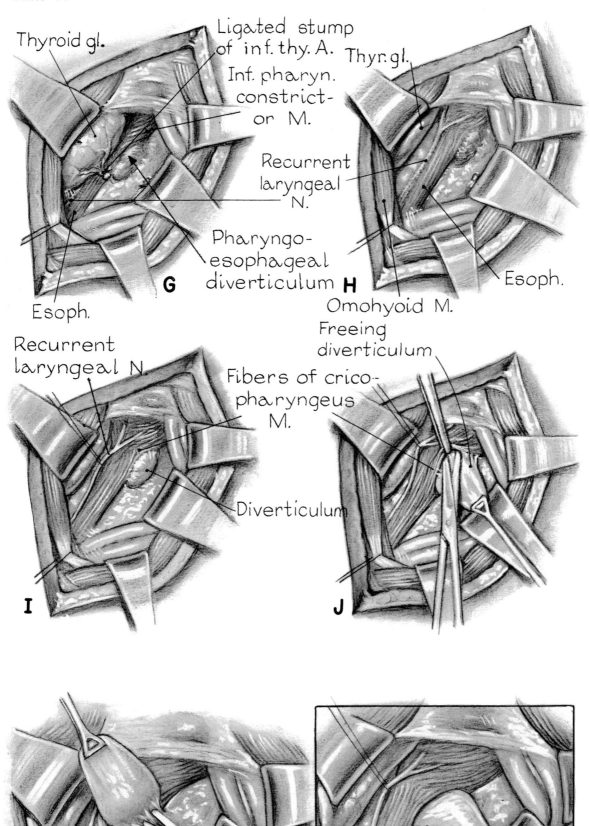

Thyroid gl.

Ligated stump
of inf. thy. A.   Thyr. gl.

Inf. pharyn.
constrict-
or M.

Recurrent
laryngeal
N.

Pharyngo-
esophageal
diverticulum

G

Esoph.

H

Esoph.

Omohyoid M.

Recurrent
laryngeal N.

Freeing
diverticulum

Fibers of crico-
pharyngeus
M.

Diverticulum

I

J

K

L   Catheter in
esophagus

M, N. Traction guy sutures of silk (000) are inserted through the neck of the diverticulum at its upper and lower borders, and the diverticulum is cross-clamped distally. The excision is begun by scissor dissection (M), and, following a partial resection, the cut margins of the mucosa and the submucosa layers of the esophagus are approximated with interrupted sutures of silk (000). In excising the diverticulum, excessive traction on its distal portion should be avoided. Otherwise, the walls of the esophagus may be tented into the line of resection with resulting constriction of the esophageal lumen.

O. The excision of the pharyngoesophageal diverticulum is completed, and the opening in the esophagus is closed with a series of interrupted sutures of silk (000).

O′. Inset to show an alternate method for the closure of the opening into the lumen of the esophagus. The interrupted sutures of silk (000) are inserted from the "inside out" to the "outside in" so that, when tied, the knots of the sutures are on the inside of the lumen.

P, Q. The defect in the musculature through which the diverticulum protruded is closed with interrupted sutures of 000 silk (P), and a Penrose (cigarette) drain is inserted into the cervical mediastinal space (Q).

R. The left sternomastoid muscle is gently retracted to show the relation of the surrounding muscles, previously labeled, to the carotid sheath and the site of drainage. The large tributary of the internal jugular vein previously mentioned is visible in the upper angle of the wound.

S. The operation is completed by closure of the skin incision about the drain, using interrupted sutures of silk (000).

DISCUSSION—DR. WARREN (cont.)

parallel to the longitudinal esophagus and that as the dissection of the sac from the esophagus is carried out, an acute angle is made by the junction of the neck of the sac with the longitudinal esophagus. If recurrence of the diverticulum is to be avoided, it is extremely important to dissect the neck of the sac completely. It is easy to misjudge the degree of thoroughness of the dissection at this point, for the neck of the sac will be completely covered by an investment of the muscle fibers of the cricopharyngeus even though the sac has been liberated so that it hangs by its neck. We have always made it a point to dissect the neck of the sac until the pale white fibers of the submucosa of the sac are clearly visible. This dissection is relatively easily achieved in the inferior, superior, and left lateral positions. Unfortunately, dissection of the right side of the neck is more difficult since the fixed position of the cricoid cartilage and of the pharynx makes it impossible to rotate the posterior wall of the pharynx sufficiently to see the right lateral wall of the sac directly, except in those instances in which the diverticulum is very small and the neck quite narrow. If this phase of the dissection is done with care and with appreciation of the anatomic relationships and of the embryology of these diverticula, there will be no difficulty in determining the site of the junction of the diverticulum with the longitudinal esophagus.

When the sac has been thoroughly mobilized as previously described, one must decide how to deal with the neck of the sac. If the diverticulum is small or only moderately large and the neck is narrow, it is reasonable to ligate the neck of the sac flush with its junction with the longitudinal esophagus, using a 00 chromic catgut ligature. A clamp is then placed distal to this ligature and the sac is amputated, leaving an adequate amount of stump to insure that it will not retract through the previously placed ligature. When the neck of the sac is broad, it is best to divide its neck slightly distal to its precise junction with the longitudinal esophagus, and to close the defect with a continuous Connell inverting suture of fine catgut reinforced by a row of interrupted sutures of the same material. It is quite permissible to close this defect with interrupted sutures but we prefer to use inverting sutures, even though they be interrupted. After amputation of the sac and closure of the esophagus either by ligature or by the inversion suture method, it is important to approximate the cricopharyngei muscles over the closed neck of the sac. We usually employ a cigarette drain and bring it out in the lower angle of the incision.

This comment has been limited to the one stage procedure. However, it is well to remember that the two stage procedure still has merit in the presence of the large pulsion diverticulum of the pharyngoesophagus when the sac extends well down into the mediastinum and when diverticulitis and peridiverticulitis are prominent features. The two stage procedure should also have considerable appeal to those surgeons with a limited experience in esophageal surgery who, nevertheless, undertake to operate on pharyngoesophageal diverticula.

Plate 78   193

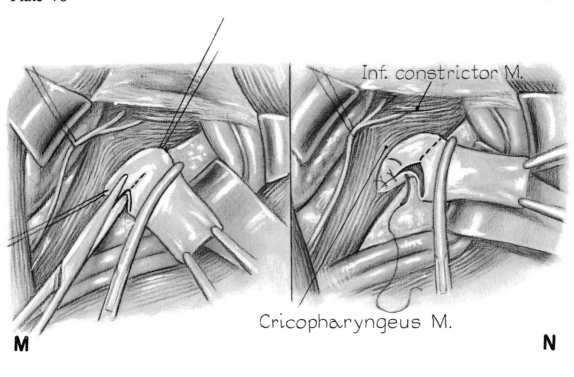

Inf. constrictor M.

Cricopharyngeus M.

M

N

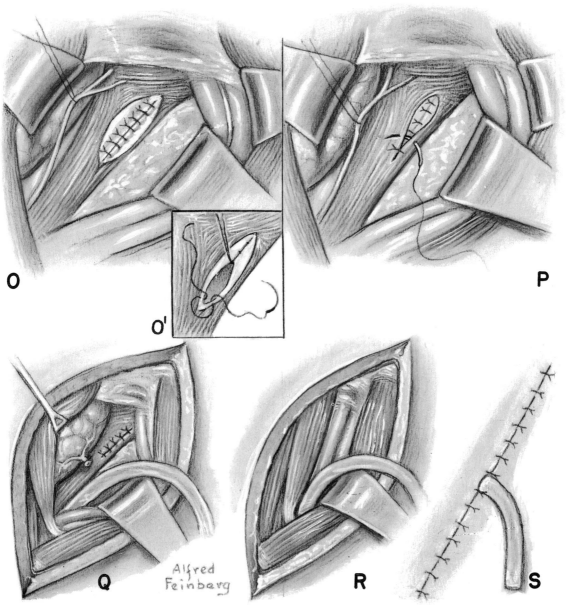

O

O'

P

Alfred
Feinberg

Q

R

S

ESOPHAGOCARDIOMYOTOMY—TRANSABDOMINAL APPROACH

A, B. The peritoneal cavity is entered through an upper left rectus muscle-splitting or muscle-retracting incision (A) and the underlying intraperitoneal viscera are demonstrable (B).

C. By manual retraction overlying a protective moist gauze pad the peritoneal attachment forming the left triangular ligament of the liver is made taut and severed as indicated by the dotted line.

D. The mobilized left lobe of the liver, covered by a moist gauze pad, is folded downward on itself and retracted medially to expose the opening in the peritoneal fascial layer overlying the esophagocardial junction. The lower end of the esophagus, the vagus nerves, and the esophageal hiatal ring formed by the superficial and deep muscle bundles of the right crus are visible. The tapered and thinned out terminal portion of the esophagus and the dilatation proximally, characteristic findings in achalasia, may also be seen.

E. By careful digital manipulation within the posterior mediastinum, the lower portion of the esophagus is mobilized and displaced downward into the peritoneal cavity.

F. The esophagus at the level of the esophagocardial junction is encircled by a tape of rubber tissue, and with downward traction maintained, a linear incision through the fibers of the longitudinal muscle layer of the esophagus and the adjoining segment of the stomach is begun.

DISCUSSION—DR. RICHARD H. SWEET. The operation of esophagomyotomy may be performed either through an abdominal incision, as originally advocated by Heller, or through a left thoracotomy incision. In my opinion the latter is preferable for the following reasons: (1) The incision through the left eighth intercostal space can be easily and quickly made and closed. (2) The exposure of the lower esophagus is more easily obtained, and access to the entire length of the lower segment is secured without dissection and mobilization which must always be employed when the abdominal approach is used. This makes it easier to avoid the vagus nerves and to minimize the amount of trauma in the lower esophageal region. (3) The fascial layers in the esophageal hiatus of the diaphragm are not greatly disturbed. (4) It is simple, using this approach, to repair a coexisting hiatus hernia with a minimum of dissection.

A technical matter which may make the difference between success and failure in the use of this operation for the treatment of megaesophagus is the length of the myotomy incision. As shown in Plate 79 (F), this incision must extend upward on the esophagus to a point where the diameter of the organ is large. It is not necessary, on the other hand, to extend the incision onto the wall of the stomach below the cardia. No hypertrophied circular muscle fibers are ever found distal to this point. It must be remembered that the abnormality is in the esophagus. The unnecessary extension of the incision into the stomach wall below the cardia usually is harmless, but because the muscular layers there are thin, it is easy to penetrate the mucosal layer. If this accident should occur, a careful closure of the opening should be made with sutures of fine silk.

The dissection between the circular muscle layer and the submucosa as shown in Plate 80 (H and I) is unnecessary and might even be harmful. It is much easier and safer merely to cut through the muscle layers with a sharp knife. It is absolutely essential, however, to divide every single circular muscle fiber in order to avoid leaving a stenotic point. Plate 80 (J) shows the appearance of the bulging mucosal layer when the division of the muscle has been completely accomplished, although in my opinion the incision as illustrated extends unnecessarily far into the wall of the stomach.

Plate 79   195

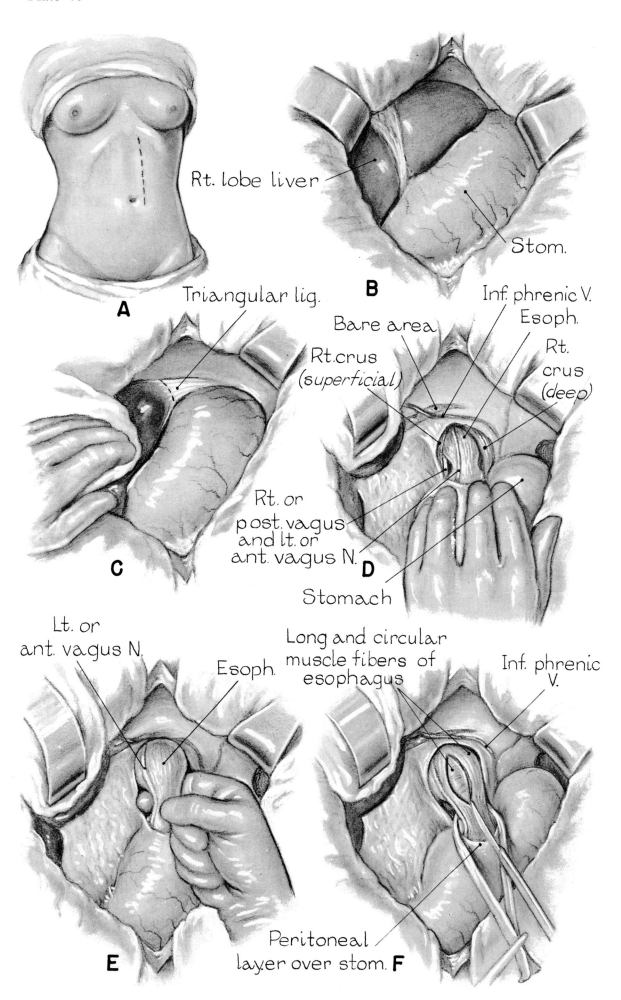

Rt. lobe liver

Stom.

A

B

Triangular lig.

Bare area

Rt. crus
(superficial)

Inf. phrenic V.
Esoph.

Rt.
crus
(deep)

Rt. or
post. vagus
and lt. or
ant. vagus N.

C

D

Stomach

Lt. or
ant. vagus N.

Esoph.

Long and circular
muscle fibers of
esophagus

Inf. phrenic
V.

E

Peritoneal
layer over stom. **F**

G. The incision through the longitudinal muscle layer of the esophagus is completed, and the underlying layer of circular muscle fibers is visible. A vessel crossing transversely at the level of the cardia is shown elevated on a clamp prior to its double ligation and severance.

H, I. Following the completion of the incision in the longitudinal muscle layers of the esophagus, the cardia, and the segment of the gastric wall immediately below the cardia, the underlying circular layers of muscle fibers are elevated in segments and severed by scissor dissection.

J, K. The esophagocardiomyotomy is completed and the herniation of portions of the mucosa of the esophagus, the cardia, and the adjacent segment of the stomach respectively are depicted. The prominence of the vessels in the submucosal layer of the stomach may also be seen.

L, M, N. The wound is closed in layers using a double strand of a continuous interlocking suture of 00 chromic catgut for the peritoneum (L), interrupted sutures of 00 silk for the fascia (M), and 000 silk for the skin (N).

DISCUSSION—DR. MARK M. RAVITCH. In many patients an oblique subcostal incision provides easy access to the esophageal hiatus. The rectus-splitting incision invariably paralyzes the portion of the rectus muscle medial to it and does not provide significantly better exposure than the rectus-retracting incision. For most gastric operations, unless the patient has a very flat costal arch, the midline incision, through the linea alba, is satisfactory and is technically the simplest. As emphasized in G through K, the esophagogastric incision is a long one, extending 5 cm. up on the esophagus and 5 cm. down on the stomach, through to the submucosa. Wangensteen suggested the passage of a balloon into the esophagus to distend it and to render this phase of the operation simpler.

It will be seen in D, E, and F that there is considerable dissection within the hiatus, and this may result in the appearance of a postoperative hiatus hernia. It is probable that a certain proportion of the unsatisfactory results following Heller's cardiomyotomy, are, in fact, due to the operative creation of a hiatus hernia. For this reason it is wise always to place one or two sutures behind the esophagus, approximating the fibers of the right crus, as in the repair of a hiatus hernia from the abdominal approach. In order further to prevent regurgitation into the esophagus and subsequent esophagitis, the bane of most other procedures for achalasia, Lortat-Jacob has emphasized the wisdom of tacking the gastric fundus up to the esophagus in order to re-create the angle of His and introduce what is almost a valvular mechanism at the esophagogastric junction, like the one produced by the normally acute angle of insertion of the esophagus into the stomach.

DISCUSSION—DR. C. ROLLINS HANLON. I prefer an upper midline approach for this type of subdiaphragmatic exposure. A transverse epigastric incision dividing both rectus muscles may be adequate in patients with flaring costal margins.

Neither of these abdominal incisions provides full access to the esophagus for an upward extension of the myotomy, which is, at times, desirable.

Conversely, it is easy to overextend the gastric portion of the muscle division, which may destroy the subdiaphragmatic portion of the esophageal sphincter. This destruction is conducive to reflux and, at times, to esophagitis.

The ability to explore the abdomen is an obvious advantage of the transabdominal approach but does not seem to be a dominant consideration.

Plate 80   197

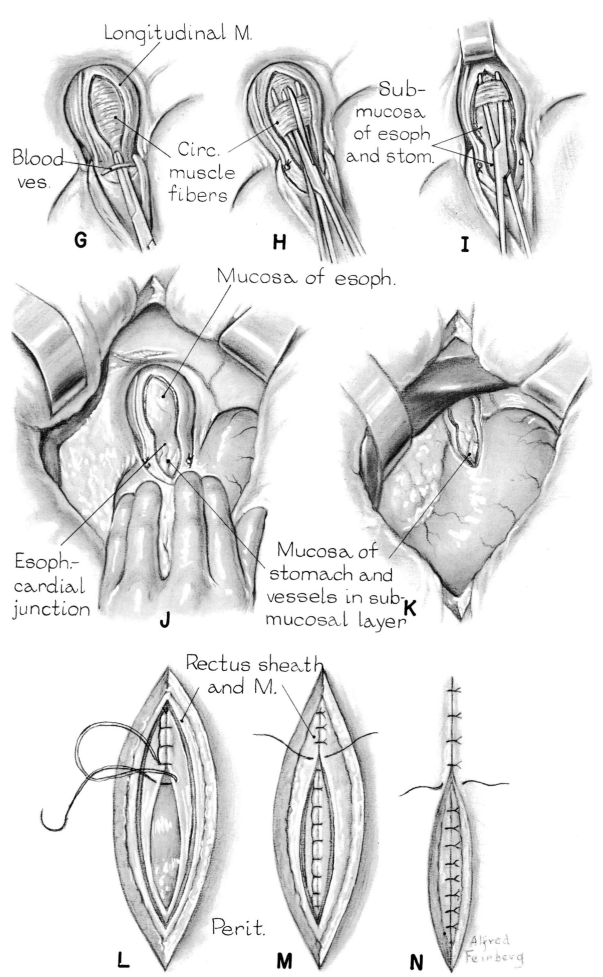

Longitudinal M.

Circ. muscle fibers

Blood ves.

Sub- mucosa of esoph and stom.

G   **H**   **I**

Mucosa of esoph.

Esoph.- cardial junction

Mucosa of stomach and vessels in sub- mucosal layer

J   **K**

Rectus sheath and M.

Perit.

L   **M**   **N**

Alfred Feinberg

ESOPHAGOCARDIOMYOTOMY—TRANSTHORACIC APPROACH

A. The patient is placed in the direct right lateral prone position. The incision overlying the eighth rib is indicated by the broken line.

B. The left pleural cavity is entered through the eighth intercostal space (Brock technic), and the related intrapleural structures are depicted. The lower lobe of the left lung, partly visible, is covered by a moist gauze pad and retracted cephalad. Sutures of 000 silk are inserted in the inferior pulmonary ligament, which is subsequently incised between the ligatures.

C. The incised margins of the inferior pulmonary ligament are retracted by sutures (000 silk), and the areolar tissue attachments about the esophagus are freed by scissor dissection.

D. The lower portion of the dilated esophagus is mobilized by blunt digital dissection from its "bed" in the posterior mediastinum.

DISCUSSION—DR. MARK M. RAVITCH. Ordinarily patients with achalasia who require operation have lost sufficient weight so that there is no difficulty in dissecting about the cardia through the transabdominal approach. It is easier, and does less violence to the hiatus, to bring the esophagus into the peritoneal cavity from below, than to bring the stomach up into the thoracic cavity from above. In either case, it is mandatory to make the esophagogastric incision a long one, and just as long (5 cm.) on the gastric side as on the esophageal side of the esophagogastric junction.

Heller originally advised two incisions, one anterior and one posterior. This would make assurance doubly sure but does not appear to be necessary. Whether the operation is done from above or from below, the hiatus should be reinforced at the conclusion of the esophagocardiomyotomy. Tacking the fundus to the side of the esophagus is as feasible in the transthoracic as in the transabdominal approach.

Plate 81

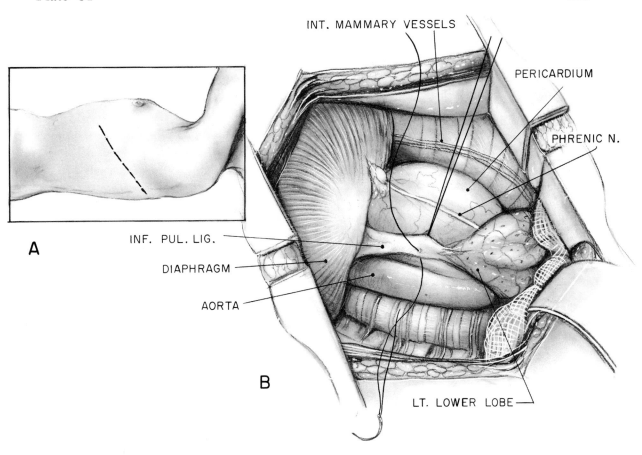

INT. MAMMARY VESSELS

PERICARDIUM

PHRENIC N.

INF. PUL. LIG.

DIAPHRAGM

AORTA

A

B

LT. LOWER LOBE

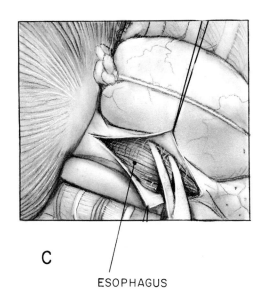

C

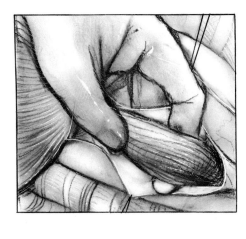

D

ESOPHAGUS

E, F, G. A rubber-tissue tape is inserted beneath the esophagus (E) to encircle it (F), and as traction on the tape is maintained, the esophagus is mobilized by scissor dissection of its areolar tissue attachments (G). The right or posterior vagus nerve in relation to the partly mobilized esophagus is visible (G).

H. A second rubber-tissue tape encircles the esophagus caudad, and as traction is maintained on the tapes, the longitudinal or outer layer of muscle fibers in the lower portion of the esophagus is incised. Through the incision some of the fibers of the underlying circular muscle layers may be seen.

I. The incision in the outer (longitudinal) muscle layer is completed, and the inner (circular) muscle layer, elevated on a curved (Kelly) clamp, is incised.

J. The circular muscle layer cephalad is similarly elevated on a Mixter clamp, and the severance of its fibers is completed (broken line).

DISCUSSION—DR. C. ROLLINS HANLON. It seems clear that esophagocardiomyotomy, omitting the posterior of the two incisions advocated by Heller, is the best treatment for achalasia of the esophagus. I prefer a transthoracic approach, despite the occasional occurrence of annoying intercostal neuralgia after this procedure. Satisfactory access may be obtained by excision of the seventh, eighth, or ninth rib; entry through the eighth intercostal space gives adequate exposure.

The technic portrayed in illustrations B through G is quite satisfactory. Particular care should be taken not to damage either vagus nerve, because vagotomy tends to aggravate the dysfunction. In contrast to use of the knife in H, I use Metzenbaum scissors to divide both layers of muscle, thus minimizing the likelihood of mucosal perforation, especially at the important lower end of the dissection. The incision is usually 10 cm. long and extends over the stomach only far enough to insure complete division of all circular esophageal muscle fibers. Excessive prolongation of the incision on the stomach or damage to the right crus may explain some cases of late, regurgitant esopha-

Plate 82   201

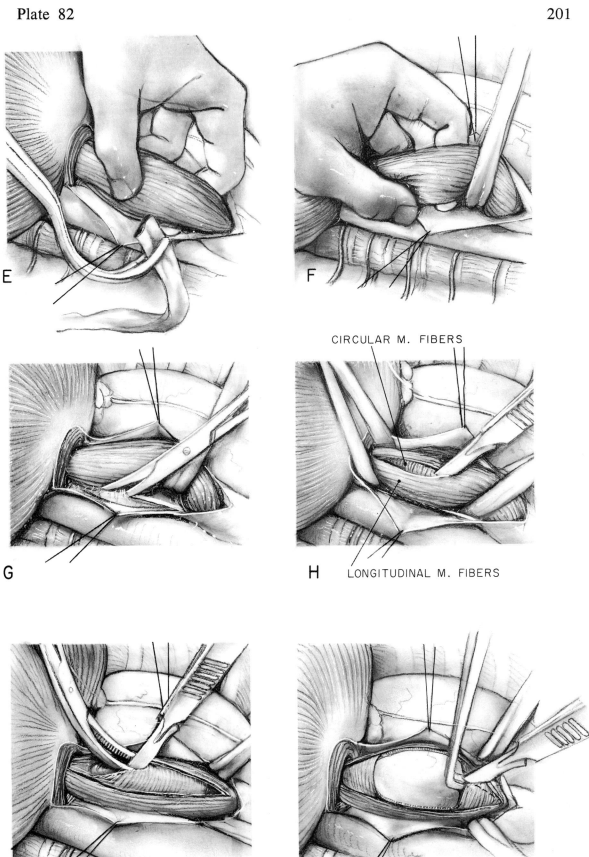

CIRCULAR M. FIBERS

LONGITUDINAL M. FIBERS

E

F

G

H

I

J

K. The fibers of the remaining and caudad segment of the circular muscle layer are transected as indicated (broken line).

L. The esophagocardiomyotomy is completed, and the herniation of the mucosal layer of the esophagus is visible. The relation of the incised margins of the muscle layers of the esophagus to the muscle fibers of the right crus of the diaphragm which form the esophageal hiatal ring is also visible.

M. A close-up view shows more clearly the relation of the lower portion of the esopha-

gus to its hiatal ring. A segment of the right (posterior) vagus nerve is also seen.

N, O. The operative field before (N) and after (O) approximation of the pleural leaflets overlying the diaphragm is shown. The mediastinal pleural leaflets are not sutured. Expansion of the lung and closure of the thoracic incision complete the operation. A waterseal drainage catheter (18 F) is used during the closure of the wound and may be removed as the final skin suture is being tied about it.

DISCUSSION—DR. HANLON (cont.)

gitis. If hiatus hernia is present or is rendered likely by the dissection, a few sutures may be placed for approximation of the fibers of the right crus posteriorly.

The mucosa should bulge over a wide area, as shown in L. Passage of a sound or easy inflation of a pneumatic dilator (60 F) by the anesthesiologist assures one that the size of the cardia is adequate. In addition, it may demonstrate persistent circular muscle fibers requiring division. Though some have advocated retrograde passage of the fingers or a balloon dilator through a gastrotomy, this seems unnecessarily complex and increases the risk of infection in the pleural space. With an incidence of mucosal perforation in the vicinity of 10 per cent, it seems safer to leave an intercostal waterseal drainage catheter in place for a day or two, especially if a recognized perforation has been sutured.

Plate 83   203

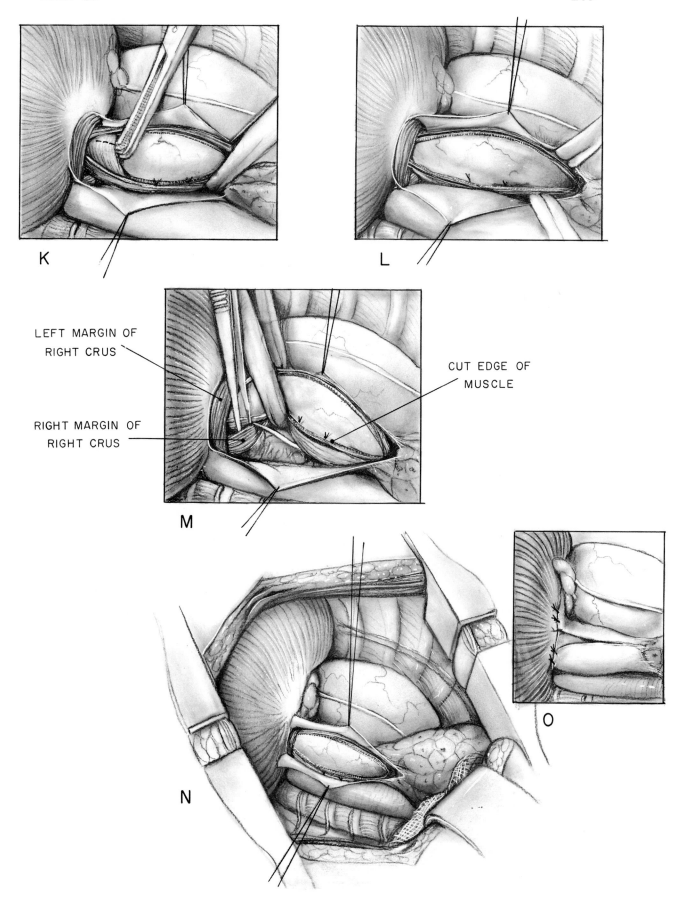

K

L

LEFT MARGIN OF
RIGHT CRUS

RIGHT MARGIN OF
RIGHT CRUS

CUT EDGE OF
MUSCLE

M

N

O

THE TRANSABDOMINAL APPROACH FOR THE REPAIR OF AN ESOPHAGEAL HIATUS HERNIA

A. The patient is placed in the supine position, and the incision of choice, a long left paramedian muscle-retracting (lateral) incision, is outlined.

B. The peritoneal cavity is entered, and the related intraperitoneal viscera are demonstrable. By manual retraction the left lobe of the liver is displaced downward toward the midline, and its mobilization is commenced by the severance of the avascular left triangular ligament. In some instances the left lobe of the liver is elongated and the left triangular ligament is markedly foreshortened. Under such circumstances the esophagocardial region is exposed by the retraction upward of the left lobe of the liver, the surface of which is protected by a moist gauze pad.

C. The mobilized left lobe of the liver is turned downward and inward on itself, and, after being covered with a moist gauze pad, it is retracted medialward. By manual traction the herniated segment of the stomach into the posterior mediastinum through the esophageal hiatus is reduced, and the layer of peritoneum overlying the esophagocardial junction is severed by scissor dissection.

D. The posterior mediastinal space is entered and the terminal portion of the esophagus, mobilized previously by digital dissection, is encircled by a rubber tissue drain for the purpose of traction.

E. The reduction of the hernia is maintained by downward traction. The terminal 4 cm. of the esophagus is exposed, and its relation to the vagus nerves and the right and left margins of the esophageal hiatus formed by the superficial and deep muscle layers respectively of the right crus of the diaphragm are demonstrated.

F. The esophagus is displaced to the left to show the enlarged esophageal hiatus and its formation by the separation of the fibers of the right crus into thin superficial (right margin) and thick deep (left margin) muscle layers.

G. The superficial and deep muscle layers of the right crus of the diaphragm, the right and left margins respectively of the hiatal ring, are approximated in a slightly oblique plane posterior to the esophagus, using two or three interrupted sutures of silk (No. 1). In this approximation, tension on the suture line should be avoided.

Plate 84

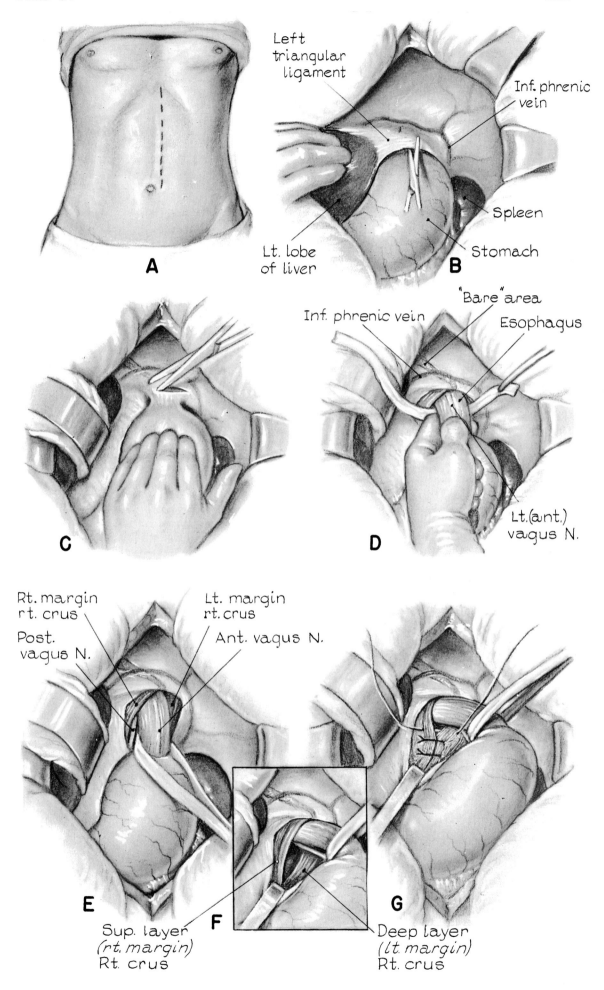

DISCUSSION—DR. DENTON A. COOLEY. Indications for the transthoracic or transabdominal approach in the repair of an esophageal hiatal hernia were not part of this presentation, yet this aspect of the technical problem is important and deserves careful consideration. After an experience with a sizable series of patients operated upon by both technics, I have concluded that the transabdominal approach should be the procedure of choice. Two exceptions to this policy would be, first, the extremely obese patient in whom surgical exposure in the upper abdomen would be difficult and, second, the patient with a recurrent hernia. Recurrence of an esophageal hiatal hernia is difficult to repair from the abdominal route, since adhesions about the hiatus and herniated stomach located in the mediastinum or pleural space are difficult to divide transabdominally. In some of the more complicated recurrences with a history of more than one attempted repair, consideration should even be given to a combined thoraco-abdominal incision so the repair can be accomplished from above and below the hiatus.

Selection of the transabdominal approach for all other elective situations depends upon a number of factors. Exposure of the anatomy about the hiatus is best demonstrated from below. Anatomists and artists support this viewpoint, since their descriptions and drawings usually emphasize this surface of the diaphragm. Avoiding the thoracotomy incision also eliminates the intercostal nerve pain or troublesome neuralgia, which may simulate the symptoms caused by the hernia. Efforts to eliminate this postoperative chest pain by technics of reapproximating the ribs, as described by Dr. Madden, are helpful but by no means completely effective. Moreover, pericostal sutures of heavy silk should probably be replaced by absorbable chromic catgut. The midline abdominal incision is less difficult than a paramedian and is easier to repair. Nonabsorbable Dacron or Mersilene sutures in the linea alba give a firm repair with a low incidence of incisional hernia.

An important step in repair of the lesion is complete reduction of the hernia and withdrawal of the esophagus well down into the subdiaphragmatic position. This can best be accomplished by the vertical downward traction from the upper abdomen with the patient lying supine. Since the muscle fibers of the crus are usually attenuated and friable, interrupted sutures have a tendency to cut through the fibers. Thus, from the transabdominal approach these sutures should be placed through the covering peritoneum for additional support. Repair of the hiatus, in my opinion, should always be done by approximating the fibers of the crus posterior and inferior to the hiatus, leaving the anterior sling unrestricted by plicating sutures. The size of the hiatus should be carefully controlled and should not be too tight because edema may cause dysphagia after operation. After the repair, the opening should accommodate an index finger easily alongside the esophagus.

When the hernia is completely reduced, a portion of 2 to 3 cm. of longitudinal muscle fibers of esophagus above the esophagogastric junction is visible below the newly repaired hiatus. Usually the phrenicoesophageal ligament, which in my opinion is overrated as a useful structure in the repair of the hernia, is located well down in the abdominal cavity. An important part of the repair is placement of a circle of interrupted 000 nonabsorbable sutures, about six or eight in number, to anchor the esophagus to the hiatal fibers. Another technical point that may be important is to place a row of interrupted sutures between the gastric cardia and the adjacent esophagus. The maneuver maintains the acute esophagogastric angle that is important to prevent esophageal reflux. The vagus nerves should not be divided or sutured into the repair unless the patient requires additional surgery for peptic ulcer or reflux esophagitis.

Perhaps the strongest argument in favor of the transabdominal approach is the opportunity afforded for exploration of the peritoneal cavity for additional pathologic lesions. Among the more common associated lesions in my experience were chronic cholecystitis with cholelithiasis and duodenal ulcer. Occasionally unsuspected retroperitoneal or intraperitoneal neoplasms have also been discovered: they were the actual cause for the patient's symptoms. Routine appendectomy was also employed in our patients.

Discussion—Dr. Richard H. Sweet. The *abdominal approach* for the repair of a hiatus hernia is well illustrated in Plate 84. Here also precise knowledge of the anatomy is absolutely essential. In fact, the failures which result from the use of this approach are undoubtedly due to inaccuracy in dealing with the structures involved. As with all surgery, a wide exposure of the operative field must be obtained. It is this aspect of the employment of the abdominal approach which creates the greatest technical problem.

The incision must be long and must reach upward to the costoxiphoid angle (Plate 84, A). So also the left lobe of the liver must be retracted away from the operative field. This step requires the division of the left triangular ligament and the folding under of the liver edge as shown in Plate 84 (B and C).

It should be stressed also that, with the abdominal approach as with the thoracic, the margins of the hiatus must be exposed to view so that sutures can be inserted in the muscle bundles. This is best accomplished by retracting the esophagus to the left (Plate 84, F and G).

Little remains of the peritoneal sac after the dissection necessary to expose the lower esophagus and the muscle bundles of the right crus has been completed, but nothing much need be done about it. Any redundant edges of peritoneum, however, can be trimmed away and the peritoneal layer closed with sutures which attach it to the undersurface of the diaphragm as an additional safeguard against recurrence.

THE TRANSTHORACIC REPAIR OF AN
ESOPHAGEAL HIATUS HERNIA

Artist's illustrations of the inferior or abdominal aspect of the diaphragm drawn from a fresh cadaver specimen. The right crus, longer, thicker, and more tendinous than the left, separates into superficial and deep muscle bundles to form completely the esophageal hiatus. The superficial layer forms the right margin and the deep layer the left margin of the hiatal ring, effecting a slinglike arrangement of the fibers of the right crus. The close relation of the tendinous portion of the diaphragm and the inferior phrenic vein to the anterior angle of the hiatal ring is depicted.

MIDDLE

A. Artist's interpretation of the anatomy of the esophageal hiatus drawn from a fresh cadaver specimen showing the esophageal hiatus from the abdominal view. The formation of the hiatal ring or sling by the muscle fibers of the right crus is depicted. The greater length and width of the right crus compared to the left are demonstrated.

B. The esophageal hiatus as it appears looking obliquely downward from the head of the cadaver specimen. The thick or deep layer of muscle fibers of the right crus which forms the left margin of the hiatal ring lies superficial to and crosses the superficial or thin layer of muscle fibers of the right crus

DISCUSSION—DR. PAUL C. SAMSON. The first plate illustrates two facts of great importance: (1) the esophageal hiatus nearly always comprises muscles fibers from the *right* crus of the diaphragm; (2) the hiatus is oval, with the long axis in a generally anteroposterior direction. The anterior "angle" is rounded and firm; the posterior angle is usually the "weak spot" and is formed by the crossing or decussation of muscle fibers from the right (or medial) and left (or lateral) margins of the hiatus.

Illustrations A through U depict a method of transthoracic repair that differs in several details from the one I usually employ. In D, resection of the eighth rib is acceptable and may give more room without undue spreading of the ribs. In E, there is no point in injecting the left phrenic nerve. In fact, I think it is contraindicated. The anesthesiologist can easily control diaphragmatic motion during operation. In addition, I have seen hours and days of phrenic paralysis from injection alone. In F, the label should read simply *"pulmonary ligament,"* since there is no *inferior* pulmonary ligament. Regarding H and I, careful dissection of the esophagus is necessary, but the vagi should *not* be separated from the esophagus and should not be put on great tension. A drain passed around the

which forms the right margin of the hiatal ring.

C. Diagrammatic representation of the slinglike arrangement of the muscle fibers of the right crus of the diaphragm in the formation of the esophageal hiatal ring.

BOTTOM

These two artist's illustrations were drawn from fresh cadaver specimens and show the variations in the anatomy of the esophageal hiatus from that previously described.

Left. The muscle fibers of the left crus are separated into superficial and deep layers. The fibers of the superficial layer cross over the deep layer of muscle fibers of the right crus, and join with the fibers of the superficial layer of the right crus to form the right margin of the esophageal hiatal ring.

Right. In this specimen a thick bundle of muscle fibers from the left crus crosses beneath the deep layer of fibers of the right crus and ultimately blends with the superior or thoracic surface of the superficial layer of muscle fibers of the right crus. This particular anatomic configuration was originally described by Low and the crossing bundle of fibers of the left crus is commonly called the band of Low.

esophagus should include both vagus nerves. Also, I carefully free the muscle fibers of the right crus circumferentially from the hernial sac for a distance of 6 or 7 mm., which prevents a "rolling in" of the muscle when the hernia is reduced. In J, my counterincision is longer and roughly parallels the curve of the left (lateral) margin of the hiatus. This is because I believe strongly in Allison's method of tacking remnants of the sac, phrenoesophageal ligament and peritoneum to the undersurface of the diaphragm (see B). Regarding K, L, and M, I do not *excise* any portion of the sac, but with a wide horizontal (anteroposterior) incision a generous cuff is left attached to the region of the esophagogastric junction. From four to six, spaced, 000 silk sutures taken in the cuff at this stage are later passed through the counterincision, reneedled, and sewn to the undersurface of the diaphragm approximately 7 to 10 mm. from the left margin of the hiatus. In passing, I must confess that most illustrators make the phrenoesophageal ligament much more easy to identify than I am frequently able to do at the operating table. In O, since the anterior rounded "angle" of the hiatus usually is firm, I doubt if I employ sutures at the anterior angle in more than 10 per cent of cases. In P and Q, the essence of repair is the

Plate 85   209

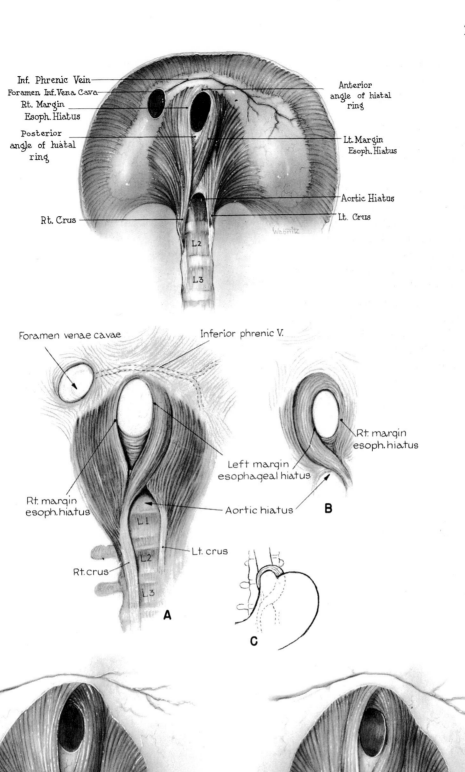

Inf. Phrenic Vein

Foramen Inf. Vena Cava

Rt. Margin Esoph. Hiatus

Posterior angle of hiatal ring

Rt. Crus

L2

L3

Anterior angle of hiatal ring

Lt. Margin Esoph. Hiatus

Aortic Hiatus

Lt. Crus

Foramen venae cavae

Inferior phrenic V.

Rt. margin esoph. hiatus

Left margin esophageal hiatus

Aortic hiatus

Rt. crus

Lt. crus

L1

L2

L3

A

B

Rt. margin esoph. hiatus

C

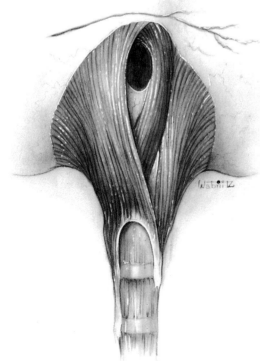

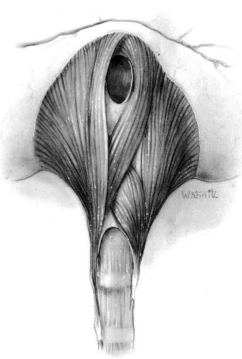

A. The patient is placed in the right lateral prone position, and the incision overlying the eighth interspace is outlined.

B, C, D. The incision is deepened through the underlying muscle layers to expose the line of incision in the eighth interspace.

E. The left pleural cavity is entered, and the wound margins are retracted with two self-retaining rib retractors of the Tuffier type. The resection of a rib is not required. The phrenic nerve is not crushed by clamping, but temporary paralysis of the diaphragm is obtained by injection of the nerve with 6 to 8 ml. of procaine solution (one per cent). Paralysis of the phrenic nerve by crushing destroys the bellowslike action of the diaphragm which is believed to predispose to postoperative pulmonary complications.

F. The deflated left lung is displaced upward and maintained in position by retraction over a moist gauze pad. This exposes the characteristic protrusion of the sliding hernia in the esophageal triangle. This triangle is bounded medially (anteriorly) by the pericardium and laterally (posteriorly) by the aorta. The base is formed by the diaphragm and the apex by the proximal portion of the inferior pulmonary ligament. The inverted T-shaped incision in the mediastinal and diaphragmatic pleura is depicted by the dotted lines. The horizontal portion of this incision extends medially (anteriorly) to the base of the pericardium and laterally (posteriorly) to a point just beyond the thoracic aorta.

G. The flaps of mediastinal pleura are retracted by guy sutures of silk (000), and the extension of the underlying muscle fibers of the diaphragm onto the base of the hernial protrusion may be seen.

DISCUSSION—DR. SAMSON (cont.)

posterior closure, where the fibers from the left (lateral) and right (medial) margins of the hiatus frequently appear to decussate. I think medium heavy silk (0 or 1), is better than fine silk. Dr. Madden rightly points out that the right marginal fibers are thin, and heavier silk will not cut. In this connection, I always seek to buttress any muscle sutures by passing the needle through pleura, peritoneum, or an available portion of the sac, which frequently I can pull up from below. The silk is tied with four throws of the knot. I am sure there have been some recurrences simply because the silk came untied early in the postoperative period. The closure usually needs only two to four sutures. With a Levin tube in the esophagus, the closure should be snug to the passage of the tip of the index finger.

In R, the closure of the counterincision must be in two layers, with interrupted silk. In all of the hernias occurring through the counterincision that I personally have seen, either single-layer silk or catgut closures had been employed. R, S, and U show a typical closure for an intercostal incision. When a rib is removed, subperiosteally, interrupted silk is used to close the pleural cavity. By taking generous bites of intercostal muscle, the intercostal nerve is protected and pain is less. No pericostal sutures are then employed.

I, II, and III illustrate well the modification described. As I have stated, I prefer to suture the cuff beneath the diaphragm. This technic is not difficult or time-consuming particularly if the counterincision is a little longer and parallels the left margin of the hiatus. It does mean that there will be several millimeters further reduction of the hernia.

The last two plates nicely illustrate an unusual problem and its solution. I think they emphasize the necessity of accurate anatomic delineation of the entire situation before repair has commenced.

The plates show clearly the steps in the trans-abdominal repair of an esophageal hiatus hernia. The end result of the repair should be the same as with the transthoracic approach. I may say that there is no uniformity of opinion regarding the method of approach. Some general surgeons believe the transthoracic approach is superior, while, conversely, some thoracic surgeons, particularly those who now perform a more complicated operation as a routine, have switched to the abdominal route. In a given case, complete familiarity with one or the other approaches should be the guiding factor. The operation from either aspect is not one of critical proportions, but there are a number of important technical details which must be remembered, and I think it is fair to say that the occasional operator will not have as high a percentage of success, as the surgeon who does the operation frequently.

If other abdominal pathologic lesions (possibly requiring surgery) are uncovered during the preoperative workup, then the operation should be performed from below. If, however, the gall bladder and stomach are not implicated, if the patient is quite fat (as many are), or if other abdominal surgery has preceded the prospective repair, then I think there is fairly general agreement that the transthoracic approach is superior.

Finally, I have encountered a rare situation when with a transthoracic approach, vagotomy and pyloroplasty seem called for. In such an instance, I have not hesitated to do the vagotomy through the chest, repair the hernia (if possible), and after closing the thoracic incision, turn the patient supine and perform a pyloroplasty through a separate small abdominal incision.

Plate 86   211

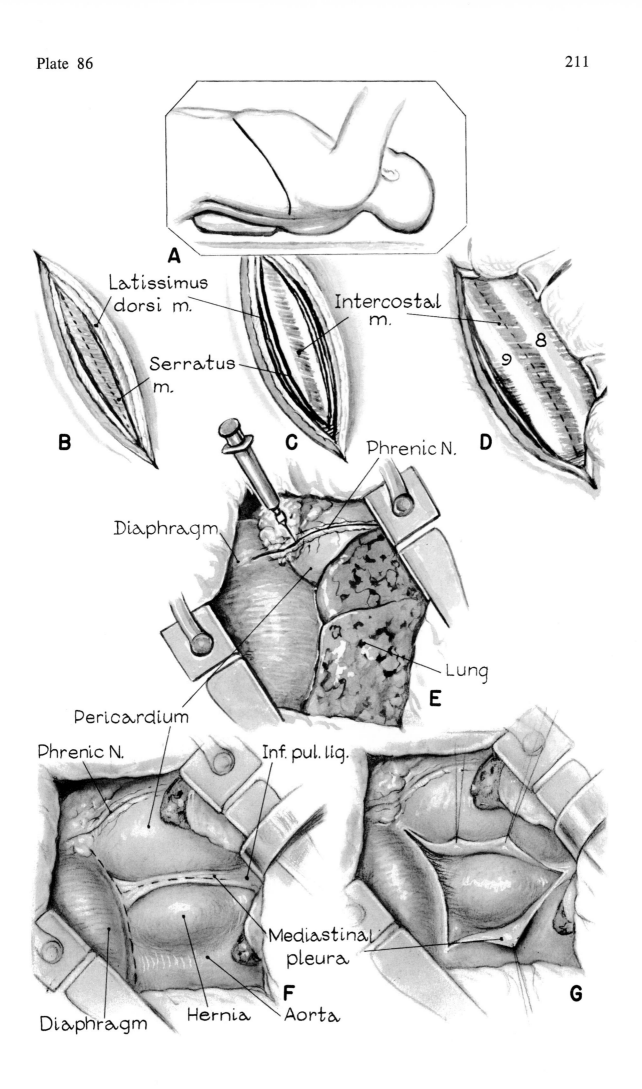

A

Latissimus dorsi m.

Serratus m.

Intercostal m.

B

C

8

9

D

Phrenic N.

Diaphragm

Lung

E

Pericardium

Phrenic N.

Inf. pul. lig.

Mediastinal pleura

Diaphragm   Hernia   Aorta

F

G

H, I. The distal portion of the esophagus is first mobilized by blunt digital dissection and then encircled by a rubber tissue drain. Traction upward on the esophagus is maintained and the hernia is mobilized by scissor dissection to expose the whole of the hiatal muscle ring which is formed completely by the muscle fibers of the right crus of the diaphragm (I). This step is considered an essential part of the operative technic. The thick layer of muscle fibers of the right crus which forms the left margin of the esophageal hiatal ring is anterior (lateral) and crosses superficial to the thin layer of muscle fibers of the right crus which is posterior (medial) and which forms the right margin of the esophageal hiatal ring.

J. A segment of the diaphragm in juxtaposition to the esophageal hiatus is tented by Babcock clamps and incised as indicated by the dotted line.

K. The left index finger of the surgeon is inserted through the incision in the diaphragm into the peritoneal cavity and then upward through the esophageal hiatus into the herneal sac. The overlying structures are tented on the index finger, and the phrenoesophageal ligament is incised to expose the underlying layer of the parietal peritoneum which forms the anterior wall of the sliding hernial sac. The area of the phrenoesophageal ligament to be excised is depicted in dotted outline. This ligament is a definite anatomic structure, possessed of good holding power and best demonstrated by elevation on the index finger as indicated.

L, M. Similarly, as in K, the peritoneum is incised and the lumen of the hernial sac is entered. This exposes the posterior wall of the hernial protrusion which is formed by the anterior wall of the stomach and thereby conforming to the definition of a sliding hernia. A sliding hernia defined is an irreducible hernia in which a portion of the wall of the sac is formed by the protruding or herniated viscus.

DISCUSSION—DR. RICHARD H. SWEET. A knowledge of the anatomy of the diaphragm and particularly of the structures in and about the esophageal hiatus is essential to an understanding of the principles involved in the successful repair of a hiatus hernia. Plate 85 (Top) shows the configuration of the muscle bundles of the right crus and the relations of the right and left crura. It should be emphasized, however, that this is a view of the inferior surface of the diaphragm. When viewed from above on the mediastinal surface, the right margin of the hiatus becomes the deep layer and the left margin is the superficial layer. This distinction is important for those who use the thoracic approach. The view in Plate 85, Top, is that of the surgeon who uses the abdominal approach. This is true also of Plate 85, Middle, A. Plate 85, Middle, B, shows the relations of these bundles as seen when the thoracic approach, which is preferred, is employed.

These relations of the muscle fibers which constitute the margin of the hiatus are of interest to the surgeon, but of even greater importance is an understanding of the disposition of the fascial layers and of the peritoneum in both the normal condition and in the presence of an esophageal hiatus hernia. One must realize that the pouch of peritoneum which comprises the hernial sac in the sliding variety in hernia pushes up in front of and to the right of the anterior surface of the herniated portion of stomach. Because of its anatomic relations it is impossible for the sac to envelop the entire circumference of the stomach, the anterior wall of which always makes up the posterior wall of the sac. Thus the term "sliding type" is the technically correct designation for this kind of herniation.

The fascial layer called by Allison the "phrenoesophageal ligament" is often so stretched out over the herniated stomach and the sac that it may not be recognized unless the surgeon realizes that this layer is always present. It is made up of a reflection of the transversalis fascia below and of the mediastinal fascia above which fuse at the margins of the hiatus to provide a loose tissue attachment for the esophagus. It is difficult to demonstrate this layer in a drawing, but it is important to place sutures in it at the operation. An impression of the relations of this layer may be gained from Plate 87, K, L, and M.

The impression is gained from Plates 87 and 88 that the cardia must always be pulled down below the hiatus by means of a sling inserted through a counter incision in the diaphragm. Although this maneuver is helpful, it is by no means always necessary. Actually the majority of hernias, excepting those which are unusually large or when the patient is excessively fat, can be handled without opening the diaphragm. This is done either by plication of the sac when it is small or by incision of the sac in the larger hernias. In the latter, additional sutures placed in the fascial layer are often needed to maintain a complete reduction of the hernia.

Plates 87 and 88 demonstrate clearly all of the steps in the repair of the hernia. The placing of sutures across the hiatus in front of the esophagus as shown in Plate 88, O, P, and Q, is essential when the shape of the hiatus is that of an ellipse, thus leaving a triangular defect in front. In the majority of instances, however, the hiatus is U or horseshoe shaped with a rounded contour in front. In these it is necessary merely to place a few sutures behind the esophagus.

The situation illustrated in Plates 91 and 92 appears to be somewhat theoretical. I have never encountered it. With any anomaly of the diaphragm at the esophageal hiatus, a thorough knowledge of the normal anatomy should make it possible to improvise a satisfactory technic for closure.

Plate 87

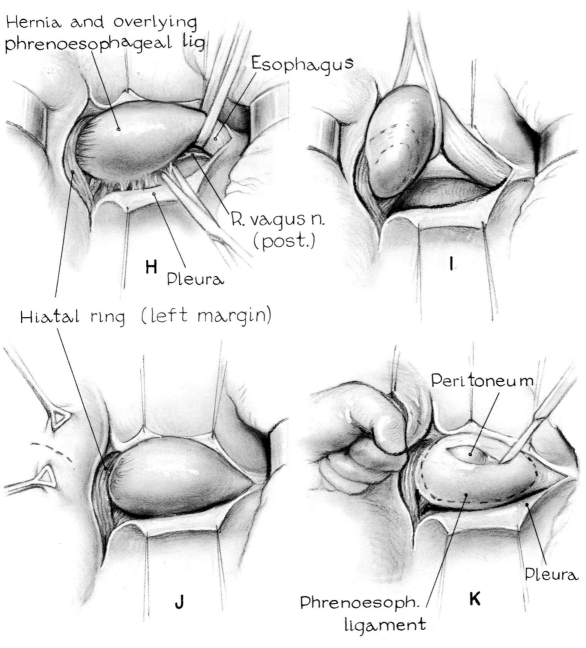

Hernia and overlying
phrenoesophageal lig

Esophagus

R. vagus n.
(post.)

H Pleura

Hiatal ring (left margin)

I

J

Peritoneum

Phrenoesoph.
ligament

Pleura

K

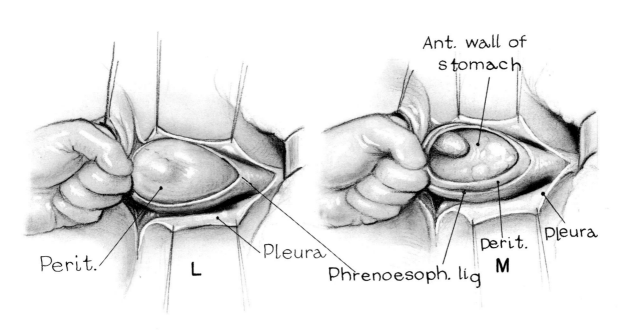

Ant. wall of
stomach

Perit.

L

Pleura

Phrenoesoph. lig

Perit.

Pleura

M

N. The hernia is reduced either by traction through the diaphragm as shown or by downward displacement with the aid of a pledget of gauze held in a ring clamp (P). If desired a combination of both maneuvers may be used.

O. After reduction of the hernia, the esophagus is retracted laterally (posteriorly) and the innermost or "crown" suture is inserted. This suture approximates the muscle fibers of the right crus which forms the medial (anterior) angle of the hiatal ring. This angle is in juxtaposition to both the tendinous portion of the diaphragm and the inferior phrenic vein. Accordingly, caution should be observed in the placement of sutures to avoid injury to the inferior phrenic vein. A second suture in this area may or may not be required.

P, Q. The esophagus is displaced medially (anteriorly) and the lateral (posterior) sutures (No. 1 silk) are inserted. These sutures approximate not the right and left crura as so commonly thought but the superficial and deep muscle layers of the right crus of the diaphragm which form the right and left margins respectively of the esophageal hiatal ring. The muscle fibers of the superficial layer (right margin of the esophageal hiatus) are frequently thinned out and have a poor holding power. Accordingly, in the suture approximation of the superficial and deep layers of the muscle fibers of the right crus, tension on the suture line should be avoided. When completed, the closure of the hiatal ring is snug but not too tight.

R. The incision in the diaphragm is closed (00 silk) and the flaps of diaphragmatic pleura are approximated with sutures of fine silk (0000). The posterior mediastinal pleura is not sutured because, in the event of an infection, the more readily treated complication, a pleural empyema, rather than a mediastinal abscess would then occur.

S, T, U. Two pericostal sutures of silk (No. 3) or, if preferred, double strands of chromic catgut (No. 2), are used to approximate the rib cage, and the muscle layers of the wound are closed with interrupted sutures of silk (000). Periosteal "windows" are formed along the inferior border of the lower rib to prevent impingement upon either the intercostal nerve or the sensitive periosteum. A water-seal catheter drainage of the pleural cavity is routinely employed. This catheter is withdrawn approximately 36 hours postoperatively.

DISCUSSION—DR. DENTON A. COOLEY. In regard to the technic described by the author for transthoracic repair of the hernia a larger secondary incision in the diaphragm should be used so the esophagus can be anchored with sutures below the diaphragm. The phrenicoesophageal ligament can be used for this purpose. Overcorrecting the hernia into the abdomen is important, since roentgenographic studies after operation may otherwise suggest an incomplete repair.

DISCUSSION—DR. JOHN ROBINSON BROOKS. In recent years at the Peter Bent Brigham Hospital, increasing use of the abdominal approach for repair of esophageal hiatus hernia has been prompted by a number of factors. It has been shown that approximately 40 per cent of patients coming to operation for esophageal hiatus hernia have some concomitant process within the abdomen, such as peptic ulcer or biliary tract disease, which may be treated at the same sitting. When gastrointestinal bleeding becomes a problem with site unknown and with both peptic ulcer and esophageal hernia present, it is almost mandatory to explore the abdomen in order to evaluate properly and correct the source of blood loss. Moreover, the abdominal approach may be said to compromise less the pulmonary reserve of patients with hiatus hernia, many of whom are elderly and have chronic lung disease. Although the pulmonary complications following subdiaphragmatic surgery do exist, there is, nevertheless, no question that pulmonary reserve is more compromised intraoperatively during a chest procedure than during an abdominal procedure. The abdominal approach confines the surgeon to one cavity. The transthoracic approach involves an incision through the diaphragm (with possible interference of the phrenic nerve in the course of this procedure), thereby opening both the pulmonary and abdominal cavities simultaneously.

Plate 88   215

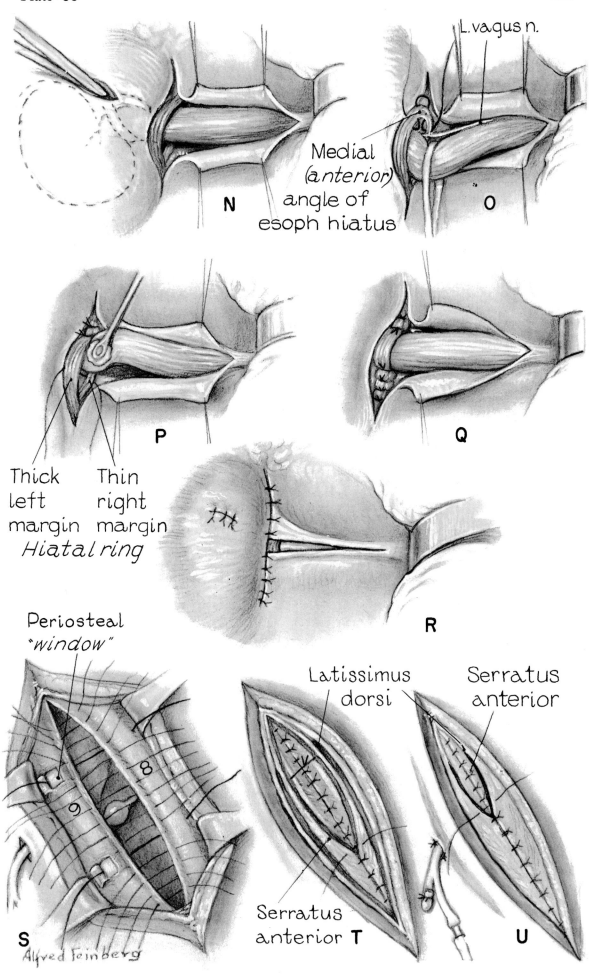

L. vagus n.

Medial
(anterior)
angle of
esoph hiatus

N

O

Thick   Thin
left   right
margin   margin
Hiatal ring

P

Q

R

Periosteal
"window"

Latissimus   Serratus
dorsi   anterior

Serratus
anterior T

U

S

Alfred Feinberg

These illustrations depict diagrammatically the three most commonly used methods in the repair of a hernia through the esophageal hiatus of the diaphragm.

I. *a.* The anatomic pathologic findings in a sliding hernia through the esophageal hiatus are shown. The posterior wall of the sac is formed by the protruding viscus, the stomach, and thereby conforms to the definition of a sliding hernia.

b. The posterior mediastinal pleura, the phrenoesophageal ligament, and the peritoneum are incised to enter the lumen of the hernial sac. The extent of the resection of the phrenoesophageal ligament and the peritoneum is indicated by the small solid black lines.

c. The herniated segment of the stomach into the posterior mediastinum is reduced, and the superficial and deep muscle layers of the right crus of the diaphragm are approximated around the esophagus just above the cardia. The diaphragmatic pleura, but not the opening in the posterior mediastinal pleura, is sutured. This method of repair of a sliding hernia is the same as shown in the preceding artist's illustrations.

II. *a, b.* These sketches demonstrate an essential step in the Allison method of repair. Following the excision of segments of the phrenoesophageal ligament and the peritoneum (anterior wall of the sac), the cuff formed by the proximal cut margins of the phrenoesophageal ligament and peritoneum is sutured to the under surface of the diaphragm. Another important step in the Allison method, although not illustrated in the sketches, is the closure of the muscular hiatal ring in a vertical plane, "with the grain," posterior to the esophagus.

III. *a, b, c.* These sketches outline the essential steps in the technic advocated by Sweet for the repair of small and medium sized hernias. A series of circumferential or longitudinal plication sutures are inserted in the overlying phrenoesophageal ligament and peritoneum to obliterate the sac. The closure of the lax muscle ring of the hiatus about the esophagus completes the repair of the hernia.

DISCUSSION—DR. BROOKS (cont.)

In preparation for hiatus herniorrhaphy, an evaluation of gastric secretion is mandatory. A high acid level in the face of coexisting esophagitis may indicate the need for concomitant vagotomy. Esophagoscopy is performed if possible to evaluate more accurately the lower esophagus and rule in or out ulceration, esophageal ring, or tumor. Finally, the presence of ulcer disease with or without pyloric stenosis may indicate the need for pyloroplasty or vagotomy and pyloroplasty at the time of hernia repair. Careful roentgenographic examination of the esophagus to rule out a diverticulum, an esophageal web, or ring is important and may be clarified by cineradiography.

The incision for the abdominal approach to hiatus herniorrhaphy can be adapted to the patient at hand. If herniorrhaphy alone is to be performed, a left rectus muscle-retracting incision is preferable and should be extended up lateral to the xiphoid, which may be removed if indicated. A right rectus "hockey stick" incision carried across the midline up to the left of the xiphoid is used if concomitant biliary tract disease is present and is to be treated.

It is characteristic of the abdominal approach that exposure becomes easier as the operation pro-

ceeds. Frequently, the most difficult aspect of the operation is with mobilization and retraction of the left lobe of the liver. In instances where that lobe is small, severance of the triangular ligament may not be necessary. In most cases, however, this must be done and may be difficult to perform in patients with a high-riding diaphragm and an overhanging costal margin. Once the triangular ligament is severed and the left lobe of the liver is retracted to the right, exposure rapidly becomes easier, and reduction of the hernia can then be carried out with ease. It is only the extremely rare, longstanding hernia with periesophageal inflammatory changes that is difficult to reduce below the diaphragm. Dissection is carried around the esophagus. The sac is excised, and an incision is made in the attenuated phrenoesophageal ligament, the proximal portion of which will later be sutured to the undersurface of the diaphragm. Approximately 2 in. of esophagus is thereby mobilized, and the vagus nerves can then be severed if indicated.

The esophagogastric junction is retracted to the left, and the two limbs of the right crus of the diaphragm located posteriorly are cleared of overlying tissue and peritoneum. The more posterior

Plate 89   217

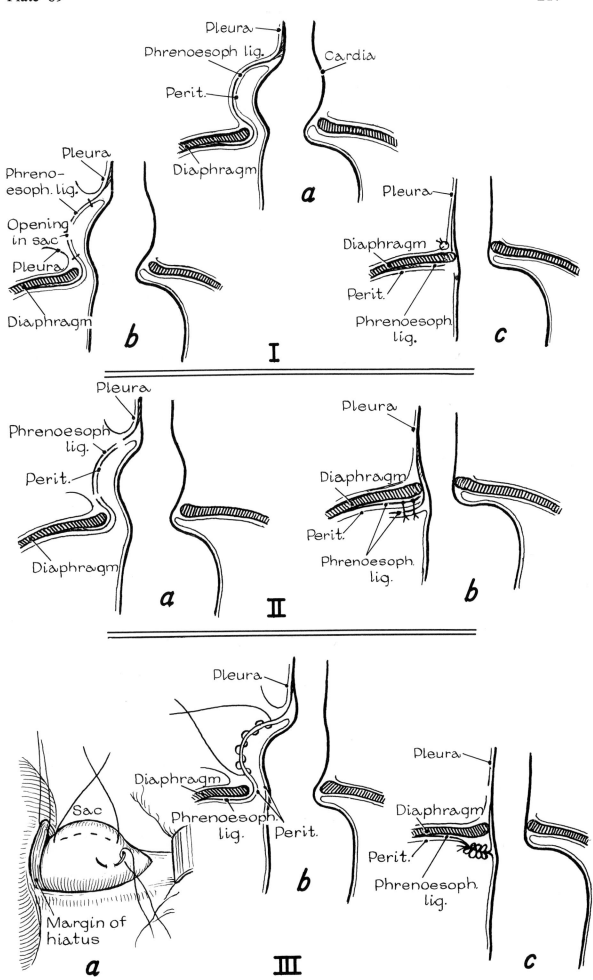

Pleura

Dhrenoesoph lig.

Perit.

Cardia

Diaphragm

a

Pleura

Phreno-
esoph. lig.

Opening
in sac

Pleura

Diaphragm

Pleura

Diaphragm

Perit.

Phrenoesoph
lig.

b   I   *c*

Pleura

Phrenoesoph
lig.

Perit.

Diaphragm

Pleura

Diaphragm

Perit.

Phrenoesoph.
lig.

a   II   *b*

Pleura

Diaphragm

Phrenoesoph.
lig.

Perit.

Sac

Margin of
hiatus

Pleura

Diaphragm

Perit.

Phrenoesoph.
lig.

a   III   *b*   *c*

The modification of the Allison method which is now used routinely as the preferred technic in the repair of an esophageal hiatus hernia is illustrated. The main modification is that the proximal cuff formed by the phrenoesophageal ligament and the peritoneum is sutured to the upper rather than the under surface of the diaphragm. Technically this is simpler, and it is believed not to lessen the anchorage effect on the esophagus.

The modification of Allison's method, recently suggested by Johnsrud, has much to recommend it. In this technic the phrenoesophageal ligament and the peritoneum forming the anterior wall of the hernial sac is not incised but instead inverted through the esophageal hiatus into the peritoneal cavity. The double thickness of the wall of the inverted hernial sac is then sutured to the under surface of the diaphragm with a series of interrupted silk sutures.

A. Through an incision in the diaphragm, the index finger is inserted into the peritoneal cavity and then through the esophageal hiatus into the lumen of the sac. The phrenoesophageal ligament is incised, and the underlying peritoneal layer is tented on the tip of the index finger.

B. The peritoneal layer which forms the anterior wall of the sac is incised, and the lumen of the hernial sac is entered. The anterior wall of the stomach which forms the posterior wall of the sac is visible. A cuff of the phrenoesophageal ligament and peritoneum is formed proximally by making the incisions indicated by the dotted lines.

C, D. The ends of the traction tape of rubber tissue which encircles the esophagus are withdrawn through the esophageal hiatus into the peritoneal cavity and then through the opening in the diaphragm into the pleural cavity. By traction on this tape the hernia is reduced into the peritoneal cavity and the muscle bundles of the right crus which form the boundaries of the esophageal hiatus are approximated both medial (anterior) and lateral (posterior) to the esophagus.

E. The proximal cuff formed by the phrenoesophageal ligament and peritoneal layers is sutured to the upper or pleural surface of the diaphragm for anchorage of the esophagus. The incision in the diaphragm is closed and the flap of diaphragmatic pleura, but not the mediastinal pleura, is sutured.

F. A diagrammatic illustration of the completed operation is shown in profile.

DISCUSSION—DR. BROOKS (cont.)

portion of these two can be felt rising up to the left of the aorta and is usually bulkier than the more anteriorly located right portion. In mobilizing these muscle bundles, care must be taken not to damage the inferior phrenic artery or the inferior vena cava. An appropriate number of braided silk interrupted sutures are taken so that the esophageal hiatus is snug. If the esophageal hiatus is made too snug, dysphagia may occur and require postoperative esophageal dilatation. As a general rule, however, most patients have some transient symptoms of esophageal hold-up for several weeks following an "adequate" repair.

Following suture of the hiatus, the phrenoesophageal ligament is sutured to the undersurface of the diaphragm if it can be obtained as a significant structure. If not, small fine silk stitches of 0000 silk are taken between the esophageal wall and the undersurface of the ring of the hiatus to secure the esophagogastric junction at this point and prevent retraction up into the mediastinum. The usual anchoring stitches of silk are then taken between the lower esophagus and the undersurface of the diaphragm and between the cardia of the stomach and the undersurface of the diaphragm. No attempt is made to reperitonize these surfaces.

A concomitant vagotomy and pyloroplasty is done if severe duodenal ulcer disease exists or if there is esophagitis with ulceration and beginning stenosis of the lower end of the esophagus. Under these circumstances, an inlying gastrostomy tube is placed, using a No. 16 Foley with a 5 cc. bag. This is brought out to the left of the incision and remains in place until the patient is eating well. In the usual patient with esophagitis without fibrosis, no vagotomy is performed.

The repair of an hiatus hernia from below the diaphragm is easily performed and can be carried out in elderly people with relatively little risk. There is less chance of impairing pulmonary reserve. A statistical evaluation of the end results shows no higher recurrence rate following repair from below than that from above, and when done from below, coexisting intra-abdominal disease can be handled at the same time.

Complicated lower esophageal strictures and problems of esophageal shortening or hernia fixation above the diaphragm can be readily handled by extending the abdominal incision across the costal margin into the left side of the chest if indicated. In my experience this is rarely required.

Plate 90   219

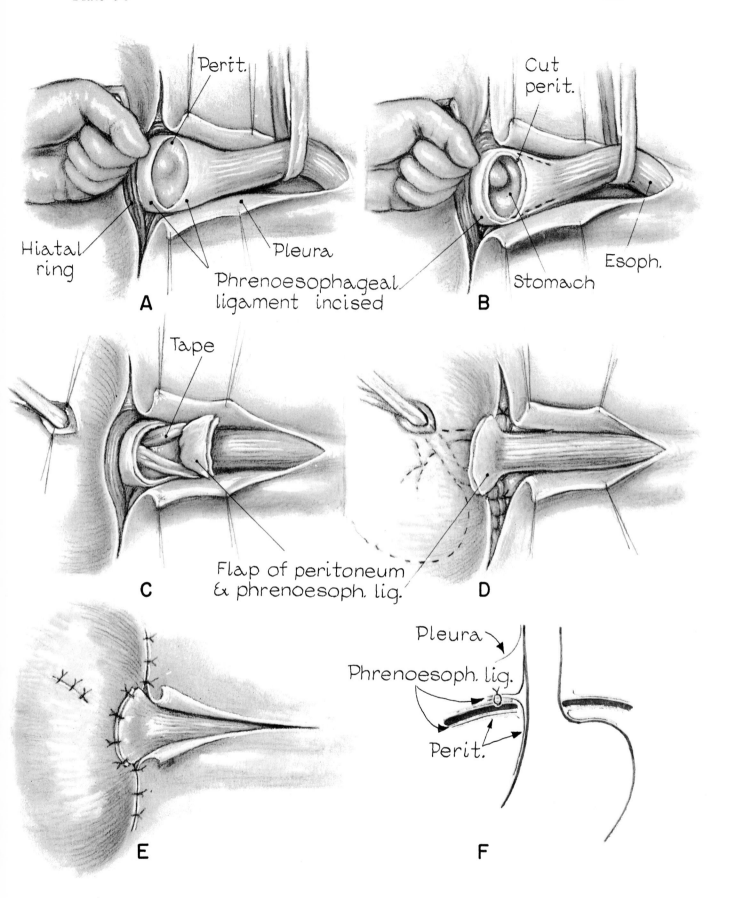

Perit.

Hiatal
ring

Pleura

Phrenoesophageal
ligament incised

A

Cut
perit.

Esoph.

Stomach

B

Tape

C

Flap of peritoneum
& phrenoesoph. lig.

D

E

Pleura

Phrenoesoph. lig.

Perit.

F

Allison emphasized the importance of closure of the hiatal ring in a vertical plane posterior to the esophagus. In the succeeding illustrations the difficulty in performing this method of closure when the long axis of the hiatus is in the transverse or horizontal plane is shown.

A. The esophageal hiatus viewed from the lower or abdominal surface of the diaphragm. The dilated hiatal ring prior to closure is demonstrated. The long axis of the ring is in a horizontal plane.

B. The excessive angulation and tension on the suture line and the inadequacy of the closure on attempted approximation of the muscle layers of the right crus in a vertical plane posterior to the esophagus are shown.

C, D. The muscle fibers of the right crus are approximated in a horizontal plane to the left of the esophagus. The closure is adequate and there is a minimum of tension on the suture line.

Although in many instances the illustrated technic has proved satisfactory, it is believed anatomically unsound. The inherent weakness in the method is the suturing of the muscle fibers of the right crus in the reconstruction of the esophageal hiatus.

Muscle tissue has a minimal "holding" power for sutures, and, as a consequence, when the muscle contracts, the sutures tear through, even though the tension on the suture line is not excessive. This occurrence has been observed repeatedly during operations, and on several occasions it was necessary to abandon the method.

The rationale of attempting to decrease the size of the hiatus is questioned. Frequently in the performance of abdominal operations the hiatus is explored digitally to estimate its size. Often it will admit three to four fingers, yet no hernia is demonstrable surgically, radiographically, or by clinical manifestations. On the contrary, a hernia may be present in a patient with a relatively small esophageal hiatus. Accordingly, the size of the hiatus is not the basic factor in the presence or absence of an esophageal hiatus hernia.

If these tenets are accepted—viz., (1) the muscle fibers of the hiatal ring should not be sutured and (2) the presence of esophageal hiatal hernia is not dependent upon the size of the hiatus—the logical question is, What operation should be performed? Admittedly, I do not know. However, it is believed that the sac should always be opened and a flap formed cephalad of peritoneum (sac) and phrenoesophageal ligament (transversalis fascia). The hernia is next reduced, and the flap previously formed is sutured to the pleural surface and tendinous portion of the diaphragm. In this manner a firm serosa-to-serosa apposition of tissues possessed of good "holding" power is obtained. Since the principle of the method is believed of basic importance, anchorage of the flap to the under or peritoneal surface of the diaphragm is not considered necessary. In fact, this procedure not only is technically more difficult but also necessitates the apposition of fascia (phrenoesophageal ligament) to serosa rather than the preferred serosa-to-serosa union that is obtained with the technic previously described. The union of serosa to serosa is a time-honored principle in intestinal surgery.

In some instances the ends of the peritoneal-fascia flaps are sutured together behind the esophagus to form a circular cuff about the esophagocardial junction. The lower margin of the cuff is then sutured in a circular manner to the adjacent cut margins of the diaphragmatic pleura and the underlying tendinous portion of the diaphragm. Again, serosa-to-serosa apposition is obtained with concomitant fascia reinforcement on each side of the suture line. This technic, from theoretical as well as practical considerations, is preferred.

In each of the technics described the transthoracic route is required. Accordingly, this route is of necessity preferred. Many surgeons elect the abdominal route so that an artificial angle of His may be more easily established by suture of the fundus of the stomach to the undersurface of the diaphragm in juxtaposition to the hiatus. The basis for this maneuver is more theoretical than real. What is more important is the reduction of the hernia and the maintenance of its reduction, which may be more ably accomplished by use of the transthoracic approach.

Plate 91

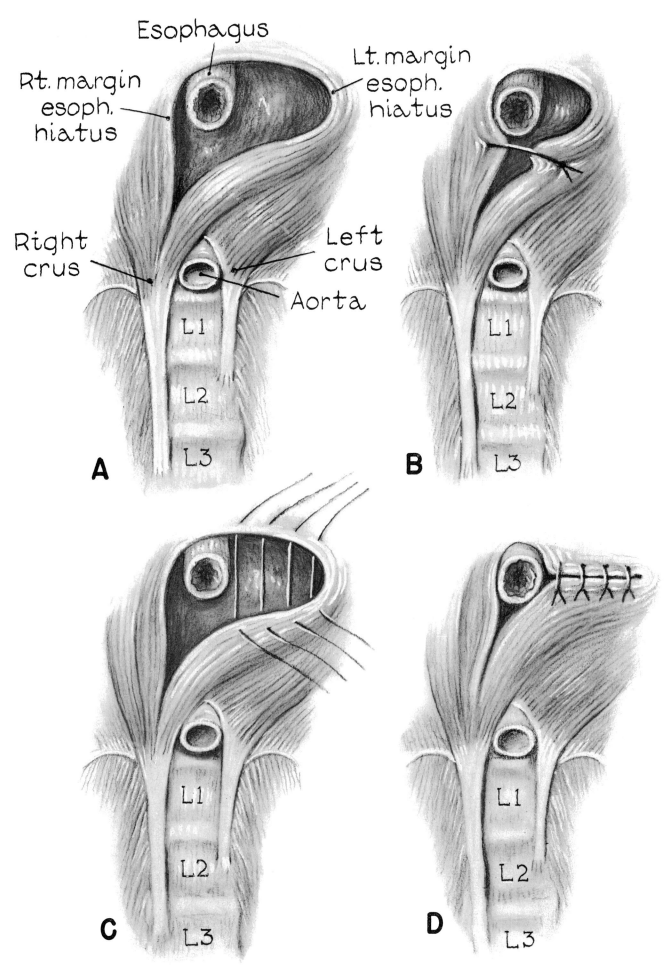

Esophagus

Rt. margin
esoph.
hiatus

Lt. margin
esoph.
hiatus

Right
crus

Left
crus

Aorta

L1

L2

L3

A

L1

L2

L3

B

L1

L2

L3

C

L1

L2

L3

D

The same illustrations as in Plate 91 when viewed from the upper or thoracic surface of the diaphragm with the patient in the direct right lateral prone position.

A. The thick layer of muscle fibers of the right crus, the left margin of the hiatal ring, crossing superficial to the thin layer of muscle fibers of the right crus, the right margin of the hiatal ring, is shown. The long axis of the hiatus is in the left lateral or horizontal plane.

B. The excessive angulation and tension on the suture line and the inadequate closure on attempted approximation of the muscle fibers of the right crus in a vertical plane posterior to the esophagus is demonstrated.

All too frequently artist's illustrations depicting the transthoracic approach for the repair of an esophageal hiatus hernia will show the thoracic incision being properly made with the patient in the right lateral prone position. But when the left pleural cavity is entered, the anatomic relations of the hiatal ring and the method for its closure are illustrated as if the patient were supine. It is believed that such illustrations are perpetuations of error which have led to needless confusion and misunderstanding of both the anatomy of the hiatal ring and the methods of surgical repair. The surgeon should remember that in the transthoracic approach, with the patient in the right lateral prone position, the posterior angle of the hiatal ring is always facing toward him. Furthermore, it is at this angle that the crossing of the fibers of the right crus occurs (A).

Commonly in the transthoracic approach, closure of the hiatal ring in the lateral plane to the left of the esophagus (C) is described as anterior to the esophagus. Similarly, closure in the opposite or right lateral plane (D) is described as posterior to the esophagus. However, a careful study of the comparative relation of the hiatal ring to the esophagus in the supine (Plate 91) and in the right lateral prone positions (Plate 92) should aid in the correction of these anatomic misinterpretations.

Plate 92

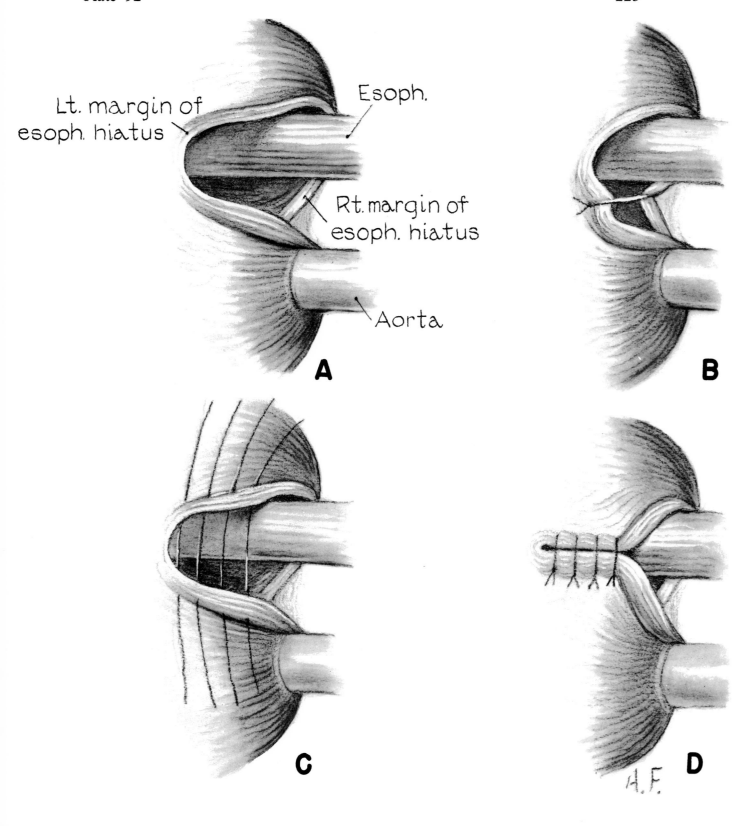

Lt. margin of
esoph. hiatus

Esoph.

Rt. margin of
esoph. hiatus

Aorta

A

B

C

D

A. F.

INFRADIAPHRAGMATIC RESECTION OF THE VAGUS NERVES
AND ANTECOLIC GASTROJEJUNOSTOMY

A, B, C. The peritoneal cavity is entered through a left paramedian muscle-retracting (lateral) incision.

D. The wound margins are retracted, and the structures in the region of the esophago-cardial junction are shown. The site of severance of the avascular left triangular ligament is shown in dotted outline. In some instances this ligament may be too short to sever. Under such circumstances, a moist protective pad is placed beneath the left lobe of the liver which is gently retracted upward.

E, F. An incision is made through the peritoneal and fascia layers overlying the lower-most portion of the esophagus, and the posterior mediastinal space is entered. The relation of the esophagus to the margins of the right crus of the diaphragm which form completely the esophageal hiatal ring is shown.

DISCUSSION—DR. LESTER R. DRAGSTEDT. In the transabdominal approach for resection of the vagus nerves, it has been my usual practice to divide the triangular ligament to the left lobe of the liver, as illustrated in D, Plate 93. I believe that this gives better access to the lower portion of the esophagus. However, some surgeons of experience, including Dr. Joseph Weinberg of Los Angeles, omit this step and retract the left lobe of the liver upward with a large broad blade retractor. In entering the mediastinum, I have found it wise to make the opening midway between the esophageal hiatus and the large inferior phrenic vein, as demonstrated in the illustrations E and F, Plate 93. I customarily do this by picking up the diaphragm with forceps with protruding teeth, making a small nick with a pair of scissors, and

Plate 93   225

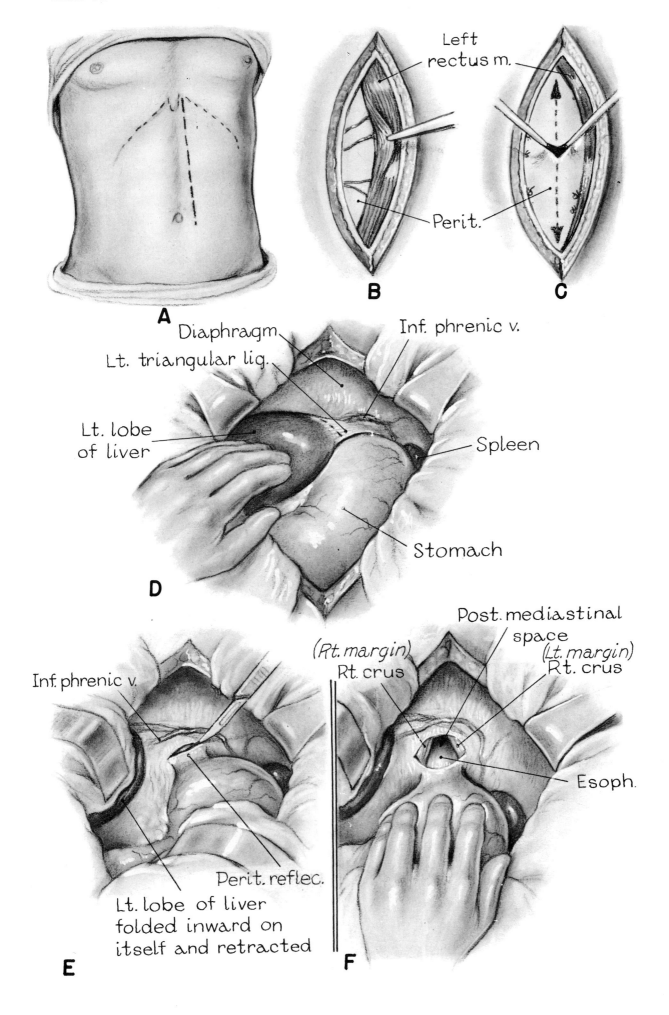

A

B

Left
rectus m.

Perit.

C

Diaphragm   Inf. phrenic v.

Lt. triangular lig.

Lt. lobe
of liver   Spleen

                                                   Stomach

D

Inf. phrenic v.

Perit. reflec.

Lt. lobe of liver
folded inward on
itself and retracted

E

Post. mediastinal
space
(Rt. margin)   (Lt. margin)
Rt. crus   Rt. crus

                                          Esoph.

F

G. The lower end of the esophagus is mobilized by blunt digital dissection and encircled by a rubber tissue traction tape. The left anterior vagus nerve which is always in close relation to the anterior surface of the esophagus is visible.

H, I. The esophagus is displaced to the left by traction, and the right or posterior vagus nerve located in the fibroareolar tissue posterior and medial to the esophagus is mobilized on the right index finger and secured on a nerve hook.

J. The right (posterior) vagus nerve is divided with scissors between a silver clip marker above and a clamp below.

K. The left (anterior) vagus nerve is similarly divided, and careful digital exploration of the periesophageal region for additional nerve fibers is being performed. This is considered a most important part of the operation. A minimum of 3 and a maximum of 13 additional nerve fibers have been identified by this maneuver.

L. The duodenojejunal junction at the base of the transverse mesocolon, as indicated by the ligament of Treitz, is visualized, and a segment of jejunum, 9 to 12 inches distally, is isolated by two guy sutures of silk.

DISCUSSION—DR. DRAGSTEDT (cont.)

then thrusting the scissors into the mediastinum, thus enlarging the opening. Sometimes I think this may avoid troublesome hemorrhage.

In mobilizing the esophagus by blunt finger dissection it is important to emphasize that this be done gently. Several cases have been reported where the esophagus has been opened with rough handling. Upon mobilization of the esophagus it is my practice to sweep the fingers of the right hand around the esophagus in an effort to include all of the vagus fibers within their grasp. The esophagus and vagus nerves are then pulled downward into the abdomen whereupon the posterior vagus nerve, which is felt against the yielding esophagus, is pulled over to the left and a segment excised between ligatures of non-absorbable suture material. The use of silver clips is equally satisfactory.

If a gastrojejunostomy rather than pyloroplasty is selected as a drainage procedure, I believe it is wise to place the gastroenterostomy stoma within five or six cm. of the pylorus. We have encountered a number of patients where a high-lying gastrojejunostomy

failed to drain adequately the antrum of the stomach, and the stasis of food in this area caused an excessive secretion of gastric juice of humoral or hormonal origin. It has also been my practice to make a small gastroenterostomy opening so that when the operation is completed the stoma is approximately one-and-one-half cm. in diameter. It is my conviction that such a small stoma decreases the incidence and severity of the dumping syndrome.

The transthoracic approach for division of the vagus nerves, such as indicated in the illustrations of this operation, was the method that I first employed. However, this operation has been very largely abandoned by me because it does not provide an opportunity to add a drainage procedure to the vagotomy, it does not permit inspection of the ulcer and possible associated pathology, and because of the frequency of postoperative intercostal pain. This approach, however, may be used for the treatment of recurrent gastrojejunal ulcers after repeated gastric resection and possibly in some other special situation.

Plate 94   227

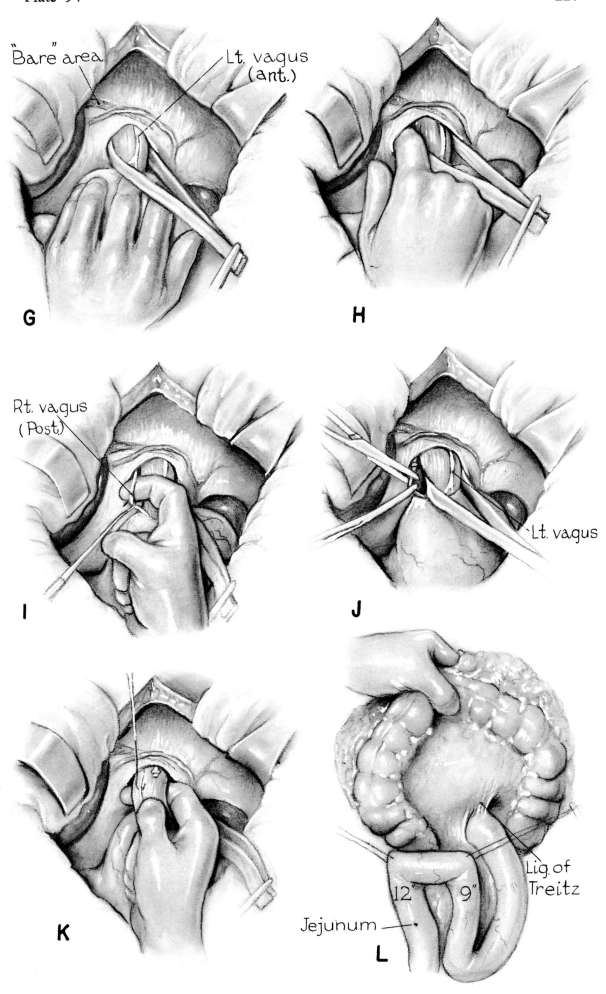

"Bare" area

Lt. vagus
(ant.)

G

H

Rt. vagus
(Post.)

I

Lt. vagus

J

K

Lig. of
Treitz

12"   9"

Jejunum

L

M, N. A segment of the anterior wall of the stomach in juxtaposition to the most dependent portion of the greater curvature is mobilized by Babcock clamps, and the anterior gastric branches of the gastroepiploic arch are serially clamped, severed, and ligated.

O. The anterior, and all but one of the posterior, gastric branches of the gastroepiploic arch have been severed and ligated, and the lesser sac is entered.

P. The segment of jejunum previously isolated is brought anterior to the transverse colon and approximated to the posterior wall of the greater curvature of the stomach by a series of interrupted silk (000) sutures. If preferred, the jejunum may be brought through an opening in an avascular portion of the transverse mesocolon and a "short loop" retrocolic gastrojejunostomy performed. The sites of incision in the jejunum and in the avascular plane of the greater curvature of the stomach are indicated in dotted outline. No clamps are used in the performance of the anastomosis. This is the preferred technic.

p'. Inset to show the relation of the first posterior layer of sutures to the mesenteric border of the jejunum.

Q. Incisions are made through the seromuscular layers of the jejunum and the greater curvature of the stomach, and the vessels in the submucosal layers are undersewn with hemostatic suture ligatures of silk (0000).

R. The lumen of the stomach is first entered by an incision with a scalpel, and the opening is extended by scissor dissection. The opening, similarly made previously into the lumen of the jejunum, is visible. Soiling of the operative field with either gastric or jejunal contents is minimized by aspiration with the suction tube.

DISCUSSION—DR. STANLEY O. HOERR. I prefer a midline incision that will extend to the left of the xiphoid and, if necessary, to the left of the umbilicus (A, B, C). It is very important for ease of exposure to go as high as possible. A self-retaining retractor of the Balfour type may be used instead of hand-held retractors (D). Exposure of the diaphragmatic reflection at the cardioesophageal may be obtained by a ribbon or malleable retractor elevating the left lobe of the liver; in my experience, division of the left triangular ligament is rarely necessary.

Instead of tugging on the esophagus with an encircling rubber tape or catheter (G, H, J), I employ traction on the stomach to make the nerve stand out like a bowstring. The first assistant is instructed to pull the stomach (grasped through a gauze pad) toward the left great toe of the patient. The surgeon may wish to do this first himself, using his right hand, while with his left forefinger he palpates the nerve. While palpating the nerve, he transfers the stomach to his assistant, who maintains the same degree of traction. A long nerve hook with a right-angle tip (rather than a curved one as shown in I and K) may be used to break through the overlying thin layer of peritoneum, thus omitting the stages shown in E and F. A second nerve hook may be used to free up a segment of nerve for easy division and removal of a segment for the pathologist. Sometimes the nerve trunk, particularly the posterior trunk, is accompanied by a small blood vessel; both cut ends should then be clipped or ligated (J). After division of the main trunks, the operator standing on the right side of the patient may encircle the esophagus with his *left* forefinger, permitting the surface to be inspected for additional fibers. The posterior (right) vagus nerve at the level of the cardioesophageal junction may lie a centimeter or more posterior to the esophagus, and characteristically overlies the aorta, coursing slightly to the left as it descends. Sometimes elevating the stomach slightly (toward the ceiling) while maintaining traction toward the feet will facilitate exposure of this trunk. Inexperienced surgeons may easily overlook even a sizable posterior vagus nerve. Reconstruction of the hiatus may be done after severance of the nerves but is rarely indicated. An exception may be the coexistence of an hiatus hernia believed to be symptomatic.

Plate 95   229

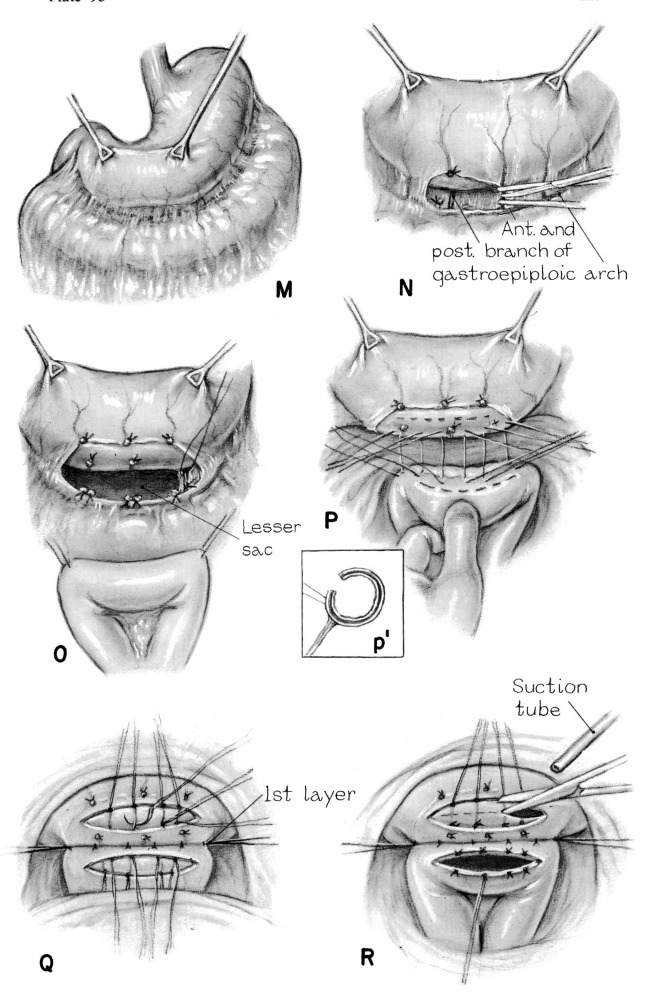

M

N

Ant. and
post. branch of
gastroepiploic arch

O

Lesser
sac

P

p'

Q

1st layer

R

Suction
tube

S. The middle hemostatic sutures on the anterior cut margins of the jejunum and stomach respectively are left long for traction, and the second posterior layer of interrupted sutures of silk (0000) are inserted. No complications have ensued from the use of silk sutures for the mucosal layer. In fact, this method of suture is preferred to the use of a continuous interlocking suture of fine chromic (00) catgut.

T. The closure of the second posterior layer is completed with a wide approximation of the adjacent posterior serosal surfaces.

U. The first anterior layer of silk sutures (0000) are inserted. The sutures at either angle are inserted from the "inside out" to the "outside in" and are tied as oblique traction is maintained on the angle sutures of the second posterior layer. This type of suture produces an inversion of the serosal surfaces with the suture knot on the inside of the lumen.

U'. Inset to show the use of interrupted inversion sutures throughout for the closure of the first anterior layer.

V. The closure of the first anterior layer with single through and through interrupted silk sutures is completed and the insertion of the second anterior layer of interrupted seromuscular sutures (Lembert) of fine silk (0000) is begun.

W. The antecolic, isoperistaltic gastrojejunostomy along the most dependent portion of the greater curvature of the stomach is completed.

X, Y. The commencement of the wound closure, using interrupted sutures of silk (00) for the peritoneum is shown. If preferred, interrupted silk sutures of the mattress variety, or a continuous chromic catgut (00) suture that is doubled, may be used. The fascia and skin layers are closed with interrupted sutures of 00 and 000 silk respectively.

DISCUSSION—DR. HOERR (cont.)

The ligament of Treitz should invariably be identified directly (L). After selecting a suitable segment of jejunum—as close as possible to the ligament of Treitz without creating tension at the proposed site of the anastomosis—the proximal end of the segment may be grasped with a "soft" Allis clamp (teeth filed off to avoid injury to the bowel), and the distal end of the segment may be grasped by a Babcock clamp. Since A comes before B in the alphabet, the mnemonic 'A' for Allis and 'B' for Babcock will identify the proximal and distal jejunum and may help avoid confusion once the ligament of Treitz is no longer in view.

The use of the greater curvature for the gastric stoma (M, N, O) is very sound practice and permits accurate placement at the most dependent portion of the stomach. I refer to this as an "antecolic dependent gastrojejunostomy" rather than as an anterior gastrojejunostomy, which may be interpreted as being to the anterior surface of the stomach.

The figures show proximal jejunum to the left of the anastomosis. Ordinarily this will be the more "comfortable" from a mechanical stand-point. The surgeon should not hesitate, however, to turn the jejunum in the opposite direction if this would seem to be more free of undesirable kinks or twists.

Interrupted silk sutures for both layers make an excellent anastomosis. I personally employ two layers of continuous 00 chromic catgut on an atraumatic needle, with emphasis on the bites being sufficiently deep into muscularis but creating minimal inversion with the outer layer. The end result with either suture material seems to be the same, but a continuous suture is a little faster. Nonabsorbable materials such as silk and cotton are not suitable for continuous sutures.

If a midline incision has been used, interrupted No. 30 stainless steel wire is a convenient mass suture for the deep layers.

The surgeon should utilize antecolic dependent gastrojejunostomy as shown in these figures when feasible, but in an occasional patient with a long transverse mesocolon and a heavy omentum, a posterior gastrojejunostomy may be simpler. It is best to remain openminded as to the type of gastrojejunostomy until the exact situation in the given patient has been assessed.

Plate 96   231

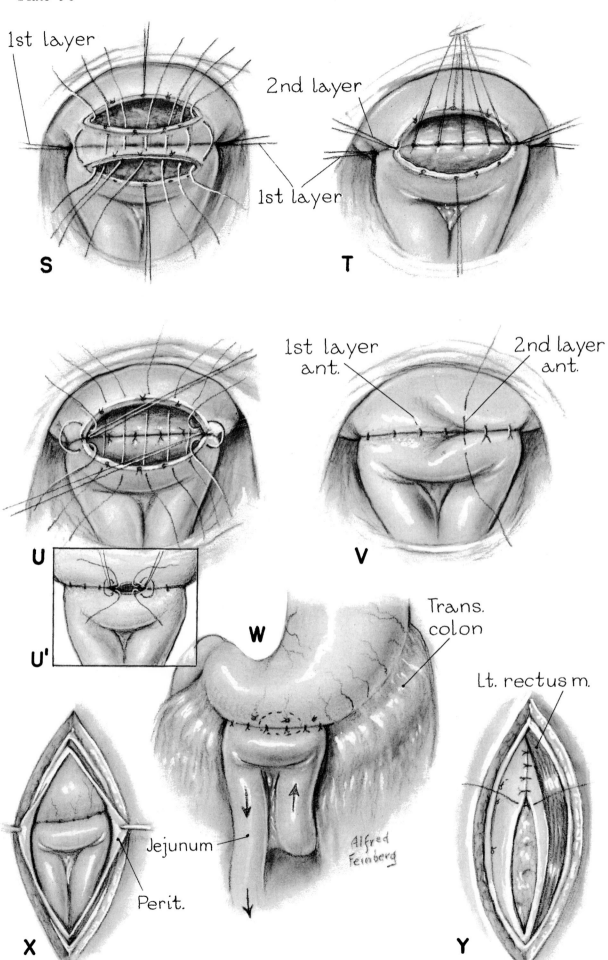

1st layer

2nd layer

1st layer

S

T

1st layer
ant.

2nd layer
ant.

U

V

U'

W

Trans.
colon

Lt. rectus m.

Jejunum

Perit.

Alfred
Feinberg

X

Y

TRANSABDOMINAL RESECTION OF THE VAGUS NERVES, PYLOROPLASTY (HEINEKE-MIKULICZ), AND GASTROSTOMY

A, B, C. The upper left paramedian incision (A) is deepened through the underlying rectus fascia and muscle layer (B) to expose the line of incision in the peritoneum (C).

D, E. The peritoneal cavity is entered, and the wound margins are retracted to expose the stomach and surrounding viscera.

DISCUSSION—DR. JOSEPH A. WEINBERG. The abdominal incision should be one which gives adequate exposure of the high-lying esophageal hiatus and at the same time provides exposure for the pyloroplasty. This may be accomplished with the paramedian incision shown (A, B, C) or with a high transverse abdominal incision with moderate convexity upward extending to the lateral border of the rectus abdominis on each side. The incision used will depend on the type the surgeon is most accustomed to in performing operations in the upper abdominal field. A large-blade retractor designed for use in this area facilitates exposure of the hiatal region without the need for accessory retractors or gauze packs to keep neighboring viscera out of the field.

Although it is common practice to divide the triangular ligament of the left hepatic lobe for exposure of the hiatal area, this maneuver is not only unnecessary but may make control of the hepatic lobe more difficult. With the ligament intact and with suitable retraction, the left hepatic lobe is easily held away from the hiatus without tending to slip back into the field of operation.

The lower mediastinal portion of the esophagus and the vagus nerves are exposed through a transverse incision about 2 cm. in length through the esophageal hiatal membrane just anterior to the esophagus. The index finger is used to enlarge the opening. The esophagus and nerves are brought into view by finger traction, and an empty gutta-percha (Penrose) tube is placed around these

Plate 97

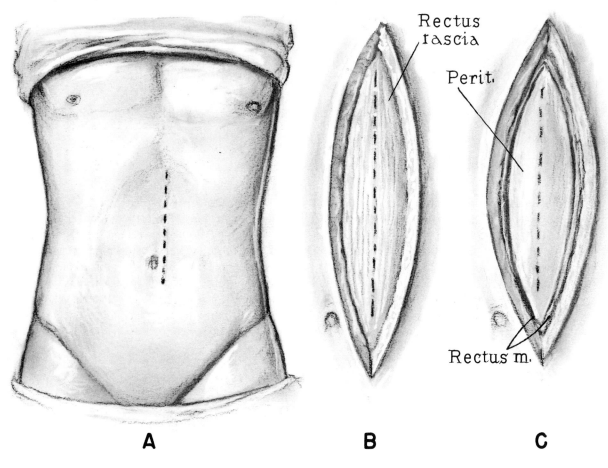

Rectus
fascia

Perit.

Rectus m.

A   **B**   **C**

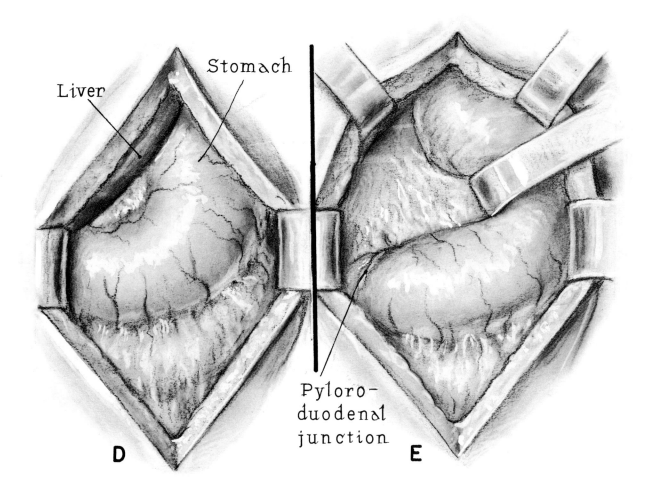

Liver

Stomach

Pyloro-
duodenal
junction

D   **E**

F. The avascular left triangular ligament is severed, and the left lobe of the liver is retracted to show the opening made into the posterior mediastinum and the related structures. Following severance of the left (anterior) vagus nerve, the right (posterior) vagus is mobilized on a nerve hook, and as upward traction is being maintained, it is encircled by the surgeon's right index finger before it is cut.

G. The vagotomy is completed, and clamps (Babcock) are placed on the anterior wall of the stomach for purpose of traction. Guy sutures of silk (0000) are inserted to indicate the center of the anterior surface of the stomach and duodenum, respectively. The longitudinal incision for the performance of a Horsley physiologic pyloroplasty is shown (broken line). Two-thirds of the incision is on the gastric side of the pyloroduodenal junction and one-third on the duodenal side, the length on this side not to exceed 1 inch.

H. The respective lumens of the stomach and duodenum are entered, and the insertion of a figure of 8 suture (00 silk) in the base of the ulcer for hemostasis is completed.

I. The suture ligature is tied, and the start of the pyloroplasty, using the Heineke-Mikulicz principle, is shown. The sutures at each cut margin of the pyloroduodenal junction are inserted from the inside-out to the outside-in (half of a Connell suture), so that, when tied, the knots are on the inside of the lumen.

DISCUSSION—DR. WEINBERG (cont.)

structures for retraction and control during transection of the nerves. The left (anterior) nerve is easily identified in its anterior position in close relationship with the esophagus. The right (posterior) nerve is more difficult to locate because of its loose attachment to the esophagus and its obscured posterior position. The nerves are transected at a level 4 to 6 cm. proximal to the junction of the stomach and esophagus, where they are compact and accessible for complete division. Accessory fibers are searched for and divided as they are exposed. It is not necessary to repair the incision in the hiatal membrane after completing the vagotomy.

The pyloroplasty is performed after completion of the vagotomy unless there is a specific reason for reversing the order. This has the theoretical advantage of avoiding contamination of the mediastinal area by intestinal content, which may escape during the performance of the pyloroplasty. Exceptions to this order are operations for massive bleeding, in which the pyloroplasty is performed first to permit early ligation of the bleeding vessel, and operations in which the preoperative diagnosis is uncertain and the surgeon wishes to inspect the mucosa of the pyloroduodenal segment for further evaluation of the disease. In the latter situation, an unnecessary vagotomy is avoided if there is insufficient evidence of disease to justify its use.

The pyloroplasty which Dr. Madden describes is the preferred emptying procedure with vagotomy for several reasons. It conforms to the physiologic concept of the operation of vagotomy in that the normal continuity of the gastrointestinal tract is retained, no part of the stomach is removed, and

Plate 98   235

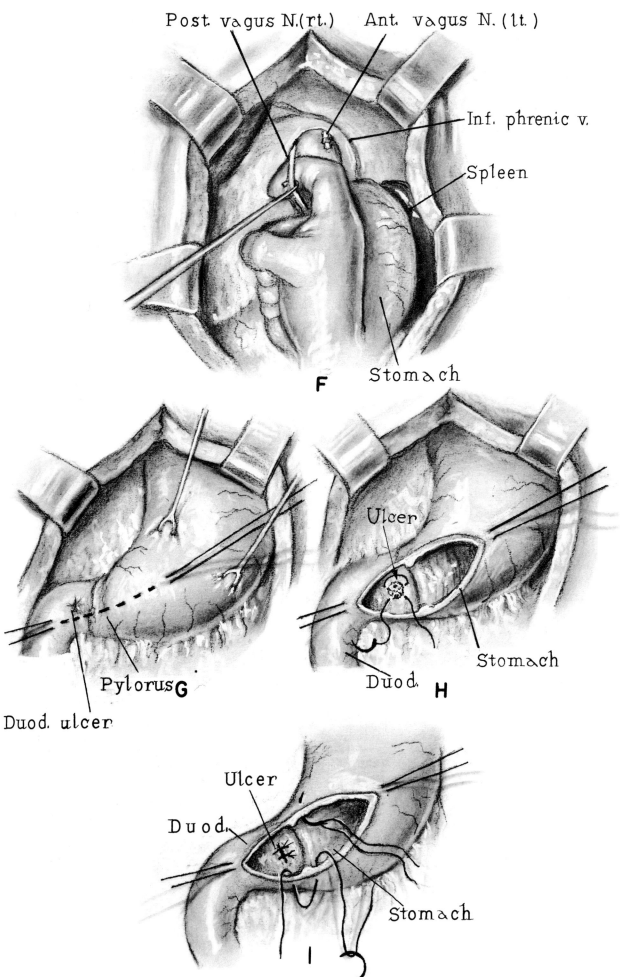

Post. vagus N.(rt.)   Ant. vagus N. (lt.)

Inf. phrenic v.

Spleen

Stomach

F

Pylorus **G**

Duod. ulcer

Ulcer

Stomach

Duod.   **H**

Ulcer

Duod.

Stomach

I

J. The sutures are inserted alternately from either end, and as each one is being tied, traction on the suture previously inserted facilitates the inversion of the cut margins.

K. The sutures terminate in the center of the line of closure and are enclosed by an untied figure of 8 mattress suture of 000 silk. A single-layer closure as depicted is entirely adequate. If preferred, simple through-and-through sutures may be employed with equally satisfactory results.

L, M. The insertion of a second layer of sutures is optional. This consists of a series of interrupted Lembert-Cushing seroserosal mattress sutures of 000 silk, the center one being inserted first (L).

N. The two-layer closure is completed, and the cut margins of the incision into the lumen of the stomach are held apart in Babcock clamps. A complementary gastrostomy is always elective and never performed as a routine.

O. The incision through an opening in the anterior wall of the stomach is closed about a Foley catheter (18 F), using interrupted through-and-through sutures of 000 silk.

P. A second or inverting layer of interrupted Lembert sutures is inserted. The first two sutures are tied, and the third suture is inserted but not tied.

DISCUSSION—DR. WEINBERG (cont.)

the operation is performed with minimal surgical mortality and morbidity because of its simplicity. Also, it permits direct inspection of the pyloroduodenal mucosa for evidence of pathologic changes. In cases in which massive bleeding is the indication for operation, it allows early ligation of the bleeding vessel through the open pyloroplasty wound.

Success with the simple pyloroplasty described here depends largely on an important modification in the method of closing the pyloroplasty wound. The original method of closing the pyloroplasty incision with two or more rows of sutures as described by Heineke and Mikulicz causes an infolding of tissues, which impairs the lumen and impedes the flow through the pyloroduodenal segment. This difficulty is avoided by using a single row of interrupted sutures (J, K, L) instead of the multiple rows (M, N, O, P). The use of a single row of sutures does not add to the risk of postoperative leakage. On the contrary, experience shows that it is at least as safe as multiple-row closure, and probably safer. There has been no clinical evidence of leakage in the more than 1,200 operations I have performed with one-row closure. Nonabsorbable suture material is used rather than gut suture because of the possibility of disruption of the latter by the lytic acid of the digestive juices.

Vagotomy and pyloroplasty combined with ligation is an effective procedure for control of the massively bleeding duodenal ulcer, as shown in I. It has obvious advantages over the more prolonged and traumatizing procedure of partial gastrectomy

Plate 99   237

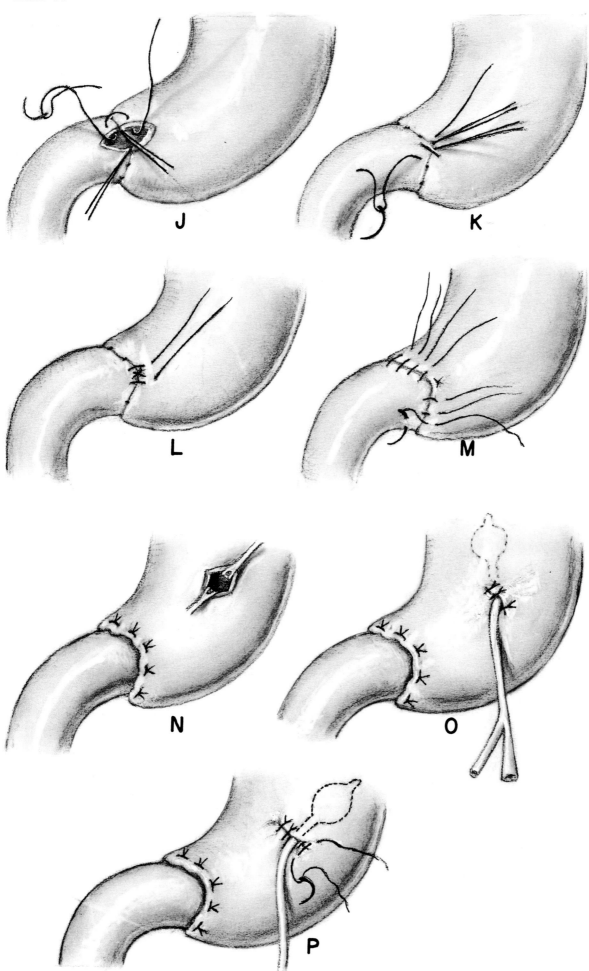

J

K

L

M

N

O

P

Q. The peritoneum is being closed, using a series of interrupted everting mattress sutures of silk (00), which are all first inserted and then tied individually. The gastrostomy tube has its exit through the central portion of the incision. If preferred, it may have its exit through a separate stab wound, and the anterior wall of the stomach may be sutured to the anterior parietal peritoneum around the catheter.

R, R₁, S. The peritoneal closure is completed, and the rectus fascia is closed about the catheter, using interrupted far-near, near-far, mattress sutures of the pulley type.

T, U. The wound is irrigated with copious quantities of hot (112° F.) saline solution (T), and the skin closure is completed about the tube, using interrupted sutures of 00 silk (U).

DISCUSSION—DR. WEINBERG (cont.)

in a situation in which minimal time and minimal trauma are important considerations. The pyloroplasty incision may be somewhat longer than the usual 6 cm. to facilitate exposure of the ulcer. The bleeding vessel is ligated with a nonabsorbable suture threaded on a half-circle needle that is stout enough to resist breakage and small enough for easy manipulation within the limited working space. Success or failure with the ligation depends upon insertion of the suture completely and immediately around the vessel at the site of bleeding. The vagotomy should be performed after the completion of the pyloroplasty in the same operative session. Postponement of the vagotomy may result in rebleeding before the vagotomy is accomplished.

The gastrostomy tube shown in O and P is an excellent means of preventing gastric distention in the first few days after operation. It is my practice to use gastric suction as illustrated here for the first five postoperative days. Nothing is given by mouth during this period. Supportive fluids are given intravenously.

Bland fluids are given orally beginning the evening of the fifth postoperative day, with gradual increase to a liberal diet by the tenth to twelfth day. The prescribed diet is high in proteins, moderately low in fats, and low in carbohydrates, with complete abstinence of free sugar for several months following the operation. This program appears to lessen the possibility of disturbing digestive symptoms in the early postoperative period.

Plate 100   239

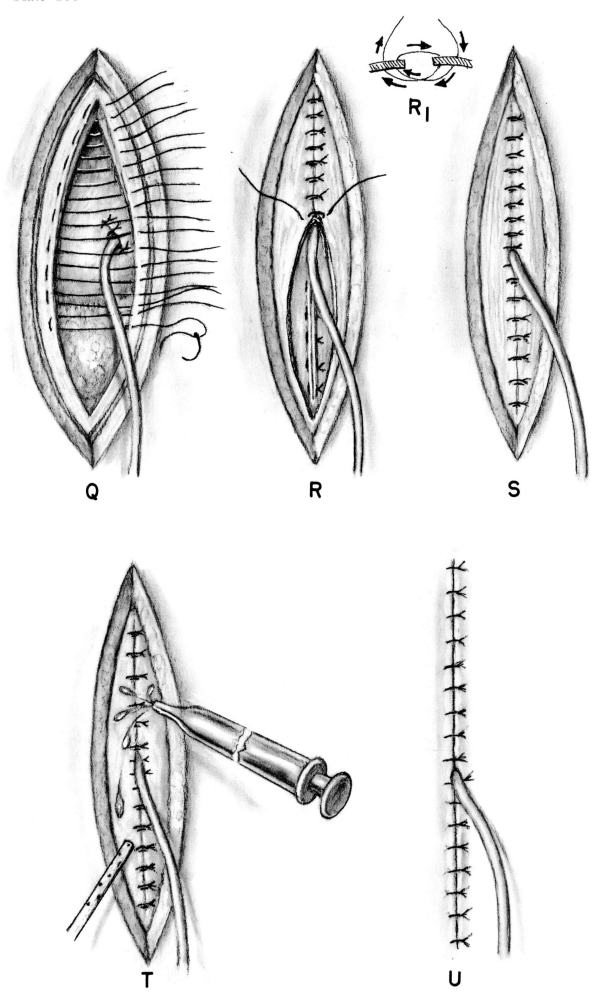

Q

R

R_1

S

T

U

SELECTIVE VAGOTOMY AND SIDE-TO-SIDE GASTRODUODENOSTOMY (JABOULAY)

A. The left paramedian incision routinely employed is indicated by the broken line. A muscle-splitting incision between the inner and middle thirds of the rectus muscle is preferred to the lateral retraction of the whole of the muscle. Admittedly, a muscle-splitting incision is less physiologic, since it destroys the innervation of the inner third of the muscle. However, this has not proved of practical significance. Furthermore, paradoxical as it seems, the strength of the wound closure seems greater with the use of the muscle-splitting incision. A further proposed advantage of the muscle retraction incision is that the rectus muscle serves as a protective "buffer" between the lines of closure of the peritoneum and fascia. However, after a thorough trial of many years with the use of the muscle retraction incision, this advantage is believed more theoretical than real.

B. The peritoneal cavity is entered, and as downward traction with a clamp is maintained on the relatively avascular left triangular ligament, it is severed with scissors. In this dissection, care should be taken to avoid injury to the adjacent inferior phrenic vein.

C. The stomach is retracted manually, and the peritoneum overlying the esophagocardial junction is incised. The relation of the "bare" area, representing the attachment of the left triangular ligament to the inferior phrenic vein, is visible.

D. The index finger is inserted anterior to the esophagus through the esophageal hiatus of the diaphragm into the posterior mediastinum, preparatory to mobilizing the esophagus from its "bed."

DISCUSSION—DR. HENRY N. HARKINS. I have not utilized the Jaboulay side-to-side gastroduodenostomy as a drainage procedure in connection with selective gastric vagotomy or truncal vagotomy. The combination sounds like a good idea in this particular patient, however, and nothing in my animal experiments or clinical experiences, both to be referred to later, would indicate otherwise.

Selective vagotomy was introduced by Jackson of Ann Arbor and Franksson of Stockholm independently in 1947 and by Francis Moore of Boston in 1948. Its early use was, in conformity with standard truncal or Dragstedian vagotomy of that time, performed *without* a drainage procedure. Possibly for this reason the method fell into disuse. It remained for Griffith (1957, 1960) and later Burge (1960), Kraft, Fry, and Ransom (1962), Smith and Farris (1963), Harkins et al. (1963), and others to revive the procedure, but this time *with* a drainage procedure—or, as in most of my patients, with antrectomy.

Stripped to its essentials, the rationale of selective gastric vagotomy is that it is unnecessary to vagotomize the major portion of the intestinal tract below the diaphragm (stomach, biliary tract, pancreas, all of small bowel, and right half of large bowel) merely to vagotomize the stomach. Selective gastric vagotomy is also believed by its advocates to reduce the incidence of certain complications of standard truncal vagotomy, especially diarrhea.

I am convinced that a quantitative assessment of each individual patient is of importance. I depend on a 12-hour night secretion study, with careful control of the position of the tip of the tube, or the augmented histamine test. Such a study will not influence the vagotomy, which should naturally be complete to the stomach, but may influence the choice between an antrectomy or pyloroplasty, as well as help rule out a Zollinger-Ellison ulcer. Also, the physical habitus of the patient, as pointed out by the Ohio State group, may help determine the type of hook-up to be used.

I have now utilized selective gastric vagotomy in about 90 patients. In substance, my technic varies from that of Dr. Madden in details rather than in principle.

I generally prefer a midline incision, believing it is not only more quickly made but more safely closed than paramedian or rectus incisions (this despite the fact that my teacher, Dr. Dallas B. Phemister, taught me to utilize a paramedian incision for most upper abdominal work). I stagger the peritoneal incision so that it is 1 or 2 cm. to the left for gastric cases and 1 or 2 cm. to the

Plate 101

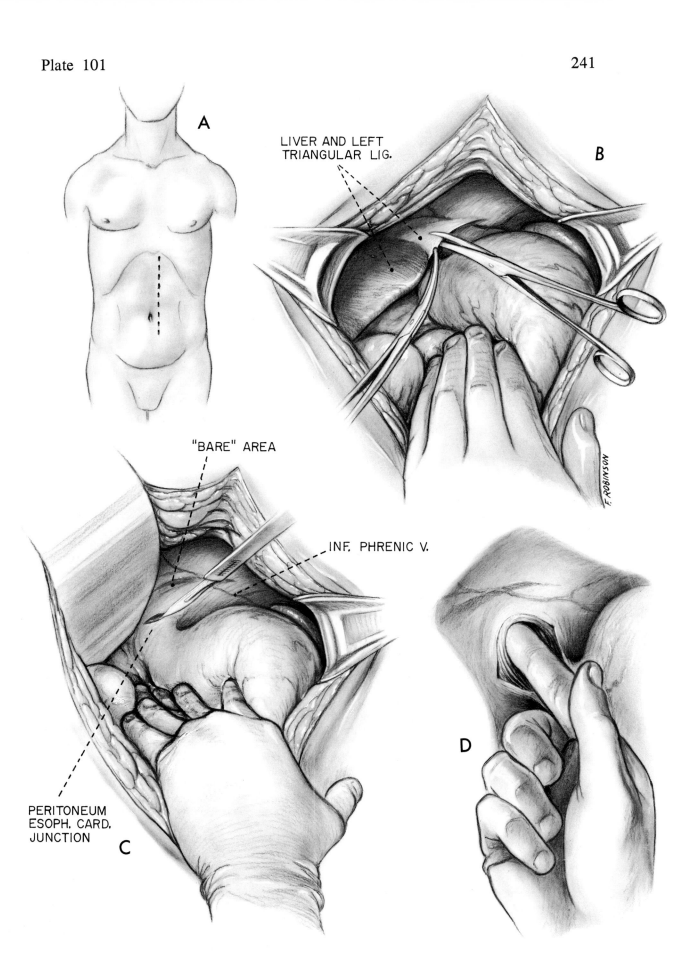

A

B

LIVER AND LEFT
TRIANGULAR LIG.

F. ROBINSON

"BARE" AREA

INF. PHRENIC V.

PERITONEUM
ESOPH. CARD.
JUNCTION

C

D

D₁. The finger is withdrawn through the hiatus and used to compress the lower end of the esophagus and accentuate the left or anterior vagus nerve, which is closely approximated to its anterior wall. The muscular ring of the esophagus, formed by the fibers of the right crus, is partly visible. The muscle fibers forming the right border of this ring are superficial and thin, whereas those of the left border are thicker and on a deeper plane.

E, F. The left or anterior vagus nerve, encircled by a guy suture of silk (00), is ele-

vated from the esophagus by gentle traction (E). The lower end of the esophagus, mobilized on the index finger, is retracted upward to expose the right or posterior vagus nerve, seen elevated on a nerve hook (F). The right or posterior vagus nerve is almost always found in the areolar tissue posterior and medial to the esophagus. Because of this location, it is frequently missed in the performance of a bilateral vagotomy. This nerve is larger than its anterior counterpart and may be more readily identified after the distal portion of the esophagus has been mobilized from its "bed."

DISCUSSION—DR. HARKINS (cont.)

right for biliary tract work. In certain instances of selective gastric vagotomy I utilize the "sabre slash" or long Kocher incision taught to me by Kraft and Fry at the University of Michigan.

I seldom cut the left triangular ligament (nor does Weinberg). If I do, I not only avoid the inferior phrenic vein, as Dr. Madden points out, but also do not cut too close to the liver for fear of sectioning invisible outpouching hepatic ducts, as Wayson (1959) has cautioned.

I usually identify a small gastric vagal branch on the anterior surface of the stomach and clamp it. As I exert gentle downward traction on it, the left trunk becomes tense and can be palpated. Thus, I use palpatory identification for the left trunk. The hepatic branch, usually a series of parallel fibrils, can be identified in almost all patients, even the most obese, immediately on retracting the left lobe of the liver. It is readily visible just under the anterior peritoneal surface of the gastrohepatic omentum. The one exception to this rule of ready visual identification of the hepatic branch is in cases with a previously perforated ulcer or another condition producing an upper abdominal peritonitis. In such instances a selective gastric vagotomy, at least of the left nerve, becomes difficult if not impossible.

The hepatic branch and the left trunk are isolated with a fine drain or suture for gentle traction. The gentleness is important, because I wish to preserve the hepatic branch, both anatomically and physiologically.

I then cut everything to the left of the arc formed by the trunk and the hepatic branch. The left vagotomy is completed by a careful search for

descending accessory branches in the region of the hiatus.

Whereas I identify the hepatic branch by sight, I use palpatory identification of the celiac branch. In fact, I have never seen the celiac branch, but I can always feel it. The index finger is hooked around the left gastric "triad" (my name for it) and pulled caudally. The "triad" is comprised of the coronary vein caudad, the left gastric artery in the middle, and the celiac vagal branch cephalad. This tenses the right vagal trunk ("Griffith maneuver"), which then can be identified by palpation.

This identification of the right vagal trunk is especially important, since in some instances the trunk is not near the esophagus. I believe that missing such an eccentrically placed right trunk (it is usually to the right of the esophagus) is the reason for most of the incomplete standard vagotomies. In my opinion, utilization of the Griffith maneuver lessens the likelihood of an incomplete vagotomy. Despite the voiced objection to selective gastric vagotomy—usually by those who have never performed the operation—that the gastric portion of the procedure, and the most important, will less likely be complete, I believe that actually the opposite is true. (Parenthetically, the mnemonic word "LARP" is a useful help in remembering left-anterior and right-posterior vagi.)

The concept of an "antiselective" vagotomy is important in another context. It should be readily evident from H, I, and J that both the hepatic and celiac branches, which are spared in selective gastric vagotomy, are in an extremely vulnerable position for inadvertent division during the course

Plate 102

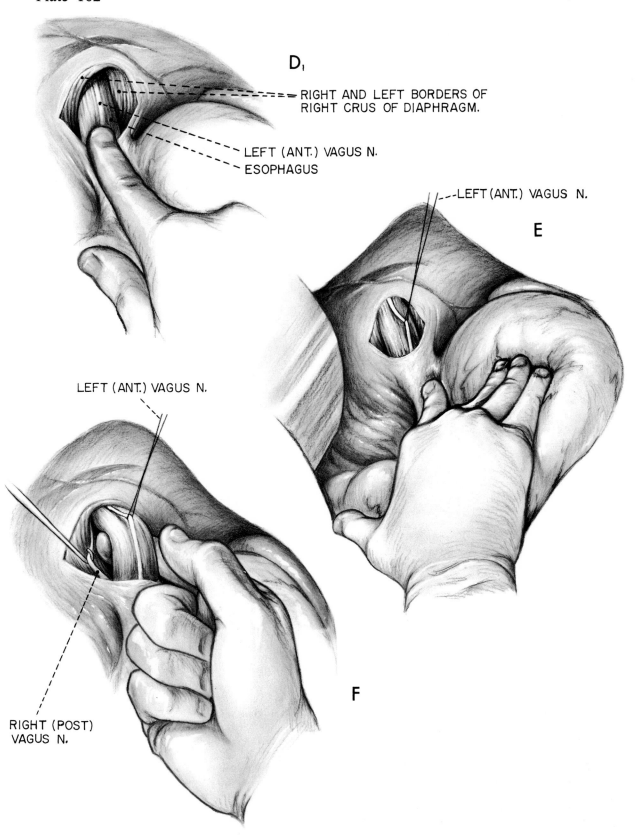

D₁

RIGHT AND LEFT BORDERS OF
RIGHT CRUS OF DIAPHRAGM.

LEFT (ANT.) VAGUS N.

ESOPHAGUS

LEFT (ANT.) VAGUS N.

E

LEFT (ANT.) VAGUS N.

RIGHT (POST)
VAGUS N.

F

G. The vague nerves, each encircled with a guy suture of silk (00), are gently retracted upward. The lesser sac is entered, and the gastrohepatic ligament at the esophagocardial junction is elevated on a clamp (Mixter) and severed, as indicated by the broken line.

H. A branch of the anterior (left) vagus to the esophagocardial junction, elevated on a clamp (Mixter), is transected with scissors. The relatively large hepatic branch, which

may be larger than its parent trunk, is partly visible.

I. The dissection of the anterior (left) vagus nerve is completed, and its branches—the gastric, hepatic, and duodenal—are depicted. The stump of the severed esophagocardial branch is also visible. The gastric and duodenal branches are severed subsequently, but the continuity of the hepatic branch is preserved. The duodenal branch that originates from the hepatic is not always demonstrable.

DISCUSSION—DR. HARKINS (cont.)

of gastric resection. This is particularly true when the surgeon, usually a better surgeon, goes high along the lesser curve. In such instances he may unwittingly section these branches, and hence some of the so-called postgastrectomy syndromes may be due to this iatrogenic, unintentional, antiselective vagotomy, with the possibilities of diarrhea, steatorrhea, etc.

I generally perform an antrectomy with my selective gastric vagotomies. I prefer this technic because of the low (0.5 per cent) secondary stomal ulcer incidence resulting from the combined operation of truncal vagotomy and antrectomy, as compared to many times that figure with truncal vagotomy and simple drainage operations. Assuming, as I do, that selective gastric vagotomy is complete to the stomach about as often as truncal vagotomy (possibly more so), comparable figures should be expected, depending on the type of hook-up selected.

When I do utilize a simple drainage procedure, I perform either a Heineke-Mikulicz or Finney pyloroplasty. It is of interest that Nyhus (1953) was the first to show experimentally on dogs that these two pyloroplasties do not have the harmful antrum-stimulating action of gastrojejunostomy (see also Harkins et al., 1954). Furthermore, the Jaboulay procedure was tested and found to be moderately stimulating, as shown in Table 1, but not when combined with vagotomy.

Table 1. Antrum-Stimulating Action of Different Gastric Drainage Procedures

(Note: The percentage figures indicate Heidenhain pouch secretion increases over control values. Values of ± 15 per cent are not significant.)

Gastrojejunostomy	+167%
Gastrojejunostomy + Vagotomy	+141%
Jaboulay	+ 50%
Jaboulay + Vagotomy	− 11%
Heineke-Mikulicz Pyloroplasty	− 17%
Heineke-Mikulicz Pyloroplasty + Vagotomy	+ 15%
Finney Pyloroplasty	− 14%
Finney Pyloroplasty + Vagotomy	− 10%

An additional point in favor of antrectomy is that one does not need to worry about the pyloric branch (I), irrespective of the uncertainty as to its importance, since it is severed when the antrectomy is performed.

When I close an upper midline abdominal incision (i.e., above the line of Douglas), I never close the peritoneum. Rather, I depend upon the flap of the peritoneum, the use of which was first demonstrated to me by K. H. Giertz (Chief of Surgery at the Sabbatsberg Hospital, Stockholm, and teacher of Clarence Crafoord) on June 6, 1939. I have utilized this technic ever since.

Plate 103   245

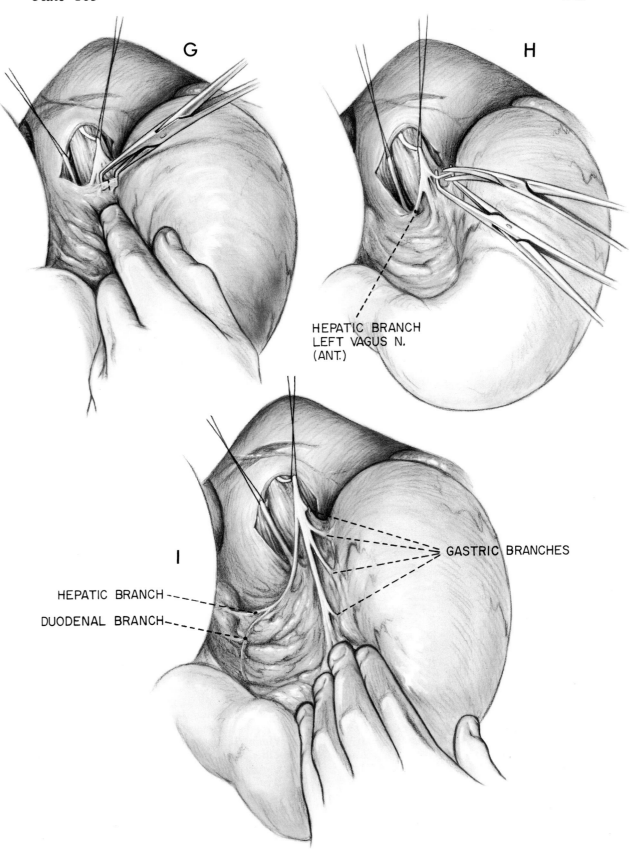

G

H

HEPATIC BRANCH
LEFT VAGUS N.
(ANT.)

I

GASTRIC BRANCHES

HEPATIC BRANCH - - - - - -

DUODENAL BRANCH - - - - - -

J, K, K₁. The transection of the gastric and duodenal branches of the left (anterior) vagus nerve being completed (J), the right (posterior) vagus nerve is withdrawn beneath the left (J) to facilitate the dissection and severance of its gastric branches (K). In this dissection the left gastric artery is a useful anatomic guide. In this patient, a celiac branch from the left vagus united with the normally present celiac branch from the right vagus to form a common celiac trunk (J, K). In K₁ the normal anatomic pattern, a celiac branch from the right (posterior) vagus and none from the left (anterior) vagus, is depicted. The large lymph node that characteristically overlies the hepatic artery at its origin may be seen in each of the illustrations. Also the formation of the esophageal hiatus by the muscle fibers of the right crus of the diaphragm is visible.

DISCUSSION—DR. JACK MATTHEWS FARRIS. Vagotomy combined with some type of drainage procedure in the surgical treatment of duodenal ulcer is gaining stature and may ultimately replace in popularity various types of gastric resection as a primary treatment for this condition. In the minds of many, division of the vagus nerves is a more subtle physiologic approach to the fundamental problem of hypersecretion of gastric juice rather than a more primitive mechanical attack designed to extirpate the end organ (stomach) of a stimulus arising in the central nervous system.

Whether to perform *total* or *selective* vagotomy in many instances becomes an academic question. The factors concerned with the total cure of the ulcer and rehabilitation of the patient are infinitely more important than the theoretic undesirable sequelae presumably due to denervation of the biliary duct system, pancreas, and small intestine in total vagotomy.

My studies indicate that approximately 28 per cent of patients who have undergone total vagotomy show some alteration in their bowel habit, which might possibly be contributed to total vagal denervation. However, most of these patients who have achieved a satisfactory result with cure of their ulcer are reluctant to place any emphasis upon this alteration, and the existence of such a change may at times be elicited only by careful questioning.

At the present time, I feel that if a *selective* vagotomy can be done easily, it may well be the ideal operation. Particularly intriguing is a possibility that preservation of the anterior nerve only (with total division of the posterior nerve) may accomplish the same result as bilateral selective operation. Furthermore, I feel that selective vagotomy should not be done where the operating time is important and certainly not by those who have not had an opportunity to familiarize them-

Plate 104   247

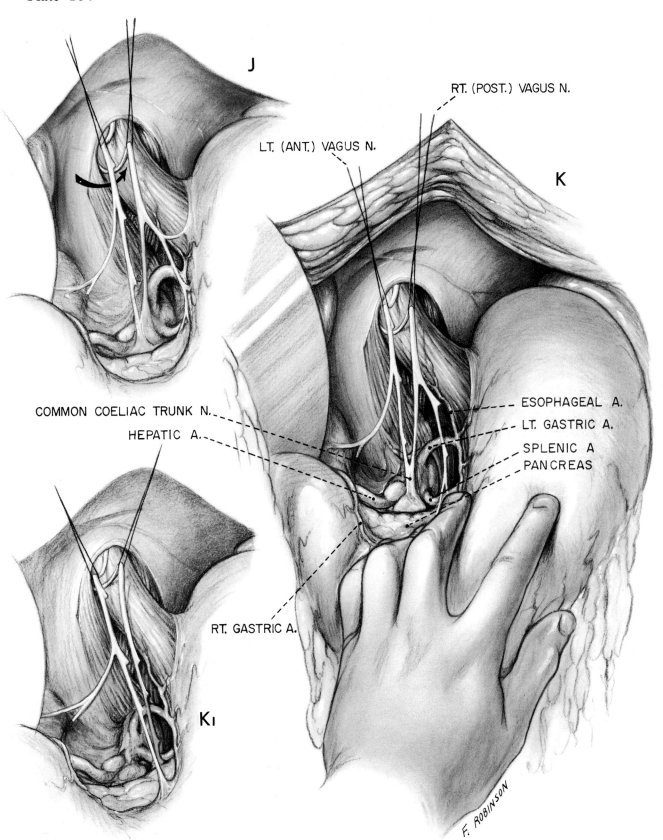

J

RT. (POST.) VAGUS N.

LT. (ANT.) VAGUS N.

K

COMMON COELIAC TRUNK N.

ESOPHAGEAL A.

HEPATIC A.

LT. GASTRIC A.

SPLENIC A

PANCREAS

RT. GASTRIC A.

K₁

F. ROBINSON

L, L₁, M. In this patient the local findings of pyloric obstruction and inflammatory edema precluded the performance of either a Heineke-Mikulicz or Finney pyloroplasty. Admittedly, a gastroenterostomy could have been done, but a gastroduodenostomy was preferred. Prior to its performance, the greater curvature of the stomach in its antral portion is skeletonized by serially clamping and severing the gastrocolic ligament cephalad to the gastroepiploic arch. Next, the posterior parietal peritoneum in juxtaposition to the duodenum is incised, and by blunt digital dissection posteriorly, the duodenum and head of the pancreas are mobilized. A clamp (Babcock) is applied to the pyloroduodenal junction, and guy sutures of silk (000) are placed equidistant on the mobilized duodenum and antrum of the stomach (L_1). By traction on the clamp and sutures, the stomach and duodenum are first triangulated (L_1) and then approximated with interrupted seroserosal sutures (Lembert) of 000 silk (L).

N, O. The seromuscular layer of the anterior wall of the duodenum is incised (N), and the vessels in the submucosal layer are undersewn with sutures of 0000 silk for hemostasis (O).

DISCUSSION—DR. FARRIS (cont.)

selves with the anatomic features of the operation in the laboratory or through experience with the conventional type of total vagotomy. Selective vagotomy is ill advised in a patient who is hemorrhaging or in one whose exposure factors could make completeness and accuracy difficult, with even a remote chance of compromising the result because of incompleteness of the vagotomy.

Where selective vagotomy is done, I prefer the transverse incision to the paramedian vertical incision illustrated in A, although this is not a particularly important point but rather a personal preference. Originally I routinely divided the left triangular ligament, as illustrated in B, but in the past 200 operations I have omitted this maneuver. I have found it completely unnecessary, and in certain instances where the left lobe of the liver is large is may actually increase its mobility to the point where it interferes with visibility of the esophageal hiatus.

The illustrations depicting the gastric branches of the anterior and posterior vagus nerves are excellent but may oversimplify. I would like to emphasize that this operation is infinitely more difficult than total vagotomy. At the present time I believe that the theoretic benefits that might accrue from selective vagotomy are not well documented, and the increased effort involved is therefore not justifiable except in ideal subjects.

Regarding the Jaboulay pyloroplasty, I have found it to be an excellent operation as an adjunct to any type of vagotomy. It actually is a way of performing the most dependent type of gastroduodenostomy possible. At the same time, it is a clever maneuver to make an anastomosis that avoids, in most instances, the area of the duodenum that may be involved in the inflammatory process accompanying a perforating or penetrating duodenal ulcer. It does possess one disadvantage, however: it does not provide an oppor-

Plate 105   249

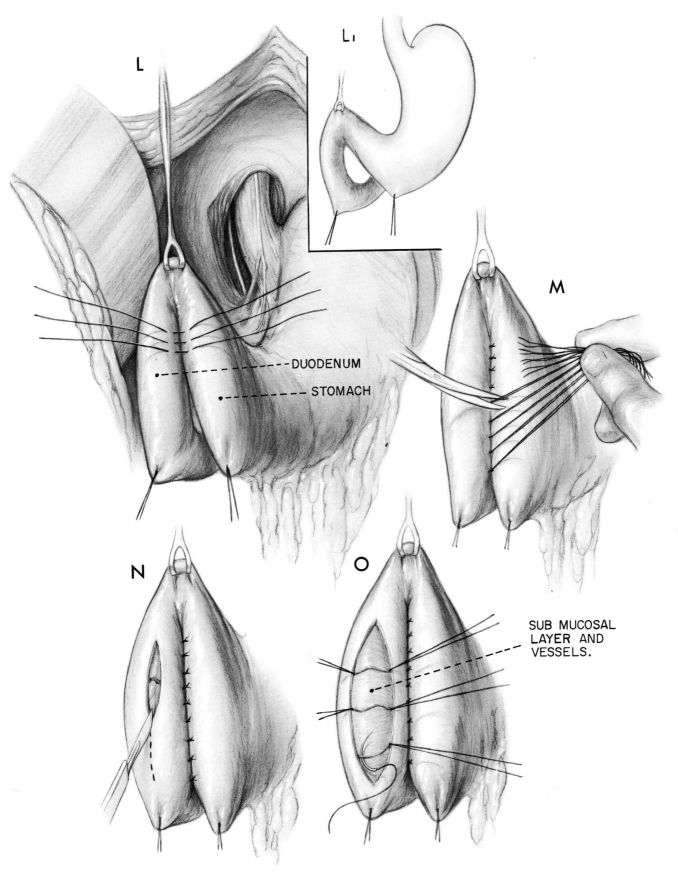

DUODENUM

STOMACH

SUB MUCOSAL
LAYER AND
VESSELS.

P, Q. Similarly, the vessels in the submucosal layer of the gastric antrum are occluded, and the opening previously made into the lumen of the stomach is enlarged by severance of the mucosal layer with scissors (P). In like manner, the lumen of the duodenum is entered (Q).

R, S. The second posterior layer of the anastomosis consists of a series of through-and-through sutures that include all the layers of the stomach and duodenum (R). These sutures are all first inserted and then tied (S).

DISCUSSION—DR. FARRIS (cont.)

tunity to visualize the ulcer crater itself. For those who employ vagotomy and pyloroplasty with suture of the ulcer base for the bleeding duodenal ulcer, the Heineke-Mikulicz type of pyloroplasty will prove to be preferable. This is done through a 10 cm. gastroduodenotomy incision parallel to long axis of the stomach and duodenum followed by reconstruction with a single row of seromuscular sutures applying the well-known Heineke-Mikulicz principle.

The Jaboulay pyloroplasty is, in my opinion, preferable to the Finney type. Converting the two parallel incisions (as shown here) into a horseshoe type of incision (as in the Finney) adds little or nothing to the ability of the stomach to empty.

In a series of considerably over 200 patients who have been treated by vagotomy and pyloroplasty for duodenal ulcer, 76—or about one out of three—were operated upon because of hemor-

rhage. In 50 of these patients the extent of the bleeding qualified as "massive," with hemoglobin levels of 8 g. per cent or less and/or requirements of at least 2000 ml. of blood to restore circulation to normotensive levels. The success depends upon an accurate vagotomy (either a total or selective), a firm ligature of the bleeding vessel, and a good functioning pyloroplasty. Only three deaths occurred in this group, and one of these could have been prevented. Data I have accumulated over a 12-year period indicate that the abnormal cephalic and humoral phases of gastric hypersecretion associated in man with chronic duodenal ulcer may be effectively corrected by vagotomy and pyloroplasty. Cognizance of this experience is important to those dealing with "poor risk" patients, who in the past felt an implied obligation to carry out a more formidable operation, such as extensive subtotal gastrectomy.

Plate 106

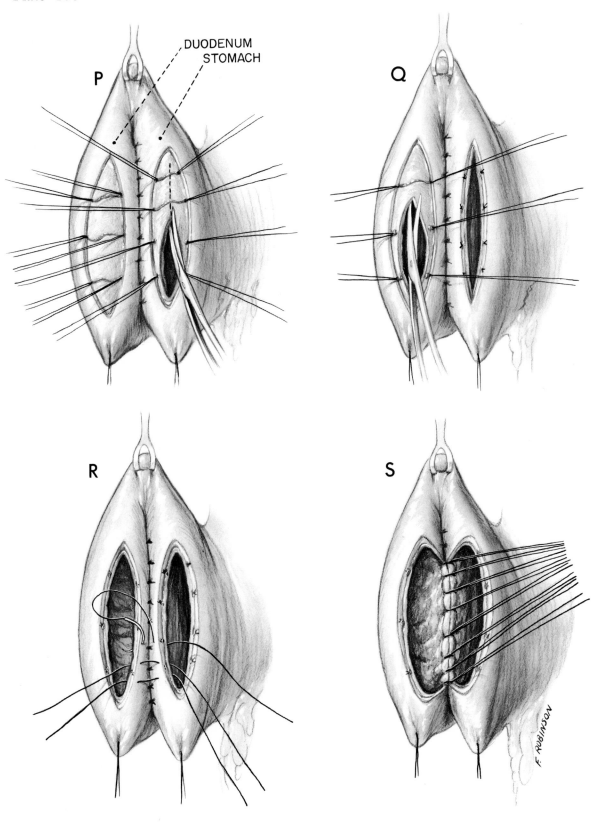

T, U. The sutures of the second posterior layer of the anastomosis are cut, and the clamp (Babcock) and triangulating sutures are removed (T). The first anterior layer of the anastomosis is begun, and at each angle of the anastomosis the suture is inserted from the inside-out on the stomach and from the outside-in on the duodenum, so that, when tied, the knot of the suture is on the inside of the lumen. These sutures effect a neat turn-in at the angles of the anastomosis. Either the remainder of the sutures comprising the first anterior layer may be of the single through-and-through type (T) or the interrupted inverting sutures first described may be continued, alternately from either angle, to terminate in the center of the anastomosis (U).

V. A reinforcing figure of 8 mattress suture (000 silk) is inserted about the terminal 2 center sutures, and, when tied, the first anterior layer of the anastomosis is completed.

W. A series of interrupted seroserosal sutures (Lembert) are inserted to complete the second anterior layer of the gastroduodenostomy.

X. The closure of the skin, using interrupted sutures of silk (000), completes the operation. The underlying peritoneum and fascia layers are approximated with interrupted everting mattress sutures (00 silk) and simple interrupted sutures (00 silk), respectively.

In a review of our own experience in the treatment of duodenal ulcer by vagus resection and gastroenterostomy, a failure rate of about 21 per cent was noted. Also, the incidence of urgent and distressing diarrhea was high (8.8 per cent). Accordingly, when Burge in England and Harkins in the United States reported their experiences with the use of selective vagotomy, the operation was undertaken with enthusiasm. Thirteen patients were operated upon, and within a two-year follow-up study there were four failures, a rate of about 30 per cent. Paradoxically, a persistent and urgent diarrhea occurred in one patient, a complication that was hoped to be avoided by the performance of a selective vagotomy. Time and further experience with this operation will determine its efficacy. Accordingly, it is believed that its use should be continued in various centers until sufficient clinical data are obtained and carefully evaluated. Technically, the operation is more "messy" and more difficult to perform. Although its use is based on excellent physiologic reasoning, a general acceptance of this operation by surgeons is doubted. In the personal experience cited, the early poor results obtained are not encouraging for its continued use.

In conjunction with the selective vagotomy, a side-to-side gastroduodenostomy (Jaboulay) was done because, as previously stated, other types of pyloroplasty were precluded by the local findings. Admittedly, a gastroenterostomy could have been done. However, our experience with gastroenterostomy has been so unsatisfactory as to preclude its use.

In 1923, the late B. O. C. Pribram stated that gastroenterostomy was a disease and not an operation. This statement is substantiated by our own experience, and it is the reason why it is not advocated, even though at times it might appear the preferred operation. It is often stated that gastroenterostomy is still a good operation if performed when properly indicated. The proper indication is repeatedly listed as: an elderly patient, with anacidity and complete pyloric obstruction. However, during the past 10 years gastroenterostomies have been performed in five patients, all over 70 years of age, in each of whom a complicating marginal ulcer occurred within a period of five years. It is believed that both mechanically and physiologically gastroenterostomy is an unsatisfactory operation. Furthermore, it is not believed that its combination with vagotomy can suddenly transform gastroenterostomy from a physiologically unacceptable to a physiologically acceptable and sound operation.

Plate 107

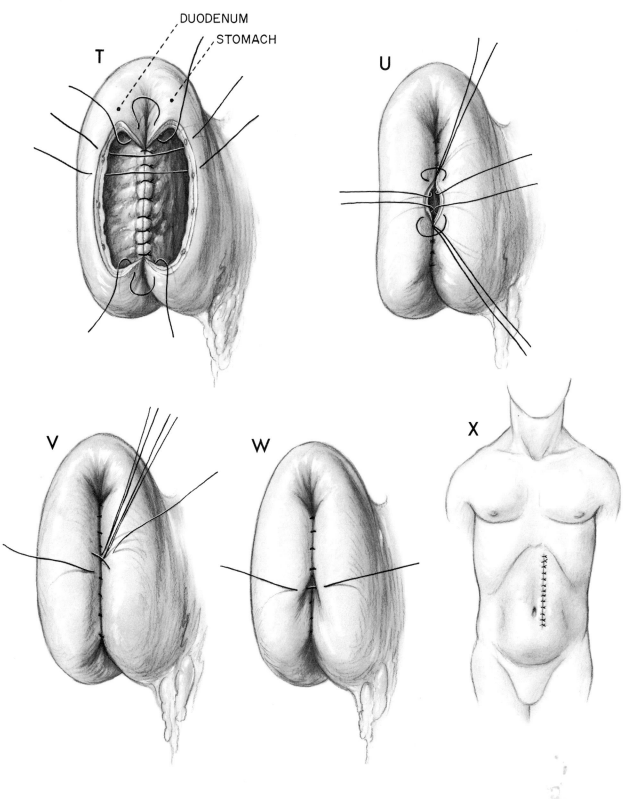

T

DUODENUM

STOMACH

U

V

W

X

DISMANTLING OF GASTROJEJUNOSTOMY AND PYLOROPLASTY (FINNEY)

The patient, a 24-year-old man, was operated upon 16 months previously, at which time an elective vagus resection and antecolic gastrojejunostomy was done for recurrent (two episodes) hemorrhage secondary to a duodenal ulcer. The postoperative course was uneventful until fourteen months preceding the second admission to the hospital, at which time moderately severe gastrointestinal bleeding occurred. The response to conservative treatment was satisfactory. The patient was then well until the day of readmission, when a second hemorrhage occurred, which was severe and characterized by hematemesis, tarry stools, and syncope. Blood replacement was begun, and concomitantly preparations were made for the performance of an emergency operation. The operation disclosed a constriction and a firm cicatrix at the site of the healed duodenal ulcer. This was in marked contrast to the huge inflammatory phlegmon surrounding the pyloroduodenal area at the time of the first operation. On the jejunal side of the efferent angle of the anastomosis there was a moderate degree of edema and induration of the tissues consistent with the presence of a marginal ulcer.

The technic of the operation performed is depicted. The healed ulcer site was too far from the pylorus to effect a satisfactory Heineke-Mikulicz type of pyloroplasty. Also, its close proximity to the common duct did not warrant a partial gastrectomy. Accordingly, a Finney type of pyloroplasty was done. It is now 19 months since the operation, and the patient has remained completely free of symptoms.

A, B. The scar of the previous operation is excised (A), and the peritoneal cavity is entered (B).

C. The indentation beyond the pylorus indicates the site of the healed duodenal ulcer. The stippled area at the efferent angle of the anastomosis (arrow) depicts the location of the anastomotic ulcer.

D. By scissor dissection openings are made through the gastrocolic ligament into the lesser sac on either side of the antecolic gastrojejunostomy. Through these openings cotton tapes are inserted and encircle the stomach for traction. The broken line indicates the incision on the gastric side of the anastomosis anteriorly for dismantling of the gastrojejunostomy. The stomal ulcer in relation to the anastomosis is shown by the stippled area.

E. The anastomosis is dismantled anteriorly, and the separation is being completed posteriorly by scissor dissection.

DISCUSSION—DR. ROBERT M. ZOLLINGER. The cause of recurrent hemorrhage after vagotomy and gastroenterostomy may be drugs rather than failure of the original surgical procedure. Such a possibility should first be ruled out, especially in those patients taking medication, either self- or physician-administered, particularly for the control of the discomfort of migraine, arthritis, or hypertension. Unfortunately, a far more common cause will be iatrogenic, resulting from an overlooked vagus nerve or a gastrojejunal stoma placed so far to the left that the distended post-vagotomy antrum is not properly drained. The location of the gastrojejunal stoma in relation to the antrum as well as proof of a marginal ulcer should be verified by barium studies before operation.

The abdominal scar shown in A should be excised, but the incision should be extended well up into the left xiphocostal angle to insure adequate exposure for evaluation of the completeness of the previous vagotomy. Removal of the xiphoid process will further assist in the exposure over the top of the left lobe of the liver. Sharp dissection should be used to free the adhesions from the liver, lest the capsule be torn and bothersome bleeding develop from the surface of the liver.

In addition to verification of a marginal ulcer, the region of the old duodenal scar should be evaluated to determine the amount of deformity as well as evidence for or against an active duodenal ulcer. Despite the presence of the anticipated mass of adhesions in the region of the esophagus, this area should be re-explored to determine the completeness of the initial vagotomy. The large posterior trunk tends to be pushed away from the esophagus, making careful exploration posterior to the esophagus essential.

The verification of a marginal ulcer makes it mandatory that the gastrojejunal anastomosis be dismantled. The possibility of involvement of the adjacent transverse colon by the inflammatory re-

Plate 108   255

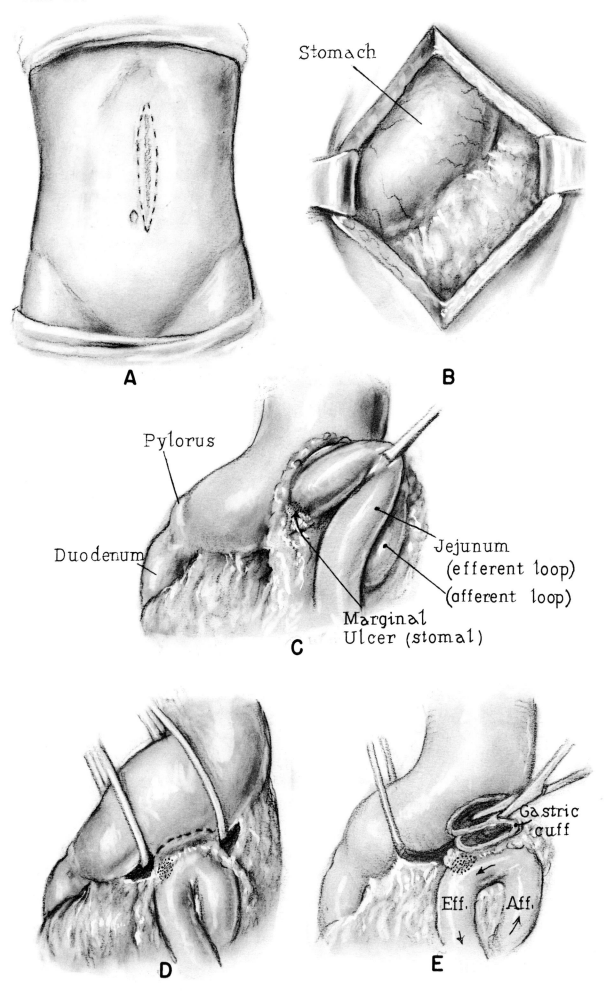

Stomach

A

B

Pylorus

Duodenum

Jejunum
(efferent loop)

(afferent loop)

Marginal
Ulcer (stomal)

C

D

Gastric
cuff

Eff.   Aff.

E

F. G. The opening on the greater curvature of the stomach is closed with a series of interrupted silk (000) sutures, which are inserted alternately from either end and pass from the inside-out to the outside-in, so that, when tied, the knots are inside the lumen (F, G). The final two sutures terminate in the center of the closure and are encircled by a figure of 8 mattress suture of 000 silk (G).

H. After the mattress suture is tied and the strands cut, a second or reinforcing layer of interrupted Lembert-Cushing seroserosal mattress sutures are all first inserted before being tied individually.

I. The gastrorrhaphy is completed, and the jejunum on either side of the enteric stoma is encircled by cotton tapes for traction. The tapes are passed through relatively avascular areas of the mesentery in juxtaposition to the bowel wall. From these sites directional incisions for the application of clamps are made through the peritoneum covering the mesentery.

J. The serial clamping, severance, and ligation of the mesentery and its vessels is completed, and the afferent limb is transected (broken line) between clamps. To avoid excess trauma, the clamp on the proximal side is not locked, the jaws being held only in firm apposition to facilitate the transection.

K, L. The mattress sutures (000 silk) at the mesenteric and antimesenteric border of the bowel lumens are inserted (K) and tied after the completion of insertion of the mattress sutures that form the first posterior layer of the anastomosis (L).

M, N. The mattress sutures, when tied, evert the posterior tissue layers into the lumen of the anastomosis (M). This facilitates the insertion of the second posterior layer, a series of interrupted through-and-through sutures of 000 silk (M, N). The first anterior layer of sutures is begun at either angle of the anastomosis, the sutures being inserted from inside-out to outside-in, so that, when tied, the tissues are inverted and the knots are on the inside of the lumen (M).

O, P. The interrupted inversion (half-Connell) sutures are inserted alternately from either end and terminate in the center of the anastomosis (O). When tied, they are encircled by a figure of 8 mattress suture (P) to reinforce the center of the anastomosis anteriorly.

Q, R. The figure of 8 suture is tied (Q), and the second anterior layer, a series of interrupted seroserosal (Lembert) sutures, is inserted (Q) and tied (R). The closure of the opening in the mesentery (R) completes the anastomosis.

DISCUSSION—DR. ZOLLINGER (cont.)

action or fistula formation should be considered at all times when the stoma is being dissected free (C). I prefer to control the bleeding from the gastric wall by the application of noncrushing clamps of the Scudder type.

After the stoma has been excised on the gastric side, the opening is invariably much larger than anticipated, and the closure results in considerably more deformity than shown in G and H. Less distortion usually results if the opening is closed at right angles to its original long axis similar to a pyloroplasty. The extent of ulceration involving the jejunum is evaluated. It is possible on occasion to close the rather long opening in the jejunum in a transverse direction without resecting the segment. In the presence of distortion of the lumen and in the case of a marked inflammatory reaction in the adjacent mesentery, it may be easier and safer to perform a wedge resection of the area, as shown in I and J. Because of the vascularity in this area and the large size of the bowel involved, little difficulty is encountered in carrying out an end-to-end anatomosis. Straight noncrushing

clamps of the Potts type are applied more on the oblique than shown in Figure J, to insure a larger lumen and a better vascular supply to the antimesenteric border. Contrary to K and R, the mesentery should be approximated before the bowel anastomosis is started, since a hematoma may develop or the blood supply become compromised when the mesentery is approximated after the anastomosis has been completed. Furthermore, the mesenteric border should be cleared of fat for a short distance (approximately 1 cm.) to insure the accurate approximation of the serosa in this critical area by interrupted silk sutures (K). A layer of 00 silk sutures on French needles is preferred for the serosal layer, and the mucosa is approximated with interrupted 0000 silk sutures. The anterior layer is more safely closed by the interrupted sutures with knots tied on the inside (N, O). Additional figure-of-8 sutures are not necessary. The adequacy of the stoma should be tested by palpation.

The possibility of an enteroenterostomy having been previously performed should also be ruled

Plate 109   257

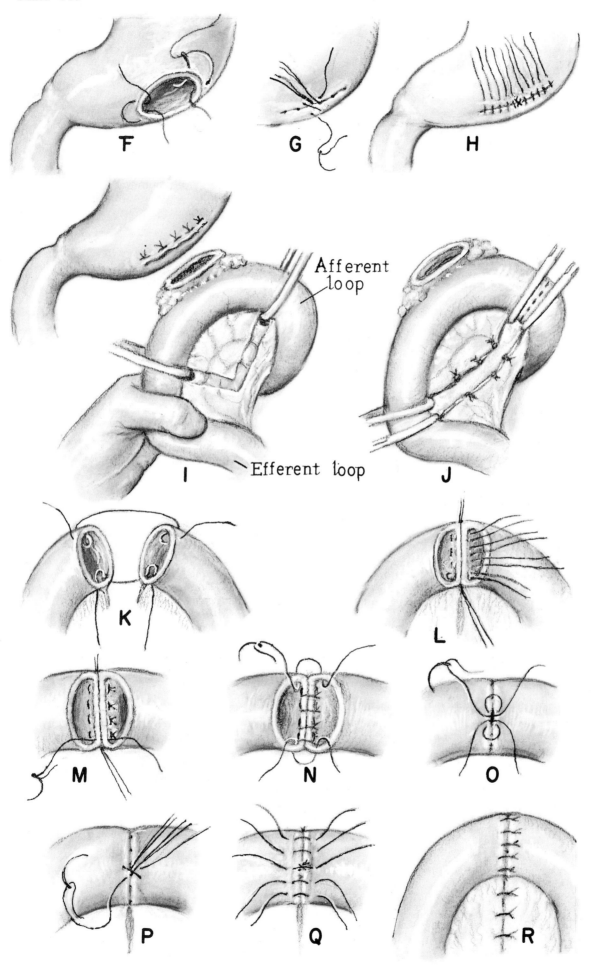

Afferent loop

Efferent loop

S. The indentation deformity of the healed ulcer is visible. The broken line indicates the incision in the posterior parietal peritoneal fusion layer for the mobilization of the retrocolic portion of the duodenum.

T. The duodenum and the head of the pancreas are mobilized and retracted medially to expose the inferior vena cava, which is crossed by an anomalous right renal artery located anterior rather than posterior to the vena cava.

U. The mobilized second portion of the duodenum and the gastric antrum are apposed by triangulating traction guy sutures, and the first posterior layer of sutures (Lembert) is inserted.

V. The sutures are tied, and all but one which is used for traction are severed (U). The inverted-U incision through all the layers of the stomach, pylorus, and duodenum is shown (V).

W. The incision through the anterior wall of the stomach and pylorus is completed, and the incision into the lumen of the duodenum is being completed by scissor dissection.

X, Y. The sutures that form the second posterior layer, a series of interrupted sutures of 000 silk through all the layers of the stomach and duodenum, are inserted (X) and tied (Y). The start of the first anterior suture layer is shown by the inversion sutures inserted at either angle of the anastomosis (Y). The subsequent sutures are inserted alternately from either end and pass from the inside-out to the outside-in, terminating in the center of the anastomosis.

Z, Z′. The first anterior suture layer is completed, and the interrupted Lembert-Cushing seroserosal mattress sutures that form the second anterior layer are all first inserted (Z) and then tied (Z′) to complete the Finney type of pyloroplasty.

It is interesting to note that in the completion of this type of pyloroplasty, the appearance is not that of a side-to-side anastomosis, which one would expect. On the contrary, it appears as if a partial gastrectomy and end-to-end gastroduodenostomy (Billroth I) has been performed.

DISCUSSION—DR. ZOLLINGER (cont.)

out by carefully visualizing the jejunum from the ligament of Treitz to well beyond the gastrojejunal anastomosis.

When the vagotomy has been found to be complete and the gastrojejunal stoma located to the left, a decision must be made as to the type of procedure safest for the particular patient and most likely to prevent recurrent ulceration. In the absence of an ulcerogenic tumor of the pancreas or a parathyroid adenoma, the secondary procedure should be as conservative as possible. Rather than perform a radical gastric resection, a more conservative procedure that insures drainage of the paralyzed antrum should be considered.

Consideration should be given to the re-establishment of a new gastrojejunal stoma within 4 cm. of the pylorus if the previously closed gastrojejunal stoma is far enough away to the left. The blood supply should be cleared from the greater curvature in the immediate prepyloric area, so that the new stoma is placed in the most dependent area of the pylorus. Occasionally the original opening in the jejunum can be used or a new stoma made just beyond the area of resection and anastomosis.

I would agree that a pyloroplasty is the preferred procedure. When the duodenum is mobilized, the middle colic vessels should be carefully swept downward to avoid their injury. To insure the maximum mobilization of the pyloric region, the peritoneal pillar forming the inferior portion of the foramen of Winslow should be divided as part of the complete Kocher maneuver. The second portion of the duodenum should be thoroughly mobilized. A Heineke-Mikulicz rather than a Finney pyloroplasty would be the desirable procedure despite the scarring some distance from the pylorus. There is less bleeding with this procedure, and it is not necessary to provide a large pyloric outlet. The omentum about the inner curvature of the first part of the duodenum can many times be cleared sufficiently to provide unexpected mobility of the duodenal wall. One suture includes the pyloric vein as near the greater curvature side as possible, and the blood supply is further controlled by another suture across the pyloric ring at the lesser curvature side. The incision is made on the gastric side of the pylorus first and curved across the thickened pyloric ring rather near the greater curvature side. The duodenum should be divided beyond the point of constriction by the ulcer. Usually an equal distance on either side of the pylorus is divided and active bleeding points ligated with 0000 silk. The opening is closed in a transverse direction to the long axis of the original opening. Inversion sutures similar to those shown in Y and Z are satisfactory. A two-layer closure is used, although some prefer only one.

The patient's postoperative comfort is enhanced and the several suture lines best protected if a temporary gastrostomy is provided. During the 10 or more days the tube is in place, the completeness of the vagotomy is checked by 12-hour overnight secretion studies. Frequent residuals after an adequate diet has begun should also be taken before the tube is removed.

Plate 110   259

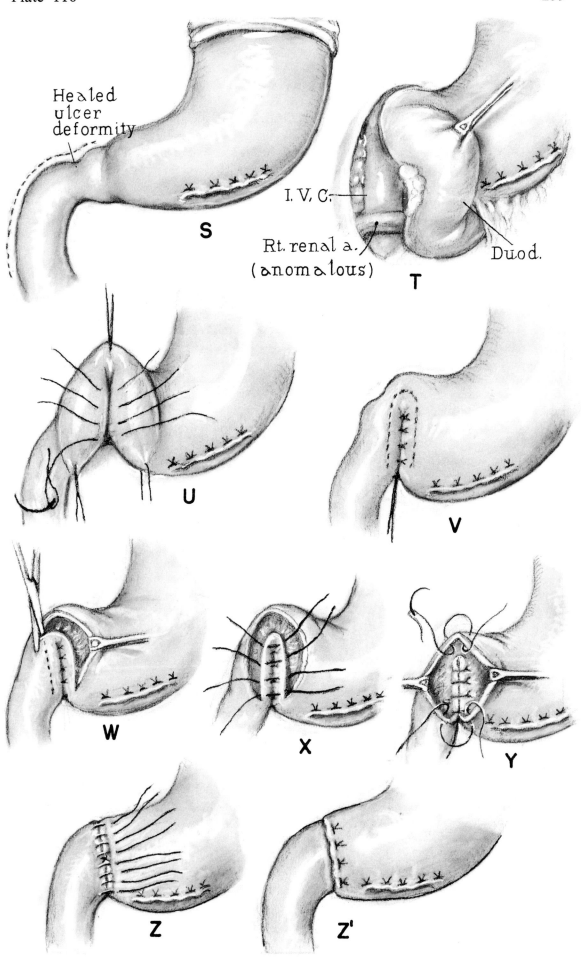

Healed
ulcer
deformity

I. V. C.

Rt. renal a.
(anomalous)

Duod.

S

T

U

V

W

X

Y

Z

Z'

PARTIAL GASTRECTOMY WITH END-TO-END GASTRODUODENOSTOMY (BILLROTH I)

A, B, C. The peritoneal cavity is entered through a right paramedian muscle-retracting (lateral) incision. Whenever concomitant severance of the vagus nerves is contemplated, and in gastric resections performed for carcinoma of the stomach, a left paramedian muscle-retracting incision is preferred.

D. The ascending colon is mobilized and the hepatic flexure is freed by incising the right phrenocolic ligament as indicated by the dotted line.

E. The ascending colon and the hepatic flexure are displaced downward and to the left to expose the retrocolic portion of the duodenum. The gallbladder and the common bile duct are also visible. The curvilinear dotted line indicates the site of the incision (Kocher) which is made in the posterior parietal peritoneum for the mobilization of the duodenum and the head of the pancreas.

F. The mobilized segment of the duodenum is displaced upward and to the left to show the inferior vena cava and its tributary, the spermatic (or ovarian) vein. The lymph node lateral to the distal portion of the common bile duct and posterior to the first part of the duodenum is a constant anatomic finding. The terminal portion of the common bile duct is located between this node laterally and the gastroduodenal artery medially which are the anatomic landmarks emphasized by Cattell for the identification of the distal portion of a previously severed bile duct.

DISCUSSION—DR. S. ARTHUR LOCALIO. The mobilization of the duodenum is of critical importance in the performance of an end-to-end gastroduodenostomy after an adequate partial gastrectomy. However, we have not found it necessary to mobilize the hepatic flexure of the colon as illustrated by the author. The peritoneum lateral to the duodenum from the foramen of Winslow to the superior mesenteric vessels may be readily incised and the duodenum elevated from the inferior vena cava. Exposure of the common duct is done from the cystic duct down to the point at which the common duct passes behind the lateral sweep of the duodenum. If the duodenum is rolled medialward, the duct will be seen to enter the pancreatic head and disappear from view, well protected by the pancreas, until it enters the ampulla about three inches from the pylorus on the posteromedial wall of the duodenum. The knowledge of these anatomic relations is important for the safe mobilization of the duodenum from its surrounding attachments.

In mobilizing the greater curvature of the stomach, the clear area devoid of blood vessels between the left gastroepiploic artery and the first short gastric vessel is an important landmark because it is the point of proximal transection of the stomach in the performance of a 65 to 75 per cent gastric resection. One or two of the short gastric vessels are severed to permit the mobilization of the proximal portion of the greater curvature of the stomach.

On the lesser curvature side of the stomach an attempt should be made to ligate the left gastric artery in its course across the dome of the lesser sac before it has divided into ascending and descending branches. The existence of two left gastric arteries, as illustrated (N'), is an unusual anomaly.

A method, which can be used as an alternate to that depicted (Plate 113, N–Q) in handling the lesser curvature, is believed of value particularly in the patient with a high lying lesser curvature ulcer. In the use of this alternate method, Kocher clamps are applied to the greater curvature of the stomach in the bare area above the entrance of the left gastroepiploic artery. The width of the bite of the Kocher clamp should approximate the width of the duodenum so that there will be a minimum of disparity in diameter between the transected ends of the stomach and duodenum at the site of anastomosis. The gastric incision is now carried cephalad across the anterior and posterior walls of the stomach to a point on the lesser curvature one to two cm. below the esophagus. This maneuver permits the resection of a high-lying lesser curvature ulcer. It also adds to the mobility of the remaining gastric pouch and tubes the stomach, making the gastroduodenostomy a simpler anastomosis. In the performance of this particular step in technic, the Von Petz clamp is of value.

In the performance of the anastomosis (Plate 115, V–X"), the surgeon must use care in closing the lesser curvature corner at its point of junction with the duodenum. This angle is best sealed by a simple seromuscular purse-string suture that includes the anterior and posterior walls of the stomach and the duodenum.

Plate 111   261

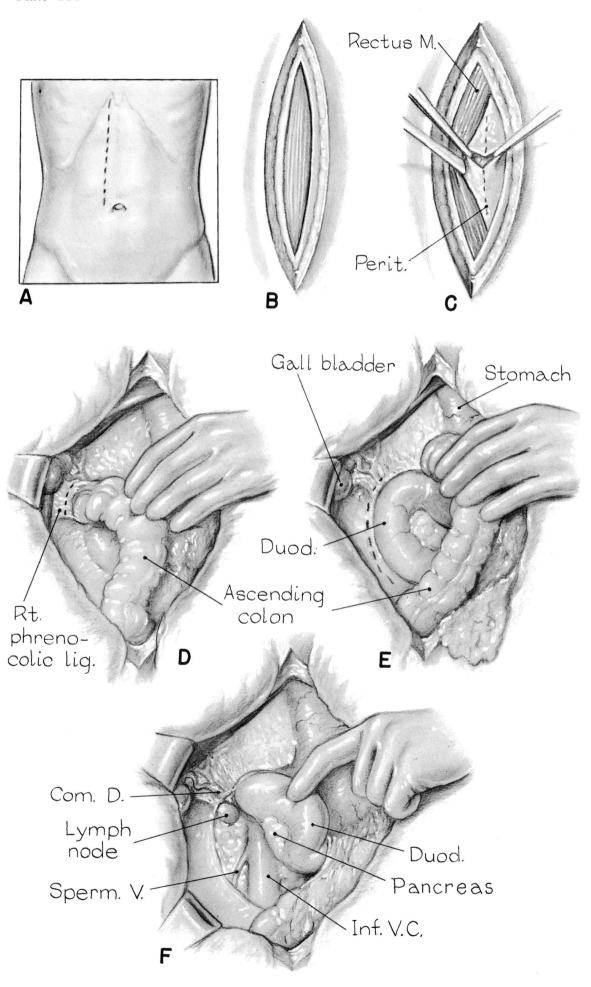

A

B

C

Rectus M.

Perit.

Gall bladder

Stomach

Duod.

Ascending colon

Rt. phreno-colic lig.

D

E

Com. D.

Lymph node

Sperm. V.

Duod.

Pancreas

Inf. V.C.

F

G, H. By blunt dissection with a clamp, an opening is made in the relatively avascular gastrohepatic ligament (G) through which the left index and middle fingers of the surgeon are inserted into the lesser sac. By blunt digital dissection in the lesser sac the posterior wall of the stomach is separated from the often adherent transverse mesocolon, and the index finger is seen to protrude through an opening in an avascular area of the gastrocolic ligament (H). This method of entrance into the lesser sac is preferred to the approach through the gastrocolic ligament because it is believed to lessen the possibility of injury to the middle colic artery with resulting segmental compromise of the circulation to the transverse colon.

I. The greater curvature of the stomach is mobilized by serially clamping and severing the gastrocolic ligament.

J, J'. The stomach is encircled by a catheter (No. 14 F) through which it is elevated by upward traction to expose the pancreas and the thin fibroareolar adhesions between the anterior surface of this organ and the stomach (J). Just beneath the inferior border of the pyloroduodenal junction, the gastroduodenal artery and its two branches, the superior pancreaticoduodenal and the right gastroepiploic arteries, may be seen. This is represented diagrammatically in J'.

The short solid black line just distal to the bifurcation of the gastroduodenal artery (J') indicates the site of severance of its superior pancreaticoduodenal branch.

K. By traction through the catheter the stomach is displaced downward, and through an opening in the gastrohepatic ligament, the right gastric artery and the branch from it to the duodenum are clamped preliminary to being severed and ligated.

L. The stomach is rotated upward and retracted cephalad, and the fibrous tissue attachments of the gastric ulcer on the posterior wall of the stomach to the anterior surface and superior border of the pancreas are being severed by scissor dissection. In this particular patient two left gastric arterial branches arising separately from the celiac axis were present as depicted. The arch formed by the bifurcation of the hepatic artery into its hepatic propria and gastroduodenal branches is clearly illustrated. This arch is an important landmark for the identification of the portal vein which passes obliquely upward beneath the arch and is covered by fatty areolar tissue. A large lymph node overlying the hepatic artery in the region of its bifurcation is a constant anatomic finding. The splenic artery and the ligated and severed ends of the superior pancreaticoduodenal artery are also visible.

DISCUSSION—DR. STANLEY O. HOERR. The principles to be followed in a gastric resection for a gastric ulcer and subsequent anastomosis are three: (1) the resection should include enough margin of normal stomach about the ulcer to suffice if later pathologic sections show malignancy, (2) blood supply at the anastomosis should be unimpaired, and (3) the anastomosis must be free of tension. The technic illustrated is a perfectly safe and satisfactory one and correctly emphasizes gentle handling of tissues. Nevertheless, many safe variations are possible and may be dictated by circumstance in the individual patient or personal preference of the surgeon.

I employ a midline incision rather than a muscle-retracting one. This permits surgery on either side (that is, incidental cholecystectomy for stones or mobilization of the spleen) to be performed with equal facility. A self-retaining retractor of the Balfour type may be used instead of manual retraction. Mobilization of the duodenum (E) should be done routinely, but it is not necessary to dissect out the vena cava, the lymph node near common bile dust, etc. (F). Frequently the finger may be introduced gently through the avascular gastrohepatic ligament rather than creating an opening with an instrument, but elevation of the stomach with a catheter (J, K) rubber drain, or

narrow-gauge sponge, contributes materially to the exposure and ease of surgery. In some patients it may be easier to remove the appropriate segment of greater omentum with the stomach rather than dividing it as in I. If a segment of greater omentum is not removed en toto, it is often possible to avoid clamping and tying the many branches at the greater curvature by finding two or three key vessels several inches away from the stomach. Removal of the greater omentum, however, does not contribute to a safer cancer operation for a lesser curvature malignant ulcer.

Though there can be no objection to dividing the duodenum without a distal clamp (M, M'), the duodenum may be divided between Kocher clamps and the crushed area preserved for hemostasis. (It is surprising how often bleeding will occur at the crushed edge after removal of the clamp, especially when used on the stomach.) However, an outer layer of sutures must be securely placed in sound tissue beyond the crushed tissue.

I personally prefer to perform a mass ligation of the left gastric vessels, with the stomach retracted to the patient's left, and cephalad rather than the procedure shown in R. In the obese patient, the thumb and forefinger of the surgeon's left hand may be used to pinch tissue together at the very

Plate 112   263

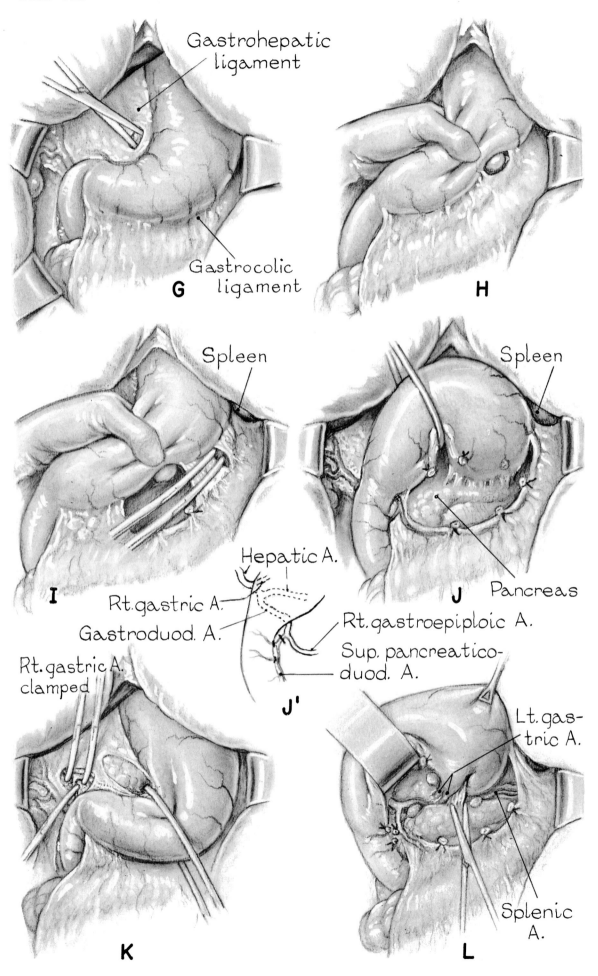

Gastrohepatic ligament

Gastrocolic ligament

G

H

Spleen

Spleen

I

J

Pancreas

Hepatic A.

Rt. gastric A.

Gastroduod. A.

Rt. gastroepiploic A.

Sup. pancreatico-
duod. A.

J'

Rt. gastric A.
clamped

Lt. gas-
tric A.

K

Splenic
A.

L

M. The pyloroduodenal region of the stomach is cross-clamped with a small Payr clamp, and two Babcock clamps are used to immobilize the duodenum as its anterior wall is transected with a scalpel. To avoid unnecessary tissue trauma the distal transected end of the duodenum is not cross-clamped.

M′. Inset to show the transection of the posterior wall of the duodenum with scissors rather than a scalpel. To prevent cutting the posterior wall shorter than the anterior, the scissors are inclined upward toward the stomach as the transection is continued.

N. The lumen of the distal transected end of the duodenum is occluded temporarily with Babcock clamps and the proximal cross-clamped end is covered by a moist gauze pad and reflected upward toward the patient's left shoulder. This upward displacement of the distal portion of the stomach exposes the gastropancreatic fold of peritoneum which contains the left gastric vessels. An opening is made in this fold, and one of

the two left gastric arteries previously mentioned is shown elevated on a clamp. The relation of the ulcer on the posterior wall of the stomach to this vessel is visible.

N′. Inset showing the uppermost of the two left gastric arteries being doubly clamped distal to the previously applied ligature (00 silk). Either the triple clamp method or the preliminary ligature and two clamp method as illustrated is used routinely for the severance of the left gastric artery.

O. The proximal portion of the lesser curvature of the stomach is cleared in preparation for the subsequent anastomosis to the duodenum by the resection of segments of the ascending and descending branches of the left gastric artery.

P, Q. The resulting "bare" area of the lesser curvature is reperitonized by interrupted seromuscular sutures (Lembert) of silk (000) which are first all inserted (P) and then tied (Q).

DISCUSSION—DR. HOERR (cont.)

edge of lesser curvature stomach wall, aiding him in finding an avascular plane between stomach and left gastric vessels for the placement of the clamps. Such mass ligation should always be double on the "business" side (toward the coeliac axis); doubled 00 silk is a sufficiently strong and convenient suture material.

While cutting the stomach without the use of clamps is artistic (although bloody), I personally use two large Kocher clamps placed along the greater curvature, the "bite" corresponding to the estimated width of the duodenal stump. A scalpel divides the stomach between these two clamps, and then two more Kocher clamps, or somewhat longer specially designed angled clamps, may be used pointing cephalad to include as much of the lesser curvature as is desired above the ulcer. The lesser curvature is then closed to accomplish the same purpose shown in V and V′. I believe it is possible to preserve more stomach along the greater curvature—always desirable—by this maneuver.

The posterior outer suture line between the gastric stoma and duodenum (V″) is ingenious and one I have never seen used. The theoretical

disadvantage of having the external row of sutures enter the lumen is neutralized by the very close and accurate approximation of the seromuscular layers it permits. This technical trick is worth noting and remembering for this and other possible applications.

Experience with one-layer pyloroplasty has given me the courage to utilize a single anterior layer of sutures—through seromuscular layers of stomach and duodenum—rather than the conventional two-layer technic. The operation is thereby shortened, and the lumen of the anastomosis may be a little larger since there is no infolding.

If a true midline incision has been made, there will be only one deep layer of the wound to close, and for this the buried mass suture of No. 30 or 31 stainless steel wire, introduced by Dr. Thomas E. Jones years ago, is probably safer, easier and quicker than other technics.

Dr. Madden undoubtedly agrees [undoubtedly —J.L.M.] that if any degree of tension is present in the completed anastomosis, the duodenal stump should be closed and a Billroth II type of gastrojejunostomy constructed instead of a Billroth I.

DISCUSSION—DR. H. WILLIAM SCOTT. Dr. Madden has depicted the technical steps of a method of very high subtotal gastrectomy that, in my opinion, has rather limited application in modern surgical practice. Such a procedure is physiologically poorly conceived in the treatment of duodenal ulcers and unnecessarily radical in the treatment of the great majority of benign gastric ulcers.

Most of the latter are located in the antrum along the lesser curvature and are readily managed by resection of the antrum with the contained ulcer without reducing the parietal cell mass and sacrificing the bulk of the gastric reservoir as does the operation indicated in these sketches. For these common gastric ulcers I prefer the Schoemaker modification of the Billroth I technic—a pro-

Plate 113   265

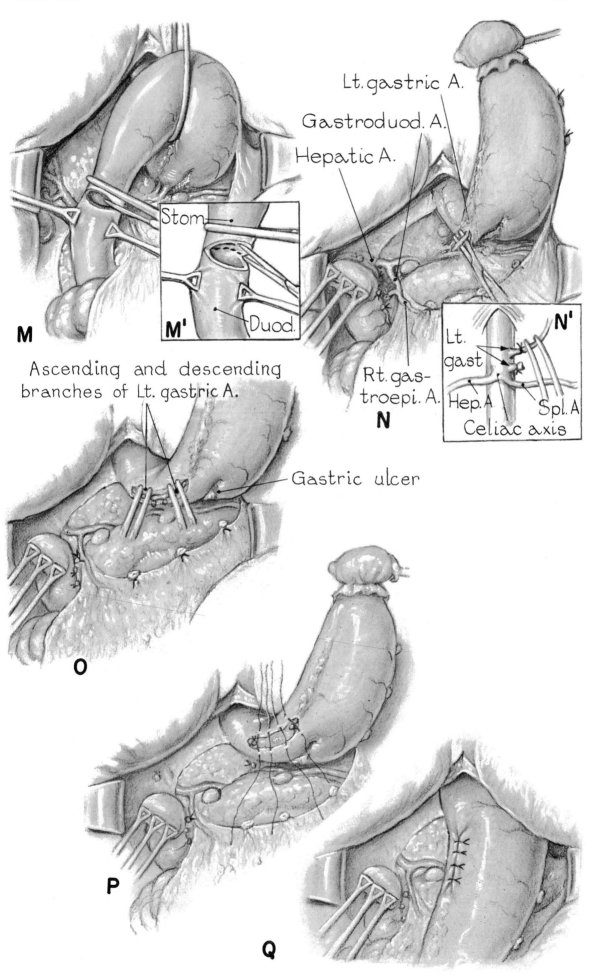

M'

Stom

Duod.

M

N

Lt. gastric A.

Gastroduod. A.

Hepatic A.

Rt. gas-
troepi. A.

N'

Lt.
gast

Hep. A

Spl. A

Celiac axis

Ascending and descending
branches of Lt. gastric A.

Gastric ulcer

O

P

Q

R. Further mobilization of the proximal portion of the greater curvature of the stomach is obtained by serially clamping and severing the gastrosplenic ligament which contains the vasa brevia.

S. Guy sutures of silk (000) are inserted at opposite sites on the lesser and greater curvatures just proximal to the site of election for transection of the stomach. The stomach is then cross-clamped distally with a large Payr clamp. An incision is made through the seromuscular layer of the proximal portion of the stomach anteriorly, and the vessels in the submucosal layer are undersewn with suture ligatures of silk (000).

T. The stomach is displaced upward, and similarly an incision is made through the seromuscular layer of the proximal portion of the stomach posteriorly, and the underlying vessels are undersewn with suture ligatures of 000 silk. The ulcer on the posterior gastric wall is now clearly visible.

U. The stomach is reflected downward, and the incision through the submucosal and mucosal layers anteriorly is being made with a scalpel. Similarly this incision will be continued posteriorly to complete the partial resection of the stomach. It may be observed that to avoid crushing trauma to the tissues, no clamps are applied to the proximal segment of the stomach which will be anastomosed to the duodenum.

DISCUSSION—DR. SCOTT (cont.)

cedure that also lends itself readily to resection of most high gastric ulcers, which are also usually located on the lesser curve.

Since 10 to 12 per cent of ulcerating lesions of the stomach that resemble benign gastric ulcers prove to be malignant, one must obviously be suspicious of carcinoma in every ulcerated gastric lesion; the gross characteristics of the ulcer should be assessed with this suspicion in mind. A high, large posterior wall lesion of the type depicted in the sketches is certainly to be considered malignant until proved otherwise. Accordingly, with such an ulcer I would very early in the operation place a generous gastrotomy incision in the anterior wall of the body of the stomach and obtain a clear view of the ulcer and a transgastric biopsy of each of its quadrants. If a frozen-section report by a well-qualified pathologist indicated carcinoma, then an extended total gastric resection with removal of the tail of the pancreas en bloc would be the chosen procedure, rather than the operation illustrated.

If, on the other hand, the ulcer is benign, alternatives to high subtotal gastrectomy may be used. These include segmental or wedge resection of the ulcer coupled either with vagotomy and pyloroplasty, as recently recommended by Farris, or with resection of the antrum, as supported by Dragstedt. Various abdominal incisions can be used in approaching a high posterior wall gastric ulcer, but the possibility of malignancy in such a lesion prompts me to prepare in every instance so that a thoracoabdominal exposure can be obtained if radical total gastrectomy proves necessary.

I use a midline linea alba-splitting incision in most operations for peptic ulcer in patients with average habitus, and if the lesion proves to be a carcinoma, I extend this incision across the left costal margin into the sixth, seventh, or eighth interspaces, with division of the diaphragm and wide thoracoabdominal exposure. In a very obese individual with a wide costal angle, the oblique upper abdominal incision carried into the chest across the left costal margin provides excellent exposure of high gastric lesions. Needless to say, careful exploration of the abdominal contents prior

to beginning the technical steps of a planned operation on the stomach is an integral part of good procedure. Certainly wide "Kocherization" of the duodenum, as indicated in the sketches, is desirable if gastroduodenostomy is to be done whether after high subtotal gastrectomy or after antral resection. However, I doubt if one often needs to take down the hepatic flexure to accomplish this maneuver.

If the surgeon has satisfied himself that the high gastric ulcer is benign and is bent on doing the radical procedure illustrated in treating a benign ulcer, the next technical step is mobilization of the lesser and greater gastric curvatures. The method illustrated is sound and is designed to avoid injury to the middle colic vessels in the transverse mesocolon. Downward traction on the transverse colon during mobilization of the greater curve provides an additional protective factor. The steps in the mobilization and division of the duodenum are clearly and accurately depicted. When mobilizing the duodenum for a duodenal ulcer, I prefer transecting the stomach above and using the distal part of the stomach as a handle during the duodenal dissection. This is much less essential in dealing with a gastric ulcer, but it not only facilitates dissection of the duodenum but also permits easy placement of a posterior layer of seromuscular sutures between the proximal stomach and the duodenal wall before the duodenum is transected—a step that Dr. Madden apparently does not use in his method of gastroduodenostomy.

The method of dividing the duodenum and elevating the stomach with traction does indeed facilitate the freeing and division of the proximal gastric attachments and permits ligation and division of the left gastric artery at its origin—a step that is important in a cancer operation but in my opinion usually unnecessary in dealing with benign gastric ulcer. Division of the ascending branches of the left gastric vessels coupled with extensive interruption of the short gastric branches of splenic origin will cause great reduction in blood supply of the proximal gastric stump in subtotal gastrectomy and may occasionally result in ischemic necrosis. In most patients, however, the

Plate 114   267

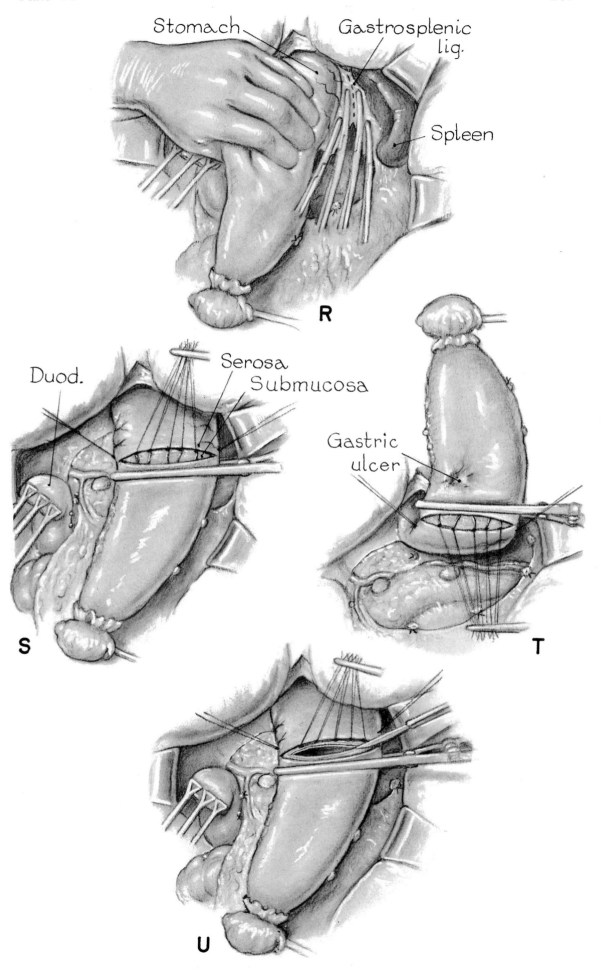

Stomach

Gastrosplenic lig.

Spleen

R

Duod.

Serosa

Submucosa

S

Gastric ulcer

T

U

V. The lumen of the proximal gastric pouch is diminished by partial closure on the lesser curvature side using inversion sutures of interrupted silk (000). These sutures are inserted from the "inside out" on one side and from the "outside in" on the other so that, when tied, the knots are on the inside of the lumen.

V'. A second layer of inversion is obtained with a series of interrupted seromuscular mattress sutures (Halsted) of silk (000).

V''. The sutures forming the first posterior layer of the anastomosis, a series of interrupted mattress sutures of silk (000), are first all inserted before being tied.

W, W', W''. The first posterior layer of mattress sutures is tied. Through and through sutures (0000), which include all the layers of the stomach and duodenum and form the second posterior layer, are being inserted. The insertion of the second posterior layer is completed (W'), and the first layer anteriorly is begun by the insertion of a coapting W-shaped mattress suture on the lesser curvature "angle" of the anastomosis (W'').

X. Subsequently the sutures which form the first anterior layer are inserted alternately from either end toward the center. Each suture is inserted from the "inside out" to the

"outside in" so that, when tied, the knots are on the inside of the lumen and the anterior layers of the stomach and duodenum are inverted.

X', X''. A through and through interrupted figure of 8 mattress suture of silk (000) is inserted in the midline about the two terminal anterior inversion sutures and, when tied, the first anterior layer of the anastomosis is completed (X''). The interrupted seromuscular mattress sutures (000 silk) forming the second anterior layer of the anastomosis are all first inserted before being tied to complete the end-to-end gastroduodenostomy.

Y. The end-to-end gastroduodenostomy is completed, and its relation to the surrounding structures is visible. A drain is not employed.

Z. The anterior parietal peritoneal layer is being closed with a continuous interlocking double strand suture of 00 chromic catgut.

Z'. The fascial layer is approximated with interrupted sutures of silk (00) and the skin is being closed with interrupted sutures of 000 silk threaded on straight milliner or Cambric needles. These needles are all first inserted, withdrawn individually, and the sutures tied.

DISCUSSION—DR. SCOTT (cont.)

esophageal and phrenic arteries provide adequate collateral to supply a small proximal gastric remnant of the type illustrated. The method of suturing the submucosal vessels on the anterior and posterior gastric walls is a good one if no clamps are to be applied to the proximal gastric stump. In a similar resection I prefer to apply paired Allen clamps first to the greater curvature segment of the gastric stump to define the size of stoma and, after transecting the stomach between them, to extend another similar pair of clamps across the lesser curvature portion. I place a running hemostatic mattress suture of chromic catgut behind the clamp on the lesser curve, remove the clamp, trim away the crushed cuff, and return the running suture as an over-and-over stitch or a continuous Cushing suture. This is then reinforced with a layer of interrupted Lembert sutures of silk. The remaining clamp on the greater curvature segment serves as a convenient handle for exposing the posterior aspect of the gastric stump for placement of the posterior seromuscular row of interrupted sutures of silk between the stomach and duodenum.

Dr. Madden's method of closure of the lesser curvature with interrupted sutures is a sound technic and avoids the hazard of damage to the esoph-

agus, which presents as a problem in a very high resection of the stomach when clamps are used, but I suspect his method is more apt to result in postoperative bleeding from the inverted cuff of gastric mucosa. The method of beginning the anastomosis between the stomach and duodenum is one which I have never used, and I much prefer the more conventional gastrointestinal anastomotic technic using an outer layer of interrupted seromuscular silk sutures and an inner layer of continuous or interrupted fine chromic catgut. The final result of this procedure is technically very satisfactory but physiologically distressing to me because of the tiny residual gastric reservoir that has resulted, which I believe to be largely unnecessary. If the high gastric ulcer indicated in this set of sketches were malignant, I would tend to carry out a total gastric resection with reconstruction of the alimentary tract using a jejunal pouch which would provide a large substitute gastric reservoir. If the ulcer were benign, a number of techniques are available to avoid this extensive sacrifice of the gastric reservoir. One can predict that the physiologic result of the procedure illustrated will be in most instances poor from the nutritional point of view, and in my opinion this is both undesirable and unnecessary.

Plate 115

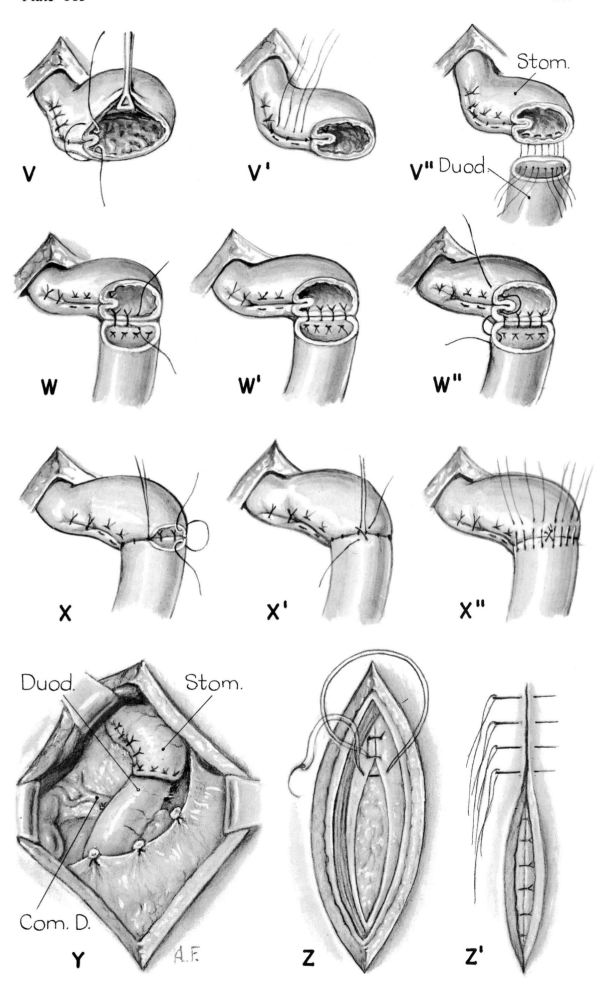

V

V'

V" Stom.

Duod.

W

W'

W"

X

X'

X"

Duod.

Stom.

Com. D.

Y

A.F.

Z

Z'

PARTIAL GASTRECTOMY FOR STOMAL (MARGINAL) ULCER WITH SEGMENTAL ENTERECTOMY, JEJUNOJEJUNOSTOMY, AND GASTROJEJUNOSTOMY (BILLROTH II)

This patient, a 64-year-old white man, was admitted to the hospital because of acute massive gastrointestinal bleeding. Three-and-one-half years previously an infradiaphragmatic partial resection of the vagus nerves and an antecolic gastrojejunostomy along the most dependent portion of the greater curvature of the stomach in close proximity to the pyloroduodenal junction was done. The indication for operation was intractable pain. At the time of operation an active chronic duodenal ulcer with extensive edema of the surrounding tissues was observed. The postoperative course was entirely satisfactory until the present admission to the hospital because of the bleeding episode. The bleeding was controlled under conservative management, and ten days following the initial hemorrhage, operation was performed as depicted in the illustrations.

A, B. The previous operative scar is excised in an elliptical manner (A), and the peritoneal cavity is entered (B).

C. The omental cuff is elevated and the cicatrix, indicative of the location of the marginal or stomal ulcer at the juncture of the stomach and efferent loop of jejunum, is visible. The extensive inflammatory reaction that was observed at the primary operation in the area surrounding the duodenal ulcer is absent. In the process of healing, a cicatrix formed which caused a constriction of the lumen of the duodenum between its first and second portion. The dotted line indicates the site of severance of the right phrenocolic ligament preparatory to mobilizing the hepatic flexure of the colon.

D. The hepatic flexure is displaced downward, and the line of the incision (Kocher) in the posterior parietal peritoneum prior to mobilizing the duodenum is depicted in dotted outline.

D¹. The retrocolic segment of the duodenum and the head of the pancreas are rotated (Moynihan rotation maneuver) toward the midline, and the related subjacent structures are depicted.

Plate 116   271

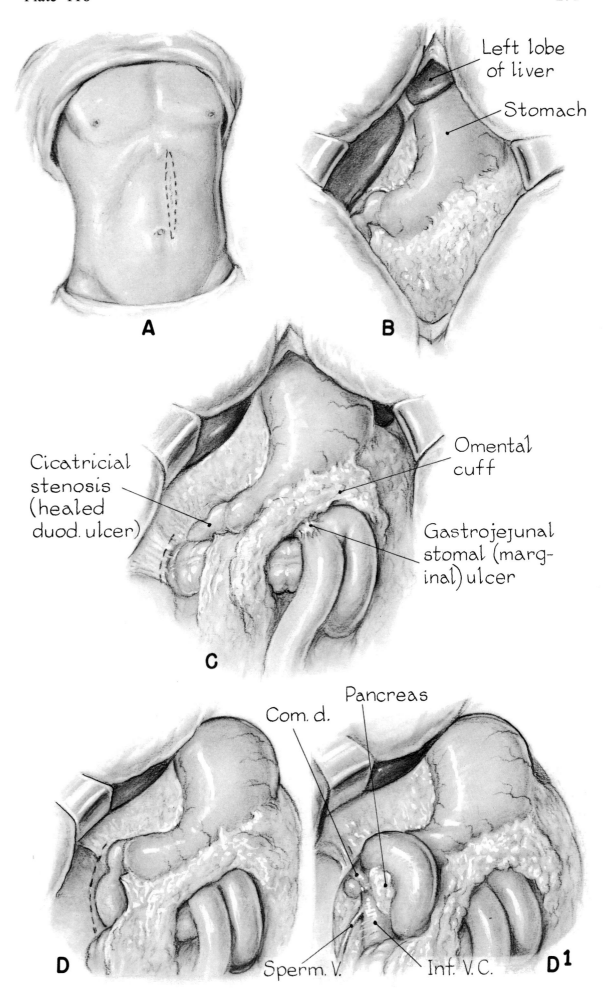

A

B

Left lobe
of liver

Stomach

C

Cicatricial
stenosis
(healed
duod. ulcer)

Omental
cuff

Gastrojejunal
stomal (marg-
inal) ulcer

D

Com. d.

Pancreas

Sperm. V.   Inf. V. C.   D¹

E, F. An opening is made by blunt dissection in the relatively avascular area of the gastrohepatic ligament (E). The index and middle fingers of the left hand of the surgeon are inserted through this opening into the lesser sac, and, by blunt dissection within the sac, the adherent transverse mesocolon is separated from the posterior wall of the stomach. The blunt dissection is continued until the fingers are finally protruded through an opening in an avascular portion of the gastrocolic ligament along the greater curvature of the stomach (F). The gastrocolic ligament is serially clamped and severed (dotted line) to mobilize partially the proximal portion of the greater curvature of the stomach (F).

F¹, G. The partial mobilization of the greater curvature of the stomach proximally is completed (F¹). The inset (G) shows an alternate method for entrance into the lesser sac in mobilizing the distal portion of the greater curvature of the stomach. Instead of severance of the gastrocolic ligament, the relatively avascular line of attachment of the greater omentum to the transverse colon is severed with a scalpel, as depicted.

H. Traction is applied to a piece of rubber tissue tape encircling the antral region of the stomach, and the right gastroepiploic artery just distal to its site of origin from the gastroduodenal artery is doubly clamped before being severed and ligated (000 silk).

Plate 117

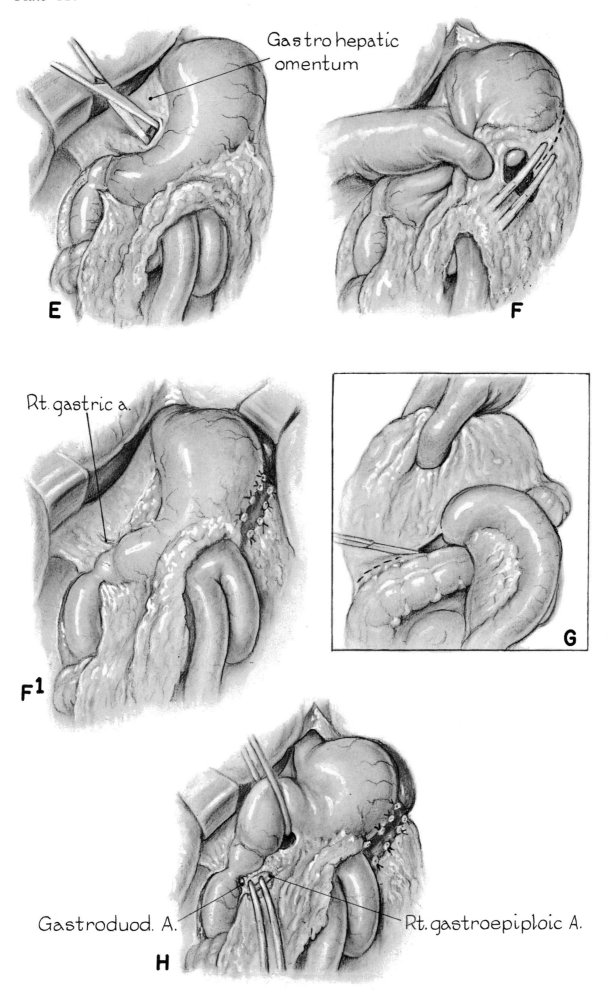

Gastrohepatic omentum

E

F

Rt. gastric a.

F¹

G

Gastroduod. A.

Rt. gastroepiploic A.

H

I. The sites of election for transection of the afferent and efferent limbs of the jejunum are encircled by catheters (12 F), and direction lines for severance of the mesentery are made through its serosal covering.

J, J¹. The remaining mesenteric attachment of the segment of bowel which is being resected is doubly clamped preparatory to severance (J). The clamps on the mesenteric side of the segment of jejunum that is removed are replaced with ligatures of silk (000) while those on the opposing mesentery are replaced with hemostatic suture ligatures of 000 silk (J¹). The jejunum is doubly cross-clamped at the sites of election for transection of the afferent and efferent limbs of the jejunum (J¹).

K. The transected ends of the segment of jejunum that is resected are covered with pieces of rubber dam and occluded with heavy ligatures (No. 1) of silk. The remaining transected ends of the jejunum are held in clamps ready to be approximated for the performance of a closed or "aseptic" end-to-end anastomosis.

K¹, K². The handles of the clamps are held downward (caudad), and a series of interrupted seromuscular mattress sutures of silk (000) are inserted but not tied (K¹). The handles of the clamps are next rotated upward (cephalad), and in like manner a second series of interrupted seromuscular mattress sutures are inserted on the opposite side of the bowel (K²).

Plate 118

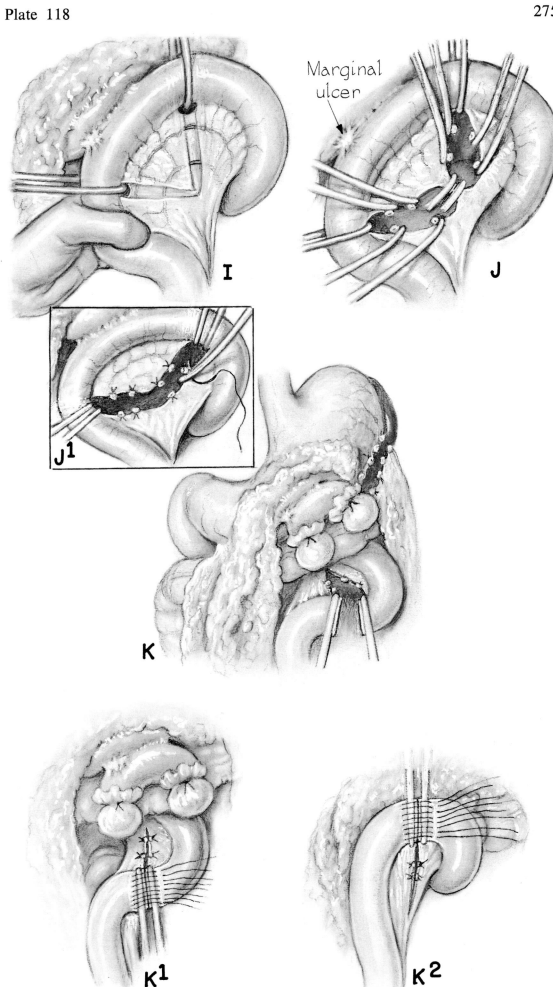

Marginal
ulcer

I

J

J¹

K

K¹

K²

K³. The strands of the untied seromuscular mattress sutures are held between the thumb and index finger of each hand of the surgeon, and traction is applied as the first assistant removes slowly the clamps from the transected ends of the jejunum.

K⁴. The mattress sutures are tied and cut with the exception of the two sutures which are immediately adjacent to either side of the mesentery. The opening remaining on the antimesenteric wall of the bowel following the removal of the clamps is to be closed with a mattress suture of 000 silk which is inserted but not tied.

K⁵. The strands of the sutures adjacent to the mesenteric sides of the bowel wall are used to rotate partially the bowel and expose the opening at its mesenteric border which is occluded when the mattress suture previously inserted is tied. The insertion of this suture, though most important, is rarely shown in illustrations depicting the closed or "aseptic" technic for bowel resection.

K⁶. Upon completion of the anastomosis, digital invagination of the bowel wall on either side of the anastomotic line is done to insure patency of the stoma. This particular step in technic cannot be overemphasized, as one of the technical hazards in this operation is the formation of a diaphragmatic occlusion of the bowel lumen. The cut margins of the mesentery are approximated with interrupted sutures of 000 silk.

L. Upon completion of the small bowel resection and anastomosis, the pyloroduodenal region of the stomach is mobilized by doubly clamping and severing the right gastric artery which is isolated through an opening made by blunt dissection in the gastrohepatic ligament.

M. The pyloroduodenal region is completely mobilized and the most distal portion of the pylorus is cross-clamped with a crushing (Payr) clamp. The duodenum is not cross-clamped. Instead it is secured with guy sutures of silk (000). A scalpel is used for the transection of the anterior wall of the duodenum immediately distal to the pyloric vein (vein of Mayo) as depicted. The constriction of the duodenum caused by the healed duodenal ulcer is readily visible. The location of this constriction, between the first and second portions of the foreshortened duodenum, is in close approximation to the entrance of the common bile duct.

M¹. Inset to show the transection of the anterior wall of the duodenum completed and its posterior wall being severed with scissors. The scissors are inclined upward on the posterior wall to assure an adequate length.

M². The transection of the duodenum is completed and its proximal cut end is covered with a thick moist gauze pad. Digital exploration of the lumen of the duodenum distally showed adequate patency at the site of constriction. Accordingly, closure of the duodenal stump proximally was believed feasible.

DISCUSSION—DR. S. ARTHUR LOCALIO. In patients, as illustrated, with a gastroenteric stomal ulcer we have found it expedient to transect and reconstruct the jejunum as illustrated in Plates 118 and 119, I–K⁶, as the first step of the operation. The operation can now proceed as a routine gastrectomy for duodenal ulcer.

The operation for a callus-penetrating duodenal ulcer presents its technical difficulties and dangers during the mobilization of the duodenum. By first transecting the stomach at the proximal line of resection, the lesser sac is widely opened, and the duodenum and the ulcer can be approached from several directions. We have used the greater curvature

clear area between the left gastroepiploic artery and the lowest short gastric artery as the proximal line of transection in order to perform a 65 to 75 per cent resection.

With the stomach transected, the duodenum and pancreas are mobilized and the common duct exposed. The surgeon can now safely proceed to dissect the duodenum and ulcer from the pancreas and to mobilize a sufficient length of normal duodenum beyond the ulcer to effect a secure closure of the duodenal stump. This is accomplished by using the common duct as a reference point and dissecting the ulcer from whichever direction it appears to proceed easily. At times it is valuable to make an incision in

Plate 119

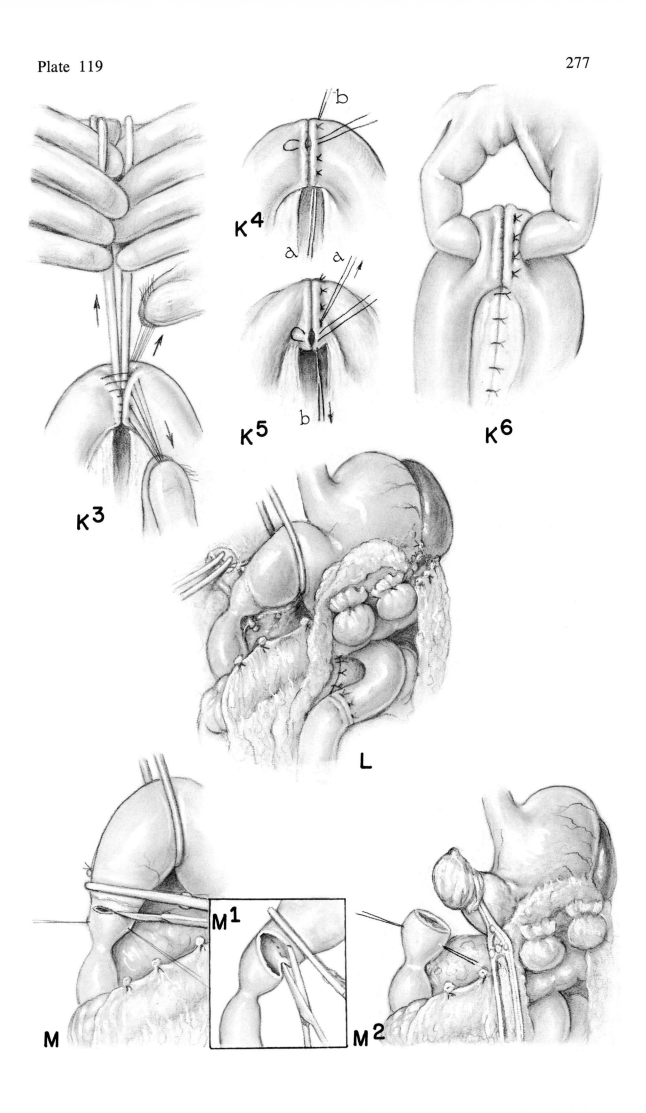

K⁴

K⁵

K⁶

K³

L

M

M¹

M²

N, N¹, N². The duodenal stump is closed with interrupted sutures of silk (000). The sutures are inserted from the "inside out" to the "outside in" so that, when tied, the tissues are inverted and the knots are on the inside of the lumen (N). The sutures are inserted alternately from either end and terminate in the center of the line of closure (N¹). The two terminal sutures are encircled by a figure of 8 mattress suture (N¹), following which the terminal sutures are cut and the reinforcing mattress suture is tied (N²). A serosal layer of interrupted seromuscular sutures is used for the closure of the duodenal stump. This suture layer is begun at either angle by the insertion of half purse-string seromuscular sutures (N²). When these sutures are tied the angles are inverted and "dog ears" are avoided.

N³, N⁴. Insets to show the completion of the second layer of the closure by the insertion of a series of seromuscular Halsted mattress sutures. These sutures are all first inserted (N³) and then tied (N⁴).

O. The closure of the duodenal stump is further reinforced by impingement against the serosal covering overlying the pancreas (posterior wall of lesser sac) with interrupted sutures of silk (000). The anchorage of the lesser curvature of the stomach by the gastropancreatic fold of peritoneum and the contained left gastric vessels is visible.

P. An opening is made in the gastropancreatic fold of peritoneum, and the exposed left gastric vessels are triply clamped and severed between the two distal clamps (solid black line).

P¹. Inset to show the occlusion of the proximal cut end of the left gastric artery by a ligature and a suture ligature respectively to replace the previously applied clamps. The bifurcation of the distal end of the severed left gastric artery into ascending and descending branches on the lesser curvature of the stomach is visible.

P², P³. The ascending and descending branches of the left gastric vessels are doubly clamped (P²). Following the severance of the vessels between clamps, the intervening segment is removed to clear the proximal portion of the lesser curvature of the stomach. The "bare" area is reperitonized with interrupted Lembert sutures of 000 silk (P³).

DISCUSSION—DR. LOCALIO (cont.)

the anterior duodenal wall close to the pylorus. The index finger of the left hand inserted into the duodenum will aid in following the contortions made by a chronic ulcer. This dissection is at times associated with very little bleeding because of the paucity of blood vessels in the fibrous tissue. The bed of the ulcer in the pancreatic head is not removed. The ulcer consists merely of a rim of duodenum. The vast percentage of duodenal ulcers occur in the first 2.5 cm. of duodenum and must therefore be removed if complete antrectomy is to be performed and a secure closure of the duodenal stump effected.

The ease of exposure of the common duct and the protection that it receives in its course in the pancreatic head can protect this structure from injury.

In our experience the accessory pancreatic duct has been more vulnerable. If this duct is transected it can be ligated with a purse-string suture of 00000 arterial silk. A sump or other suitable drain should be placed down to the pancreatic head for six to seven days in the event that subsequent leakage from the ligated duct should occur.

The final gastrojejunostomy may be performed, antecolic or retrocolic, antiperistaltic or isoperistaltic, and to the whole of or to a portion of the proximal cut end of the stomach. The main factors of importance are an adequate resection, the complete removal of the antrum, and the use of a short jejunal loop.

Plate 120

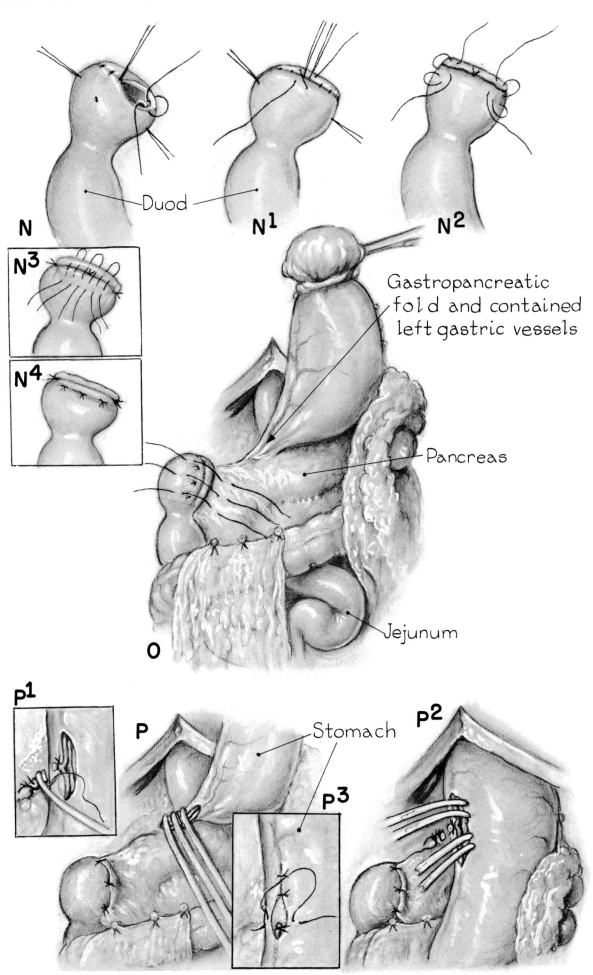

N

N1

N2

N3

N4

Duod

Gastropancreatic
fold and contained
left gastric vessels

Pancreas

Jejunum

O

P1

P

Stomach

P2

P3

Q. The stomach is cross-clamped with a large Payr clamp just below the site of election for its transection and then reflected upward and to the left to demonstrate the insertion of the first posterior layer of the side-to-side antecolic gastrojejunostomy (Reichel–Polya). This layer consists of interrupted 000 silk sutures which approximates the proximal (afferent) limb of jejunum to the lesser curvature and the distal (efferent) limb to the greater curvature of the stomach.

Q[1]. An incision is made through the seromuscular layer of the jejunum, and the vessels in the submucosal layer are undersewn with suture ligatures of silk (0000). The incision to be made through the seromuscular layer of the posterior wall of the stomach is indicated by the dotted line.

Q[2]. The insertion of the hemostatic suture ligatures is completed. Only one line of such sutures is required on the gastric side as the clamp distally prevents retrograde bleeding.

Q[3]. The opening previously made into the lumen of the stomach with a scalpel is enlarged by scissor dissection. In like manner an opening was previously made in the jejunal segment and covered with a warm moist pad.

R. The stomach is turned downward, and an incision is being made through the seromuscular layer anteriorly to expose the vessels in the submucosa.

R[1]. A row of hemostatic suture ligatures of silk are inserted proximally and the transection of the stomach anteriorly is being completed by scissor dissection.

S. A partial gastrectomy (70 per cent) is completed and the second posterior layer of the anastomosis is being inserted. This consists of a continuous interlocking suture of 00 chromic catgut swedged on minimum trauma needles at either end. The suture starts in the midline posteriorly and continues to the right with one needle and then to the left with the other. This particular technic avoids terminating the closure at the angles of the anastomosis. Interrupted through and through sutures of silk (000) may be used, and generally this is the preferred method.

S[1], S[2]. The sutures "turn the angles" as depicted (S[1]) and continue from either end toward the center as inverting (Connell, "loop on the mucosa") sutures which form the first anterior layer (S[2]).

DISCUSSION—DRS. CHARLES MARKS AND EDWIN H. ELLISON. In considering the best surgical procedure for the cure of a stomal ulcer consequent to a previous vagotomy and gastroenterostomy, certain aspects of the situation require careful analysis before one proceeds with reoperation:

In examining the etiology of gastrojejunal ulceration following vagotomy and gastrojejunostomy, three possibilities must be considered. First, the vagotomy may have been inadequate and incomplete: preliminary study of overnight gastric secretion utilizing the Hollander and augmented histamine tests will provide pointers in this direction. Secondly, technical errors in construction of the gastrojejunostomy may have occurred. Dr. Marks and others feel that the use of nonabsorbable sutures in the mucosal anastomosis may provide a site for ulcer formation. Finally, the presence of an ulcerogenic tumor in the pancreas or elsewhere should always be considered, and careful preoperative consideration should be given to this possibility. A large volume of overnight secretion with high acidity, which is maximal and not increased by histamine stimulation or decreased significantly with anticholinergics, will help determine the need to search for a pancreatic tumor at operation (Zollinger-Ellison Syndrome). Frozen-section biopsies of lymph nodes and of nodules in the duodenal wall may result in an accurate diagnosis. When the surgeon is highly suspicious of a tumor and none is found, then the presence of small islet cell tumors or hyperplasia may be found in the resected tail of the pancreas. This finding, or the presence of a malignant tumor, will indicate the need for a total gastrectomy.

In the type of problem presented, jejunal resection and restoration of continuity by an end-to-end jejunostomy is a necessary procedure, but utilization of a closed aseptic technic seems an unnecessary refinement. We would perform an open anastomosis, thus obviating the risk of diaphragmatic occlusion of the bowel lumen without really increasing the risks of infection. Partial gastrectomy is certainly necessary in most of these cases; however, the finding of an intact and an overlooked nerve trunk, thought to represent either the right or left vagus, might influence one to limit the procedure to vagotomy alone. If this is not the case, then at least 50 per cent gastric resection would be in order. Dr. Ellison would prefer restoration by means of a gastroduodenostomy if technically feasible; however, the close proximity of the biliary tract resulting from cicatrical healing of the old duodenal ulcer would possibly influence one to do a Billroth II type reconstruction.

Though it is aesthetically more desirable to excise an old scar in providing surgical access, there are occasions when the nature of the scar, the possibility of a subsequent incisional hernia, and the anticipation of technical embarrassment by massive adhesions at this site will lead the operator to choose a virgin area for incision and approach.

A thorough intraperitoneal inspection and palpation is indicated to rule out concomitant or unexpected pathologic lesions, such as gallbladder disease or hiatus hernia, that may require repair. As indicated previously, a careful search for a possible ulcerogenic tumor should be accomplished in appropriate cases.

Plate 121   281

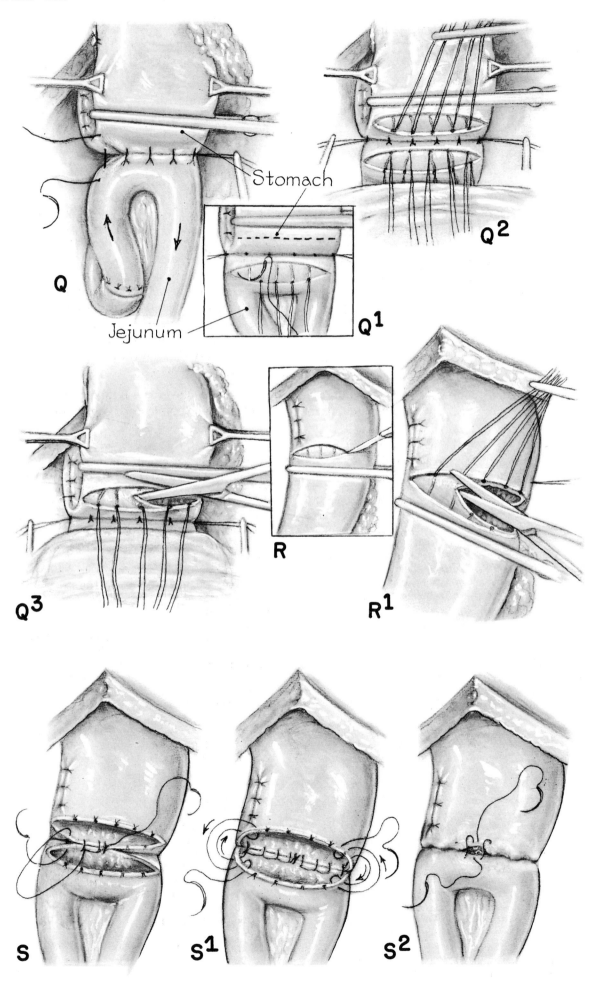

Stomach

Jejunum

Q

Q¹

Q²

Q³

R

R¹

S

S¹

S²

S³. The needle of the suture which terminates in the center on the gastric side is inserted into the lumen of the jejunum and out through its anterior wall. Conversely, the needle of the suture which terminates in the center of the jejunal side is inserted into the lumen of the stomach and out through its anterior wall. When tied, these sutures complete the closure of the first layer anteriorly.

S⁴. The second anterior layer, a series of interrupted 0000 silk sutures, is inserted, and all the sutures are tied with the exception of the suture inserted for the closure of the "angle of leakage." This suture, a modified pursestring, includes a "bite" in the anterior and posterior walls of the stomach at the "angle" of the anastomosis on the lesser curvature and abuts the afferent limb of the jejunum into the "angle" to reinforce the closure.

T. This is a view of the operative field following the completion of the operation. closed and "buried" duodenal stump, the end-to-end anastomosis of the jejunum, and the end-to-side antecolic gastrojejunostomy (Reichel–Polya) are visible.

U. The artist's sketch of the operative specimen after it was opened along the wall of the jejunum opposite the stoma is shown. The ulcer is located on the margin of the anastomosis at its efferent end. Approximately two thirds of the ulcer projected onto the jejunal side and one third onto the gastric side of the stoma.

V, W. The wound is closed according to the technic described by the late T. E. Jones of Cleveland, using interrupted sutures of 0 silk. For a paramedian muscle-retracting incision each suture is first inserted through fascia, muscle, and peritoneum on one side and then through the peritoneal and fascial layers on the other (V). The suture is then reinserted on either side through the fascial layers only (V). The completed closure is illustrated in W.

X. The skin closure with interrupted sutures of 000 silk completes the operation.

DISCUSSION—DRS. MARKS AND ELLISON (cont.)

Whether to clamp, ligate and divide the gastrocolic omentum or to separate the omentum from its avascular colic attachment is a matter of personal preference in the individual case, but at all times it is important to separate the gastrocolic omentum from the mesocolon and to identify the middle colic artery in the latter, since the accidental ligation of same would result in subsequent gangrene of the transverse colon. We would also underline as an important point of technic the author's reperitonealization of the lesser curve "bare" area after division and ligation of the branches of the left gastric artery.

It is our practice to free the duodenum for at least ¼ in. beyond the area of duodenal ulceration or fibrosis so as to provide sufficient healthy tissue for inversion of the cut end.

After applying two straight clamps to the duodenum, the bowel is divided between them. The clamp on the gastric side is covered and drawn well to the left, the other clamp is rotated laterally to expose the undersurface of the duodenal stump, which is then closed by Dr. Marks with a continuous over-and-over 00 chromic catgut stitch on an atraumatic needle. The suture is then drawn tightly as the clamp is released. Dr. Ellison would prefer to close the stump with interrupted silk sutures. The suture is then carried back to the starting point, where it is tied firmly and provides added insurance against bleeding from this area. A layer of interrupted 000 silk seromuscular sutures reinforces the closure, and a few interrupted silk sutures incorporating pads of omental tissue on either side further consolidate this area.

There are many variations of the Billroth II or Polya operation and our preference is for the Polya-Hofmeister type of anastomosis, fashioning a valve on the lesser curvature and leaving a 3-5 cm. stoma on the greater curvature. The immediate and late functional results are usually good, and in our opinion such an anastomosis minimizes the incidence of postgastrectomy "Dumping Syndrome." A short loop of jejunum—that is, 3-4 in. —from the ligament of Treitz, should be employed, and Lane's twin bladed gastrojejunostomy clamp makes for an easy anastomosis. Furthermore, this clamp can be loosened after completion of the posterior anastomotic layer so that any residual bleeding can be dealt with before completing the anterior layer.

Dr. Marks would use a continuous chromic catgut suture for the mucosal anastomosis and interrupted silk for the seromuscular layer. Dr. Ellison would prefer to use interrupted silk sutures throughout.

Dr. Marks prefers an antecolic anastomosis, which eliminates kinking of the jejunum at or through the mesocolon or when there is need to suture the mesocolic edges to the afferent and efferent limbs of jejunum. Dr. Ellison would prefer the retrocolic anastomosis to help avoid duodenal stump leakage and afferent loop stasis and obstruction. Both of us agree that use of good surgical technique will probably prevent most of such complications regardless of the position of the jejunum.

Though it is generally unnecessary to drain the peritoneal cavity, if we have any doubts about the duodenal stump closure, then a rubber drain will be placed in the subhepatic pouch; on occasions with a friable duodenal stump, it will be closed about a catheter and the subhepatic pouch drained. Dr. Ellison would resort to a complementary jejunostomy.

A good abdominal wound closure is important, and variations on the theme, as described by Dr. Madden, are myriad. Whether one uses 0 silk or monofilamentous wire, it is important to repair the peritoneum, the posterior rectus sheath, and the anterior rectus sheath as individual layers, using interrupted 000 silk for the skin. Dr. Marks would only rarely find need for retention sutures; in contrast, Dr. Ellison would use them routinely.

Plate 122

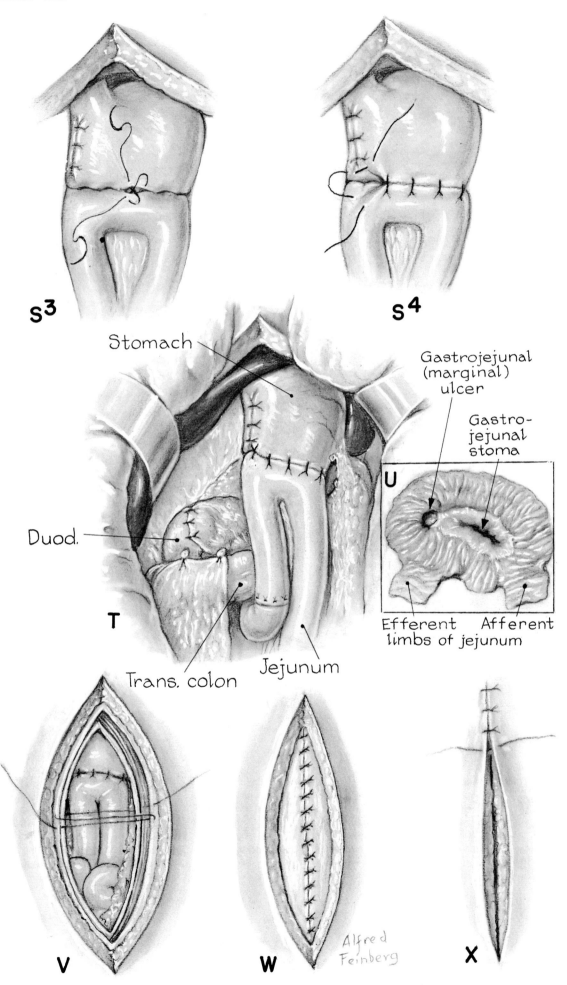

S³

S⁴

Stomach

Duod.

Trans. colon

Jejunum

Gastrojejunal
(marginal)
ulcer

Gastro-
jejunal
stoma

U

Efferent   Afferent
limbs of jejunum

T

Alfred
Feinberg

V

W

X

TOTAL GASTRECTOMY, SPLENECTOMY, AND PARTIAL PANCREATECTOMY

A. The solid black line indicates the left paramedian muscle-retracting (lateral) incision that is employed. Other types of incisions that may be preferred are in dotted outline.

B, C, D. The anterior rectus sheath is incised, the rectus muscle is mobilized laterally from its midline attachment, and the peritoneal cavity is entered. The blood vessels and their relation to the tendinous inscriptions are visible.

E. The left lobe of the liver is mobilized by severance of the avascular left triangular ligament.

F. The mobilized left lobe of the liver is turned inward on itself. covered by a moist gauze pad, and retracted toward the midline. The peritoneal reflection overlying the esophagocardial junction, the inferior phrenic vein, and the "bare" area of the diaphragm may be clearly seen.

G. The stomach is displaced medialward to demonstrate the gastrosplenic ligament with its contained vasa brevia and the line of incision in the posterior layer of the lienorenal ligament for the mobilization of the spleen and the tail of the pancreas.

DISCUSSION—DR. GEORGE T. PACK. In all instances of gastric cancer the abdominal incision should be done first, thereby permitting abdominal exploration. If the cancer be inoperable, the laparotomy would be enough. The surgeon may decide that it is technically feasible to do an abdominal total gastrectomy. However, the abdominal incision is planned so that if the exposure is better facilitated by a thoracic extension, the upper abdominal oblique or vertical epigastric incisions may be prolonged into the left thorax either intercostally or through a rib bed after excision of the rib. Also the left Marwedel paracostal incision permits an inverted T-prolongation into the chest.

In earlier years all of our total gastrectomies were done by the abdominal route, and our patients experienced fewer pulmonary complications. In spite of the longer incision and the greater time required for wound closure, the actual resection and anastomosis can be done more quickly thereby saving total time. In many of our patients the operation has been technically easier to perform through an abdominothoracic exposure. This has been an important advantage in difficult cases, especially those of borderline operability and when the gastric cancer is situated high in the gastric cardia. Gastric adenocarcinomas can and do invade the abdominal esophagus and may extend above the diaphragmatic level. Al-

Plate 123

285

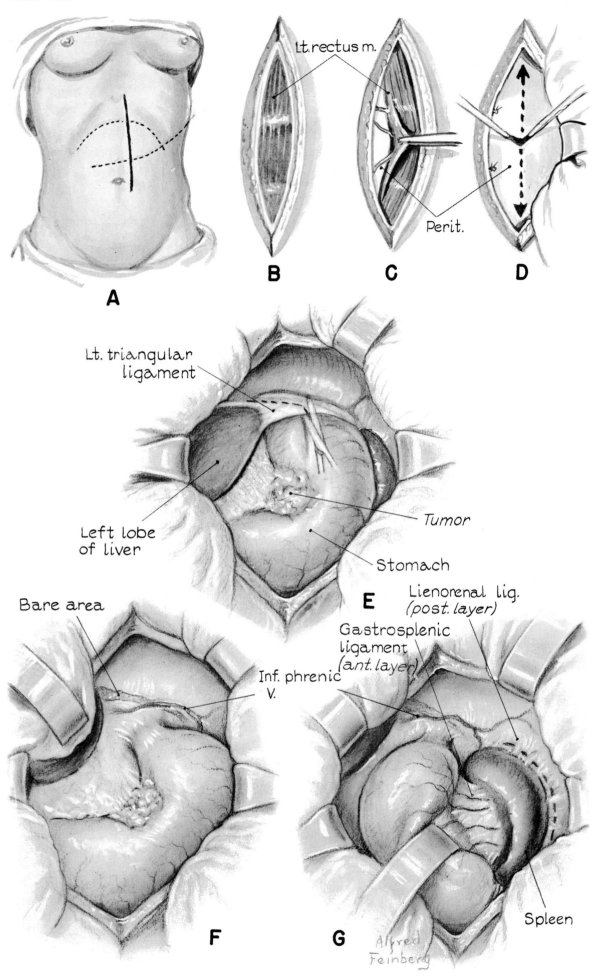

Lt. rectus m.

B

Perit.

C

D

A

Lt. triangular
ligament

Left lobe
of liver

Tumor

Stomach

E

Lienorenal lig.
(post. layer)

Gastrosplenic
ligament
(ant. layer)

Inf. phrenic
V.

Bare area

F

G

Spleen

Alfred
Feinberg

H. The mobilization of the spleen posteriorly is completed, and the freeing of the splenic flexure of the colon by severance of the left phrenocolic ligament is shown in dotted outline. One may prefer to mobilize the spleen in a later stage of the operation because of the potential risk of excessive blood loss from a tear in the splenic capsule or from the raw area of the splenic bed.

I. The apron of greater omentum which is removed in continuity with the tumor is freed by scalpel dissection from its relatively avascular attachment to the transverse colon.

J. The hepatic flexure of the colon is mobilized by scissor dissection along the fascial fusion layer of Toldt ("white line") and the right phrenocolic ligament.

K. The right and transverse colon are retracted downward and to the left to expose the retrocolic portion of the duodenal loop and the enclosed head of the pancreas. The incision (Kocher) in the posterior parietal peritoneum preparatory to the mobilization of the duodenum and head of the pancreas is shown in dotted outline.

K[1]. Through an opening in the gastrohepatic ligament, the right gastric artery is doubly clamped prior to its severance.

DISCUSSION—DR. PACK (cont.)

though the thoracic esophagus may be mobilized from below and drawn down into the abdomen for an added four to six cm. of length, there is some hazard of too much tension on the anastomosis. Furthermore, transection of the esophagus with abdominal anastomosis (below the diaphragm) may not be adequately high to ensure against recurrence in the proximal esophagus. In earlier years we were frequently disappointed to receive reports from the pathologist that the transection through the esophagus was above grossly visible cancer but microscopically detected cancer was found at the line of excision. In consequence of this denouement, we consistently have requested frozen section microscopic analysis of the esophageal end of the surgical specimen before proceeding with the anastomosis. In our experience, leaks in the anastomoses have occurred more commonly when the total gastrectomy is done solely from the abdominal approach.

With an abdominothoracic incision, the diaphragm may be radially severed partway just for added exposure to enable mobilization of the thoracic esophagus and to construct an intrathoracic anastomosis, or it may be completely incised radially to permit an even wider exposure and mobilization of the entire esophagogastric segment.

If the left lobe of the liver be invaded by continuity with a gastric cancer on the lesser curvature side of the gastric cardia, one may perform a left hepatic lobectomy en masse with the stomach, spleen and distal pancreas.

In the performance of a total gastrectomy, I dissect the inferior connections first, leaving the great omentum intact with the surgical specimen and freeing it completely from the transverse colon and the hepatic and splenic flexures which then can be packed downward and out of the way. The mobilization from left to right is the same as shown in the illustrations, except for occasional differences. The body of the pancreas is transected and the stump closed at the end of this left to right maneuver, with the specimen reflected toward the right side of the patient. The transection of the duodenum and ligation of the right gastric and right gastroduodenal vessels are not done in patients whose cancers are of questionable operability until the surgeon is reasonably sure that the operation can be accomplished. The stomach will survive with intact esophagus and duodenum and with preservation of only the right gastric vessels. Elevation of the stomach specimen out of the abdomen and over the left costal arch (Moynihan maneuver) has the advantage of getting the specimen out of the way, facilitating the exposure of and placing

Plate 124 287

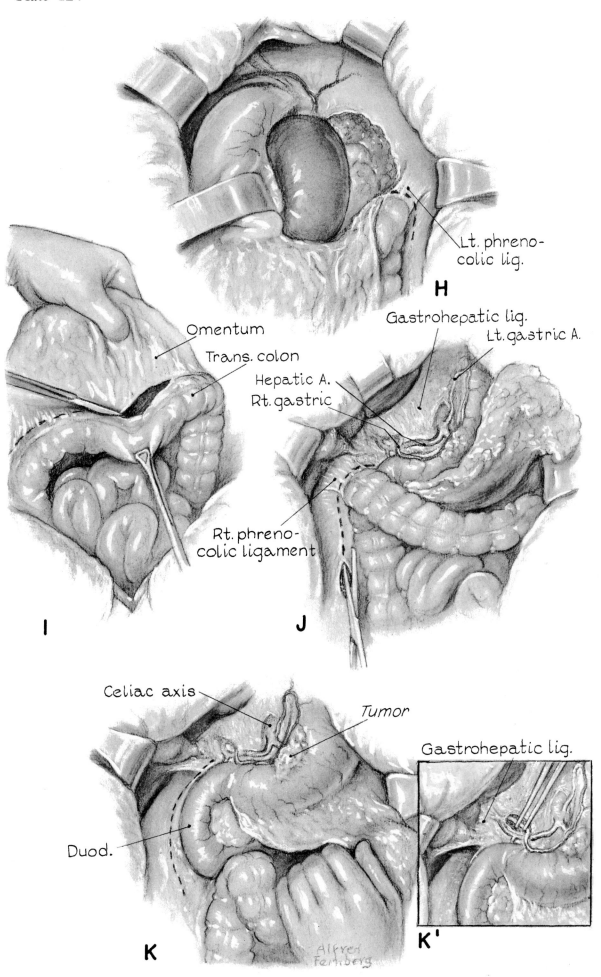

Lt. phreno-
colic lig.

H

Omentum

Trans. colon

Gastrohepatic lig.

Lt. gastric A.

Hepatic A.
Rt. gastric

Rt. phreno-
colic ligament

I

J

Celiac axis

Tumor

Gastrohepatic lig.

Duod.

K

K'

Alfred
Feinberg

L, L¹. The duodenum and the head of the pancreas are mobilized and retracted upward and medialward to expose the related retroperitoneal structures. The distribution of the lymph nodes in relation to the aorta, the inferior vena cava, the left renal vein, and the common bile duct are shown. When an esophagoduodenostomy is planned following total gastrectomy for carcinoma of the stomach, the exposure and removal of the lymph nodes depicted is routinely done (L′). This does not usually obtain when an esophagojejunostomy is performed. Accordingly, when an esophagoduodenostomy is done, one performs not a less but, on the contrary, a more radical operation.

M. The pyloroduodenal area is retracted upward by a rubber tissue traction tape inserted through the lesser sac, and the gastroduodenal artery and its two branches, the superior pancreaticoduodenal artery, and the severed right gastroepiploic artery, are demonstrated. The inferior pancreaticoduodenal artery, a branch of the superior mesenteric artery, is visible.

N, N¹. The stomach is displaced downward, and the exposed reflected layer of peritoneum overlying the esophagocardial junction is severed by scissor dissection to show the lower end of the esophagus and a portion of the hiatal ring. (N′).

O. The lower end of the esophagus is first mobilized by digital dissection and encircled by a rubber tissue traction tape. With traction maintained, resection of the gastrohepatic omentum is performed, and the right (posterior) and left (anterior) vagus nerves are individually mobilized on a nerve hook and severed. Upon completion of this dissection the distal 5 to 8 cm. of the esophagus is freely mobile.

DISCUSSION—DR. PACK (cont.)

the esophagus on a stretch, but a residual stomach tube should be thoroughly aspirated before this procedure, then withdrawn so the tip is in the lower esophagus, after which a large right angled clamp is placed across the esophagus below the level of transection in order to avoid possible flooding of the esophagus and trachea with a sudden upward gush of stomach contents.

In the restoration of continuity of the alimentary tract, although it is technically possible to anastomose the esophagus and duodenum in many cases (and I have done it within the thoracic cavity), the risk of leakage due to ischemic necrosis and/or tension on the suture line is greater than for esophagojejunostomy. Theoretically, and based on animal experimentation, the direct passage of food into the duodenum stimulates greater external pancreatic secretion than when the duodenum is bypassed by an esophagojejunostomy; an advantage of this naturally would be less steatorrhea and creatorrhea after total gastrectomy. Whenever the esophagoduodenal or esophagojejunal anastomosis is done below the diaphragm, an elevated peritoneal flap may be sutured over the anastomosis, a procedure which reinforces it and also serves as an additional suspension to relieve the weight and tension. The jejunojejunostomy (Braun supplementary anastomosis) may be enlarged to include the greater length of the jejunal limbs, thereby constructing a reservoir as a substitute stomach which may have some advantages in delaying the onset or lessening the degree of the occasional dumping syndrome which may follow total gastrectomy. Substitutive stomachs have been constructed by the use of interposed segments of the jejunum or the transverse colon or the right colon with contained ileocecal valve between the esophagus and duodenum or esophagus and jejunum in an attempt to afford a temporary reservoir and to avoid some of the unpleasant sequels of total gastrectomy, notably the dumping syndrome. In our hands the employment of these substitute stomachs has merely delayed and not lessened the frequency or severity of the post total gastrectomy syndrome. The vasomotor phenomena characteristic of this symptom complex, such as a feeling of weakness, collapse, pallor, sweating, palpitation, and cardiovascular changes typical on the electrocardiogram and suggestive of coronary spasm may be delayed postprandially for 30 to 90 minutes longer than obtains with the conventional esophagoduodenostomy or esophagojejunostomy.

Plate 125   289

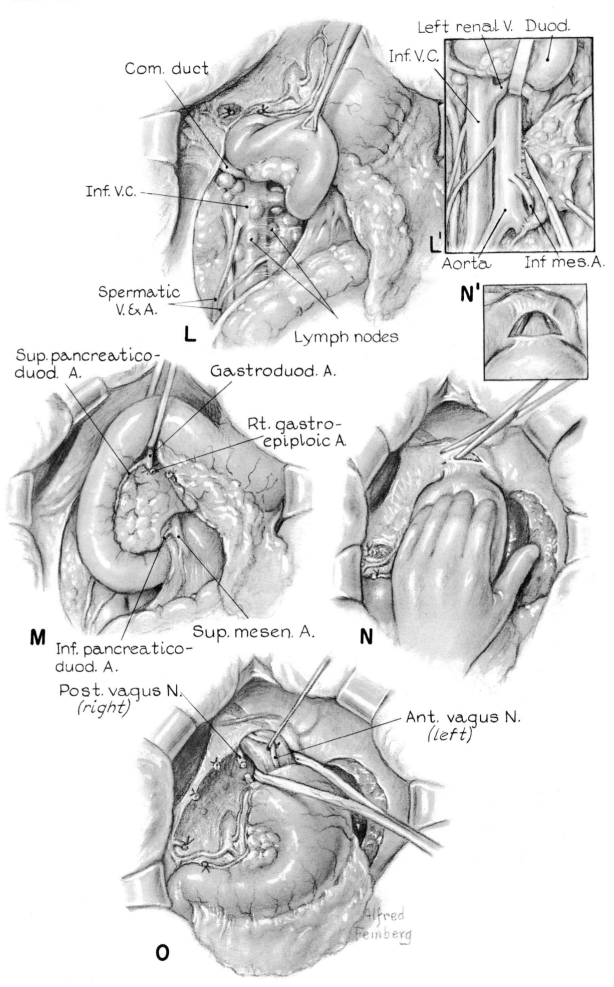

Com. duct

Inf. V.C.

Spermatic
V. & A.

Lymph nodes

L

Left renal V. Duod.

Inf. V.C.

L'

Aorta   Inf mes. A.

N'

Sup. pancreatico-
duod. A.

Gastroduod. A.

Rt. gastro-
epiploic A.

Sup. mesen. A.

M

Inf. pancreatico-
duod. A.

N

Post. vagus N.
(right)

Ant. vagus N.
(left)

Alfred
Feinberg

O

P. A Payr clamp is placed across the proximal portion of the duodenum, and two Babcock clamps are used to immobilize the duodenum distally. The duodenum is transected distal to the Payr clamp and approximately 4 cm. below the pyloroduodenal junction. A wide cuff of the duodenum is resected to encompass the zone of potential submucosal spread of the tumor. To avoid crushing trauma and the unnecessary sacrifice of tissue, the distal segment of the duodenum is not cross-clamped.

Q. To prevent soiling of the operative field, the open end of the duodenum is temporarily occluded by the approximation of its cut margins with Babcock clamps and then covered with a moist gauze pad. The index finger is inserted into a plane of cleavage between the pancreas anteriorly and the portal vein posteriorly prior to transection of the pancreas at the site indicated by the dotted line.

R. Inset showing the pancreas being transected

and a Babcock clamp in readiness to compress the cut margins of the pancreas. The eccentric location of the orifice of the pancreatic duct is also visible.

S. The division of the pancreas is completed, and for temporary hemostasis the cut margins are approximated by a series of Babcock clamps. The portal vein, formed by the junction of the superior mesenteric and splenic veins, may be seen passing obliquely upward beneath the arch formed by the hepatic artery and its gastroduodenal branch. This vascular arch is a useful landmark for the location of the underlying portal vein. The line of division of the peritoneal attachment of the inferior border of the pancreas is shown in dotted outline.

T. The operative field, essentially as in S, with the cut margins of the pancreas now approximated with mattress sutures of silk (00) and the mobilization of the inferior border of the pancreas completed.

DISCUSSION—DR. KOMEI NAKAYAMA. The line of the incision in the triangular ligament can be closer to the edge of the liver, since this part of the ligament can be used later for the reinforcement of the esophagojejunostomy. In many cases where the lesion is localized in the cardiac segment of the stomach, a portion of the gastric antrum can be and should be preserved, since it plays an important role in hormonal gastric secretion. The preserved gastric antrum is also used for the insertion of the temporary gastrostomy tube. In most cases, esophagogastrostomy is not advised even though the gastric antrum is preserved, for the reason that regurgitant esophagitis and stricture at the anastomotic site is a frequent postoperative complication.

All of the dissections illustrated are excellent, and I have nothing further to add. However, in some instances the dissection, such as that shown in the area about the portal vein, may be too radical. When the lesion is localized rather low on the lesser curvature, a subtotal gastrectomy is preferred to a total gastrectomy. Retaining a small portion of the stomach in its cardiac portion makes a tremendous difference in the postoperative status of the patient.

In the restoration of continuity of the alimentary canal following total gastrectomy, it is believed extremely important to employ some method that prevents the regurgitation of bile into the anastomotic stoma. Accordingly, the inter-

position of a jejunal loop as described by Longmire and also myself or the use of the Roux "en Y" principle are the best choices. A new type of anastomosis making this entire procedure simpler was recently devised here in Japan and will be published soon. In the use of the jejunal interposition operation, one must be extremely careful to maintain an adequate blood supply to the end of the jejunum that is to be anastomosed to the esophagus. I have made it a rule to "bend" the end of the jejunum so that the esophagus will be anastomosed to the side of the jejunal segment rather than performing an end-to-end anastomosis as illustrated (Z''', Z'''').

To complete the operation, it is suggested that the jejunal serosa be anastomosed to the crus of the diaphragm so that the anastomotic site will be completely covered with a serosal layer. This step is used to compensate for the absence of a serosa layer in the esophagus. When anyone deals with the esophagus, the idea of accomplishing a satisfactory anastomosis by use of the esophageal muscle layer will lead only to an increased incidence of anastomotic leakage. One should cover the anastomotic site with every possible structure available in the region of the anastomosis.

In general, the technical steps of the operation are well illustrated. The removal of the tail of the pancreas and the spleen can and should be accomplished when such an operation is indicated.

Plate 126   291

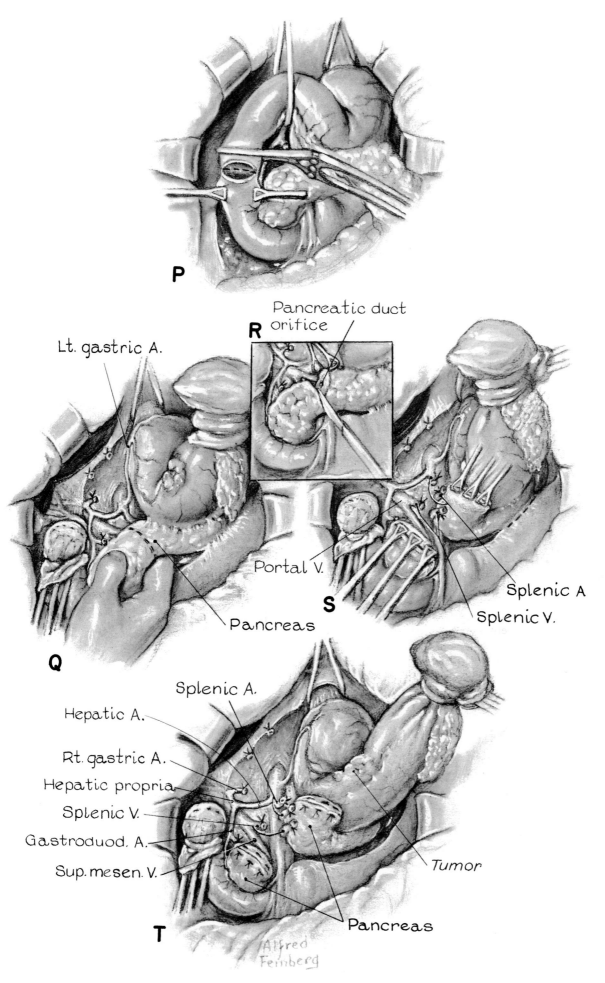

P

Pancreatic duct orifice

R

Lt. gastric A.

Portal V.

S

Splenic A

Splenic V.

Pancreas

Q

Splenic A.

Hepatic A.

Rt. gastric A.

Hepatic propria

Splenic V.

Gastroduod. A.

Sup. mesen. V.

Tumor

Pancreas

T

Alfred
Feinberg

U. The surgical specimen is elevated upward and to the left to place on tension the remaining vascular attachments of the stomach, the left gastric vessels. These vessels are triply clamped close to the celiac axis to include the lymphatic drain, and the line of severance between the two distal clamps is indicated.

V. The surgical specimen is further elevated, and two guy sutures of silk are inserted through either side of the lower portion of the esophagus. The whole of the related retroperitoneal structures is now visible.

W. The bulky specimen is removed as it is a hindrance rather than a traction aid in the performance of the anastomosis. The duodenum and esophagus are now ready for their approximation by sutures.

X. *1.* The first layer posteriorly of interrupted sutures of silk (000).
2. Alternate and frequently preferred method of using interrupted through and through mattress sutures of silk (000) for the first layer posteriorly.
3. The second layer posteriorly of interrupted through and through sutures of silk (000).

Y. *1.* The first layer anteriorly using interrupted sutures of silk (000). The two angle sutures are inserted from "inside out" to "outside in" to place the knots on the inside of the lumen.
2. The first layer anteriorly is completed.
3. The completion of the second layer anteriorly with interrupted mattress sutures of silk (000).
4, 5, 6, 7. Alternate method for the insertion of sutures anteriorly.
4, 5. The first layer of sutures which are inserted from the "inside out to outside in" to place the knots on the inside of the lumen.
6. The completion of the first anterior layer of sutures, the centermost one being a figure of 8 mattress suture with the knot on the outside.
7. The completion of the second layer of sutures using interrupted mattress sutures of silk (000).

Z. The anastomosis between the esophagus and duodenum is completed. The common bile duct, though abnormally displaced, is unobstructed. A drain is inserted into the left subphrenic space and a layer closure of the wound completes the operation. The use of a flap of peritoneum to suspend the site of anastomosis and take tension off the suture line is frequently recommended. In my own experience in the majority of patients this has not proved technically feasible and, accordingly, its applicability has been limited.

DISCUSSION—DR. PIETRO VALDONI. I would rather distinguish between total gastrectomy for cancer and total gastrectomy associated with pancreatic resection and splenectomy.

In the last decade the improvements in operative technics has permitted an extension of the indications for total gastrectomy in the treatment of cancer of the stomach. In my opinion, the indication for gastrectomy associated with pancreatic resection and splenectomy should be confined to those patients in whom the cancer is located on the posterior wall of the stomach with spread to the pancreas or on the greater curvature with invasion of the gastrolienal ligament. The combination of pancreatic resection and splenectomy is traumatizing, the mortality rate is high, and frequently the cancer is in an advanced stage in a patient who is a poor surgical risk.

An abdominal incision is usually performed when the cancer is limited to the cardia. Only when there is an invasion of the esophagus, as established preoperatively by roentgenographic examination and esophagoscopy, should a thoracicolaparotomy incision be performed. The surgical prognosis is worse when the thorax is opened simultaneously with the abdomen. In a review of my own statistics for the past several years, I have observed that subtotal gastrectomy is commonly limited to cancers of the prepyloric antral region, whereas total gastrectomies are performed when the cancer is located more proximally.

In performing a total gastrectomy I prefer a long midline incision that extends from the xiphoid to a point midway between the umbilicus and the pubis. I begin the operation by exposing and dividing between ligatures the right gastric artery. Next I dissect the horizontal portion of the hepatic artery and expose the portal vein. The hepatogastric ligament and the triangular ligament of the left lobe of the liver are divided, and with

Plate 127   293

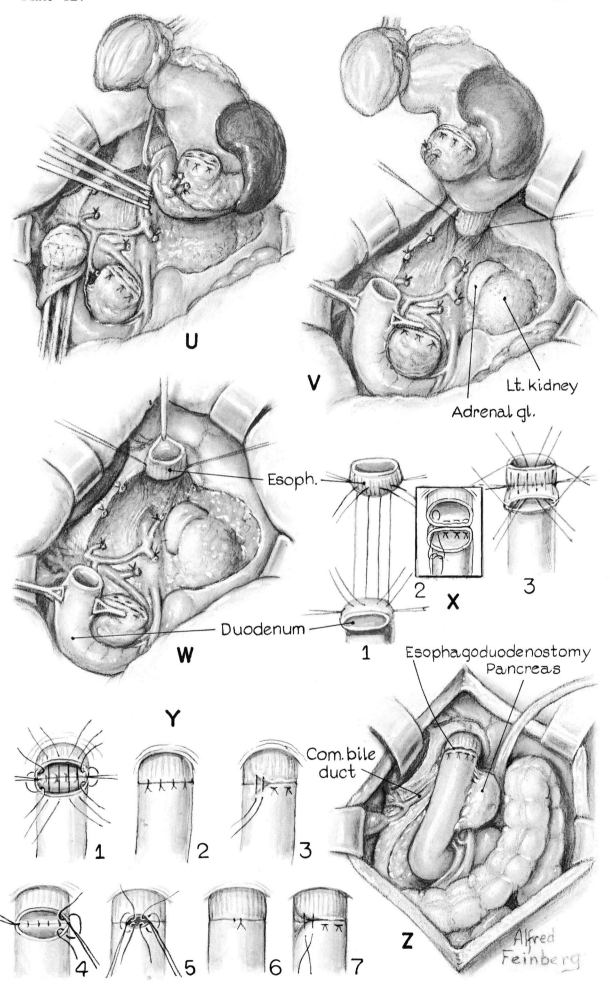

U

V

Lt. kidney

Adrenal gl.

Esoph.

2

X

3

Duodenum

W

1

Y

Esophagoduodenostomy

Pancreas

Com. bile
duct

1

2

3

4

5

6

7

Z

Alfred
Feinberg

Z′, Z″, Z‴, Z⁗. Alternate methods of anastomosis, using jejunum rather than duodenum:

Z′. Antecolic end-to-side esophagojejunostomy.

Z″. Retrocolic end-to-side esophagojejunostomy and jejunojejunostomy.

Z‴, Z⁗. End-to-end antecolic (Z‴) or retrocolic (Z⁗) esophagojejunostomy and end-to-side jejunojejunostomy.

The interposition of ileocolic, colic, or jejunal segments for restoration of alimentary continuity is not practiced. The only apparent advantage of such procedures is that they restore direct continuity between the stomach and duodenum which is more readily and easily accomplished by a direct end-to-end esophagoduodenostomy as illustrated. The value of interposed segments in the establishment of artificial gastric reservoirs and the prevention of symptoms relative to the dumping syndrome is seriously questioned.

DISCUSSION—DR. VALDONI (cont.)

the aid of an abdominal retractor the left lobe is displaced to the right.

It is important to recognize and isolate the hepatic branch of the left gastric artery, the so-called artery of Hyrtl, which in some patients may be unusually large. Therefore the severance of the left gastric artery should be distal to the origin of its hepatic branch. I then expose the right crus of the diaphragm and the splenic artery. In this dissection, the lymph nodes along the hepatic artery and the superior edge of the pancreas are removed. The left gastric vein, near the portal vein, is doubly ligated and severed between the ligatures. At this point I proceed to the colo-epiploic (omental) detachment. This starts on the left side and is progressively completed to the right colic flexure. It seems to me important to expose the gastroduodenal artery and its relation to the pancreas, colon, and duodenum, in order to sever the gastroepiploic artery at its origin. In this way, and without further dissection, the subpyloric and retropyloric lymph nodes, which remain in continuity with the pylorus, are resected en bloc. I then incise the peritoneum at the esophagocardial junction and continue the dissection along the left crus of the diaphgram. Both vagus nerves are transected in order to mobilize the terminal esophagus into the abdomen. Next, the left gastric artery (distal to its hepatic branch) and the splenic artery are isolated at their origins from the celiac axis and then doubly clamped, severed, and ligated. The vasa brevia are now secured and divided between ligatures to mobilize completely the greater curvature. At this stage the stomach is completely freed from its vascular attachments. The duodenum is divided beyond the pylorus, and the stump is closed and inverted. Finally, the esophagus is transected 2 cm. cephalad to the cardia, and the surgical specimen is removed.

The duodenal "C" and the head of the pancreas are mobilized only in thin patients with a mobile duodenum. This will frequently permit the performance of an esophagoduodenostomy by direct end-to-end anastomosis. Since this anastomosis is performed between a viscus with a partial or no peritoneal covering and one with a peritoneal covering, there is a risk of leakage at the suture line. Therefore, I usually prefer to establish an end-to-end esophagojejunal anastomosis on the Roux "en Y" principle, the jejunum being transected 10 cm. below the ligament of Treitz. The anastomosis is then inverted into the jejunum for several centimeters. After completion of the anastomosis, it is transferred through the esophageal hiatus into the posterior mediastinum. I should add that the efferent jejunal limb is passed through the transverse mesocolon. I prefer to leave the arterial arcade intact, as the vessels in each limb should be pulsating nicely. However, the efferent limb may at times be short and conceivably could exert a pulling action on the anastomosis. In order to avoid this, I detach the cecum and the last loop of ileum from the posterior abdominal wall in order to clear off completely the superior mesenteric artery in its terminal course. Thus one can gain at least 10 cm. of length for the efferent jejunal limb. The efferent jejunal limb is fixed to the mesocolic opening and the severed end of the afferent limb is inverted. A large side-to-side anastomosis is then performed between the afferent and efferent limbs of the jejunum below the transverse mesocolon. Before closing the abdomen, I pass a long soft rubber tube from the nose down the esophagus beyond the "Y" anastomosis for a distance of 40 to 50 cm. The tube assures the decompression and at the same time it permits feeding of the patient for 10 days.

When pancreatic resection is necessary, I prefer to divide the pancreas at the level of the portal vein. The dissection of the pancreatic stump to the left will expose the splenic vein, which is secured between ligatures. There are also a number of small pancreatic veins emptying into the portal vein. Since these may tear easily, they should be dissected individually and doubly ligated before division.

After the portal vein has been cleared, I proceed to perform splenectomy from the left to the right by dividing first the posterior parietal peritoneum (posterior layer of the lienorenal ligament) and then mobilizing manually the spleen together with the tail of the pancreas. The frequent presence of a bridge of pancreatic tissue behind the portal vein and the entrance of the inferior mesenteric vein tributary oftentimes presents a difficult problem. The remainder of the steps in the operative technic corresponds exactly to those described and illustrated in the text.

Plate 128 295

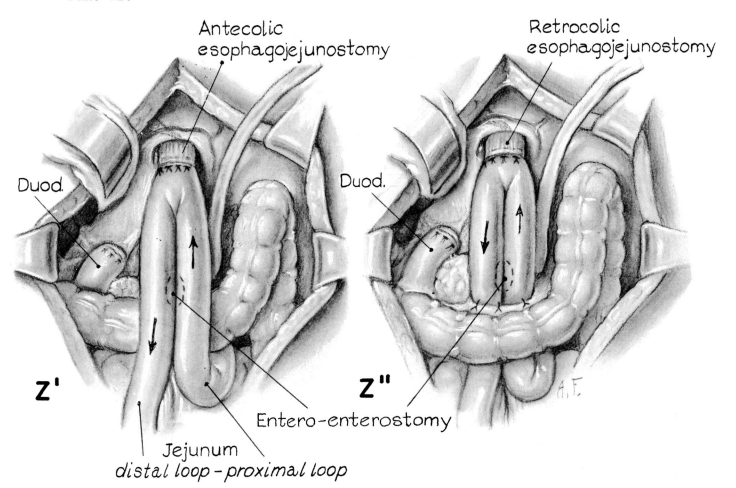

Antecolic esophagojejunostomy

Retrocolic esophagojejunostomy

Duod.

Duod.

Z'

Z"

Entero-enterostomy

Jejunum
distal loop - proximal loop

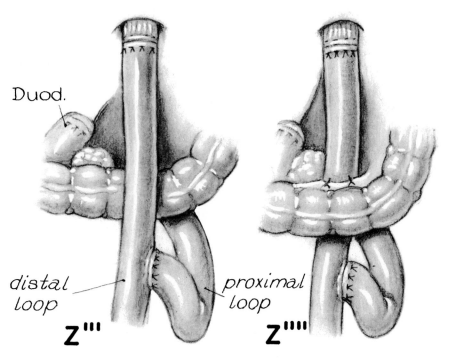

Duod.

distal loop

proximal loop

Z'''

Z''''

PYLOROMYOTOMY (FREDET–WEBER–RAMSTEDT OPERATION)

A. The right upper quadrant paramedian muscle-splitting incision utilized is depicted in dotted outline. If preferred, a transverse incision may be used. The shadowed area between the lower end of the incision and the umbilicus is indicative of a peristaltic wave, proceding obliquely downward from left to right and visible at the time of operation.

B. The incised margins of the posterior rectus sheath and the anterior parietal peritoneum are grasped in clamps, and the opening into the peritoneal cavity is extended upward by scissor dissection and downward with a scalpel.

C. The wound margins are retracted, and, first, the transverse colon and the transparent omentum overlying are withdrawn from the peritoneal cavity. Next, by manual traction the stomach is displaced upward into the wound and the pyloric tumor, the pathognomonic characteristic of infantile pyloric stenosis, is readily visible.

D. The pyloric tumor is immobilized securely between the thumb and the index finger of the left hand of the surgeon, and in the relatively avascular plane midway anteriorly, a longitudinal incision is made. To minimize the possibility of entrance into the lumen of the duodenum the direction of the incision is always from the duodenum toward the stomach. It is not the opening into the duodenum but the failure of its recognition that is dangerous. It may be recognized by the sudden appearance of bile-stained foam. Satisfactory closure is obtained with usually one, or at the most two, interrupted silk (0000) sutures.

E, F. The relatively superficial seromuscular incision overlying the pyloric tumor is deepened gradually by blunt dissection with a fine curved clamp, and the underlying layer of circular muscular fibers is exposed. During this dissection toward the pyloroduodenal junction, caution again must be observed to prevent accidental perforation into the lumen of the duodenum.

G. The layer of circular muscle fibers, mobilized on a clamp, is being severed by scissor dissection. In this dissection it is most important to sever all of the constricting fibers to permit a satisfactory herniation of the underlying mucosa.

H. Following the severance of all constricting fibers, blunt tissue dissection with a clamp is continued in the plane between the mucosa and the hypertrophied muscle layers, first on one and then on the other side of the pyloromyotomy incision. This is done to assure the severance of all constricting muscle fibers.

I. The Ramstedt pyloromyotomy is completed, and the mucosa is seen herniated through the incision.

J. A cross-section diagram of the completed operation depicting the herniation of the mucosa between the severed fibers of the hypertrophied muscle layers.

K. The incision is closed in layers using interrupted horizontal everting mattress sutures of silk (0000) for the peritoneum and interrupted sutures of silk (000) for both the fascia and skin.

Plate 129

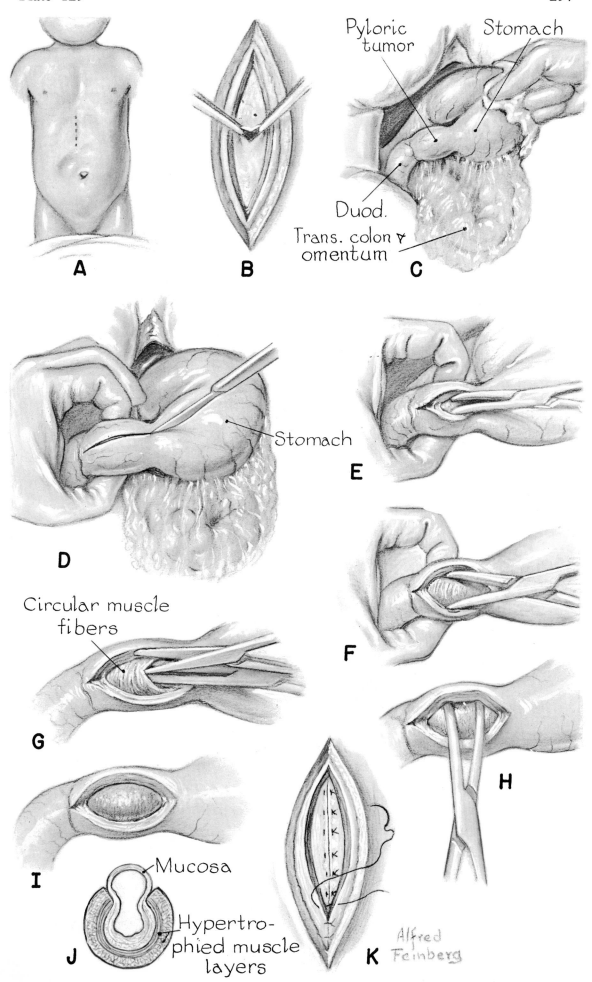

Pyloric tumor

Stomach

Duod.

Trans. colon &
omentum

A

B

C

Stomach

D

E

F

Circular muscle
fibers

G

H

Mucosa

Hypertro-
phied muscle
layers

I

J

K

Alfred
Feinberg

DISCUSSION—DR. EDWARD J. DONOVAN. In doing a Fredet–Ramstedt operation for congenital pyloric stenosis, I prefer to use a much shorter incision and place it higher than the one depicted here for the following reasons:

1. I wish to have the incision one cm. lateral to the xiphoid process and seven cm. long so that the right lobe of the liver completely covers it on the inside and has to be retracted upward to expose the pylorus. The liver then makes a splendid buffer for the incision and aids greatly in preventing disruption of the incision, which occurs quite frequently in these poorly nourished infants.

2. One need only deliver the pylorus into the incision in performing this operation. The transverse colon and the omentum need not be seen, thereby eliminating the trauma of replacing these structures in the peritoneal cavity.

The pyloric vein shows very well in D. This is a very important landmark showing the junction of pylorus and duodenum and is very constant in its location. If the incision in the pylorus goes beyond the pyloric vein one is very apt to open the duodenum, since the pyloric tumor projects into the duodenum as the cervix does into the vagina. Plate 129, G, shows the circular muscle of the pylorus being cut with scissors as a separate layer. I believe that this is unnecessary and possibly dangerous and could result in injury to the mucous membrane. If the incision in the pylorus is made just a little deeper with the scalpel, the cut edges of the circular muscle will spread easily with the clamp as shown in F. Use of the clamp as depicted in H is not believed necessary.

The Fredet–Ramstedt operation is a very simple one, but it must be done carefully. Opening into the duodenum is preventable if the proper precautionary measures are observed during the operation. Perforation of the duodenum may result in the child's death from peritonitis. Pyloromyotomy is one of the most satisfactory operations in infant surgery, and, when properly performed, effects a complete and permanent cure. This is proved by the multiple long range follow-up studies reported in the medical literature.

DISCUSSION—DR. W. H. SNYDER, JR. A general anesthetic is usually indicated. Local infiltration with 0.25 per cent novocain, however, is preferable in the marasmic or very ill baby.

I prefer a much shorter incision, 4 to 5 cm., placed just below the costal margin. The liver is lifted upward and the stomach exposed adjacent to the pylorus. The stomach is then gently grasped with a Babcock clamp and lifted into the incision. It is then held by the fingers and pulled to the left, exposing only the pylorus within the wound. The colon is left within the abdomen. There is always a thin white line at the junction of the pylorus and the duodenum, and this may be a better guide to the division between the pylorus and duodenum than the pyloric vein.

It is very important to make the incision longitudinally over the pylorus as indicated in D. If it is carried even slightly in a transverse direction, the muscle fibers do not separate satisfactorily and the stenosis may recur. Separation or splitting of the longitudinal *and circular* muscle fibers down to the mucosa is accomplished by the maneuver indicated in E. It has never, in my experience, been necessary or wise to transect the circular fibers separately as indicated in G. The longitudinal and circular fibers are so agglutinated that they react as a single unit; when, therefore, the separating force is applied by spreading of the hemostat, as indicated in E, both layers separate cleanly from the mucosa below and allow it to pout forward, as indicated in J.

The incision on the pylorus should be carried well on to the stomach. If this is done, undermining the muscular layer laterally, as indicated in H, is not, in my opinion, necessary or wise.

Silk mattress sutures are used to close the muscle and fascial layer of the abdominal incision. If this is done and a shorter incision is used than that indicated in A, I believe these measures will almost completely eliminate evisceration as a complication.

REPAIR OF PERFORATED DUODENAL ULCER

The technic of closure illustrated is a modification of the method described by the late Roscoe Graham of Canada. In Graham's technic the tab of omentum is used as a plug and is anchored into the site of perforation by the sutures which were previously inserted but not tied.

In the surgical management of perforated duodenal ulcers, it is the general practice of the author to employ simple suture closure of the perforation. Admittedly, 60 to 70 per cent of the patients so treated will have recurrent ulcer symptoms at varying intervals following the operation. However, subsequent treatment, either medical or surgical, may be prescribed on a purely elective basis according to the individual needs of the patient.

Partial gastrectomy as a primary definitive procedure was stressed in particular by Von Haberer in 1919. Although popular amongst surgeons on the Continent for many years, it has assumed popularity in the United States only in relatively recent years. Admittedly in some instances partial gastrectomy may be performed, either as a procedure of choice or as a mandatory operation according to the operative findings in the particular patient. However, its use as a routine procedure is not considered advisable.

In some patients with acutely perforated duodenal ulcers, conservative management by nasogastric suction, parenteral alimentation, and antibiotic therapy may be prescribed. This method, reported upon by the author in 1943, is used as a selective rather than routine method of treatment. Prior to 1943, Wangensteen and others were advocates of its use. More recently Taylor of England and Seeley of the United States have been its staunchest proponents.

In summary the choice of treatment for an acute perforated duodenal ulcer is dependent upon the particular findings, both clinical and operative, in the individual patient, and upon the judgment of the surgeon based upon his technical skill and experience. In general simple closure of the perforation is preferred.

A. The right upper quadrant paramedian muscle-retracting (lateral) incision employed is indicated by the dotted line.

B. The peritoneal cavity is entered and by manual retraction on the stomach, the site of perforation in the first portion of the duodenum is exposed.

C. Close-up view showing the insertion of the interrupted silk (00) sutures swedged on minimum trauma needles for the closure of the perforation. In the large perforations, the needle is first inserted well back on the gastric side and has its exit through the site of perforation. The needle is then reinserted through the perforation and has its exit on the duodenal side as depicted. In the small perforations, adequate closure is obtained with a single rather than double insertion of each suture needle.

D, E, F. The sutures are all first inserted and tied individually (D). In tying the sutures, tension on the suture line is avoided because the sutures easily pull through the friable and edematous tissue surrounding the perforation. Following the completion of the closure of the perforation, the long strands of the sutures are separated and subsequently tied about a piece of omental fat which is drawn up to reinforce the line of closure (E, F).

Plate 130   301

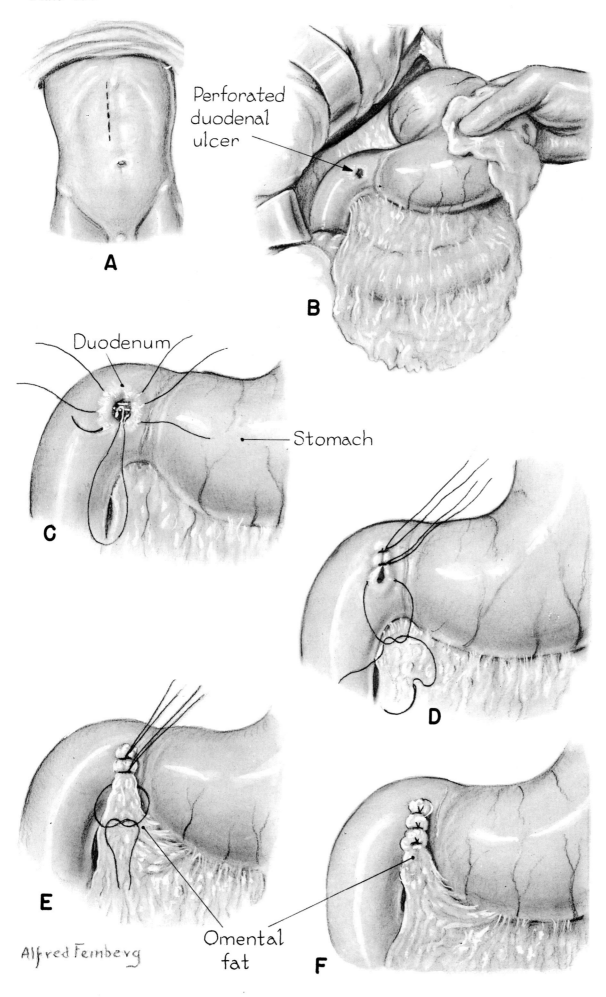

Perforated duodenal ulcer

A

B

Duodenum

Stomach

C

D

E

Omental fat

F

Alfred Feinberg

DISCUSSION—DR. AUBRE DE L. MAYNARD. I must commend the author for a lucid presentation of his subject, the excellent illustrations, and the concise but substantial text. My initial comment shall relate to the steps of the author's procedure as they are outlined.

The right upper quadrant muscle-retracting incision (A), though commonly used, is rarely my choice. For the very ill patient, it is tedious and time consuming. I prefer rapid entry into the abdomen by way of a midline incision with its minimum of bleeding. I must emphasize that to get the full benefit of this incision, it must be accurately midline. Extending from xiphoid to umbilicus, it gives excellent exposure and permits the carrying out of gastric resection with facility should this be necessary.

Manual retraction of the stomach, forward, to the left, and slightly downward (B), is the key maneuver in the exposure of the perforation. It brings into the operative field, with a minimum of trauma, the area that is the usual seat of involvement, namely the anterosuperior surface of the duodenum, pylorus, and juxtaposed stomach. Infrequently, a tiny perforation, temporarily obturated or undergoing spontaneous closure, may be obscure and difficult to detect. But in most cases the perforation is quite obvious or easily detected. Preliminary to suture closure, the perforation, with its surrounding inflammatory zone, should be freed from any contiguous protective attachments.

The author sets forth his modification of the classic technic of Roscoe Graham. The placement and number of sutures is in the Graham manner (C), except that silk (00) is used instead of catgut. Unlike the Graham technic, in which the omentum is used as a plug without approximation of the margins of the perforation, the author favors closure through approximation of those margins (D), applying the attached omentum over the site as shown (E, F). By his own admission, the sutures traverse the zone of edema and inflammatory infiltration surrounding the perforation and, in effecting a closure without tension, cut through the friable edematous tissue.

That this is sound or desirable surgical practice is at least debatable. That it has been effective surgical practice is inherent in the author's successful use of the technic. Of the many varieties of surgical closure, I have never used Dr. Madden's method, but have confined myself in difficult closures to Graham's technic, using catgut sutures. It has been consistently effective. Whenever I have employed a free omental graft, I have subsequently mantled the entire area with attached, viable gastrocolic omentum, fixed at focal points with fine silk sutures (0000). This provides added protection and further stimulates fibrin deposition and fibrogenesis over the site.

I would like to stress that, concomitant with surgical closure, continuous nasogastric suction is an indispensable ancillary measure. It should be instituted as soon as the diagnosis is made and maintained through and beyond operation, for as long as indicated. In my opinion, this measure is an important contribution to the success of any method of closure and to the eventual outcome.

In making further comment, it might be of interest to state our present attitude about the problem of the perforated ulcer.

In so far as immediate prognosis is concerned, one cannot dispute the fact that suture closure is a satisfactory method of treatment. It stops the peritoneal contamination and ordinarily controls the threat to life, but it does not, per se, influence the underlying ulcer pathology. In most instances, with the addition of nasogastric suction to immobilize the inflamed area and defunctionalize the stomach, healing does take place and recovery ensues. But the method is plagued with a high incidence of late poor results; 40 per cent to 70 per cent of the patients have the unhappy sequelae of reactivation of ulcer activity, reperforation, pyloric stenosis, and hemorrhage.

In November, 1953, trying to come to grips with this disturbing reality, we introduced emergency gastric resection for use in selected cases. There was initial difficulty in establishing positive criteria for its use, but we eventually settled on the following.

Gastric resection could justifiably be applied in cases of:

1. Perforation in a gastric ulcer that from size, situation, and character was suspect of malignancy.
2. Peptic ulcers that had a long history (certainly more than a year), and a pathology of unmistakable chronicity—
   (a) the presence of pyloric stenosis;
   (b) multiple ulcers;
   (c) perforation associated with bleeding;
   (d) reperforation;
   (e) a non-recent adhesive pathology about the involved pyloroduodenal segment.
3. The occasional perforation with callus and indurated margins and with such an intense and extensive inflammatory reaction around it that closure, even by the Graham technic appeared hazardous. It is quite possible also that this type of severe reaction may offer as much danger as the perforation, therefore the lesion would be better out by resection than left in by closure.

Within that general framework, primary gastric resection, identical with the procedure in elective cases, was applied by a number of senior residents under the supervision of a team of competent gastric surgeons with commendable results. In a group of 84 patients to date, 42 were treated by emergency gastric resection with 1 death, 40 were treated by suture closure with 4 deaths, and 2 were treated by nasogastric suction with 2 deaths. The mortality in the resection group came from delirium tremens and not peritonitis. The 4 mortalities in the closure group were attributed to peritonitis and sepsis in 2 cases and delirium tremens in 2 cases. Nasogastric suction was reserved for two types:

1. The "formes frustes" type described by Singer and associates, in which the catastrophe is short-lived, the course exceedingly mild and non-progressive, suggesting that control has taken place either by spontaneous closure or through a sealing off of the perforation by contiguous structures.
2. Patients so perilously ill from toxemia and/or bacterial peritonitis as to preclude surgical intervention of any sort.

Our results with primary gastric resection have so far been heartening and have convinced us that there is a place for this major procedure in treating this emergency. We are hopeful that over a longer period of time, with a much larger volume of cases, it will be possible to arrive at unassailable criteria for its use in selected cases.

STENOSIS, ATRESIA, AND DIAPHRAGMATIC OCCLUSION OF THE DUODENUM

This plate depicts diagrammatically the analogy between the congenital defects of the duodenum and those in the region of the aortic arch. In each, the congenital defect occurs at the site of an embryologic event. Moreover the comparative anatomic similarity is striking despite the fact that in the development of the aortic arch there is no solid phase. This similarity is particularly well illustrated between diaphragmatic occlusion of the duodenum and coarctation of the aorta of the "adult" type (C and C¹).

The exact mechanism for the occurrence of congenital anomalies of the duodenum and, in particular, of diaphragmatic occlusion is unknown. Although many hypotheses have been proposed, the two that are believed to merit discussion most are those of Bland-Sutton and Tandler.

In 1889 John Bland-Sutton reported a case of small bowel obstruction caused by a complete diaphragmatic occlusion of the ileum. The diaphragm was located in the ileum at the site corresponding to the entrance of the vitelline duct in the embryo. Accordingly it was stated that congenital obstruction and narrowing of the alimentary canal was always found at the site of embryologic events. To substantiate this hypothesis Bland-Sutton cited the following anomalies of the gastrointestinal tract: (1) an imperforate pharynx occurs at the site where the foregut and the stomadeum come into contact, (2) an imperforate or septate duodenum occurs in the region of the papilla of Vater where the diverticula issue to form the liver and the pancreas, (3) imperforate rectum and anus are due to imperfect union of the hindgut and the proctodeum, and (4) an imperforate ileum occurs in the region where the primitive alimentary canal is in communication with the yolk sac by means of the vitelline duct.

In 1900 Tandler, working with embryos of 30 to 60 days obtained by operations for ectopic pregnancies, stated that during this period of development the lumen of the duodenum is "more or less completely" obliterated and in the so-called "solid" stage. It was further stated that subsequent to the tenth week, vacuoles appear which coalesce and ultimately reestablish the continuity of the lumen. From this study it was postulated that arrests in development occurring during this transitional phase (second to third months) were a logical explanation for the occurrence of atresias, stenoses, and diaphragmatic occlusions of the duodenum. This study was confirmed by both Kreuter and by Forssner. Furthermore, Kreuter was of the opinion that the stage of epithelial occlusion was not limited to the vaterian segment of the duodenum, as Tandler concluded, but that it extended throughout the whole of the small intestine.

The hypothesis of Bland-Sutton is believed to be the most logical and acceptable of any that have been promulgated. It is particularly adaptable to congenital anomalies of the duodenum. Furthermore, it offers a satisfactory explanation for the occurrence of congenital anomalies other than in the gastrointestinal tract. In the duodenum, atresias, stenoses, and diaphragms occur almost invariably in the vaterian segment. This segment is the site of origin of the anlage of the liver, biliary tract, and pancreas, and also the site of junction of the foregut and the midgut. The main objection to this hypothesis, voiced by many, is that similar anomalies occur, either alone or concomitantly, in other parts of the intestines which are not the site of embryologic events.

The hypothesis of Tandler is believed less tenable than that of Bland-Sutton. This, however, is a minority opinion. Schridde (1909) in an examination of 50 human embryos in stages of development corresponding to that described by Tandler, Kreuter, and Forssner, was unable to demonstrate epithelial occlusions in any portion of the intestinal tract. More recently Schwegler and Boyden have questioned the presence of a "solid" phase during the development of the duodenum. Although admittedly less frequent, atresias, stenoses, and

Plate 131   305

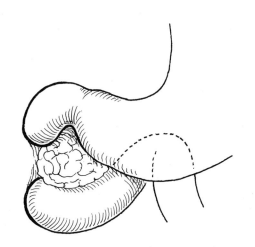

ATRESIA OF DUODENUM
A

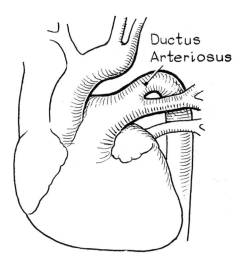

Ductus
Arteriosus

ATRESIA OF AORTA
A'

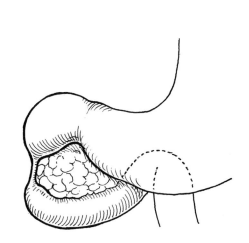

STENOSIS OF DUODENUM

B

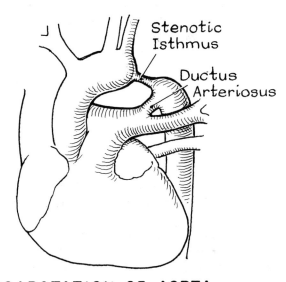

Stenotic
Isthmus

Ductus
Arteriosus

COARCTATION OF AORTA
Infantile Type
B'

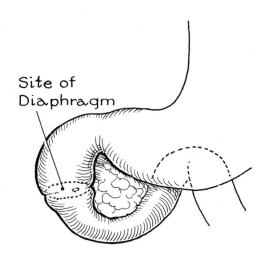

Site of
Diaphragm

DIAPHRAGM OF DUODENUM

C

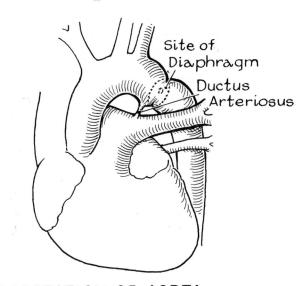

Site of
Diaphragm

Ductus
Arteriosus

COARCTATION OF AORTA
Adult Type
C'

diaphragms occur in the colon despite the fact that a "solid" phase does not occur in the development of the large bowel. Furthermore, similar anomalies occur in areas other than the gastrointestinal tract, in which there are no preexisting "solid" phases in development but which are the sites of embryologic events. This is most notably exemplified in the arch of the aorta. Despite the absence of a "solid" phase the congenital anomalies of the aortic arch are believed analogous to those that occur in the duodenum and are depicted in Plate 131. This analogy tends to negate the hypothesis of Tandler and to lend credence to the one of Bland-Sutton.

Atresia and stenosis (coarctation of the "infantile" or "adult" type) of the aorta occur at the site of an embryologic event, namely, the region of the juncture of the third and fourth aortic arches. This region is also the site of communication between the pulmonary artery and the aorta through the ductus arteriosus (Botalli). Coarctation of the "adult" type simulates closely congenital diaphragmatic occlusion of the duodenum (Plate 131, C, C'). In each, a diaphragm placed obliquely across the lumen is present. The diaphragm may or may not be perforated, but if a perforation is present, it is usually eccentric. Finally, the site of the diaphragm is indicated externally by a constriction or slight indentation of the wall.

In summary, one may state that the exact mechanism for the developmental anomalies of the gastrointestinal tract is unknown. However, from the knowledge that is available, it is believed that the concept expressed by Bland-Sutton is the most logical and the one that is the most universally applicable.

The type of operation and the order of preference in the treatment of duodenal atresia (A) and duodenal stenosis (B) are depicted.

A. This is a diagrammatic representation of an atresia of the duodenum seen at operation. It is characterized by a discontinuity of tissue in the second portion of the duodenum distal to the site of entrance of the papilla of Vater.

a 1. The ideal operation for atresia, one which relieves the obstruction and restores the continuity of the duodenum, is an end-to-end duodenoduodenostomy as depicted. *a 2.* In the event that the restoration of direct continuity of the duodenum is not feasible, either an antecolic duodenojejunostomy, as illustrated (*a 2*) or a retrocolic duodenojejunostomy may be performed. In fact, a duodenojejunostomy is the operation most commonly performed in the surgical management of duodenal atresia.

a 3. In some instances the performance of the least acceptable, but at times life saving operation, namely, gastrojejunostomy, may be required. The disadvantage of a gastrojejunostomy is the fact that adequate decompression of the "blind" duodenal segment is not obtained. Accordingly, when it is filled, retrograde regurgitation into the stomach occurs with repeated cyclic attacks of vomiting. In the inset (*a, b*) the technic for enlarging the lumen of the collapsed jejunum, by the injection of sterile saline solution preparatory to anastomosis, is shown.

B. In like manner duodenojejunostomy (*b 1*) or gastrojejunostomy (*b 2*) may be performed in the treatment of duodenal stenosis. Of the two operations duodenojejunostomy, retrocolic or antecolic (*b 1*), is preferred. The objection to gastrojejunostomy (*b 2*) is the same as previously stated: namely, recurrent attacks of vomiting, secondary to regurgitation of the obstructed duodenal contents into the stomach.

Plate 132   307

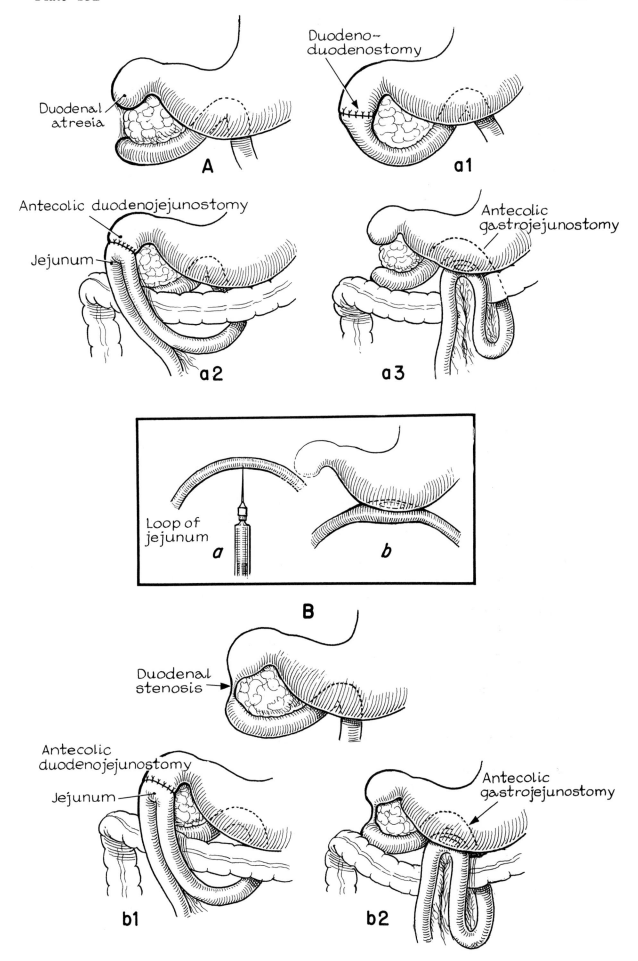

Duodenal atresia

Duodeno-duodenostomy

A

a1

Antecolic duodenojejunostomy

Jejunum

a2

Antecolic gastrojejunostomy

a3

Loop of jejunum

a

b

B

Duodenal stenosis

Antecolic duodenojejunostomy

Jejunum

b1

Antecolic gastrojejunostomy

b2

This plate depicts the direct (A – Morton, B – Peterson) and indirect (C) approaches in the surgical management of diaphragmatic occlusion of the duodenum.

A. The diaphragmatic occlusion of the duodenum is depicted. The indentation of the outside wall of the duodenum at the level of the papilla of Vater corresponds to the site of the diaphragm. The eccentric orifice in the diaphragm is visible.

a1, a2, a3, a4. This series of illustrations demonstrates the technic described by Morton for the treatment of diaphragmatic occlusion of the duodenum. The method is simple, direct, and effective. The hepatic flexure of the colon is mobilized, and the whole of the duodenal loop is exposed. A longitudinal incision is made in the anterior wall of the duodenum at the site of the diaphragm, above and below which it extends into the lumen of the duodenum (*a 1*). The diaphragm is secured in tissue forceps and transected ("bivalved") by scissor dissection (*a 2*). Each half of the transected diaphragm is excised, and the closure of the duodenum in a plane transverse to its longitudinal axis is begun (*a 3*). A two layer closure with interrupted silk (0000) sutures completes the operation (*a 4*). The enlargement of the diameter of the lumen of the duodenum by the transverse closure is demonstrable (*a 4*). In using this method one should refrain from inserting ligatures in the cut margins of the diaphragm because of danger of occlusion of either or both the common and pancreatic ducts. These structures course between the mucosal layers of the diaphragm and may be occluded by a suture, particularly one of the continuous type.

B, *b1, b2, b3.* The technic for the surgical treatment of diaphragmatic occlusion of the duodenum recommended by Peterson is illustrated. Similarly, as in the technic described by Morton, a longitudinal incision is made into the lumen of the duodenum and the diaphragm is simply transected (*b 1*). This provides an adequate lumen and does not require the resection of any portion of the diaphragm. In preparation for closure of the duodenotomy incision at right angles to its long axis, the midportions of the cut margin of the longitudinal incision are grasped in clamps (Babcock) or, preferably, traction guy sutures of 00 silk. Traction is maintained in a plane at right angles to the long axis of the bowel (*b 1*), and a suture to approximate the proximal and distal points of the linear incision is inserted (*b 1*) and tied (*b 2*). Similarly, as in the technic described by Morton (*a 1–a 4*) a two layer transverse closure of the duodenum with interrupted sutures of silk (000) is performed (*b 3*).

C, *c1, c2.* In addition to the direct approaches of Morton (A) and Peterson (B) in the treatment of diaphragmatic occlusion of the duodenum, an indirect operative procedure may be employed (*c 1, c2*). This may consist of either a side-to-side duodenojejunostomy (*c 1*) or a side-to-side gastrojejunostomy (*c 2*). The first of these operations, namely, duodenojejunostomy, is an acceptable substitute to either transduodenal excision (Morton) or transection (Peterson) of the diaphragm. However, gastrojejunostomy, as an elective operation, should not be performed because the duodenum proximal to the diaphragm may become enormously dilated. Consequently, regurgitation of large quantities of ingested foodstuffs into the stomach occurs and incites chronic recurrent attacks of vomiting. A gastrojejunostomy should only be employed if considered mandatory in saving the life of the patient. In the recorded instances in which this operation was used as a primary method of treatment, secondary corrective procedures, either duodenoduodenostomy, duodenojejunostomy, or duodenotomy with incision or excision of the diaphragm, have been required.

Plate 133   309

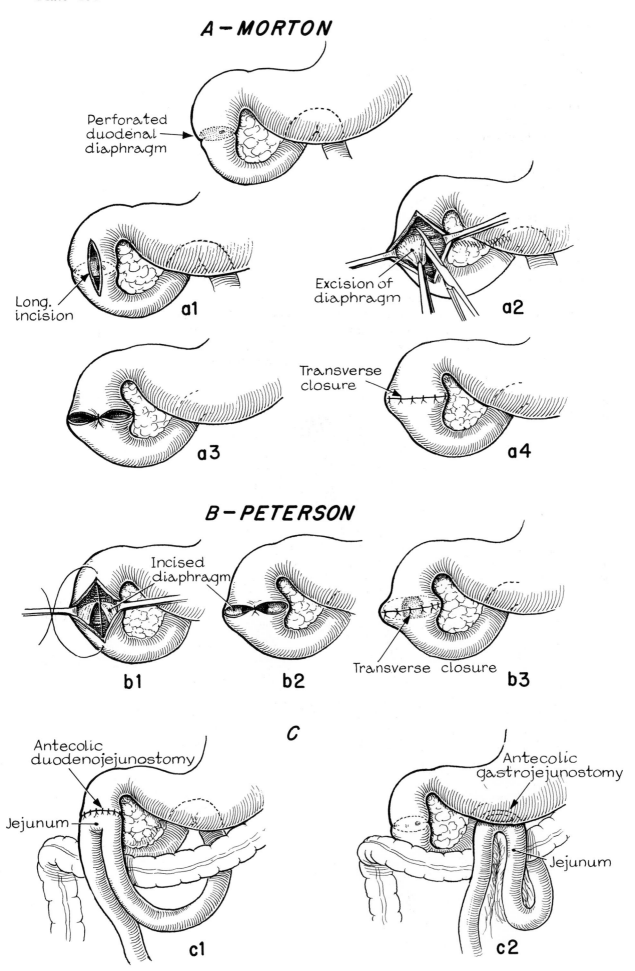

A – MORTON

Perforated duodenal diaphragm

Long. incision   a1

Excision of diaphragm   a2

a3

Transverse closure   a4

B – PETERSON

Incised diaphragm

b1   b2   Transverse closure   b3

C

Antecolic duodenojejunostomy

Jejunum

c1

Antecolic gastrojejunostomy

Jejunum

c2

A. Artist's illustrations of findings at operation in a patient with an intrinsic obstruction of the duodenum secondary to a diaphragm. The symmetrical dilatation both above and below the level of the diaphragm and the indentation of the wall of the duodenum corresponding to the site of attachment of the obliquely placed diaphragm are visible. The uniformity in the caliber of the duodenum proximal and distal to the diaphragm is a characteristic finding and frequently the reason for failure of making the diagnosis at operation. All too frequently the presence of an innocuous peritoneal membrane is incorrectly considered the cause of the obstructive symptoms that are manifest.

B. Artist's illustration of findings in a second patient in whom a diaphragmatic occlusion of the duodenum was present. In infancy a retrocolic gastrojejunostomy was performed. The postoperative course was complicated by the occurrence of intermittent attacks of vomiting of progressive severity. Finally at the age of ten years, exploratory laparotomy was performed. The symmetrical dilatation of the duodenum above and below the diaphragm, the eccentric perforation, the constriction or indentation of the wall of the duodenum at the site of attachment of the diaphragm, and the retrocolic gastrojejunostomy performed previously are shown. The illustration in the inset depicts the oblique position (45 degree angle) of the diaphragm.

C. This is a drawing to show the operation performed in this patient, namely, a side-to-side duodenoduodenostomy to bypass the obstruction caused by the diaphragm. Because of the redundancy and dilatation of the duodenum that was present, the type of bypass anastomosis depicted was easily accomplished.

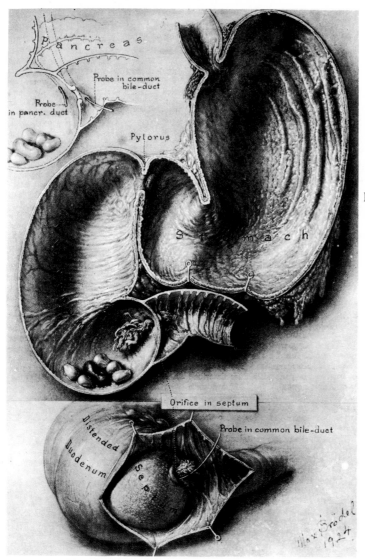

D. "Upper sketch: esophagus, stomach, and duodenum opened after fixation in formalin.

"Lower sketch: duodenal lumen with septum shown from the jejunal side.

"Drawing in upper left corner: diagrammatic representation of the course of the biliary and pancreatic ducts in relation to the duodenal septum, its surfaces and orifice." (Courtesy of S. M. Seidlin, M. D., and Bull. Johns Hopkins Hosp.)

Plate 134

A

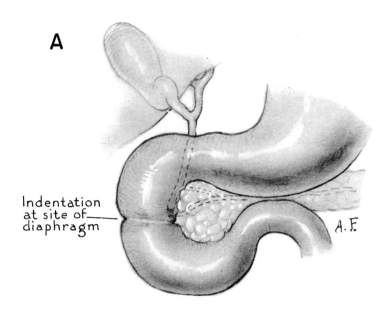

Indentation at site of diaphragm

A.F.

B

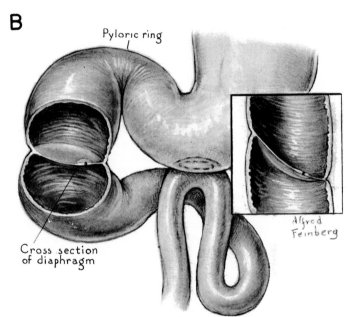

Pyloric ring

Cross section of diaphragm

Alfred Feinberg

C

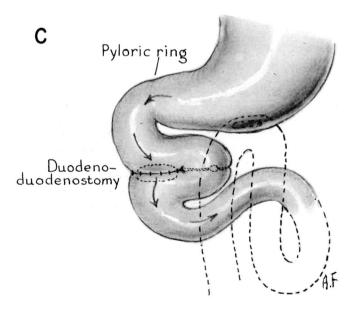

Pyloric ring

Duodeno-duodenostomy

A.F.

In patients with intrinsic obstructions of the duodenum, the primary symptom is persistent vomiting. Characteristically the vomitus contains bile, but bile may be absent, as its presence depends upon the site of entrance of the common bile duct relative to the obstruction. The vomitus is frequently "coffee ground" and oftentimes frankly bloody.

A deep icterus is commonly present. In fact, the combination of icterus and bloody vomitus occurs so frequently that it has been considered diagnostic of congenital obstructive anomalies of the duodenum. Reportedly in such cases the incidence of icterus is 40 to 45 per cent and that of bloody vomitus is 60 to 85 per cent. Furthermore, it is frequently stated that there is an increase in other congenital malformations in association with intrinsic obstructions of the duodenum, particularly mongolism. This was first mentioned by Fanconi and subsequently observed by others.

Epigastric distention and visible gastric peristalsis are prominent objective symptoms. The dilated first portion of the duodenum may be easily felt and it is frequently misinterpreted as a "palpable tumor."

If the correct diagnosis is not made and the proper treatment is not given, in the majority of patients the symptoms are progressive and are associated with rapid and pronounced weight loss, severe fluid and electrolyte imbalance, and ultimately the death of the patient.

In every newborn with persistent vomiting, the diagnosis of duodenal obstruction must be considered and either confirmed or negated as quickly as possible. This is most important when one considers the fact that the condition of infants with obstructive anomalies of the duodenum deteriorates rapidly. Accordingly, if the diagnosis is unduly delayed, the patient becomes an extremely poor surgical risk.

In addition to the symptoms previously mentioned, a careful study of the plain or "scout" roentgenograms of the abdomen taken in both the upright and inverted positions is a valuable aid in diagnosis. Characteristically, these films demonstrate a gas-filled stomach and first portion of the duodenum with little or no gas shadows in the remainder of the intestines. Unfortunately and too frequently, such findings have been considered diagnostic only in retrospect. In the event that the diagnosis still remains in doubt, the instillation of small amounts (30 to 60 ml.) of warm iodized oil (lipiodol) or a light barium mixture through a nasogastric tube (No. 8F) is almost invariably confirmatory. Although both oil and barium have been used, the oil is preferred in the newborn because of the ever present danger of the aspiration of regurgitant gastric contents and resultant pulmonary complications.

The two main conditions which should be differentiated from congenital obstructive anomalies of the duodenum are esophageal atresia and infantile pyloric stenosis.

Esophageal atresia. In atresia of the esophagus vomiting occurs during rather than after each feeding and is associated with varying degrees of cyanosis. The vomitus consists of the unchanged feeding and does not contain bile. Salivation between each feeding is excessive. "Scout" roentgenograms of the abdomen will show either abundant gas shadows throughout the whole of the gastrointestinal tract or none at all, as the shadows depend upon the presence or absence of an associated tracheoesophageal fistula. A nasogastric tube (No. 8 F) may be inserted only a short distance before an obstruction is met. Finally, the instillation of two to three ml. of warm iodized oil (lipiodol) followed by a roentgenogram of the chest, including the cervical region, will depict clearly the cul-de-sac of the proximal segment of the esophagus.

In *infantile pyloric stenosis* the vomiting is usually delayed until the third or fourth week and the vomitus does not contain bile. The fact that the vomiting is projectile is not of differential diagnostic aid since the same may occur with obstructive anomalies in the duodenum. Furthermore, the absence of bile is not an absolute differential aid because the same may obtain in intrinsic obstructions of the duodenum when the entrance of the bile into the lumen of the duodenum is below the site of obstruction. In pyloric stenosis there is a preliminary progressive gain in weight and maintenance of adequate nutrition, whereas in duodenal obstruction the progress from birth is in general one of rapid deterioration. Finally, roentgenograms of the abdomen, both plain and with the aid of contrast media (lipiodol), will aid in making the proper diagnosis.

As an aid in the diagnosis of duodenal atresia, Walz, in 1906, suggested examination of the meconium for lanugo hair and skin remnants. Since these do not appear before the fourth month of fetal life, failure to find them in the meconium would imply a preexisting and complete luminal obstruction. Subsequently Farber, in 1933, described a test founded on the same principle. This test is based on the fact that microscopic examination of the smears of normal meconium, when treated with ether, stained with Sterling's gentian violet, and decolorized by acid alcohol, reveals large numbers of cornified epithelial cells which retain the stain. The absence of cornified epithelial cells in microscopic examination of smears of meconium is indicative of congenital atresia of the gastrointestinal tract.

In the newborn the differential diagnosis of atresia, stenosis, and diaphragmatic occlusion of the duodenum is believed of academic rather than of practical importance. However, it has been repeatedly demonstrated that infants with stenoses and perforate diaphragms of the duodenum have survived through childhood and late adulthood without corrective operations. This does not obtain in infants with atresias, severe stenoses, and complete or imperforate diaphragms of the duodenum.

The two most important factors in the treatment of duodenal obstruction in the newborn are early diagnosis and early operation. One cannot be too emphatic in restating the fact that in patients with duodenal atresias, complete stenoses, and imperforate diaphragms the clinical course is one of rapid and progressive deterioration. These patients withstand the loss of fluids poorly and even in their optimum state one may not consider them good surgical risks.

In obstructive anomalies of the duodenum, the type of corrective operation is dependent upon the type of anomaly that is present. In duodenal atresia one of three operations may be selected (Plate 132, A, *a 1, a 2, a 3*): (1) duodenoduodenostomy, (2) duodenojejunostomy, or (3) gastrojejunostomy. It may be of interest to note that the first successful operation for duodenal obstruction in the newborn was a side-to-side duodenoduodenostomy performed by Fockens in 1911 for an atresia of the duodenum. If a direct anastomosis is not feasible, a duodenojejunostomy is preferred. Ernst, in 1916, employed an antecolic duodenojejunostomy in performing the second successful operation for obstruction of the duodenum, also an atresia. Finally, because of technical considerations and/or the critical condition of the patient, a lifesaving gastrojejunostomy, preferably antecolic, may be done. A retrocolic gastrojejunostomy was used by Richter in performing the third successful operation for congenital obstruction of the duodenum. The obstruction was due to stenosis. The main objection to a gastrojejunostomy is that vomiting may persist with varying degrees of severity because of the regurgitation of the blocked duodenal contents into the stomach. This obtained in the infant reported by Sweet and Robertson (1927) upon whom the fourth successful operation was performed for obstruction of the duodenum. Ladd (1937) reported a similar experience in an infant upon whom a posterior gastrojejunostomy was performed for a duodenal obstruction.

In the treatment of stenosis of the duodenum, the same operations as described may be employed. However, an antecolic duodenojejunostomy is preferred (Plate 132, B, b1).

In the surgical management of diaphragmatic occlusions of the duodenum, three other operations, in addition to the three previously described, are available. In two the operative approach is direct and in one it is indirect. The one of choice, from both the theoretical and practical viewpoints, consists of a duodenotomy and excision of the diaphragm (Plate 133, A—Morton).

A second type of direct approach is based on the principle of a Horsley pyloroplasty (Plate 133, B —Peterson). A longitudinal incision is made in the duodenum across the diaphragm, and a transverse closure of the incision is performed.

In utilizing the direct method for either excision or incision of the diaphragm, one must remember that both the bile and the pancreatic ducts frequently course within the membrane. In the perforate diaphragms the ducts frequently open at the margin of an eccentrically placed orifice. Accordingly, the use of sutures, particularly the continuous type, to control bleeding from the cut margins of the diaphragm may endanger the patency of the ducts.

Finally, a duodenoduodenostomy, the indirect approach, may be performed.

DISCUSSION—DR. HUGH B. LYNN. One preliminary comment seems justified on the basis of my long-standing interest in this problem. No one explanation for these malfunctions will cover the entire field, and certainly many vascular accidents and similar conditions occur much later and produce similar results. These developments are substantiated by the fact that in a large percentage of cases the meconium is heavily stained with bile.

The descending portion of the duodenum is to me one of the most vital regions of the body. It is the main alimentary channel, and it also contains the entrance of both the pancreatic and biliary ducts in a multitude of forms and locations. It is the site of many abnormalities that are fascinating in their variations and require some meticulous and prolonged surgical dissections.

While theoretically the ideal operation for atresia or stenosis would be resection and primary end-to-end anastomosis, even the most experienced surgeons sooner or later come to grief in attempting such operations in this region. Consequently, I feel that duodenojejunostomy is the treatment of choice and should be performed with minimal exploration and dissection. In my experience, whether the anastomosis is antecolic or retrocolic has proved to be relatively unimportant, although a retrocolic isoperistaltic anastomosis is theoretically desirable. In a fairly good percentage of these cases of duodenal obstruction the association of incomplete rotation (with the duodenum descending completely on the right side) eliminates any decision for antecolic versus retrocolic anastomosis after completion of Ladd's procedure.

Gastrojejunostomy has been emphasized as the least acceptable procedure, and I agree. Nevertheless, it has been pointed out wisely that in an occasional rare case this procedure is necessary and that it is wholly acceptable as a lifesaving measure. I must admit, however, that I have found it necessary on only one occasion to perform gastrojejunostomy; in all other cases I have been able to anastomose the proximal portion of the duodenum, thereby giving more adequate drainage and retaining some semblance of normal intestinal physiology. Every effort should be made to avoid gastrojejunostomy. The few patients having this procedure whom I have seen have experienced periodic vomiting, failure to thrive, intestinal bleeding, partial closure of the stoma, and signs of irritability and discomfort.

As already indicated, I am strongly opposed to any unnecessary dissection in the region of the biliary and pancreatic ducts and avoid treating annular pancreas with anything other than a shunting procedure. For this reason I cannot subscribe to the procedure of either Morton or Peterson, since the dangers involved in such a dissection far outweigh the advantages to be gained. Moreover, although a duodenotomy with excision of the diaphragm makes a pretty operation, the follow-up unfortunately has all too frequently been one of recurrent stenosis with chronic bouts of obstruction because of the constriction created by the contraction of the congenital annulus or periphery of the diaphragm.

While I subscribe to the principle of duodenoduodenostomy in preference to duodenojejunostomy whenever possible, it is imperative that the duodenoduodenostomy be constructed on the anterolateral aspect. This is obvious when one follows the broken lines of pancreatic and common bile ducts in A. I must emphasize that the use of some curd-free formula, such as Nutramigen, probably does more to insure the success of the surgical procedure than any selection of suture materials or special operative technics. My own selection of material is that of 00000 chromic catgut sutures for the inner layer and of 00000 arterial silk for the outer layer. The only other technical point that I feel needs stressing is that in retrocolic anastomosis it is important to place sutures to maintain the mesocolon in firm approximation to the proximal duodenum so as to prevent sagging of the mesocolon with constriction of the two limbs of jejunum; if this is not done, those portions of the jejunum appear to have herniated up through the defect and may become a troublesome source of partial obstruction.

MALROTATION OF THE COLON AND VOLVULUS OF THE MIDGUT

This patient, a full-term Negro female infant, whose birth weight was five pounds, eight ounces, was seen in surgical consultation 36 hours after a normal spontaneous delivery because of rectal bleeding. On examination the infant was listless and moderately dehydrated but in no acute distress. The abdomen was soft and no masses or viscera were palpable. On digital rectal examination there were no abnormal findings. On the second day following birth, vomiting shortly after each feeding was observed. However, there was no recurrence of rectal bleeding. Because of the persistent vomiting a roentgenographic study following the ingestion of a thin barium mixture was obtained. This showed evidence of partial obstruction in the mid-descending portion of the duodenum with moderate stasis proximally. A diagnosis of intrinsic obstruction of the duodenum caused by diaphragmatic occlusion was made and operation was advised. An alternate diagnosis was annular pancreas. The findings at the time of abdominal operation and the operative procedures performed are illustrated.

This particular case serves to emphasize the fact that when an exploratory laparotomy is performed in the newborn for an obstruction of the duodenum, one should always suspect an occult intraluminal obstruction even though there are specific factors (malrotation of intestines and peritoneal membranes) to account for the clinical manifestations present.

A. The right paramedian muscle-retracting (lateral) incision employed is indicated by the solid black line.

B. In this patient, because of the primary preoperative diagnosis of an intrinsic obstruction of the duodenum due to a diaphragmatic occlusion, the incision is made in the mid-descending portion of the duodenum, as denoted by the linear dotted line. This incision overlies the site of the obstruction depicted by the preoperative roentgenograms. The "transverse" colon depicted was subsequently shown to be the ascending colon.

C. The incised margins of the duodenum are secured by guy sutures of silk (000) and retracted transversely. The exploration of the lumen of the duodenum at the site of the duodenotomy failed to reveal an occluding diaphragm. A catheter (No. 12 F) was then inserted to determine the patency of the duodenum distally.

D. Despite repeated attempts the catheter could not be inserted beyond a distance of 5 cm. It was then decided to expose the ligament of Treitz and determine the cause of the intervening obstruction. In doing this the malrotation of the colon and the volvulus of the midgut about its mesenteric vascular stalk were demonstrated. The volvulus of the midgut adequately explained the presenting but temporary symptom of rectal bleeding. The dotted line indicates the site of severance of the peritoneal membrane between the cecum and the posteriolateral abdominal wall.

E. Detorsion (anticlockwise) of the volvulus is being performed. The relation of the ileocecal junction to the duodenojejunal segment is visible.

E¹. Inset to show an artist's illustration made from a photograph of the findings at operation in another newborn in whom volvulus of the midgut (clockwise rotation) with duodenal obstruction and reversible compromise of the circulation of the greater portion of the midgut was present.

DISCUSSION—DR. THOMAS V. SANTULLI. The history in this infant is highly suggestive of intestinal obstruction due to malrotation with midgut volvulus. In a small percentage of these cases, the presenting symptom may be the passage of dark red blood by rectum. If this is accompanied or followed by bile-stained vomiting, duodenal obstruction from midgut volvulus is probably the underlying cause. The bleeding results from venous stasis in the small intestine and is probably indicative of pressure on the superior mesenteric vessels at the base of the volvulus. The great danger lies in occlusion of these vessels with ensuing gangrene of the entire midgut segment. If the diagnosis is suspected, plain three-position x-rays of the abdomen may reveal distention of the stomach and duodenum with a normal distribution, or a small amount, of air in the small intestine below. A barium enema will show malrotation of the colon and serves to confirm the diagnosis. It is rarely necessary to give a contrast agent orally for a gastrointestinal series in this type of case; however, with intermittent, low grade obstruction it may be necessary.

Once the diagnosis is suspected and there has been blood passed by rectum, immediate operation should

Plate 135

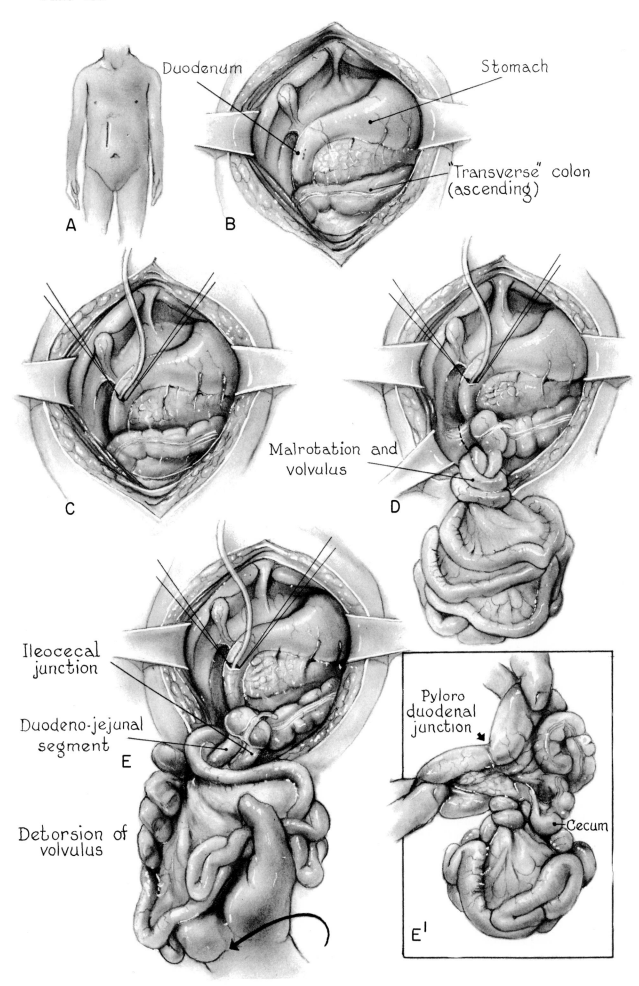

Duodenum

Stomach

"Transverse" colon
(ascending)

A

B

C

Malrotation and
volvulus

D

Ileocecal
junction

Duodeno-jejunal
segment

E

Detorsion of
volvulus

Pyloro
duodenal
junction

Cecum

E¹

F. The detorsion of the volvulus is completed, and the recommendation of Ladd to leave the duodenum on the right side and the ileocecal and cecoascending colon segments on the left side is followed.

G. The catheter is withdrawn and the linear incision in the duodenum is closed in a horizontal plane using two layers of interrupted silk (0000) sutures.

H. After the operation illustrated, obstructive symptoms remained manifest and a gastrointestinal series following a barium meal was repeated. The roentgenograms again showed evidence of duodenal stasis and partial obstruction in the region of the mid-descending portion of the duodenum. Four days following the first operation a second abdominal exploration was performed. The incision in the duodenum was reopened and on attempting a retrograde passage of the catheter (12 F) into the stomach an obstruction within a distance of 3 cm. was observed. A second incision was then made in the anterior wall of the antral region of the stomach through which a second catheter was inserted toward the opening in the duodenum. Similarly an intraluminal duodenal obstruction was present at approximately the same level as previously noted on retrograde passage of the catheter through the duodenal incision.

I, J, K. The catheters were withdrawn and a curved (Kelly) clamp was inserted through the gastric incision into the lumen of the duodenum. In so doing there was a sudden "give" felt through the clamp which then passed easily through the duodenal incision (I). In performing this maneuver no undue force was used. In fact the ease with which the obstruction was relieved made one doubt the existence of a typical intraluminal diaphragm with mucous membrane covering on either side. Instead it felt as if a thin veil of tissue was broken through. Subsequently the catheter (No. 12 F) was inserted through the gastric opening into the lumen of the duodenum to a level beyond the incision in its mid-descending portion. The incisions in the stomach and duodenum respectively were then closed in two layers using interrupted sutures of silk (0000) (J). The closure of the gastric incision was made about the catheter which was subsequently brought through the line of closure of the abdominal incision (K). The catheter was removed on the seventh day after operation, and the recovery of the patient was without incident.

DISCUSSION—DR. SANTULLI (cont.)

be done. The incision shown in Plate 135, A, is probably too small for adequate exposure. When operating for intestinal obstruction in infancy, a long paramedian incision or upper transverse incision is necessary in order to adequately visualize the pathology. In cases of malrotation or other forms of neonatal obstruction, it is mandatory to eviscerate all of the small intestine in order to be able to adequately visualize the pathology.

The midgut volvulus illustrated in Plate 135, D and E, is the usual form found in this age group. The volvulus is almost always in the clockwise direction, and reduction is accomplished by turning the bowel in the counterclockwise direction. In some cases there have been four complete turns of the intestine.

After reduction of the volvulus, the commonly associated congenital peritoneal bands should be divided so that the duodenum is completely freed. In Plate 136, F, the duodenum is seen to lie entirely on the right side as in the usual case, and the cecum will come to lie in the left lower quadrant when it is completely freed. If all of the peritoneal bands are freed, it is not essential to fix the cecum to the right lower quadrant, although some surgeons prefer to do this.

The question of intrinsic duodenal obstruction associated with malrotation and midgut volvulus is interesting. Undoubtedly, a certain percentage of cases of malrotation with midgut volvulus have an associated stenosis (diaphragm) of the duodenum.

In Plate 135, B and C, the incision in the duodenum did not disclose a diaphragm which apparently existed in this particular case. If the surgeon suspects intrinsic duodenal obstruction, after having reduced the volvulus and divided all of the congenital peritoneal bands, it is probably best to open the stomach and pass a catheter down the duodenum in order to find a diaphragm. Some pediatric surgeons routinely perform this maneuver in all patients with malrotation after having reduced the volvulus. This may be a wise precaution before terminating the procedure. A small opening made in the stomach in order to pass a catheter down the duodenum to rule out the presence of a diaphragm adds very little to the procedure.

The intrinsic obstruction which was missed at the first operation was found at the second operation by the maneuvers depicted in Plate 136, H and I. The clamp apparently perforated a duodenal diaphragm and cleared this part of the obstruction. The catheter shown in Plate 136, J, seems to be a wise precaution in such a procedure.

It should be pointed out, however, that these diaphragmatic types of obstruction anywhere in the intestinal tract are very rarely successfully treated by perforation of the diaphragm with a clamp or by any other type of plastic procedure which directly attacks the occluding membrane. It is always preferable to perform an anastomosis above and below the level of the diaphragm.

Plate 136   317

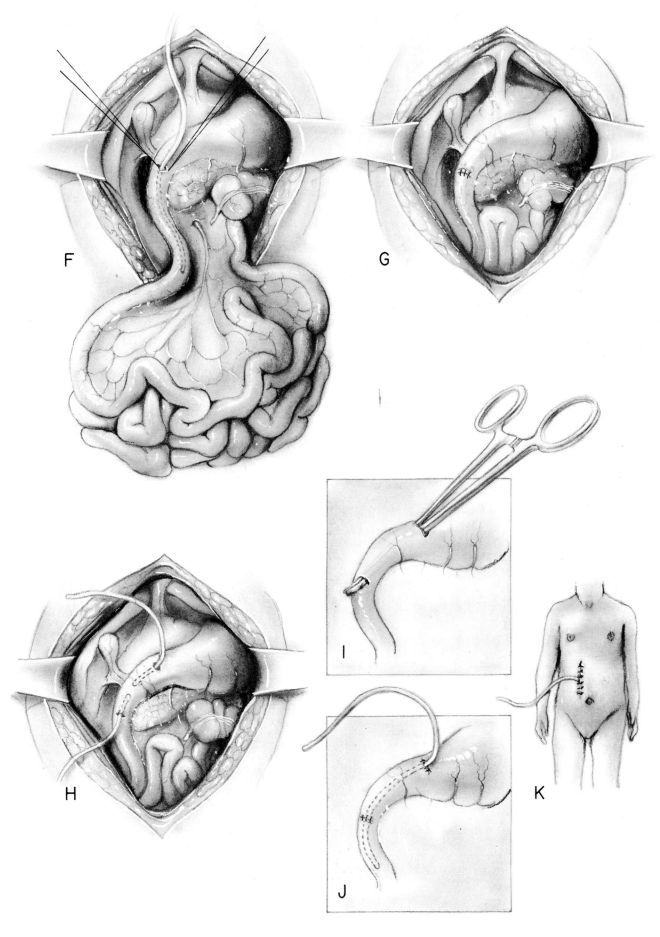

F

G

H

I

J

K

DISCUSSION—DR. HUGH B. LYNN. A movement is underway to discard the term "malrotation" of the colon in favor of the term "incomplete rotation," since the colon rarely undergoes actual malrotation. An upper abdominal transverse incision is perfectly satisfactory for exploration and is preferred by many.

The diagnosis of intrinsic versus extrinsic obstruction in the region of the duodenum has appeared for years to be strictly academic. It seems to me that the surgeon and not the patient profits by prolonged efforts to define the lesion more accurately. I no longer perform duodenotomies in an attempt to identify and possibly attack intrinsic lesions. This is based on bitter experience with removing the diaphragm and having the congenital annulus snug down and lead to a recurrence of partial obstruction. Any peritoneal folds should be divided, but I am no longer satisfied to stop after completing Ladd's procedure. In practically all cases with duodenal obstruction I now identify the region of obstruction, select the dilated duodenum above this region, and perform some type of duodenoenterostomy.

To the best of my knowledge I have never encountered a volvulus of the midgut that has not occurred in a clockwise fashion. In other words, after evisceration, untwisting of the volvulus has always been carried out in a counterclockwise direction. Should such a maneuver appear to be tightening the volvulus, the alert surgeon should recognize readily that he is dealing with a rare form of volvulus.

Once the volvulus has been corrected, some surgeons feel that gastrostomy is indicated; this, however, would depend to a large extent on the nursing care and house staff available. I have made a practice of trying to establish early alimentation by the oral route or by gastrostomy after 36 to 48 hours of nasogastric suction or drainage by open gastrostomy tube. Once sugar water is assimilated, I give Nutramigen as quickly as possible. I have felt that this formula makes its way through edematous intestine, a fresh anastomosis, and kinked bowel when curd-producing formulas would have led to much difficulty, if not to disaster.

DISCUSSION—DR. ORVAR SWENSON. It would seem to me that the title of this set of illustrations is a little misleading. Though in the strictest sense of the word the patient may have had malrotation of the colon and volvulus of the midgut with intrinsic obstruction of the duodenum, the term "malrotation of the colon" suggests a situation in which the cecum is adherent over the second portion of the duodenum, and the first step in this operation is to free the duodenum, after which one investigates the patency of the duodenum. The preferred way to do this, rather than opening the lumen, is to direct a large nasogastric tube down through the pylorus and then through the duodenum. Often this can be accomplished quite readily by the anesthesiologist with the surgeon directing the tube. This obviates the necessity of opening the duodenum when no obstruction is present. In situations where this is not possible, one should always open into the dilated portion of the duodenum above the obstruction, probing from this point downward. If it is necessary to leave a tube in place, it would seem preferable to try to feed the nasogastric tube down through and into the jejunum, thus obviating the necessity of opening and contaminating the peritoneal cavity.

EXCISION OF DUODENAL DIVERTICULA

A, A₁. The peritoneal cavity is entered (A) through an upper right rectus paramedian incision, as indicated by the broken line (A₁). In this patient a cholecystectomy was first performed for chronic cholecystitis and cholelithiasis. The ligated stumps of the cystic duct and cystic artery are visible. The origin of the cystic artery from the convex arch of the right hepatic artery, posterior to the common hepatic duct, is clearly shown. The gallbladder "bed" is usually not reperitonized, and hemostasis is therein obtained with suture ligatures of 000 silk. This is preferred to the use of compression with gauze packs, moistened in hot saline solution.

B. Following the cholecystectomy the second portion of the duodenum is mobilized by digital dissection after severance of the adjacent posterior parietal peritoneum. This maneuver is generally and incorrectly referred to as the Kocher or rotation maneuver. It was first described in 1895 by Jourdan of France and subsequently by Vautrin (1896) and Wiart (1899), also French surgeons. The mobilized second portion of the duodenum is grasped in vascular type clamps * and rotated toward the midline to show the diverticulum and related structures. The recognition of the. diverticulum is frequently difficult because of its areolar tissue covering and intimate relation to the pancreas. In one patient the diverticulum was anterior, and in the remaining 12 it was posterior, as demonstrated.

C. By blunt dissection the areolar tissue is separated from the diverticulum and severed (broken line).

D, E. The neck of the partly mobilized diverticulum is being encircled by a cotton tape (D), and as traction is maintained through the tape (E), its mobilization is being completed by scissor dissection. Frequently the summit of the diverticulum is "capped" by multiple and transparent bullae. This obtained in the present patient.

* Manufactured by Edward Weck & Co., Long Island City, N.Y.

Diverticula of the duodenum may be conveniently classified as primary and secondary. Primary diverticula occur most commonly in the region of the papilla of Vater (perivaterian). Less frequently they are located in the third and fourth portions of the duodenum. Primary duodenal diverticula are all false in that they do not contain all the coats of the bowel wall. The mucosa is herniated at its mesenteric border between the fibers of the muscle layers and is covered only by a thinned out serosal layer. When completely mobilized, the wall of the summit of the diverticulum is usually thin and transparent and frequently exhibits a multiloculated appearance. In fact, the wall of the summit of the diverticulum may be readily torn by a Babcock clamp even though lightly applied.

Secondary diverticula, as the name implies, are generally secondary to a chronic duodenal ulcer. These are true diverticula in that they contain all the layers of the wall of the duodenum. They are located on the inferior (mesenteric) border of the first portion of the duodenum at a site opposite a cicatricial duodenal ulcer.

Primary, or false, diverticula are most commonly asymptomatic, and surgical treatment is not indicated. However, in some instances a diverticulum may be the basic cause of the patient's complaints and accordingly operation is advised. The main indication for operation is abdominal pain persistently localized over the site of the diverticulum and associated with local, deepseated tenderness in the same area. Furthermore, the absence of concomitant disease in the stomach, duodenum, or biliary tract should be demonstrated. A prolonged retention of barium within the diverticulum is in itself not considered an indication for operation. In the 11 patients operated upon to date in whom duodenal diverticula were excised the results have been satisfactory. There were no complications, such as wound infection or duodenal fistula, and there were no operative deaths.

The treatment of secondary, or true, diverticula is the treatment of the primary cause, namely, chronic cicatricial duodenal ulcer.

Plate 137

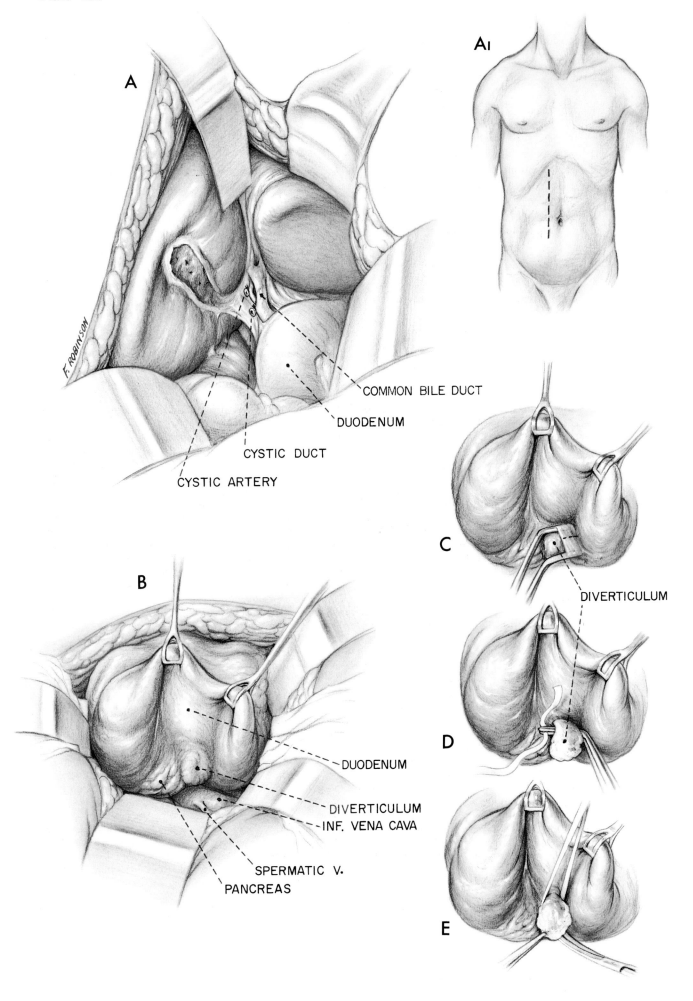

A

F. ROBINSON

COMMON BILE DUCT

DUODENUM

CYSTIC DUCT

CYSTIC ARTERY

A₁

C

DIVERTICULUM

D

E

B

DUODENUM

DIVERTICULUM

INF. VENA CAVA

SPERMATIC V.

PANCREAS

F. When the mobilization of the diverticulum is completed, it is excised in a manner similar to the removal of a hernial sac. Guy sutures of silk are used to stabilize the diverticulum as the sac is first bisected with scissors (vertical broken line) and subsequently transected (horizontal broken line). This technic, whereby the lumen of the sac is first widely entered, permits the identification of the papilla of Vater in relation to the walls of the diverticulum and should preclude its injury when the diverticulum is excised. When the diverticulum is small, simple inversion is of proved merit.

G, H, I. The opening in the duodenum is elongated transversely (right angle) to the longitudinal axis of the duodenum by trac-tion sutures of silk (0000) as the first angle inversion suture is being inserted. This suture passes from the inside-out on one side (G) and from the outside-in on the other (H), so that, when tied, the knot of the suture is on the inside of the lumen. Similarly, the opposite angle inversion suture is inserted (I). Tension on the respective traction sutures as depicted (H, I) facilitates the inversion as the angle sutures are tied.

J, K. A figure of 8 suture is inserted about the termination of the inversion suture in the center of the closure (J), and, after being tied, the second layer of closure, a series of horizontal mattress sutures (Halsted), is inserted to complete the closure of the duodenum (K).

DISCUSSION—DR. HOWARD MAHORNER. The paramedian right rectus incision for a combination cholecystectomy and duodenal diverticulum is satisfactory. However, the approach also may be advantageously made through a Mayo-Robson ("hockey stick") incision.

It is true that the duodenal diverticula, because of their frequent posterior position, are sometimes obscure and difficult to locate. Their identification at the time of operation can be facilitated by injecting 20 cc. of air through a needle inserted into the duodenum. This pumps up the diverticulum and it becomes apparent. Even when the diverticulum is in the head of the pancreas, this may be a helpful guide.

When the duodenal diverticula have been affected by complications, or when they are so large that they retain barium and cause the patient really troublesome symptoms, surgery is indicated. This occurs in a very small percentage of duodenal diverticula. Excision and a meticulous inverting-type suture closure is always acceptable when the rim of the defect is covered by peritoneum. On the other hand, many duodenal diverticula arise from an area of the duodenum partially covered by the pancreas. This is the only part of the duodenum that is not peritonealized; even the posterior surface of the second portion of the duodenum is covered by peritoneum.

When the diverticulum in any way is wholly or partially between the pancreas and the duodenum, its excision and attempted closure without complete peritoneal covering becomes difficult and dangerous, analogous in minor respects to attempting the impossible task of getting an annular pancreas off the duodenum. Therefore, safety measures have to be considered when the defect is so positioned that its entire circumference is not covered by peritoneum. The diverticulum may be in-verted after mobilization, and the defect closed with interrupted, nonabsorbable sutures; this measure at least tends to prevent a duodenal fistula, should the suture approximation of the fenestra fail. In certain instances where the diverticula are in very close approximation to the ampulla of Vater, it may not be necessary to try to obliterate them, unless they are large or unless there is a stone in them, such as I have encountered. If they are attacked directly, however, it is most important to put a T-tube in the common duct as a guide. (In two of 26 operations for duodenal diverticula on a private service, choledochostomy was a very helpful maneuver.) Otherwise, the closure in close proximity to the lower end of the common duct may compromise the duct.

In some fairly large diverticula near the outlet of the common duct between the pancreas and the duodenum (partially or completely intrapancreatic), an indirect operation is not only justified but is, in many instances, the operation of choice. The indirect operation is a partial gastrectomy associated with a vagotomy. This, then, bypasses the diverticulum and also bypasses the danger of a duodenal fistula.

After the perivaterian area, the second place of predilection for duodenal diverticula is the third part of the duodenum. Here they arise in a cascade fashion on either side of the superior mesenteric vessels and are often very large. The one to the right of the vessels is best approached from above and through the superior peritoneal surface of the transverse mesocolon; whereas the diverticula to the left of the vessels can most easily be exposed through the inferior peritoneal surface of the transverse mesocolon. The duodenal surfaces here are peritonealized, and excision and closure of the defect is proper.

Plate 138

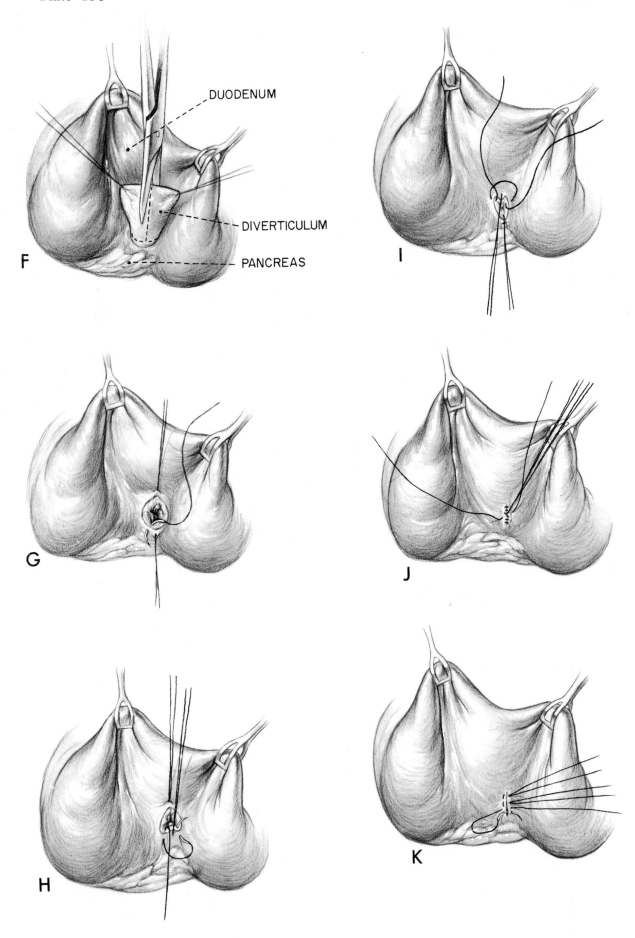

F
DUODENUM
DIVERTICULUM
PANCREAS

G

H

I

J

K

This plate depicts the various locations of duodenal diverticula demonstrated by the surgeon to the artist at the time of operation.

N. The whole of the duodenal loop is mobilized to show a diverticulum at the angle of junction of the second (descending) and third (horizontal or transverse) portions of the duodenum.

O. The apex of the diverticulum is grasped in a Babcock clamp, and with upward traction through the clamp maintained, it is severed from the surrounding attachments by scissor dissection as depicted.

P. The completely mobilized diverticulum is secured in Babcock clamps (two), and with scissors it is bisected from the apex to the base as indicated by the dotted line. The respective halves are elliptically excised at their bases, as previously shown (H).

Q. This is a demonstration of a partially mobilized perivaterian diverticulum in which intrapancreatic dissection was required for its removal.

R. This illustration depicts a diverticulum of the fourth portion of the duodenum underlying the base of the transverse mesocolon. Its relation to the ligament of Treitz and the superior mesenteric vascular stalk is visible. The incision in the serosal covering of the transverse mesocolon overlying the diverticulum is indicated by the curved dotted line.

S. The serosa covering of the base of the transverse mesocolon is incised and the diverticulum is mobilized. The resection of the diverticulum and the closure of the opening in the duodenum proceeds as previously demonstrated.

DISCUSSION—DR. RUSSEL H. PATTERSON. For the patient with a long narrow abdomen and long slanting ribs, we prefer a vertical muscle-splitting or muscle-retracting incision. The subcostal or oblique incision is used for the short broad abdomen. We have found the vertical incision more comfortable postoperatively for the patient, and also, if drainage is necessary, a lateral stab wound is easily made permitting primary closure of the operative wound.

Upon opening the abdomen the surgeon has two immediate observations to make. First, since with the majority of diverticula which produce symptoms there are other lesions present, these lesions must be carefully examined and their status in the symptom complex determined. Second, the duodenal diverticulum itself must be exposed and its relation to surrounding structures must be defined. Since these diverticula are often multiple, a decision has to be made as to the treatment of each one. Duodenal diverticula may be very difficult to find. It is helpful to appreciate, however, that the great majority of primary diverticula are in the second portion of the duodenum and often near the ampulla of Vater. To identify the diverticulum, the duodenum may be inflated or bismuth may be given by mouth prior to operation.

For most diverticula quite satisfactory exposure is obtained by mobilizing the duodenum as shown in (C–F). For exposure of those diverticula in the third part of the duodenum, the transverse colon is elevated and the peritoneum over the duodenum is opened between the midcolic and the superior mesenteric arteries. The ligament of Treitz may be carefully divided if necessary. In exceptional circumstances it may be necessary to open the duodenum and feel for the diverticulum with the fingers. In such cases it is sometimes possible to invaginate the diverticulum and remove it from the inside of the bowel.

In removing a perivaterian diverticulum one has to be certain about the integrity of the ampulla of Vater. The following maneuvers are helpful to this end: The common duct may be catheterized; the ampulla may be inspected through the stump of the excised diverticulum; a separate opening may be made in the duodenum.

When the duodenum is opened, unless the common duct has been catheterized, it is not an easy matter to immediately identify the ampulla. Though some anatomy books state that the ampulla is 7.5 to 10 cm. from the pylorus, in a series of studies we found that the ampulla was more nearly 10 cm. from the pylorus in every case. Pressure on the gallbladder will often force bile out of the ampulla. The ampulla is slightly elevated, and the duodenal transverse rugae curve up over the ampulla in such a manner as to simulate a frenum.

Though a diverticulum may be inverted it is rather generally agreed that excision is the procedure of choice (J, K). We never clamp the base of the neck of the diverticulum. We try to leave a cuff of mucosa which we close with fine catgut sutures following with interrupted single or mattress sutures in the outer bowel layers.

Following excision of a diverticulum, drainage is rarely necessary, but if there is any doubt about the integrity of the duodenal closure we would not hesitate to place a cigarette drain to the site and bring it out through a stab wound lateral to the abdominal incision.

The clinical evaluation of the radiographically established diverticulum, in relation to the symptoms, presents a difficult problem. However, when the diverticulum is the offending agent in one or more of the following complications, surgery is required: (1) obstruction of bile or pancreatic ducts with jaundice or pancreatitis; (2) obstruction of duodenum with partial or complete blocking; (3) inflammation in the form of diverticulitis, ulcer, perforation, or enterolith formation; (4) neoplastic change with leiomyosarcoma or carcinoma developing in the diverticulum; (5) hemorrhage, small or massive, resulting from ulcer or breaking of thin walled capillaries or blood vessels.

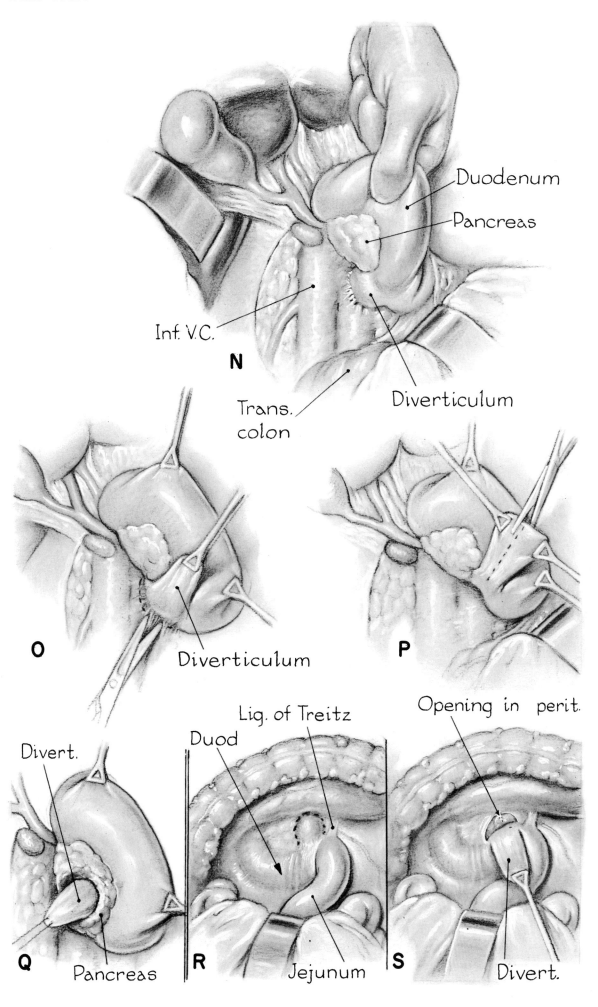

Duodenum

Pancreas

Inf. V.C.

N

Trans.
colon

Diverticulum

O

Diverticulum

P

Lig. of Treitz

Opening in perit.

Divert.

Duod

Q

Pancreas

R

Jejunum

S

Divert.

SEGMENTAL RESECTION OF THE SMALL INTESTINE AND "OPEN" END-TO-END ANASTOMOSIS

A. The irreversible compromise of the circulation to a segment of the small intestine is shown, and the lines of transection of the bowel and the subjacent mesentery are indicated by the dotted lines.

B, C. By blunt dissection with a small clamp (B), an opening is made in an avascular portion of the mesentery immediately subjacent to the bowel wall at the site elected for its transection. Through this opening a catheter (14 F) is withdrawn (C).

D. Similarly a second catheter (14 F) is used to encircle the bowel distally, and direction lines for transection of the mesentery are made through its serosal layer.

DISCUSSION—DR. ISIDORE COHN, JR. Rather than rubber catheters to encircle the bowel and outline the prospective site of resection, I far prefer to use noncrushing intestinal clamps, believing they are safer, less traumatic, and more effective. In selecting noncrushing intestinal clamps, I believe they should have longitudinal ridges (that is, running in the long axis of the clamp) and that the commonly used "rubber shoe" should be eliminated. One has only to place his own finger between the same clamp with and without the "rubber shoes" to detect the difference in pressure exerted on the bowel under these circumstances. It should be obvious that a noncrushing clamp that really deserves that name should be closed only tightly enough to prevent leakage of bowel contents, which generally means that only the first or second ratchet should be engaged.

The importance of small bites of tissue in the small bowel mesentery and the use of suture ligatures in the fatty areolar tissue, particularly in an individual with an unusually fatty mesentery, cannot be emphasized sufficiently.

Dr. Madden has stressed the importance of declaring the field contaminated when the bowel is opened, and to emphasize this has suggested the use of a "red flag" to signal this event. Too many surgeons and operating room nurses have come to assume that the availability of antibiotics have made such precautions merely the hangovers of a bygone day. No quantity of antibiotics will serve to replace proper attention to good surgical technic.

Instead of placing two clamps at each proposed site of resection and noncrushing clamps distal and proximal to this, I would prefer to place one clamp on each side of the proposed site of resection, angling them so that when the bowel was divided immediately adjacent to a clamp, the clamp would remain on the specimen to be removed. Contamination should be avoided by milking bowel contents away from this clamp to beyond the point where the noncrushing clamp would be placed, thus leaving a relatively clean field through which the bowel could be divided. By using a single clamp at each end of the bowel, the trauma to the proposed anastomotic area is prevented, and, even though Dr. Madden has suggested that this second clamp not be locked, there is always the possibility that this will be done inadvertently.

In neither the open nor the closed technic has the artist shown any clearing of mesenteric fat away from the edges to be approximated. A large area should not be denuded of mesenteric fat because of the danger to the blood supply to the bowel, but if some of the fat is not removed, the anastomosis may become unnecessarily difficult, and the approximation of bowel wall may be interfered with by interposed bits of fat.

I prefer an inner layer of chromic catgut rather than silk, probably more because I prefer to use a continuous suture than because of fear of difficulty

Plate 139

327

A

B

C

D

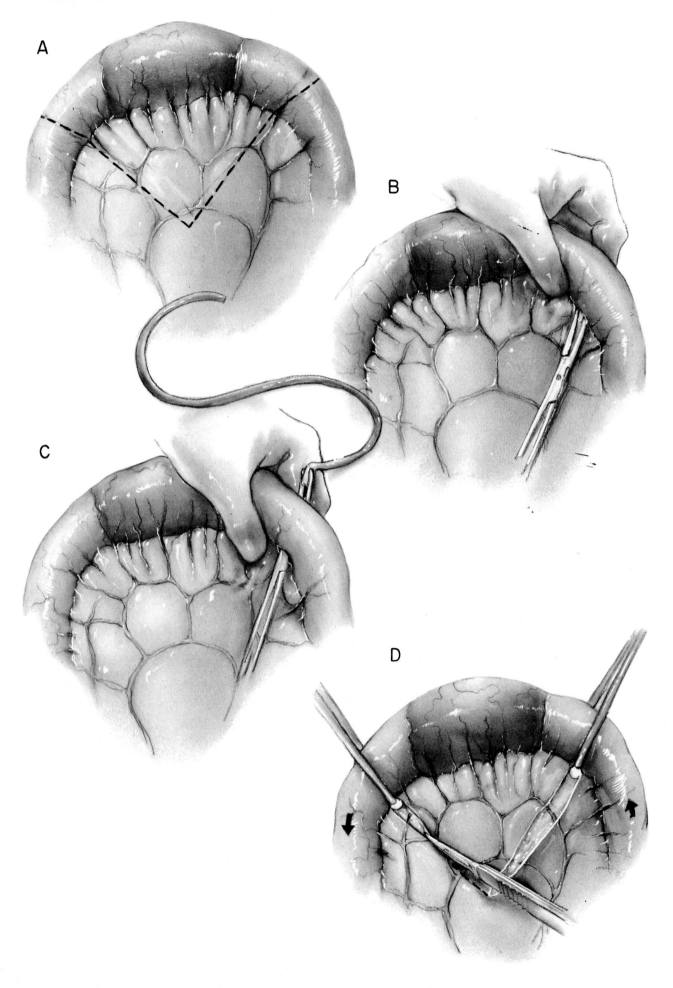

E, F. The mesentery is serially clamped and severed by scissor dissection (E), and hemostasis is obtained with suture ligatures of 000 silk (F). In the application of clamps to the mesentery, small bites of tissue should be taken and the clamps tightly locked to prevent slipping and resulting hemorrhage. In fatty areolar tissue, suture ligatures are used routinely for hemostasis.

G. The clamps on the cut margins of the mesentery of the bowel that is to remain are replaced by suture ligatures of silk (000), and those on the segment of mesentery that is resected are replaced by simple ligatures of silk (000). The remaining attachment of the mesentery is doubly clamped, and its severance is indicated by the dotted line.

H. Following the completion of the transec-tion of the mesentery and the ligation of its vessels, the operative field is declared contaminated. The field of contamination is defined by the use of moist toweling and an appropriately colored (red) laparotomy sheet. The lumen of the bowel proximally is occluded with a rubber covered intestinal clamp, and the bowel at the sites of election for its transection is doubly clamped. The transection of the bowel proximally is completed, and its severance distally with a scalpel is shown. The clamps are applied across the bowel at an approximate 60 degree angle obliquity to assure adequacy of the blood supply to the antimesenteric cut margin. The jaws of the clamps on the cut margins of the small intestine to be anastomosed are held in approximation but not locked. This is done to avoid unnecessary crushing trauma to the tissues.

DISCUSSION—DR. COHN (cont.)

arising from the use of a nonabsorbable suture. I would place two guy-wire sutures of catgut just as shown in I and J. Then I would start with another catgut suture in the middle of the posterior row, and use a continuous, locking suture toward either the mesenteric or antimesenteric border, and continue this anteriorly as a Connell suture. As soon as one angle is reached, the other suture should be placed posteriorly, tied to the first suture, and then run in the opposite direction, again as a running lock stitch on the posterior side, and brought arteriorly as a Connell suture. These two sutures should meet at approximately the midpoint anteriorly and be tied together.

If I read the text correctly, it seems to me that the posterior row of the anastomosis is a three-layer anastomosis. Since there is really very little difference between the posterior and the anterior surface of the small bowel, and since the blood supply of the small bowel is relatively good, this seems to be an unnecessary precaution, and one that may not be as effective as it seems on paper, since it only gives added protection to one-half the circumference of the anastomosis. The running lock stitch described above should serve the purpose of both of the inner layers of interrupted silk preferred by Dr. Madden.

As an outer layer, I prefer interrupted mattress sutures of silk such as those shown in the technic for an "aseptic" anastomosis. I believe the mattress sutures coapt a larger surface of bowel and therefore make a more secure anastomosis. They also invert a smaller diaphragm and thus make a larger lumen.

Recently there has been some interest in the use of plastic adhesives for the performance of "non-suture" anastomoses. In approximately 100 such end-to-end anastomosis of both small and large bowels in dogs, we found the adhesive to be satisfactory only about two-thirds of the time. In view of the known safety of suture anastomoses of any type, it would seem that the adhesive anastomosis should not be employed until better adhesives have been evolved. One of the supposed advantages of the adhesive technic is its greater speed, but, even after experience with 100 such anastomoses, I do not find it that much quicker than the suture anastomoses and therefore would not recommend it.

Most of the differences that have been pointed out are those that have evolved more on a basis of personal preference and personal experience rather than on a basis of demonstrated superiority. Each operator will use most frequently that technic with which he has the most familiarity and with which he has obtained the best results. This is as it should be.

Plate 140

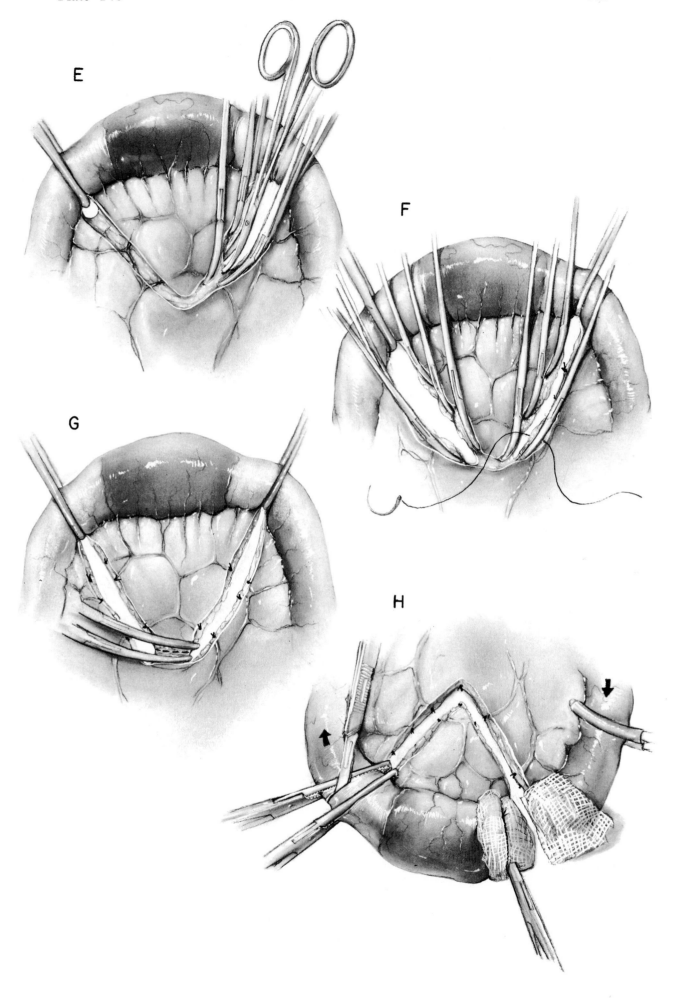

I. The end-to-end "open" anastomosis, the preferred technic, is begun. Prior to the anastomosis, adequacy of the circulation to the cut margins must be assured. This is indicated by the occurrence of fresh bleeding from and the healthy appearance of the unclamped cut margins. The antimesenteric margins of the transected small intestine are secured in Babcock clamps, and the mesenteric coaptation mattress suture of fine (0000) silk is inserted.

J. Similarly a coaptation mattress suture of silk (0000) with its "loop on the mucosa" is inserted for the approximation of the antimesenteric cut margins.

K. By traction on the coaptation sutures, the cut margins of the bowel are apposed, and a series of interrupted through and through everting mattress sutures of silk are inserted.

L. The mattress sutures are tied, and the everted layers of the bowel wall are firmly approximated with simple interrupted sutures of fine (0000) silk. Although the use of silk rather than fine (000) catgut for the inner or mucosal layer of the anastomosis is frequently condemned, no difficulty has been observed with its routine use.

M. The interrupted sutures of silk (0000) are continued anteriorly and are inserted from the "inside out" to the "outside in" so that, when tied, the knots of these sutures are on the inside of the lumen and inversion of the bowel wall is obtained.

DISCUSSION—DR. JOHN H. ECKEL. The success of an anastomosis, by whatever method, depends on close observance of three fundamental principles of intestinal surgery, well defined by Whipple as: (1) the maintenance of an adequate blood supply to the zone of the anastomosis by the careful preservation of the continuity of the blood vessels in the mesentery supplying the zone; (2) the placing of an accurate seromuscular suture to provide an adequate apposition of peritoneum on either side of the suture line; and (3) the prevention of tension on the suture line with its accompanying tissue necrosis. Tension on the suture line can be prevented by the avoidance of tying the sutures too tightly and by keeping the proximal segment of bowel empty of gas and fecal content by some form of decompression. These principles are carefully adhered to in both of the methods which are illustrated.

An "open" intestinal anastomosis is always secure and affords the surgeon the opportunity to observe the size of the lumen at the anastomotic site (Plate 141, I–M). When a "closed" or "aseptic" anastomosis is carried out (Plate 143), it is of extreme importance to test the patency of the anastomotic lumen as demonstrated (Plate 143, G).

Small bowel resection is performed in many conditions, the most common being the loss of viability due to irreversible compromise of the

Plate 141

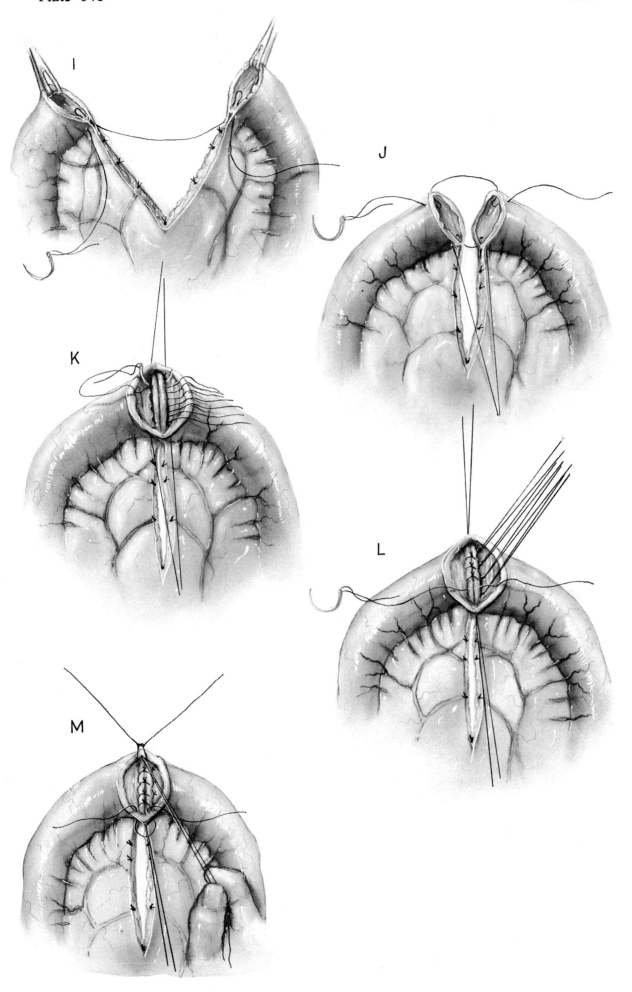

N. The sutures are inserted alternately from the mesenteric and antimesenteric borders toward the midline to avoid an angle closure. If traction on the previously inserted and tied suture is maintained toward the lumen as each succeeding suture is tied, inversion of the bowel wall is facilitated. The last two sutures have been inserted, and when they are tied, the first layer of the closure anteriorly is completed.

O. The last two sutures of the first layer anteriorly are tied and encircled by a reinforcing figure of 8 mattress suture to assure both an air tight and water tight closure.

P, Q. The second layer of sutures anteriorly, a series of interrupted seromuscular sutures (Lembert), is inserted (P) and continued as an additional reinforcing layer posteriorly (Q).

R_1. In those instances in which a linear circumferential and irreversible compromise of the circulation of the bowel caused by a constricting adhesive band is present, simple inversion by a series of interrupted seromuscular Lembert sutures may be employed. This technic is frequently referred to as the "Summers' stitch."

R, S. Traction on the circumferential layer of seromuscular sutures is maintained (R) as each suture is tied to complete the anastomosis (S). The operative field is then declared clean, and after a change of gloves by the surgical team and with a clean set of instruments, the opening in the mesentery is closed using interrupted sutures of fine (0000) silk (S). Wound closure in layers as previously depicted completes the operation.

DISCUSSION—DR. ECKEL (cont.)

circulation by strangulation. In such instances there is always a marked discrepancy in the size of the distended and obstructed bowel proximally and the collapsed bowel distally. This discrepancy may be so marked that an end-to-end anastomosis is contraindicated, and a side-to-side anastomosis must of necessity be performed. However, this is rare.

Halsted proposed an aseptic type of end-to-end anastomosis performed over Kocher clamps, and most of his three generations of disciples have continued to employ this method. Although this procedure may be more painstaking than an "open" type of anastomosis, it minimizes contamination by spillage and reduces the incidence of wound infection. In our experience postoperative peritoneal hemorrhage has not been a complicating factor.

The method described in Plate 143 (aseptic end-to-end anastomosis) is the one first worked out ex-

perimentally by Halsted and has proved satisfactory to a large group in the Department of Surgery at the New York Hospital. Person and O'Neill described a method to compensate for the disparity between the dilated proximal and collapsed distal loops by applying the distal clamps in an oblique manner. This is facilitated by employing calibrated Kocher or Allen clamps. When an "open" end-to-end anastomosis is performed, the disparity is less troublesome.

Finally, in rare instances where there is extreme disparity in the size of the loops of bowel, one may feel more secure by performing an "open" side-to-side anastomosis. In this type of anastomosis it is important that no proximal jejunum or ileum be allowed to extend distal to the anastomosis, since such a pouch may perforate or become gradually enlarged and produce symptoms of indigestion, abdominal pain, and distention.

Plate 142

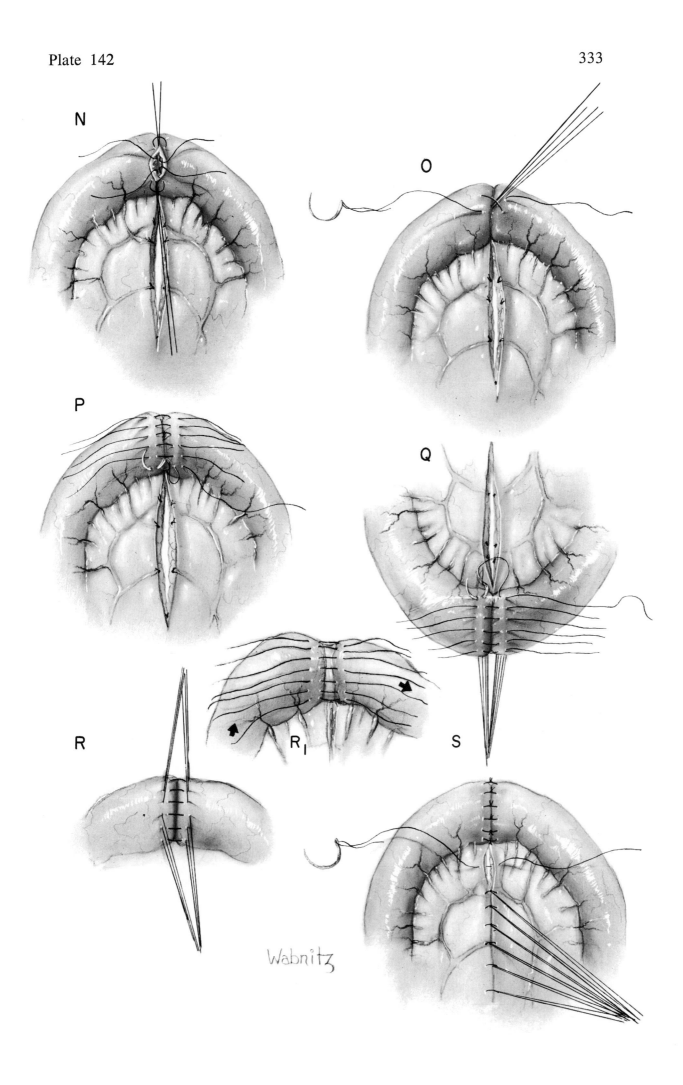

N

O

P

Q

R

R₁

S

Wabnitz

SEGMENTAL RESECTION OF THE SMALL INTESTINE AND "ASEPTIC" END-TO-END ANASTOMOSIS

Although this technic is a rapid and effective method for the performance of an end-to-end anastomosis, the "open" technic is preferred. The hazards of this method are: (1) hemorrhage; (2) inversion of an excessive amount of tissue with the formation of an obstructive diaphragm.

A. The bowel on either side of the segment to be resected is doubly clamped, and the sites of transection of the bowel and its subjacent mesentery are indicated by the dotted lines.

B, C. The segmental resection of the small intestine is completed (B), and with the occluding clamps firmly locked and carefully approximated, a series of interrupted seromuscular mattress sutures of silk (000) are inserted anteriorly (C).

D. The handles of the clamps are turned downward to rotate the bowel 180 degrees on its longitudinal axis, and a series of interrupted seromuscular mattress sutures of silk (000) are inserted posteriorly.

E. Traction is maintained on the circumferentially placed, interrupted seromuscular mattress sutures as the clamps are carefully and slowly withdrawn.

F. The mattress sutures are tied, and the opening on the antimesenteric surface of the bowel through which the clamps were withdrawn is closed with a seromuscular mattress suture of 000 silk.

G. The "aseptic" anastomosis is completed, and the opening in the mesentery is closed. By digital manipulation the agglutinated cut margins of the bowel are separated and its lumen is restored. The importance of this maneuver in the avoidance of postoperative intestinal obstruction cannot be overemphasized. Furthermore, careful inspection of the line of anastomosis, particularly along its mesenteric aspect, should be done to be sure that there is no leakage.

DISCUSSION—DR. ISIDORE COHN, JR. I would agree thoroughly with Dr. Madden that the "open" technic is preferred, and do not remember having used the "aseptic" technic for a small intestinal anastomosis. The indications for such an anastomotic technic are much clearer in surgery of the colon, though even there I have not used the "aseptic" technic. Some recent experimental work has suggested the value of a closed anastomosis in malignancy of the bowel, but malignancy is so uncommon in the small bowel as to relegate the "closed" technic to comparative obscurity in dealing with small-intestinal problems.

There is one additional hazard of the "aseptic" technic not mentioned by Dr. Madden. This is the danger of putting a suture through both anterior and posterior walls of one side of the anastomosis and thus inadvertently providing a diaphragm across the anastomosis. While it always seems as though this should not happen, I am sure everyone has had the unfortunate experience of placing sutures across both walls of the stomach while inverting the outer layer of the gastrojejunostomy sutures, and then having to remove this suture after the stomach was opened for completion of the anastomosis.

In the discussion of the "open" method, Dr. Madden has rightly emphasized the importance of cutting the small bowel on an angle to prevent devascularization of the antimesenteric side of the bowel. Similarly, the bowel must be cut on the same angle of obliquity for the "aseptic" anastomosis, and I would prefer more of an angle than the artist has shown in the pictures of the "closed" anastomosis. It is important that the angle selected for placing the clamp not be too oblique; otherwise, when the bowel ends are brought together they may provide an acute angulation and thus tend to produce an intestinal obstruction unless one limb is rotated so that the mesenteric borders are not together.

Plate 143

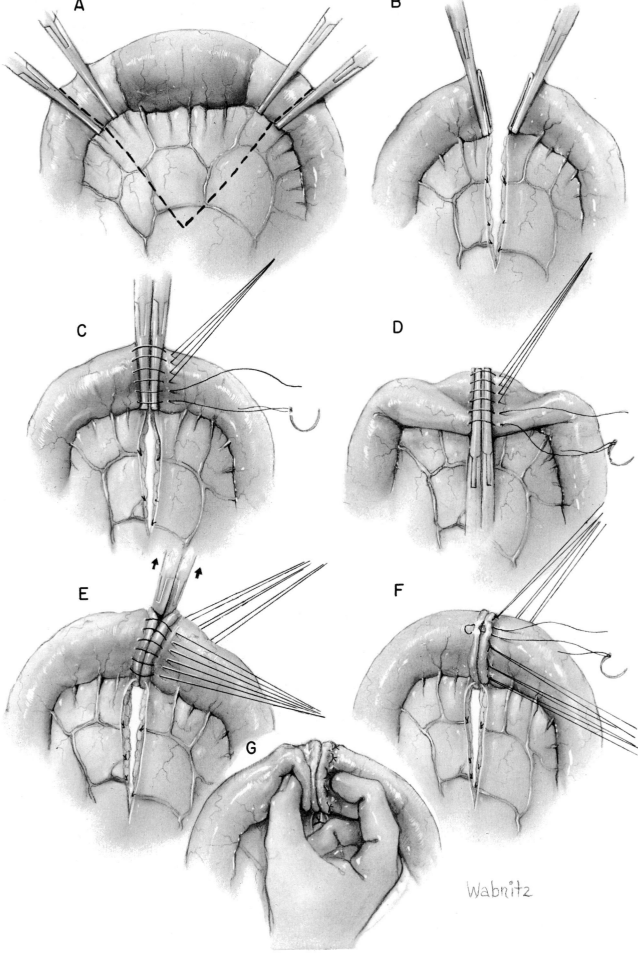

A B C D E F G

Wabnitz

DISCUSSION—DR. CLARENCE DENNIS. Experience in many Centers has shown that resection with primary end-to-end anastomosis is a practicable and safe method even in dealing with small bowel obstructions in which nonviable intestine is found. In the hands of Owings and Smith (*Ann. Surg.*, 95:840, 1932) 19 out of 31 dogs subjected to reanastomosis after two to five days of intestinal obstruction died. In contrast, Dennis (*Surg., Gynec. & Obst.*, 77:225, 1943) reported survival of 15 out of 16 similar animals reanastomosed by closed end-to-end anastomosis. Max Gaspar, in reporting 204 open anastomoses as compared to 139 closed anastomoses in clinical patients at Los Angeles County Hospital, found 29 per cent of the "open" anastomoses to be unsatisfactory, as compared to 18.7 per cent of the closed anastomoses.

The anastomosis may be performed after the pattern of Martzloff and Burget (*Arch. Surg.*, 23: 26, 1931), or, if the discrepancy in diameter of the two segments is great or if the diameter is less than 2.5 cm., an oblique type of anastomosis with a temporary basting stitch to minimize the amount of inversion may better be employed. The relative hazards of the two methods are (1) hemorrhage is more frequent in the "open" anastomosis than in the "closed," (2) inversion of an excessive amount of tissue is a greater problem with the "open" anastomosis than with the "closed," and (3) failure to recognize inadvertent suture closure of the lumen is a hazard seen with the "closed" anastomosis but not with the "open."

Inasmuch as the chief dangers and the chief advantages of the "closed" of anastomosis are seen in procedures performed in the presence of established obstruction and therefore of well-developed distention, the procedure as described is used in that circumstance.

1. Placement of the first anastomosis clamp * on the distended bowel above the point of obstruction. The clamp crosses the bowel at an angle of 75° and at the mesenteric border about 6 mm. from the edge of the unremoved mesentery. The bowel has been milked back and a rubber-shod clamp has been applied to prevent spillage.

2. Placement of the second anastomosis clamp on the contracted bowel below the point of obstruction. The line of crush begins 6 mm. from the unremoved mesentery, crosses obliquely two thirds of the bowel, and passes for a distance parallel with the antimesenteric border before crossing the remaining one third of the bowel.

2a. This length of crushed tissue, equal to that on the left, is obtained by distorting the bowel with Allis forceps. This clamp is placed from the mesenteric border. (From *Surg., Gynec. & Obst.*, 77:225, 1943.)

3. Cutting the bowel between the clamps described in Figures 1 and 2 with the cautery. To prevent spillage, additional clamps are placed between those applied for anastomosis and the specimen to be removed.

4. Placement of the posterior running fine catgut suture. The clamps are held side-by-side, so that the bowel ends are brought together with 180° rotation of one with respect to the others; thus, there will be minimal angulation. The suture is laid with the clamps rolled away from each other as shown. The bites are 5 mm. long, and the gaps between bites are 4 mm.

4a. Placement of each end bite parallel with the long axis of the gut assures good inversion later. This suture is left loose until removal of the clamps as shown in Figure 6. For very edematous bowel, 00 or 000 atraumatic catgut is safer than 0000. (From *Surg., Gynec. & Obst.*, 77:225, 1943.)

* The clamps are manufactured by the V. Mueller Co., Chicago.

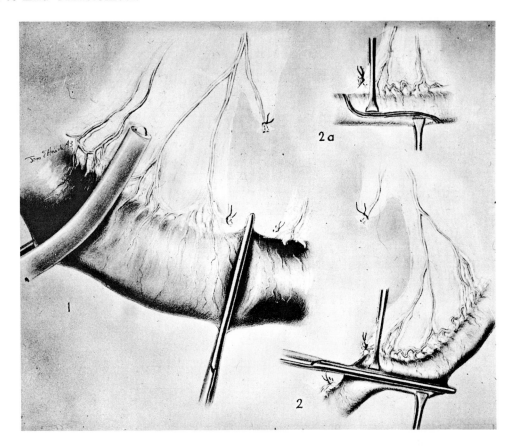

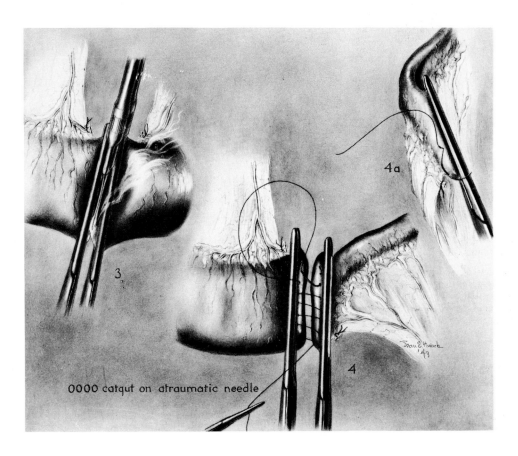

0000 catgut on atraumatic needle

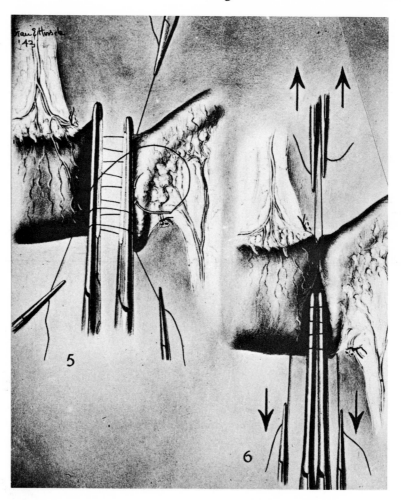

5. Placement of the anterior running catgut suture. The clamps have been rolled together.

6. Tension is applied to the two ends of each of the running sutures, the clamps are carefully loosened until the tips are spread 1 or 2 mm., and the clamps are cautiously removed. (From *Surg., Gynec. & Obst.*, 77:225, 1943.)

7. The ends of the posterior running stitch have been tied to the corresponding ends of the anterior strand, and tension has been maintained during placement of Halsted mattress sutures or of simple Lembert sutures of 2½ pound test silk. With the placement of the last silk suture, but prior to tying of this last suture, it is well to cut away the knot of the catgut basting stitch and to with-

draw the basting stitch from the other end of the anastomosis. Studies have shown that such removal of the catgut strand from the healing area usually renders the shoulder of inverted tissue temporary rather than permanent.

8. Rear view of anastomosis, showing placement of stitch to close the mesenteric defect. (From *Surg., Gynec. & Obst.*, 77:225, 1943.)

9. a, Schematic drawing to illustrate the angulation resulting from end-to-end anastomosis of bowel cut at 45° and apposed without rotation. b, The obviation of angulation accomplished by rotation of one segment with respect to the other is apparent. (From *Surgery*, 5:548, 1939.)

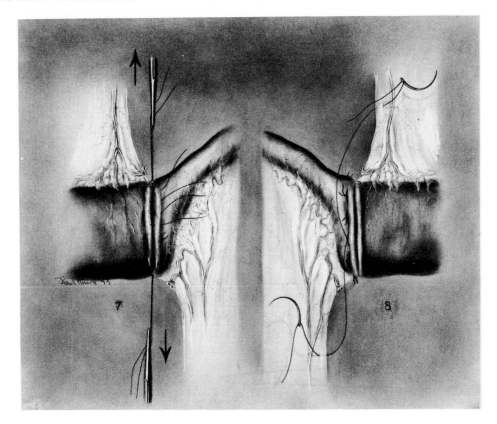

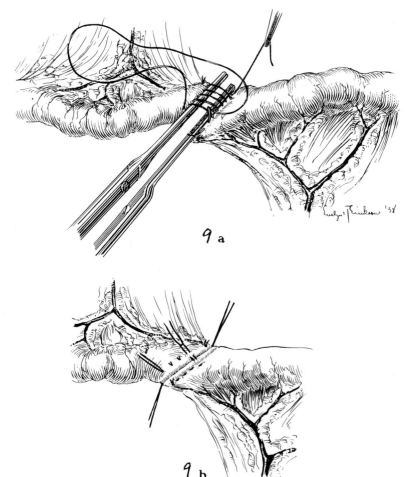

9 a

9 b

ILEO-ENTECTROPY

The title for this operation, ileo-entectropy, is derived from the Greek [ileo (εἰλεός), terminal part of small bowel, + ent (ἐντός), inside, + ec (ἐκ), outside, + tropy (τρόπος), a turning], meaning to turn the ileum inside out. The operation, originated by Charles G. Neumann of New York, was first used in the experimental animal in the treatment of ascites produced by partial occlusion of the thoracic segment of the inferior vena cava. The experimental results obtained encouraged the employment clinically of ileo-entectropy in a small select group of patients with intractable ascites. At the present writing a positive opinion cannot be formulated relative to the therapeutic efficacy of this operation because the number of patients operated upon is too small and the period of follow-up is too short. The inclusion in the Atlas of the technic for the performance of ileo-entectropy is on the basis of the interest which it has provoked and its originality. However, one cannot emphasize too strongly the fact that the merits of this particular operation remain to be proved.

A. The right lower paramedian muscle-splitting incision is outlined.

B. The peritoneal cavity is entered, and the incision in the posterior parietal peritoneum below the cecum is begun by scissor dissection.

C, D, E. The terminal ileum is encircled by catheters (No. 12 F) at the sites for its transection proximally and distally, and, with a scalpel, directional lines for the application of clamps are made through the serosa of the mesentery of the small bowel (C). The mesentery is serially clamped and severed (D), and hemostasis is obtained with suture ligatures of silk (000) as each clamp is removed (E).

Plate 144

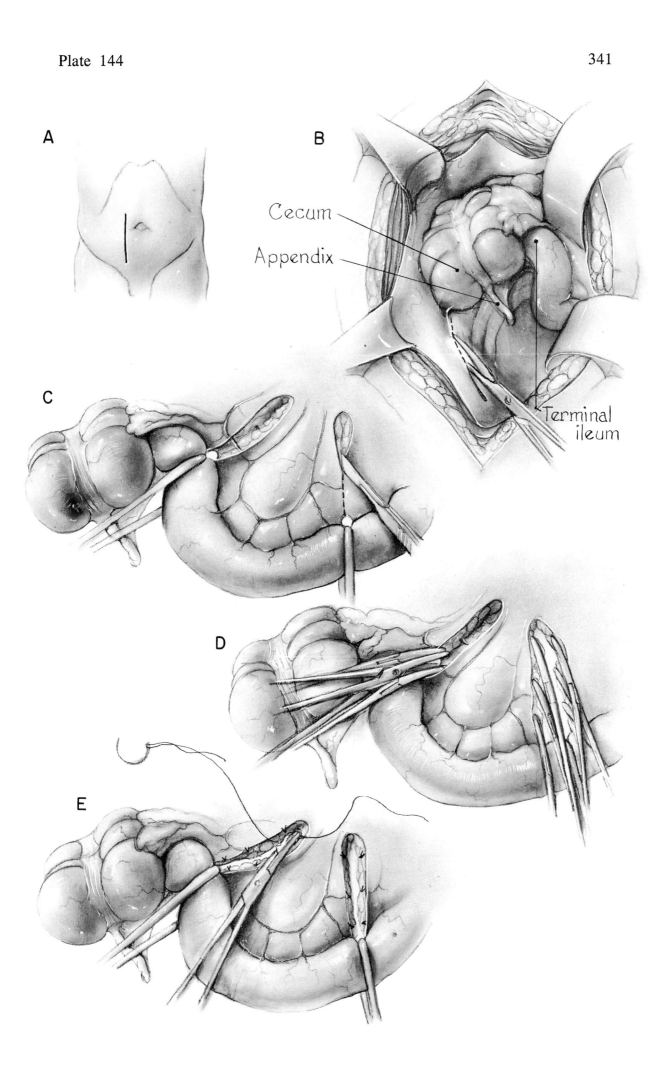

A

B

Cecum

Appendix

Terminal
ileum

C

D

E

F. The transected ends of the ileum proximally are occluded with Babcock clamps, and, with a scalpel, the transection of the ileum distally is being completed between clamps. The jaws of the clamps are approximated but not locked to avoid crushing trauma to the tissues.

G. The transection of the ileum both proximally and distally is completed and a segment 15 to 17 cm. in length, attached by its mesentery, is isolated.

H. The end-to-end anastomosis anterior to the isolated segment of ileum is begun by first inserting the mesenteric and antimesenteric approximation sutures.

I. The insertion of the first posterior suture layer, a series of interrupted everting mattress sutures, is completed. For technical expediency the sutures are all first inserted before being tied.

Plate 145   343

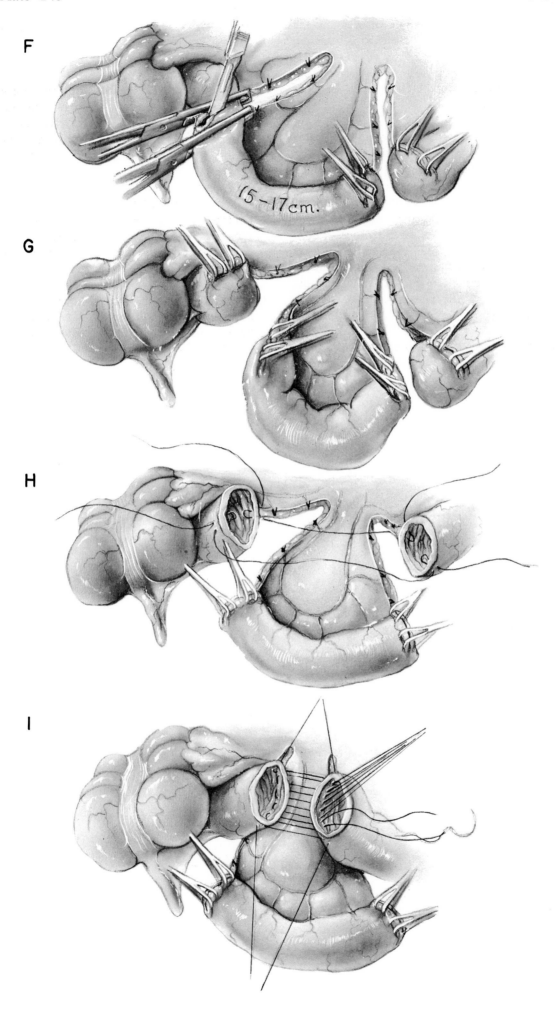

F

15—17cm.

G

H

I

J. The approximating angle sutures and the first posterior layer of mattress sutures are tied, and the long ends are cut. The insertion of the second posterior layer, a series of interrupted silk (000) sutures, is being completed.

K, L. The two layer closure posteriorly is completed, and the insertion of the first layer of sutures anteriorly is begun (K). This layer consists of a series of interrupted inverting sutures of silk (000) which are inserted from the "inside out" on one side and from the "outside in" on the other so that, when tied, the knots of the sutures are on the inside of the lumen. To facilitate the inversion of the anterior layer, traction medially is maintained on the previously inserted suture as the succeeding suture is tied (L).

M. The sutures are inserted alternately from either side and terminate in the midline anteriorly at which point the closure is reinforced by a figure of 8 mattress suture of silk (000).

N, O. The second layer of sutures anteriorly is inserted. This layer consists of a central seromuscular mattress suture (N) and a series of simple interrupted seromuscular sutures (Lembert) of silk (000) on either side (O).

P. The end-to-end "open" anastomosis is completed, and the incision through the serosal layer of the isolated segment of the terminal ileum close to its mesenteric border is being made.

Q. The incision in the serosal layer is made, and the vessels in the submucosal layer are being undersewn with hemostatic suture ligatures of silk (0000).

Plate 146

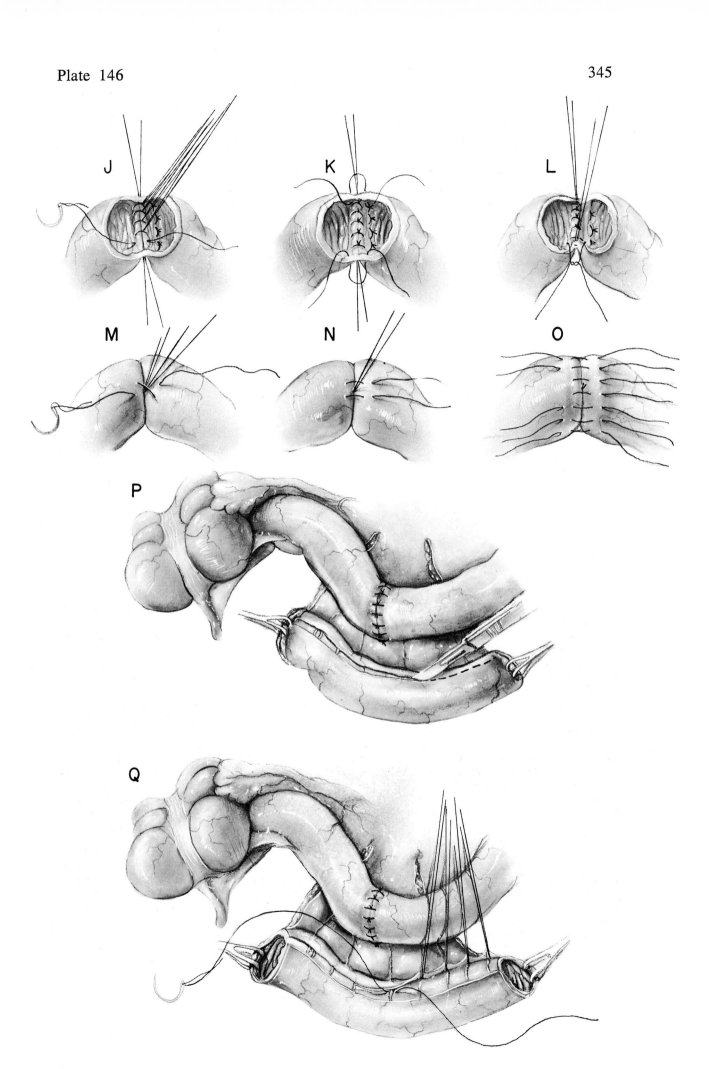

R. Two rows of hemostatic suture ligatures are inserted, and the opening into the lumen of the ileum is being made by scissor dissection.

S. An incision is made through the full length of the bowel wall of the isolated ileal segment, and one of its cut margins is being approximated to the lateral cut margin of the incision previously made in the posterior parietal peritoneum.

T. The ileo-entectropy is completed, and its relation to the adjacent intraperitoneal viscera is visible.

DISCUSSION—DR. CHARLES GEORGE NEUMANN. The operation of ileo-entectropy was designed to permit the intestinal mucosa to absorb excess fluid such as occurs in ascites of any origin (cirrhosis, nephrosis) or in hydrocephalus. Clinical trials in cirrhotics with ascites have demonstrated the ability of the mucosa to function effectively, but it can not be stressed too strongly that, in the use of ileo-entectropy for ascites, the patient's general condition must be such as to permit him to survive the trauma of the necessary surgical and anesthetic experience. Usually the very condition, namely intractable ascites, for which the operation may be beneficial, has imposed such a drain on the patient's resources that every effort must be made to qualify the patient as a surgical risk and to support him during the postoperative period.

With an understanding of the principles involved in ileo-entectropy for ascites, quite a series of modifications of the operation can be devised. Basic to any modification are sterilization of the bowel to avoid peritonitis, omentectomy to guard against encapsulation of the opened segment by the omentum, provision to minimize danger of rupture of esophageal varices (in cirrhotics) as by prolonged use of a Levin tube, and attachment of the serosa of the opened segment (in cirrhotics) to the parietal peritoneum to permit development of anastomoses between the portal and parietal circulations.

There is no valid reason for using one segment of ileum in favor of another except that surgical expediency suggests the use of the terminal ileum. Instead of reestablishing intestinal continuity by end-to-end anastomosis of the ileum, it is possible to discard the cecum and ascending colon and perform an ileo-colostomy. In this way a large area of the posterior parietes is made available for reception of the serosa of the opened ileal segment.

As for the length of segment to be opened, little can be said. Obviously, the longer the segment, the more fluid can be absorbed but also the surgical problem of placing the segment to advantage is greater. A length of 15 to 17 cm. should be adequate except in those few patients who produce prodigious quantities of ascitic fluid.

Theoretically, the possibility of the continued production of mucus by the exposed mucosa could lead to the accumulation of a disturbingly large quantity of mucus within the peritoneal cavity. Apparently mucus is secreted in very small amounts for several weeks after operation, but both in experimental animals and in patients (who have been observed up to one and one-half years without abdominal distention), the secretion of mucus ceases.

Plate 147 347

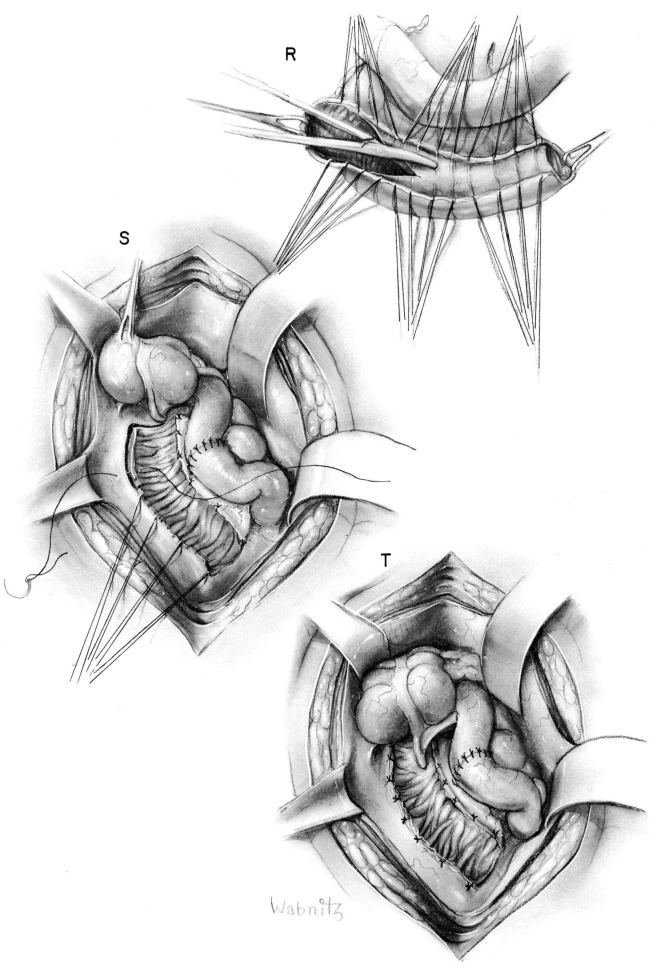

Wabnitz

INTUSSUSCEPTION

A. The right paramedian midabdominal incision employed is depicted by the solid line.

B. The peritoneal cavity is more widely exposed than usually obtains at operation to show the location of the distal portion of the tumefaction in the region of the midtransverse colon.

C. A sagittal section of the region of the intussusception is shown to depict the anatomic pathologic characteristics.

D. Manual reduction of the intussusception is initiated by a gentle retrograde "milking" maneuver.

E. The reduction of the intussusception is completed to the region of the cecoascending colon. It is in this area that further reduction may be most difficult and at times impossible. One cannot emphasize too frequently the importance of gentleness and the avoidance of trauma during the reduction of the intussusception. The exertion of a traction force on the ileum proximally, though often tempting, should not be done. In the event that the intussusception is either irreducible and/or gangrenous, ileocolic segmental resection and primary ileocolostomy is preferred to a multistage exteriorization operation.

F. The reduction of the intussusception is completed. The invaginated area on the anterior wall of the terminal ileum, frequently observed, is visible and denotes the "head" of the intussusceptum. A layer closure of the wound is subsequently performed using a continuous interlocking double strand suture of 00 catgut for the peritoneum and interrupted 000 silk sutures for the fascia and skin.

A six months old colored female infant was admitted to the hospital with the history that, 24 hours previously, the passage per rectum of blood-stained mucus occurred, subsequent to which there was no bowel movement. There was no nausea or vomiting, and at no time did the patient cry out in apparent pain.

On examination the infant was quiet, well nourished, and well hydrated. The abdomen was slightly distended but there was no evident tenderness or palpable masses. On digital rectal examination, no abnormalities were observed. On auscultation of the abdomen, intermittent high pitched metallic "tinkles" were heard, consistent with an obstruction of the small bowel. A "scout" film of the abdomen showed gaseous obstruction of the small intestines.

Operation was performed within six hours after admission; both the operative findings and the method of surgical management are shown in the illustrations. Postoperative convalescence was without incident.

Plate 148   349

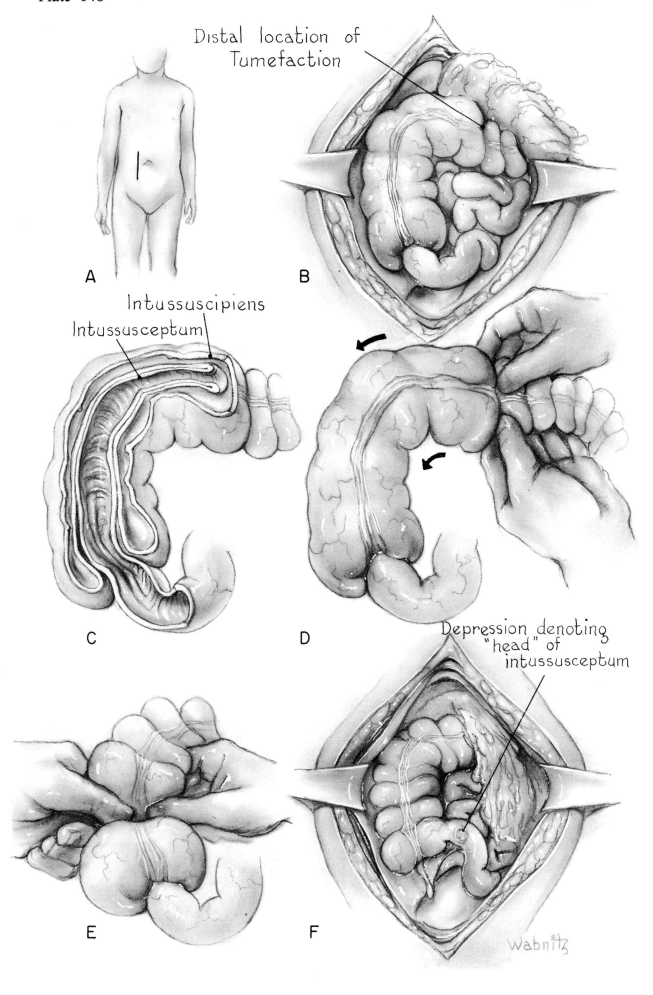

Distal location of
Tumefaction

A

B

Intussuscipiens
Intussusceptum

C

D

Depression denoting
"head" of
intussusceptum

E

F

Wabnitz

DISCUSSION—DR. ROWENA SPENCER. Diagnosis of the typical cases of intussusception requires only an awareness of the existence of the condition. In a suspected atypical case, the finding of at least one "sausage-shaped" loop of gas-filled bowel on the scout film of the abdomen indicates intestinal obstruction until proved otherwise, and a diagnosis of intestinal obstruction of undetermined cause is a sufficient indication for operation.

If the patient has been ill for more than a few hours, preoperative fluid (and blood) replacement is mandatory. The infant who is wide-eyed and staring and who submits without complaint to manipulation and venipuncture is not a "good" baby but a desperately ill one who will not tolerate operation without proper preparation. It may sometimes be necessary to gamble on continued viability of obstructed or intussuscepted bowel to assure viability of the patient for the duration of the operation.

Unless the patient is virtually moribund, general anesthesia is indicated. Use of an endotracheal tube will assure airway control and minimize reflux of gastric contents into the trachea.

Unless otherwise indicated, the incision should be on the right side of the abdomen, as most intussusceptions are ileocolic, and the proximal portion (in the right colon and terminal ileum) is the most difficult to reduce. Either vertical or transverse incision may be used, but the latter offers several advantages: it may be extended across the midline to give access to the opposite side of the abdomen if the diagnosis is changed or modified; it may be closed with subcutaneous sutures, obviating the need for placing and later removing conventional skin sutures, and it heals with a more cosmetically acceptable scar; and it probably results in a lower incidence of incisional hernia.

Reduction of the intussusception employs the technic of taxis, as opposed to traction. Pulling on the proximal ileum may result in complete disruption of the bowel. Gentle but steady compression of the distal segment of the intussusception will slowly force the intussusceptum from the intussuscipiens. This pressure is obtained by squeezing the bowel with both hands, thus distributing the pressure through the entire circumference of a long segment of intestine. It is mandatory that the reducing end of the intussusception be inspected frequently—preferably continuously—for it is here that rupture occurs. Small lacerations of the serosa in this area indicate that intraluminal pressure is too great and that reduction is too rapid. The entire process should be unhurried and atraumatic.

When reduction has successfully been accomplished, the bowel is inspected for viability and damage. Gangrenous intestine must be resected, but hemorrhagic and edematous bowel will often become obviously viable after a short period of warm saline packs. Serosal tears can be repaired with fine interrupted sutures to minimize subsequent adhesions.

Excision of a precipitating lesion, such as a Meckel's diverticulum or an intramural or intraluminal tumor, is usually contraindicated. The leading point of the intussusception is the most severely damaged and so edematous and friable that sutures cut through the tissue. Rather than risk a leak at the suture line, elective operation is planned for a later date. Appendectomy, also, is generally not advisable, for the cecum and appendix involved in an intussusception are edematous and hemorrhagic. Incidental appendectomy should not be considered unless the wall of the cecum is normally thin, soft, and pliable.

The surgeon should be aware of the existence of the "head" or leading point of the intussusception, which forms a thick, edematous, rigid plaque in the wall of the bowel and which should not be resected with the erroneous diagnosis of intramural tumor.

DISCUSSION—DR. THOMAS V. SANTULLI. The typical lesion of intussusception in this age group is well illustrated with the head of the intussusception in the right side of the transverse colon. Some of the cases present a mass which lies in the transverse direction, as part of the ascending colon rises out of the right lower quadrant.

In spite of the long incision that is usually made, the surgeon will need to reduce the most distal portion of the intussusception with one hand since it is not possible to deliver the mass at this point. By gentle retrograde "milking" starting at the head of the mass, the intussusception can usually be reduced until it reaches the cecum, when the mass can be delivered out of the wound. Here, the reduction can be completed by using both hands and continuing the gentle retrograde "milking" maneuver as shown in E. As emphasized, this is the most difficult part of the procedure and requires careful and gentle manipulation. The dimple which is the head of the intussusception is well shown in F.

In those cases in which the intussusception is irreducible, or if there is gangrenous bowel, ileocolic resection is mandatory. If the patient's condition is poor and he is not able to tolerate a primary anastomosis, exteriorization of the mass with subsequent anastomosis may be lifesaving.

We do not hesitate to remove the appendix in those cases where the reduction has been easily accomplished and where there is no undue edema of the cecum. Actually, many of the cases of intussusception in this age group have numerous congenital peritoneal bands between the ileum and cecum involving a portion of the mesoappendix. The division of these bands and complete freeing of the ileocecal area is often best accomplished by dividing the mesoappendix and performing an appendectomy. Appendectomy should not be done if there is reason to think that appreciable risk will be added in any individual case.

The history is not typical of the usual case of intussusception in the age group presented. Characteristically, there is severe abdominal pain which is periodic. Vomiting may follow, and there is the passage of blood by rectum. Physical examination will disclose the presence of a mass in the right side of the abdomen. The triad of abdominal pain, the passage of blood by rectum, and the palpation of an abdominal mass is characteristic. A barium enema will confirm the diagnosis.

We use the barium enema to reduce the intussusception in selected cases. These are cases in which the illness in under 24 hours *and* in which there is no clinical evidence of peritoneal irritation suggesting the presence of compromised bowel (fever, elevated pulse rate, abdominal tenderness and rigidity, leukocytosis). With definite precautions and under fluoroscopic control, about 75 per cent of our cases of intussusception in recent years have been successfully reduced by hydrostatic pressure with the barium enema.

Operation is immediately undertaken if the reduction is unsuccessful. It is indicated for those patients in whom there is a high suspicion of a specific lesion causing the intussusception, and it is the treatment of choice if there is any question of compromised bowel.

RESECTION OF MECKEL'S DIVERTICULUM

Meckel's diverticulum is an embryonic remnant of the vitelline duct and indicates the site of the communication in the embryo between the yolk sac and the midgut. Characteristically it is located in the segment of the ileum one to three feet from the ileocecal junction. It is classified as a true diverticulum because: (1) it contains all of the coats of the bowel wall; (2) it is located on the antimesenteric surface of the bowel; (3) it has a mesentery and blood supply of its own (mesenteriolum). However, not infrequently the mesenteriolum is absent. Furthermore, the mucosa of the diverticulum may be either partially or completely replaced by ectopic gastric, duodenal, pancreatic, or colonic tissue.

A, B, C. If a mesenteriolum is present (A), it is doubly clamped (B), severed, and the ends ligated (C) to mobilize the diverticulum.

D. Traction with a Babcock intestinal clamp is maintained upward on the diverticulum, and the circular incision about its base is begun.

E, F, G, H, I. The incision, deepened through the seromuscular layer, is completed about the whole of the circumference of the base of the diverticulum. The vessels in the submucosa are undersewn and ligated with suture ligatures of fine (0000) silk.

DISCUSSION—DR. PAUL C. KIERNAN. Meckel's diverticula are variable in size, and may contain ectopic gastric, duodenal, pancreatic or colonic tissue in either the tip or the base of the diverticulum and in the ileum adjacent to the base. Accordingly, the exact technical procedure to employ for the resection of a Meckel's diverticulum may vary. In general, several important points are to be remembered and practiced: (1) division and ligation of the mesentery and its contained blood supply; (2) complete excision of the base of the diverticulum; (3) closure of the opening in the ileum in a line at right angles to its long axis to avoid encroachment upon the lumen.

It is not necessary to remove all Meckel's diverticula which are found during the performance of an exploratory laparotomy. The resection of a small diverticulum with a wide base in an older individual who has had no evidence of intestinal bleeding would seem to add an unnecessary risk to the procedure for which the exploration is primarily undertaken. In the young individual, although no symptoms seem to be caused by its presence, and even if small, the diverticulum should be removed. Small diverticula may be the initiating cause of an intussusception. Furthermore, whenever the diverticulum is in continuity with the anterior abdominal wall, either with or without a fistula, in all instances of intestinal bleeding of undetermined origin, and when a Meckel's diverticulum coexists with a duodenal ulcer or any other lesion which may be the source of bleeding, the diverticulum should be excised.

Dr. Madden's technic for the resection of a Meckel's diverticulum certainly is excellently portrayed. However, in my opinion, it is unnecessary to make a circular incision through the seromuscular layer about the base of the diverticulum as indicated in Plate 149, D. Furthermore, I believe it is unnecessary to undersew and ligate the vessels of the wall of the bowel separately as shown in G, H, and I, Plate 149. My preference is to apply a thin bladed crushing clamp to the base of the Meckel's diverticulum, excise the diverticulum, and with a suitable suture invert the crushed segment into the lumen of the ileum, taking care to apply the clamp, as emphasized previously, at right angles to the long axis of the ileum.

Plate 149   353

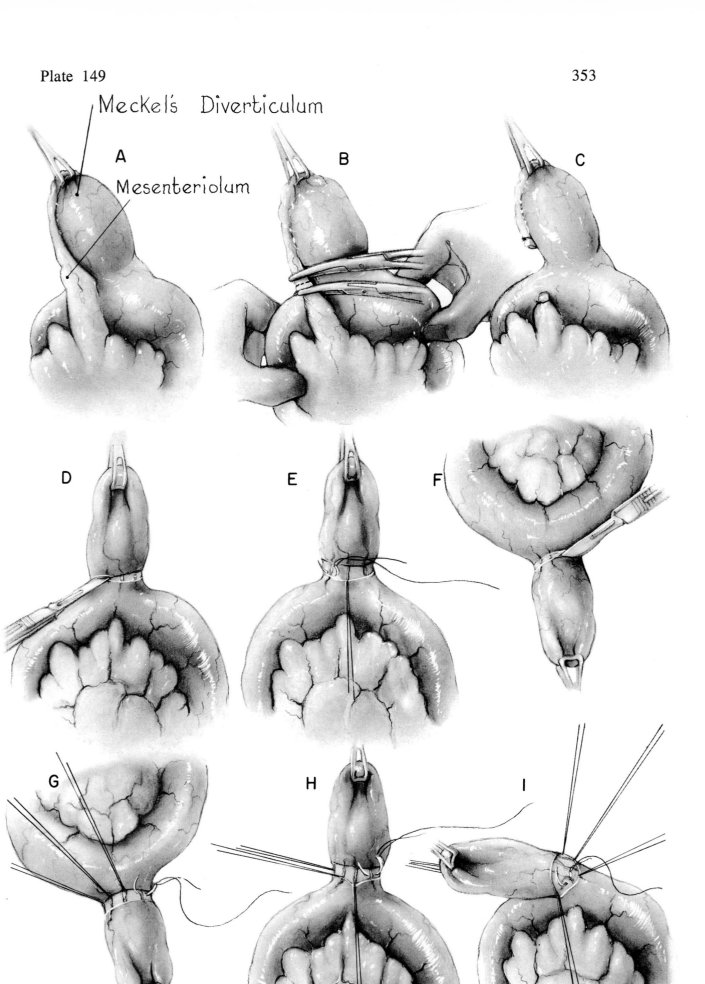

Meckel's Diverticulum

Mesenteriolum

A   B   C

D   E   F

G   H   I

J, K, L. The ligation in continuity of the vessels in the submucosa is completed (J). The lumen of the proximal segment of the ileum is occluded with a rubber covered intestinal clamp, and a crushing (Kocher) clamp is applied across the base of the diverticulum (J). An opening is made into the lumen of the bowel with a No. 15 scalpel blade (J) and the resection of the diverticulum is continued by scissor dissection (K, L).

M. The amputation of the diverticulum is completed, and the hemostatic suture ligatures on either side of the opening in the bowel are cut.

N. The polar ligatures are used for traction to convert the circular opening to a longitudinal one transverse to the long axis of the bowel (ileum).

O. An enterorrhaphy is performed, using interrupted sutures of fine (0000) silk which are inserted from the "inside out" to the "outside in" so that, when tied, the knots are on the inside of the lumen.

P. A figure of 8 suture of 0000 silk is inserted about the terminal midline suture of the first layer to assure both an air-tight and a water-tight closure.

Q, R. A second reinforcing layer of interrupted seromuscular sutures (Lembert) of fine (0000) silk is inserted (Q) and tied (R) to complete the closure of the opening in the lumen of the bowel. The line of closure, at right angles to the long axis of the bowel, avoids encroachment upon and resulting constriction of the lumen.

Plate 150

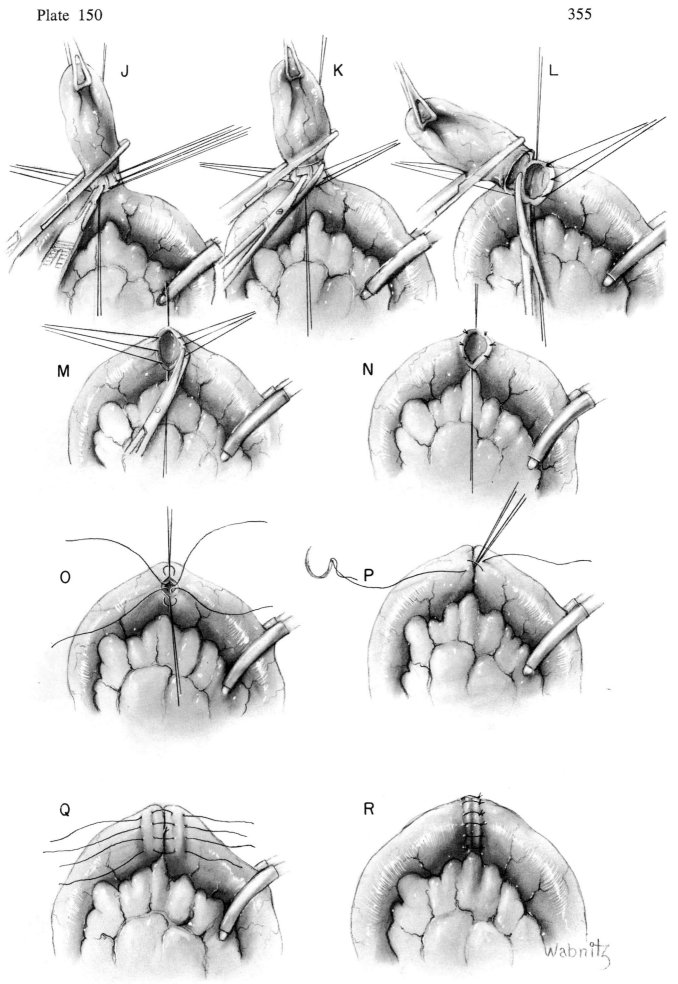

Wabnitz

APPENDECTOMY

In the performance of an appendectomy any one of a variety of incisions, depending upon the preference of the surgeon, may be used. In general either a right lower paramedian muscle-retracting (lateral) or muscle-splitting incision is preferred.

A. The tip of the mesoappendix is grasped in a curved clamp (Kelly) and mobilized, with the cecum and the terminal ileum, into the operative wound. The related anatomic structures are depicted.

B, B₁. The appendix is mobilized by severance of the attached mesoappendix. An opening may be made through an avascular portion of the base of the mesoappendix through which a ligature of silk (00) is withdrawn (B). The ligature, when tied, occludes the appendicular artery, and the site of severance of the mesoappendix distally is indicated by the dotted line. The objections to this method are the inclusion of an excess amount of fatty areolar tissue in the hemostatic ligature and the potential "slipping" of the ligature with secondary hemorrhage.

The preferred method for mobilization of the appendix is to serially clamp and sever the mesoappendix, the beginning of which is indicated in B₁.

C, D. The severance of the mesoappendix is completed as indicated.

E. The mobilization of the appendix is completed, and the clamps on the proximal cut margin of the mesoappendix are replaced with suture ligatures of silk (000). A purse-string suture of silk (00) is inserted in the wall of the cecum about the base of the appendix, and one loop of the pursestring is held in a Babcock clamp for subsequent countertraction when the stump of the appendix is inverted.

DISCUSSION—DR. PAUL C. KIERNAN. In this procedure the abdominal incision which affords the best exposure is determined by the individual surgeon. However, in most instances when an appendectomy is done as a primary procedure, a low paramedian or McBurney type of muscle-splitting incision is adequate. If the latter is used and additional pathology requires a more adequate exposure, a second incision is preferred to one which enlarges the muscle-splitting type.

Identification of the appendix, usually not difficult, may be aided by tracing the taenia coli of the cecum to their point of confluence. If retrocecal, the appendix is more easily reached and removed by first dividing the lateral peritoneal attachment of the cecum and ascending colon and mobilizing the right colon medially.

Depending upon the degree of inflammation present, either the appendix or its mesentery may be grasped. Whether or not the mesoappendix is ligated and divided in toto or segmentally is dependent upon several factors, e.g. size, amount of contained fat, edema, or other associated inflammatory changes. If it is thin and short, the entire mesoappendix may be included in a single clamp, divided and ligated. However, if marked edema and induration are present, the mesoappendix may be better clamped, severed, and ligated in segments.

In spite of all that is written relative to the treatment of the appendiceal stump either by ligation alone or inversion with or without concomitant ligation, the results seem to indicate that it makes little or no difference how the stump is treated as long as fundamental surgical practices are followed. In simple ligation of the base of the appendix, it is important that the ligature be placed proximal to any crushed portion of the wall of the appendix. If the ligature is placed in the crushed groove, the tissue may necrose too rapidly and cause a "blowout" of the wall of the cecum. Medicinal treatment of the base of the appendix, whether the stump is or is not inverted, is of no practical importance. In particular,

Plate 151   357

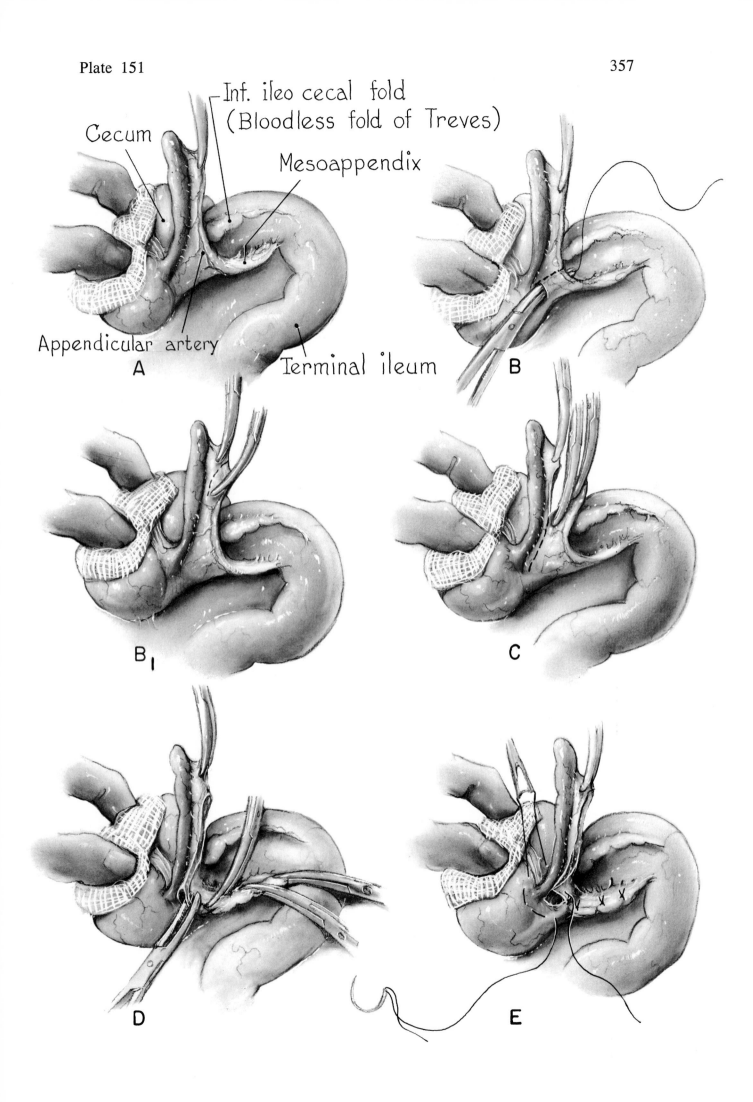

Cecum

Inf. ileo cecal fold
(Bloodless fold of Treves)

Mesoappendix

Appendicular artery

Terminal ileum

A

B

B₁

C

D

E

F, G. The base and proximal portion of the appendix is "milked" distally prior to locking the clamp (F), and a ligature of silk is placed around the base of the appendix (G). The placement of this ligature in a groove formed by crushing the appendix with a clamp is neither practiced nor recommended because it leaves an area of devitalized tissue proximal to the site of the ligature.

H. The ligature (00 silk) is tied and anatomic forceps (without "teeth") are used to hold the base of the appendix at the site of its ligation.

I. A square piece of gauze split halfway and moistened in sterile saline is placed about the appendix overlying the anatomic forceps but beneath the occluded clamp. The base of the appendix is then severed with a scalpel just beneath the clamp.

J. The severed and ligated proximal stump of the appendix is wiped with a piece of moistened gauze prior to its inversion. The scalpel used to sever the appendix is not dipped in phenol prior to use, nor is the stump "treated" with cotton applicators moistened with phenol and alcohol. This ritual, although a common practice, is not recommended.

K. The stump of the appendix is inverted with the aid of countertraction on the loop of the pursestring suture held in the Babcock clamp, and direct inversion with the anatomic forceps is obtained as the pursestring suture is drawn taut.

L. The inversion pursestring suture is tied, and a second reinforcing figure N or Z suture (000 silk) is inserted. The old axiom "If you invert the appendiceal stump, don't ligate, and if you ligate the stump, don't invert," is not followed. The objection to ligation and inversion, namely, that you invert an infected stump into a closed peritoneal space and thereby predispose to the occurrence of a complicating abscess in the cecal wall, is not believed of practical importance. This complication, though admittedly a possibility, has not been observed by the author.

The indication for drainage following appendectomy is not "When in doubt, drain." In the presence of a complicating abscess, drainage is always practiced. In the absence of an abscess the indication for drainage following the removal of an acutely suppurative or gangrenous appendix is dependent upon the appearance of the adjacent peritoneum. If the peritoneum is glistening and healthy in appearance, drains are not used. However, if the peritoneum is edematous, studded with petechiae, and lacking its normal luster, drainage is performed because these findings are believed to indicate that the protective mechanism of the peritoneum is compromised and drainage is needed. The drain should not be removed before the seventh postoperative day. Furthermore, whether a drain is or is not used, if "diarrhea" should occur between the fifth and eighth days postoperatively, the first thing a surgeon should do is a digital rectal examination to rule out the presence of a pelvic abscess. All too frequently medication to control the irritative pseudodiarrhea is empirically prescribed and continued for varying periods of time before the correct diagnosis is made.

DISCUSSION—DR. KIERNAN (cont.)
carbolic acid or other caustic solutions should not be used. However, the use of a cautery to sever the base of the appendix is practiced with success by many surgeons. The contamination of the peritoneum which may result from an infected base of the appendix is well tolerated so long as the source of the contamination is controlled, i.e., adequate ligation or inversion of the stump of the appendix.

In the absence of a localized abscess, drainage of the peritoneal cavity is rarely needed. However, when there is gross contamination of the wound, the avoidance of necrosis of the abdominal wall and resultant hernia may be assured by closure of only the peritoneum and by the insertion of sutures which are untied through the skin, subcutaneous fat, and fascia layers. The open wound is loosely packed with sterile gauze, which is removed in 24 to 36 hours, and the wound closed secondarily with the previously inserted but untied sutures.

Plate 152   359

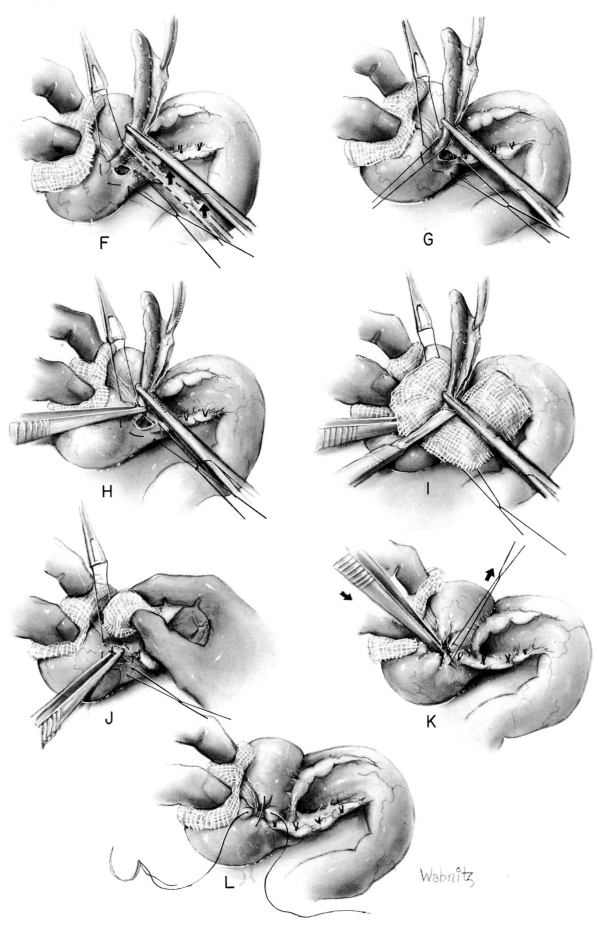

ILEOSTOMY AND SUBTOTAL COLECTOMY

A. The sites of the ileostomy stoma in the right lower quadrant and the left paramedian muscle-splitting incision are depicted in dotted outline.

B. The peritoneal cavity is entered, and the wound margins are retracted to expose the subjacent viscera.

C. Manual traction is maintained upward on the omentum and downward on the transverse colon as the relatively avascular attachments of the omentum to the colon are separated by scalpel dissection.

D. Upon completion of the detachment of the omentum, the transverse colon is mobilized and the lesser peritoneal sac is entered.

E. The ascending colon is manually retracted toward the midline, and the mobilization of the right side of the colon is commenced by scissor dissection along the "white line," the fascia fusion layer of Toldt.

DISCUSSION—DR. CLARENCE DENNIS. In reference to Plate 153, A, if the ileostomy is made precisely in the belt line and in the midportion of the belly of the right rectus muscle, the intact skin around it provides a smooth and slightly convex flexible surface for the later adhesion of an ileostomy bag. It is wise to note the position of the transverse creases which form across the abdomen when the patient bends over. These creases should be avoided in placing the ileostomy for they make secure cementing of an ileostomy bag impossible.

In a considerable number of my first twenty-odd colectomies, careful preservation of the omentum (Plate 153, C) was followed by distressing evidence of adhesive obstruction. Since that time the omentum has been completely removed routinely with the specimen, and gratifying freedom from such complications has been observed. This experience covers a total of more than 100 colectomies.

It is usually preferable to commence the intra-abdominal dissection by freeing the cecum and ascending colon (Plate 153, E) together with the very terminal ileum. This is done because it is not possible to determine the exact level of invasion of

Plate 153

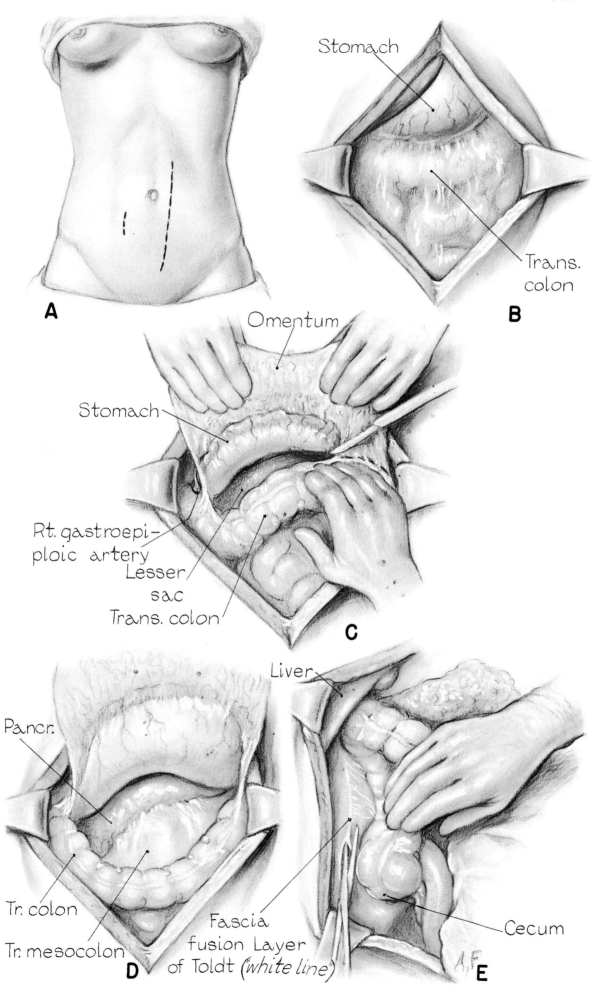

A

Stomach

Trans. colon

B

Omentum

Stomach

Rt. gastroepi-
ploic artery

Lesser
sac

Trans. colon

C

Pancr.

Tr. colon

Tr. mesocolon

D

Fascia
fusion Layer
of Toldt (white line)

Liver

Cecum

E

F, G. The hepatic flexure of the colon is mobilized by severance of the right phrenocolic ligament (dotted outline), and the retrocolic portion of the duodenum is exposed (G).

H. The right side of the colon, completely mobilized, is rotated toward the midline, and the related structures in the retroperitoneal area are visible. In this mobilization one must be careful to avoid injury to the spermatic or ovarian vessels, the right ureter, the inferior vena cava, and the retrocolic portion of the duodenum.

I. The descending colon is manually retracted toward the midline, and its mobilization, similar to that on the right side, is commenced by scissor dissection along the fascia fusion layer of Toldt ("white line").

DISCUSSION—DR. DENNIS (cont.)

the inflammatory process into the terminal ileum by gross examination of either the serosal or the mucosal surfaces. Since it is of paramount importance that the ileostomy be fashioned from the lowest normal segment of ileum, it is worthwhile to remove a short segment of the lowest area of the terminal ileum which appears normal and have rapid frozen sections prepared. The further dissection in the abdomen can be pursued while the pathologist is examining the specimen. Cellular infiltration of the submucosa or muscularis is an indication that the segment under consideration is involved with the process and that it would be wise to resect a few centimeters more of the terminal ileum. The precise level at which the ileostomy is to be made is of extreme importance in the subsequent maintenance of satisfactory water balance because the lowest portion of the terminal ileum is extremely important in water reabsorption. Furthermore, the utilization of inflamed intestine to make an ileostomy is productive of a high incidence of late ileostomy complications. It is, therefore, essential to control the level of division by the study of rapid frozen section preparations of excised portions of the terminal ileum.

A smoother surface of skin about the ileostomy can be achieved if one utilizes a circular incision rather than the simple longitudinal one illustrated (Plate 156, P). The circular incision is very satisfactory if made essentially as one would make it with a cork borer. The hemostasis must be meticulous, and the burial of suture material in the substance of the abdominal wall at this point should be minimized. Very fine catgut, or better, the utilization of the coagulation current in extremely careful fashion is worthwhile. It is my preference to preserve as much of the mesentery of the resected terminal ileum as possible, and to have the mesenteric margin of the terminal ileum directed laterally rather than cephalad as shown (Plate 156, R). The purpose of saving this mesentery is to simplify the construction of a complete diaphragm bounded by the anterior, lateral, and posterior abdominal walls and the segment of ileum forming

Plate 154   363

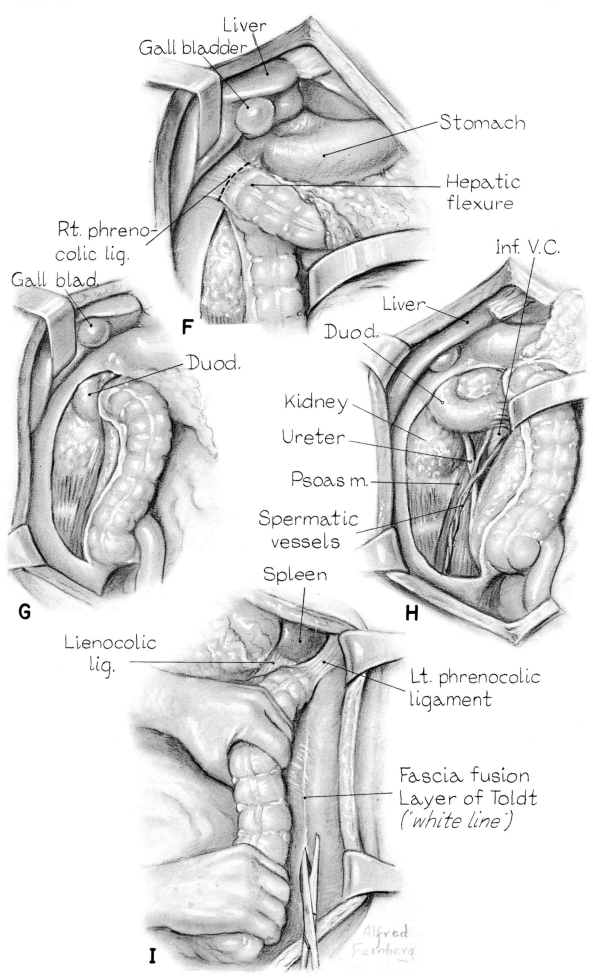

Liver

Gall bladder

Stomach

Hepatic
flexure

Rt. phreno-
colic lig.

Inf. V.C.

Gall blad.

Liver

Duod.

Duod.

Kidney

Ureter

Psoas m.

Spermatic
vessels

Spleen

F

G

H

Lienocolic
lig.

Lt. phrenocolic
ligament

Fascia fusion
Layer of Toldt
("white line")

I

Alfred
Feinberg

J. The mobilized descending colon is displaced medially, and the left phrenocolic ligament is severed. The mobilization of the left side of the colon is completed after severance of the lienocolic ligament as indicated in dotted outline.

K. The vascular pattern of the right side of the colon is demonstrated, and the levels for division of the terminal ileum and the sigmoid colon are indicated by encircling traction tapes of rubber tissue.

L. An incision is made through the serosal covering of the mesentery of the terminal ileum as a guide tract for the serial clamping and division of the mesentery.

M. The division of the mesentery of the terminal ileum is completed, and clamps are applied to the ileocolic and middle colic branches of the superior mesenteric artery prior to their severance.

N. The severance of the mesenteric vascular attachment to the colon is completed to the left colic artery, the first branch of the inferior mesenteric artery. The guide tract for the division of the mesentery of the sigmoid colon and its contained left colic artery is depicted.

O. The sigmoid colon is doubly clamped at the junction of its middle and lower thirds and divided as indicated in dotted outline. The handle of the distal clamp is directed toward the center of the abdomen to facilitate its support when the wound dressing is applied.

DISCUSSION—DR. DENNIS (cont.)

the ileostomy. Only by meticulous closure of the defect lateral to the ileostomy may one be assured that whole segments of the intestinal tract will not wrap around the segment of ileum and cause a strangulating intestinal obstruction. In my experience this happened six times prior to the construction of a hemidiaphragm as described.

The incidence of late hernia formation, stenosis, or prolapse of the ileostomy can be markedly reduced by the very careful suture of the ileum to the posterior rectus sheath and peritoneum as it passes through the abdominal wall. For this purpose my preference is to use about 15 silk sutures (0000). The proper placement of these sutures is most important. The bite upon the peritoneal surface of the ileum must be precisely parallel to the one in the posterior rectus sheath and peritoneum. The suture must not penetrate into the mucosa and it must not be tied tightly enough to cause strangulation. Although I have seen three instances in which fistulas formed about such sutures placed at the time of ileostomy, I personally have had none in the performance of over 125 ileostomies with the placement of sutures as described. Furthermore, in this series prolapse did not occur in any patient in whom the ileum was normal at the level at which the ileostomy was performed.

In the early cases in the series performed at the University of Minnesota, the parietal reperitonization was performed similarly to that indicated (Plate 156, S), but the incidence of complications was high. In the last more than 100 cases, this reperitonization has not been done in either the right or the left gutter and no drains have been used. There has been no recognized complication from pursuit of this course.

In patients who are critically ill, it is appropriate to bring out the distal segment of colon through the bottom end of the abdominal incision (Plate 156, T). Frequency of retrograde purulent drainage onto the abdominal wall and secondary pyoderma are symptoms distressing enough to lead to the decision to remove the rectum at the time of total colectomy in those patients who are not too ill to have the two operations completed in one stage. It is my personal preference to utilize the technic of B. N. Brooke of London, England (Plate 157, F), of everting the ileum routinely so as not to leave any uncovered serosa exposed to drainage from the terminal ileum. In those cases in which the level of the ileostomy has been carefully controlled by rapid frozen section studies and this technic employed, the passage of formed stools within the first four or five days is usually observed.

In the re-explorations of patients following ile-

Plate 155

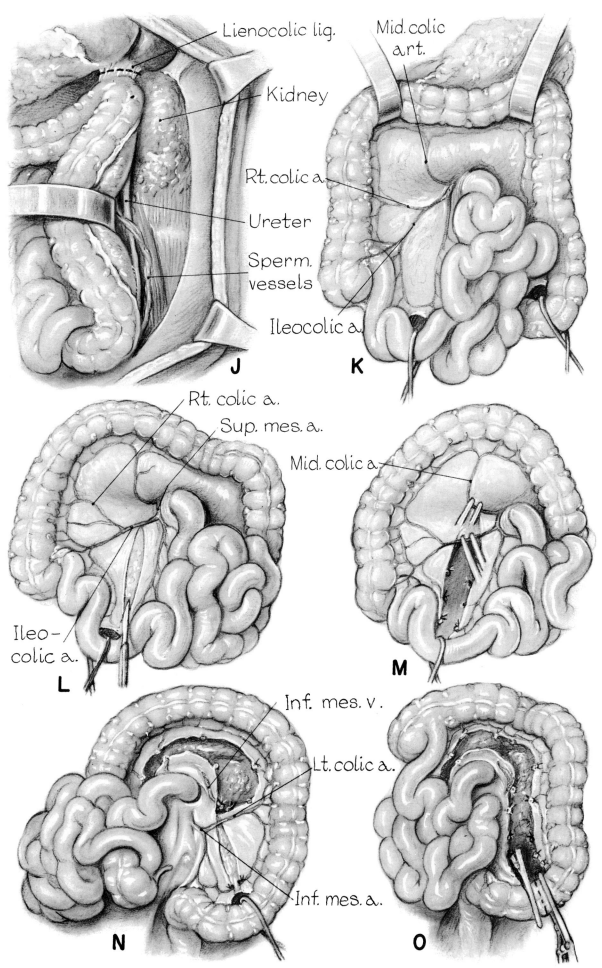

Lienocolic lig.

Kidney

Rt. colic a.

Ureter

Sperm. vessels

Ileocolic a.

Mid. colic art.

J

K

Rt. colic a.

Sup. mes. a.

Mid. colic a.

Ileo-colic a.

L

M

Inf. mes. v.

Lt. colic a.

Inf. mes. a.

N

O

P, Q. Through a small incision, to the right of and below the umbilicus, a clamp is applied to the proximal portion of the distal segment of the ileum. A second clamp is applied through the laparotomy incision to the ileum immediately distal to the first, and the ileum is severed between the clamps.

R. The distal cut end of the ileum is covered with a rubber diaphragm, and the proximal cut end is brought out through the small incision to the right of and below the umbilicus. To lessen the tendency for mucosal prolapse of the ileum, the cut margin of the ileal mesentery is sutured to the anterior parietal peritoneum.

S. The operative field, following completion of the operation, is shown. A partial reperitonization is performed, and a drain is inserted into the retroperitoneal area. Prior to closure of the incision the omentum is replaced over the small intestines.

T. The wound closure is completed about the retroperitoneal drain and the terminal portion of the sigmoid colon. To minimize the incidence of fistula formation, no sutures are used to anchor the ileum to any portion of the abdominal wall. A tube is secured in the lumen of the ileum to permit escape of the ileal contents into a bedside receptacle. The tube is ejected spontaneously between the fifth and seventh days when the retaining necrosing ligature sloughs through.

DISCUSSION—DR. DENNIS (cont.)

ostomy and either subtotal or total colectomy, I have been deeply impressed with the paucity of complications in those cases in which, at the primary operation, gentleness in the handling of tissues, meticulous hemostasis, the use of the finest and the least possible amount of suture material, and rigid adherence to strict aseptic surgical technic were practiced. If, in the performance of a colectomy, the utmost case is utilized to prevent drying, excoriation, or other trauma to the ileum, exploration at a later date reveals routinely the complete absence of any adhesions whatsoever in the abdominal cavity. The utilization, therefore, of the Noble plication technic (Plate 157, E) appears to me unnecessary. Leland S. McKittrick has emphasized that the development of enteritis above ileostomies that are properly prepared is almost never observed unless there is some obstruction at the ileostomy. In the re-explorations previously mentioned, the ileostomies which were considered truly satisfactory were only those in which the ileum just proximal to its passage through the abdominal wall was neither hypertrophied nor dilated.

The variance of these comments from the technic illustrated is an indication of the frequency with which a desired result may be obtained by a variety of successful maneuvers.

DISCUSSION—MR. BRYAN N. BROOKE. Since ulcerative colitis is not often confined to the colon and in all but 5 per cent or less of cases the rectum is involved, the condition cannot be said to be cured until the whole of the large intestine is removed. This is best done in one stage, panproctocolectomy, which as an elective procedure (and it should not be undertaken otherwise) has a mortality of 3 per cent or less. Removal of the bowel in two stages has a limited place, and primary colectomy to be followed by rectal excision is undertaken when the patient is too ill to withstand the major one-stage operation. In colectomy special technical difficulties that are not encountered in proctocolectomy, therefore present themselves, for it is in the really sick patient that bowel disintegration takes place, leading to flaccid dilatation of the dependent parts of the colon, transverse, sigmoid, and caecal areas, which are then particularly friable and prone to rupture on handling and soiling of the peritoneal cavity. Moreover, as disintegration proceeds, any area may be sealed off by adjacent intestine, or in the ascending and descending areas by adherence to the parietal peritoneum, thus obliterating the paracolic spaces and thereby the tissue planes convenient for mobilization. Therefore, whereas removal of the large intestine as an elective procedure is "child's play," as A to J indicate, in acute cases colectomy may present one of the most difficult and formidable operations.

To overcome the possibilities of soiling, it is wise in the acute case first to empty the large intestine of its contents by sucking out the transverse, sigmoid, and cecal segments before proceeding with the mobilization. The difficulty here lies in closing the hole in the colon wall made for the passage of the sucker before starting mobilization, for it is so friable that stitches frequently fail to hold. The solution lies in providing a firm ground through which sutures can be passed into the intestinal wall and back over which they can be tied. Advantage can be taken of adherence to the parietal peritoneum, since where this has occurred mobilization of the large intestine can be achieved only by extraperitoneal dissection and include that

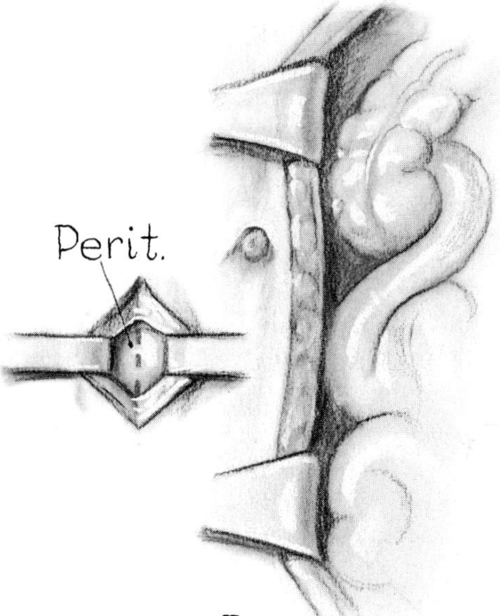

Plate 156

Perit.

P

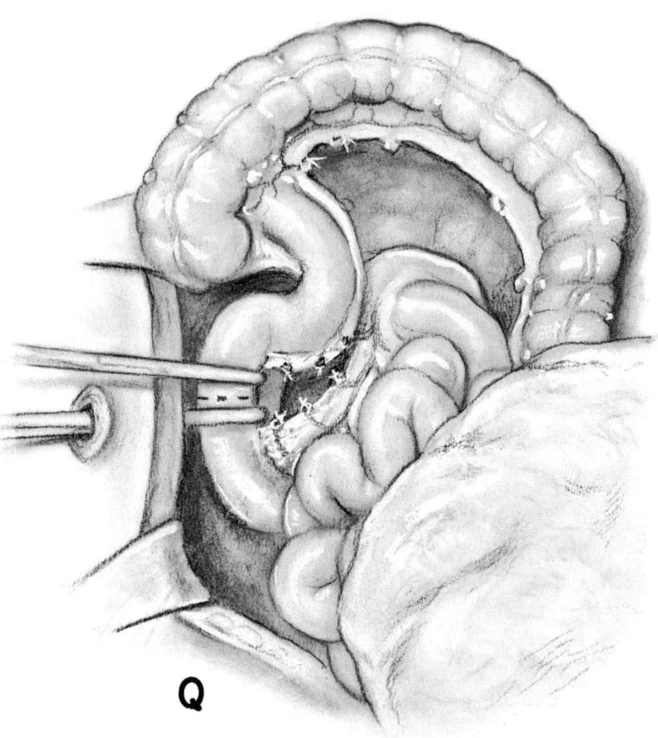

Q

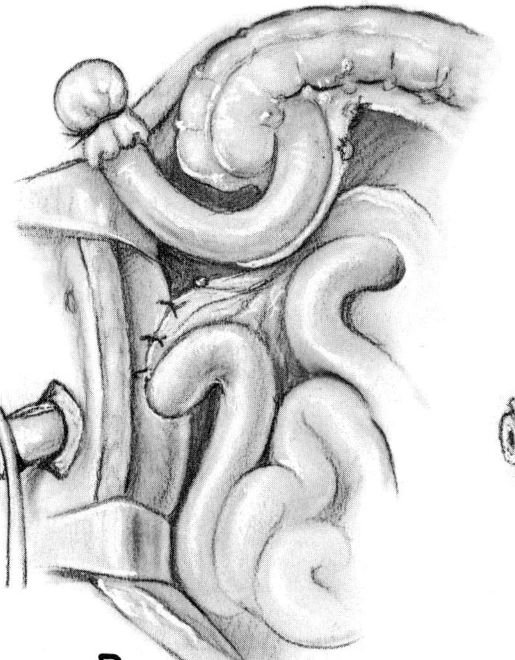

R

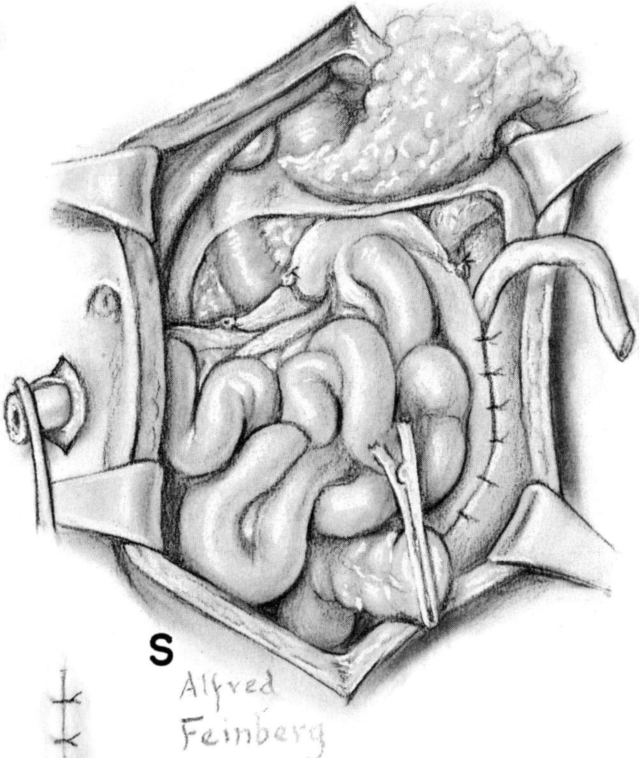

S

Alfred
Feinberg

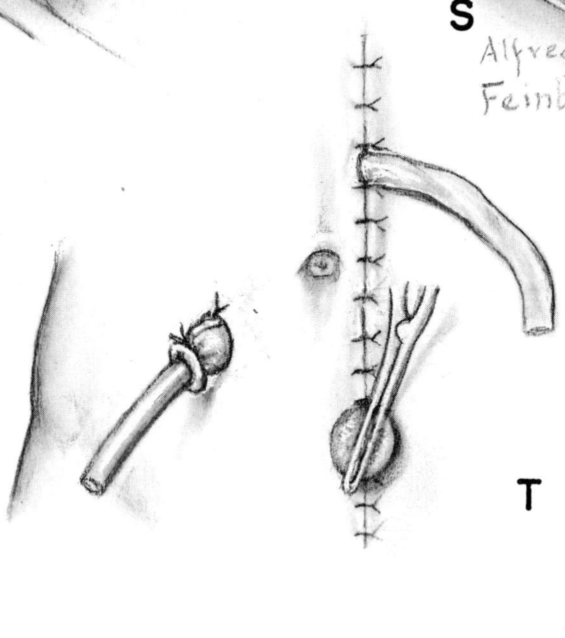

T

This plate illustrates the combination of four procedures suggested by Garlock to prevent ileal dysfunction. During the past two years, all or several of the methods illustrated have been used with excellent results. Accordingly, this is now the preferred technic in the establishment of the ileostomy stoma.

A, B, C. An opening is made into the peritoneal cavity after the removal of a wafer of skin, as advocated by Dennis to avoid scar contracture of the skin at the site of the ileostomy.

D. The attachment of the cut margin of the mesentery of the ileum to the anterior parietal peritoneum is depicted.

E. Plication (Noble) of the terminal portion of the ileum, recommended by Lichtenstein and Herzikoff for the prevention of ileal prolapse.

F, G. The immediate suturing of the whole thickness of the wall of the ileostomy stoma to the skin margin. Prior to suturing, the terminal ileum projects approximately 4 cm.

from the skin surface. Four cardinal sutures of silk (000) are first inserted (F) and held taut but not tied. In between these sutures a series of interrupted silk sutures are inserted to complete the eversion of the ileal stoma (G). This procedure, suggested by Brooke, is used routinely to prevent stenosis and dysfunction of the ileostomy which frequently occur following simple exteriorization with spontaneous eversion of the terminal ileum.

H. Appearance of the ileostomy and colostomy stomata five weeks postoperatively. One may note the spoutlike projection of the terminal ileum at this stage compared to its flat appearance immediately postoperative (G).

DISCUSSION—DR. BROOKE (cont.)

part of the peritoneum attached to and now forming the wall of the bowel. To gain access to the extraperitoneal plane, an incision from within the abdomen through the parietal peritoneum parallel to the intestine can be made 2 to 3 cm. from their point of fusion. This then provides a flap or hood of peritoneum that may be drawn down upon a hole made through the colon wall underlying it. A mattress suture passed through the outer surface of the peritoneal flap, through the colon wall to enclose the hole, and back through the flap will hold when tied on this outer surface. In the transverse colon area omentum can be used in the same way. Once the colon is empty and the suction port sealed, it is safe to proceed with mobilization, since overwhelming contamination cannot then occur if the bowel wall ruptures.

Though it is tempting in such cases to make the operation as short as possible and to save time by making no attempt to do more than withdraw the ileum through a stab incision and leave it thus (R, S, T), this temptation should be vigorously resisted. Indeed, there is now no excuse for such a measure. It can only lead to ileostomy dysfunction and a stoma that in all probability will require a further operation to make it efficient and adaptable to a bag. It must be borne in mind that though subtotal colectomy is being undertaken to save life, that life must be worth living after saving; it will only be so with an efficient stoma, and it is therefore as important to concentrate attention upon its formation as to remove the dangerously

offending bowel. Mucosal eversion (H) not only achieves a flexible stoma and precludes skin level stenosis but also avoids serositis—a most important consideration, since exposure of the serosa is thus conducive to ileostomy dysfunction with excessive loss of fluid, sodium, and potassium in the immediate postoperative period. Patients for whom subtotal colectomy is appropriate are already in a precarious state of biochemical disturbance through potassium, sodium, and water lack as a result of severe diarrhoea. An eversion ileostomy is therefore more imperative in the urgent than in the elective case if dangerous postoperative hypotensive episodes are to be avoided.

A tube placed in the stoma (T) tends to cause mucosal irritation and ulceration and so promote dysfunction. Its value is doubtful, since a polythene bag with adherent seal can be placed over the stoma to contain its exudate when bowel movement begins. Care must be taken to cut the hole in the bag so as to allow for some swelling of the stoma to occur in the first three or four days; otherwise, it may become chaffed by the edge of the bag and a fistula thus form. Edema has usually subsided by the end of a week. It is wise also to "splint" the stoma with cotton wool placed around it within the bag for the first 48 hours, to prevent the walls of the bag pressing upon the stoma and causing recession before the outgoing and returning layers have become firmly adherent to one another.

Plate 157

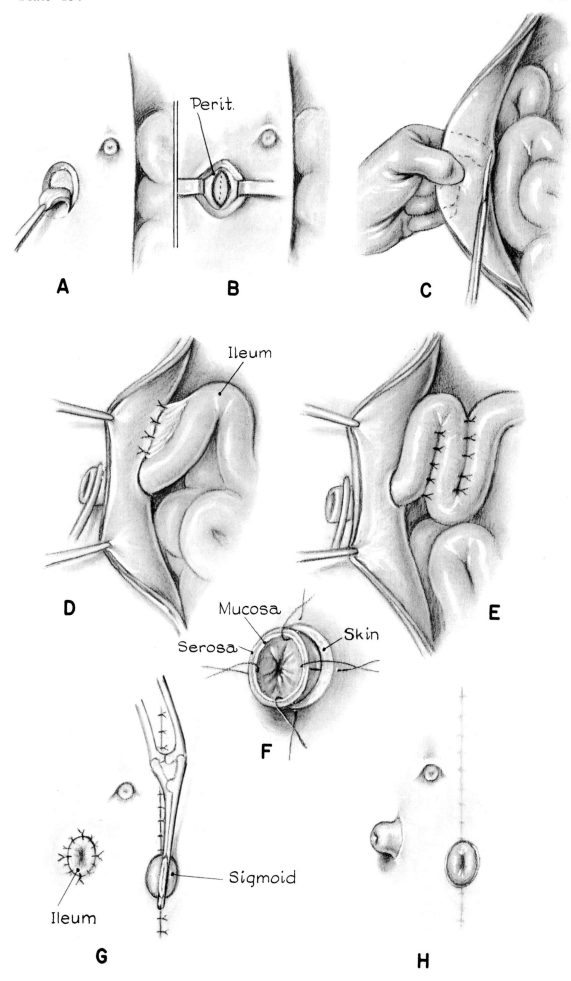

A

Perit.

B

C

Ileum

D

E

Mucosa

Serosa

Skin

F

Sigmoid

Ileum

G

H

COLOTOMY, COLOSCOPY, AND EXCISION OF POLYP

Preparation of the patient is begun four days before operation at which time magnesium sulfate is prescribed in the dosage of 1 dram (4 cc.) every four hours during the day. Warm soda bicarbonate enemas are administered each night and morning. This regimen is continued until the day preceding operation when the saline catharsis is discontinued and the patient is placed on a full liquid diet only. Castor oil (2 oz.) is given at 2:00 P.M., and cleansing enemas (soda bicarbonate) are prescribed the evening before and the morning of the operation. Chemotherapeutic or antibiotic drugs are not employed.

A. The left paramedian, muscle-splitting incision is outlined.

B, C. The sigmoid colon is withdrawn from the peritoneal cavity and surrounded with moist gauze pads. Two Babcock clamps modified on the Potts principle * are applied to the anterior taenia or band at separate sites proximal and distal to the location of the polyp (B). Between the clamps a stab wound incision is made into the lumen of the colon (B) and extended both proximally and distally by scissor dissection (C).

D. The cut margins of the sigmoid colon are grasped in clamps,* retracted, and the polyp is seen elevated on its pedunculated stalk.

E, F, G. The mucosa at the base of the polyp is circumcised (E), and the vessels in the submucosal layer are undersewn with ligatures of 000 silk (F) preparatory to excision of the polyp by scissor dissection (G).

* Manufactured by Edward Weck & Co., Long Island City, N.Y.

Plate 158

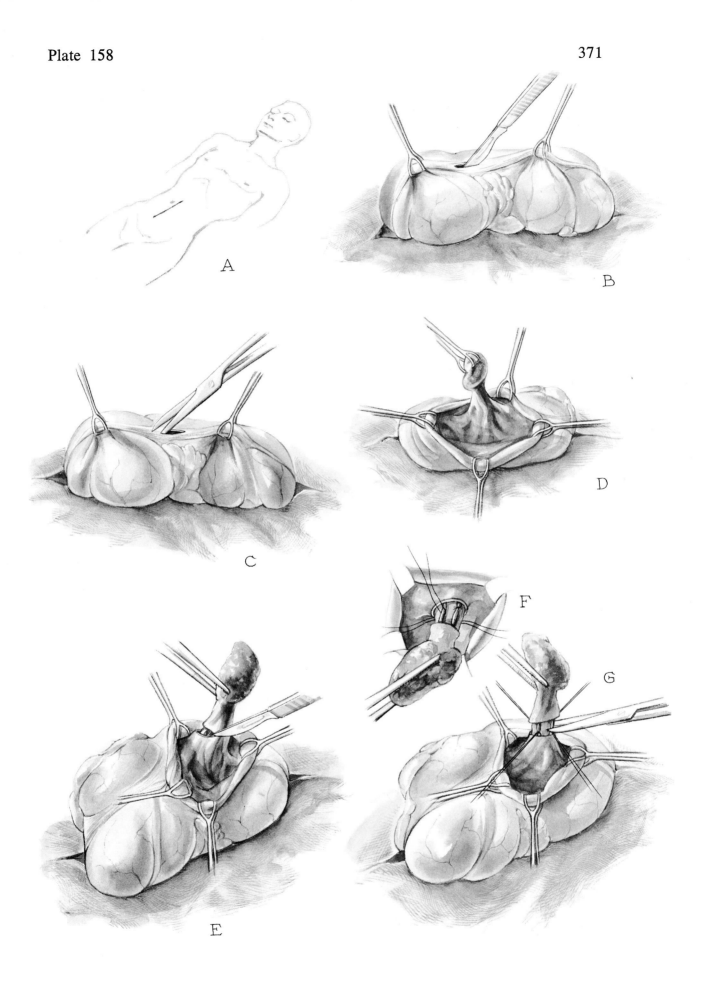

A

B

C

D

E

F

G

H, I. After excision of the polyp, the opening in the mucosa is closed, using interrupted sutures of 000 silk.

J. Prior to closure of the colotomy, a coloscopy, both proximally and distally, is performed to determine the presence or absence of additional polyps. This has proved a simple and most satisfying method of examination.

K, K$_1$. The opening in the colon is closed with a single layer of interrupted sutures (000 silk). In the insertion of these sutures a large "bite" is taken in the serosa and a small "bite" in the mucosa (K). This is more clearly shown in a close-up view (K$_1$).

L. The sutures are all first inserted, tied individually, and then cut to complete the operation.

DISCUSSION—DR. ROBERT TURELL. I would prefer preparation of the bowel with fewer laxatives and enemas but with a poorly or nonabsorbable antibiotic agent in order to avoid, among other factors, possible depletion of electrolytes, notably potassium.

The described technic is commendable and is especially useful for short-pedicled adenomas. For long pedicles, however, it is safer, and certainly, simpler, merely to clamp or crush the stalk at the base to form a groove in which a silk ligature is tied. For additional safety, a suture may be placed distal to the ligature. This maneuver prevents the inadvertent formation of a submucous hematoma and its consequences. It is because of this possibility that one may argue against the circumcision of the mucosal base (E) and the subsequent suture of the mucosa (H). This opinion is based on experience with a similar operative procedure.

Coloscopy, despite all its pitfalls, is an accepted procedure. However, I would prefer to perform endoscopy before removing the adenoma. To accelerate the value of this diagnostic procedure insufflation, as suggested by Shackelford, may be added. When the adenoma is of the sessile type and located beyond the reach of the sigmoidoscope, resection of the adenoma-bearing segment of the colon is invariably employed.

Plate 159   373

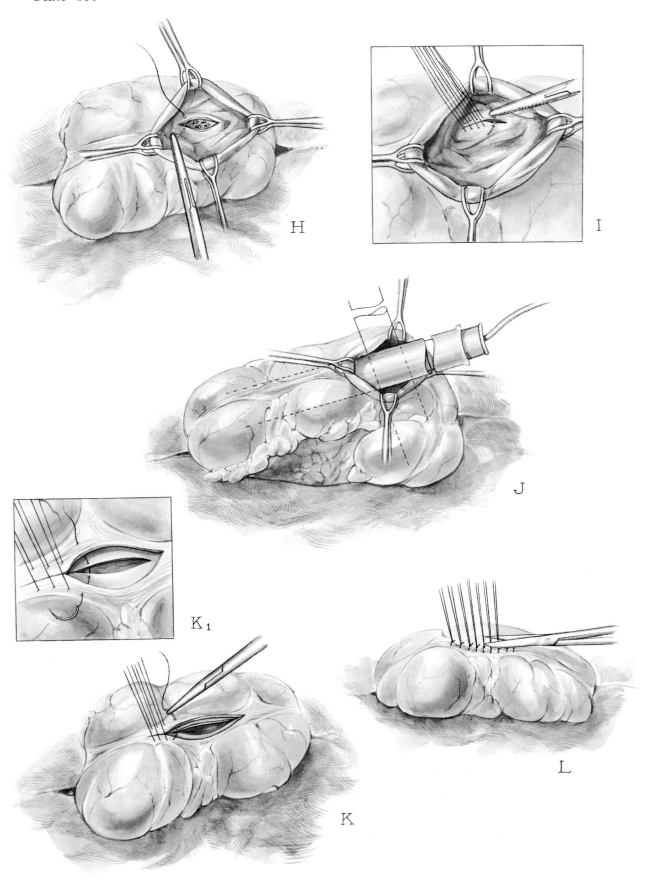

H

I

J

K₁

K

L

DISCUSSION—DR. PHILIP COOPER. There is basis for valid differences of opinion regarding the type and extent of preparation of the large bowel that is to be incised or resected. It is probably true that preparation of the bowel by dietary restriction, cathartics, and enemas alone will be satisfactory if the preparation is adequately supervised and carefully accomplished and the surgery is performed in an expeditious and skillful manner.

In the usual hospital practice, particularly in those hospitals where the surgeons do colonic operations infrequently, it seems reasonable and is probably safer to add chemotherapeutic agents to the measures noted above for the preoperative preparation of the bowel. Sulfathaladine and succinylsulfathiazole are both acceptable, and neomycin or kanamycin and possibly other antibiotics can be used with good results. This discussion is limited to comments on resection of a polyp or polyps through a colotomy in a bowel that has minimal or no obstruction. I will therefore omit from the discussion a review of the problems involved in the preparation of the bowel that is significantly obstructed.

My preoperative plan is to place the patient on a low residue diet two to three days before surgery, changing to a clear liquid diet the day before the operation. Instead of giving magnesium sulphate as recommended by Dr. Madden and others, I prefer citrate of magnesia, an effective cathartic, not unpleasant to take. Six fluid ounces is given during each of the two mornings prior to the day of operation. Cleansing saline or tap water enemas are given until returns are clear, during the two evenings before surgery. Neomycin, 1 g. every hour for four doses followed by 1 g. every four hours, is given within the 20-24 hour period before operation. Sulfathaladine (1.5 g.) is given with each dose of neomycin.

In the morning of the day of operation, a Levin tube is inserted and the stomach is lavaged and emptied of its contents. I have not felt it necessary to insert a long intestinal tube preoperatively with a nonobstructing lesion but may use it for the lesion that has produced partial obstruction.

It should be emphasized that an excellent air contrast-barium enema should be obtained, preoperatively, in all patients with polyps of the colon, so that one can more accurately identify all the polyps present and to determine, if possible, whether any have a demonstrable stalk. In general, polyps should be demonstrated on two successive air contrast-barium enemas to establish the diagnosis. The presence of a stalk with a "smooth" polyp that measures less than 1 to 1.5 cm. in diameter is fairly good evidence that the polyp is probably benign, and one may proceed with the colotomy.

The abdominal incision used should be the one most suited for exposure of the involved bowel and one that can be readily extended if necessary.

A paramedian incision, on the appropriate side, provides an approach to any part of the colon or rectum. However, if one is convinced that there is a single polyp, an oblique or transverse incision may be adequate.

The legends show the steps recommended by Dr. Madden for the excision of a polyp in the sigmoid colon. This technic could also be employed for polyps in other parts of the colon that can be mobilized and delivered onto the abdominal wall. If the segment of colon does not have a free mesentery and the bowel is not mobilized, the colotomy must of necessity be done with the bowel in situ; otherwise, if one chooses, he may mobilize the bowel by standard technics. It may be advisable to free the greater omentum, by sharp dissection, if the transverse colon is involved.

The bowel to be incised should be properly sequestrated from the abdominal wall and nearby intra-abdominal structures by adequate draping. The bowel is always incised through a taenia.

When the bowel has been opened, the polyp located, and the decision made to do a polypectomy, I would avoid grasping the body of the polyp with any instrument. Even though special grasping instruments have been made for this purpose, I would rather hold the polyp either by a piece of gauze or by applying a forceps or clamp to normal appearing mucosa on the stalk of a pedunculated polyp, or near the body of a sessile polyp. This precaution is taken to avoid, as much as possible, fragmentation of the polyp, and to decrease the likelihood of tumor cells being implanted on the surgically created raw surfaces.

If the stalk is narrow and long, a suture ligature of catgut placed through and around the base of the stalk, with sectioning of the stalk distal to the suture, may be adequate. In general, however, it is preferable to excise most lesions, as shown in the illustrations. The mucosal incision should be an adequate distance from the body of the polyp (at least 2-3 mm.). Care is taken not to section the bowel wall too deeply when the base of the polyp is severed, in order to avoid penetrating the serosa, particularly when the polyp is on the mesenteric side of the bowel. The mucosal defect at the site of the polyp is closed with interrupted 000 atraumatic catgut or 0000 silk.

I prefer a two-layer closure of the colotomy, the inner layer being of interrupted 000 atraumatic catgut or 0000 silk. The knots of the inner layer are preferably tied so that they fall within the lumen of the bowel. If the sutures are placed fairly close to each other, it is not necessary to invert much of the bowel wall. The first row of sutures is placed through the entire thickness of the bowel wall, the second row only through the seromuscular layer. I feel that a two-layer closure offers more assurance against leakage at the closure site, since the wall of the colon is relatively thin.

Even though a careful preoperative preparation

DR. PHILIP COOPER (cont.)

of bowel was accomplished, it is advisable that a "clean" and "dirty" technic, established so well by the older generation of surgeons, be carefully followed. These involve additional draping when a viscus is open, the cleansing of soiled viscera, and the aspiration of all contaminated material from the peritoneal cavity prior to closure of the wound. Instruments used on open viscera should be placed on a "dirty" or contaminated field, which is represented by a towel placed over the patient's thighs. The nurse should not handle contaminated instruments with her gloved hands, but should pass them to the operator by holding them with forceps. The nurse places each needle into a needle holder held by the operator. Needles should be retained with the "dirty" field. When the operator returns to a "clean" dissection within the abdominal cavity, the instruments on the "dirty" field should be removed, or temporarily covered, if a "dirty" field is to be re-established for a later incision or anastomosis of a viscus. Gloves are changed by those who worked within the "dirty" field. Contaminated towels or pads used for draping purposes are removed prior to the change of gloves, and clean towels or pads are applied after the gloves are changed. "Dirty" instruments should be removed from the field prior to the closure of the abdominal wound.

Coloscopy has value, but one must recognize its limitations and its hazards. Since the large bowel wall cannot be readily distended without increasing the likelihood of contaminating neighboring structures by intestinal contents when the insufflated air is allowed to escape, I prefer to avoid air insufflation. Some authors have suggested a probable increase in morbidity and mortality if coloscopy is done. It is difficult to understand why this should be so, unless the bowel was not well prepared preoperatively, and/or multiple colotomies were done. Poor draping around the bowel may contribute to the problem. Careful preoperative air contrast-barium enemas, operative inspection and palpation, and on occasion transillumination of the bowel will demonstrate most polyps. Inspection of the interior of the bowel by gentle retraction using ribbon or narrow Deaver retractors may also be of value. The newer scopes with fiber optics may improve the efficiency of coloscopy.

Some comments should be made about the problems involved in determining whether simple excision of the polyp is the procedure of choice for the patient.

In general, no serious concern arises in regard to the excision of a smooth polyp with a well-developed stalk by the transcolonic approach, as long as there is no ulceration of the body of the lesion and no induration or thickening of the tissue at the base of the stalk. Even when "cell atypia" or "carcinoma in situ" is found in the body

of a pedunculated polyp, excision with an adequate border of normal mucosa at the base of the stalk will almost invariably result in cure. If ulceration of the body of the polyp or induration at the base of the stalk is found, one would have to accept the possible presence of invasive carcinoma, and a bowel resection should be done. Careful judgment must be used in determining the extent of the resection, for if the presence of an invasive carcinoma is a remote possibility, it is probably best to do a segmental resection of the bowel and its adjacent mesentery. If this is done and the histologic sections establish a diagnosis of invasive carcinoma, a standard radical bowel resection can be accomplished within a week or ten days. If such a diagnosis is not established, the patient has been spared the increased morbidity associated with radical surgery. The impression one gains from the examination of the lesion in situ must be the determining factor in the choice of the immediate appropriate surgical procedure.

If a sessile polyp is found the problem may be more difficult. If the lesion is smooth and limited in size (less than 1-1.5 cm.), it may be excised with an adequate border of normal mucosa (at least 2 mm.). If the sessile polyp has a granular or papillary appearance and is less than 1-1.5 cm. in diameter, a total biopsy may be considered, but it would probably be wise to proceed with an excision of a segment of bowel. Sessile polyps larger than 1-1.5 cm. in diameter should always be removed with a segment of bowel. If there is the slightest possibility of neoplastic involvement of the submucosa, a bowel resection should be done.

Frozen-section studies of biopsied polyps may be misleading and could result in too limited or too extensive surgery. Total excision of the polyp rather than limited biopsy and frozen section is therefore preferred.

Villous adenomas, in general, can be recognized grossly. Although usually present in the rectum, they rarely occur elsewhere in the colon. Management of such adenomas in the rectum is not included in the subject matter of this chapter. Lesions above the peritoneal reflection should be removed with a segment of bowel. Invasion of the submucosa or histologic evidence of cellular change consistent with malignancy would demand a radical resection of the bowel as a primary procedure, or as a secondary procedure if a limited bowel resection had already been accomplished.

If more than five or six scattered polyps are present in the colon above the peritoneal reflection, consideration should be given to the advisability of doing a subtotal colectomy. This is a controversial issue. The presence of an arbitrary number of polyps cannot be used as a definite indication for such surgery. We as yet do not have enough information to make a specific recommendation on this point.

TRANSVERSE COLON COLOSTOMY

A. The transverse incision in the right upper quadrant of the abdomen is outlined and crosshatched to facilitate later closure.

B, C. The wound margins are retracted, and the underlying anterior rectus sheath and the rectus muscle are incised transversely to expose the transversus abdominis muscle and the transversalis fascia.

D. The transversalis fascia is incised, and a portion of the anterior parietal peritoneum is tented preparatory to its incision.

E. The opening in the peritoneum is extended both medially and laterally by scissor dissection to expose the underlying intraperitoneal viscera.

F, G. The greater omentum is mobilized by scissor dissection from its relatively avascular attachment to the transverse colon (F).

The dotted line (F) depicts the site of the opening to be made in the greater omentum through which the transverse colon is withdrawn (G).

It should be emphasized that, in those instances in which the obstructed colon is tensely dilated, a preliminary suction decompression with a 19 gauge needle should be done before attempting to mobilize the transverse colon. Otherwise, there is the danger of perforating the thin and distended bowel wall. Following the decompression, a pursestring suture is inserted in the wall of the decompressed and thickened bowel about the needle and the suture is tied as the needle is withdrawn. The pursestring suture should not be inserted prior to the needle decompression because of the increased likelihood of gross contamination of the wound through the sites of the needle punctures.

DISCUSSION—DR. J. ENGLEBERT DUNPHY. The transverse incision shown in Plate 160, A, is an excellent choice, particularly as the supporting glass rod under the colostomy lies at a right angle to the incision. There are disadvantages, however, and, before selecting the transverse incision, it is well to be sure of the position of the colon. This can frequently be accurately ascertained by a review of plain films taken prior to operation.

Once the peritoneal cavity is opened, it is always a difficult decision as to whether or not any exploration should be done through the transverse colostomy incision. In semielective cases where the condition of the patient is good and the degree of intestinal obstruction not extreme, it is desirable to explore the abdomen, particularly the liver and gallbladder regions, since it will not be as easy to explore this area through a lower abdominal incision once the colostomy has been made.

It is not always necessary to free the omentum from the colon as shown in Plate 160, F. Frequently, and particularly in thin patients, the colon may be brought through the omentum in an avascular area, thus avoiding the delivery of most of the omentum into the wound. This is a particularly advantageous step if the patient is quite ill and the procedure is done under local anesthesia.

It is very important, as emphasized, not to at-

Plate 160   377

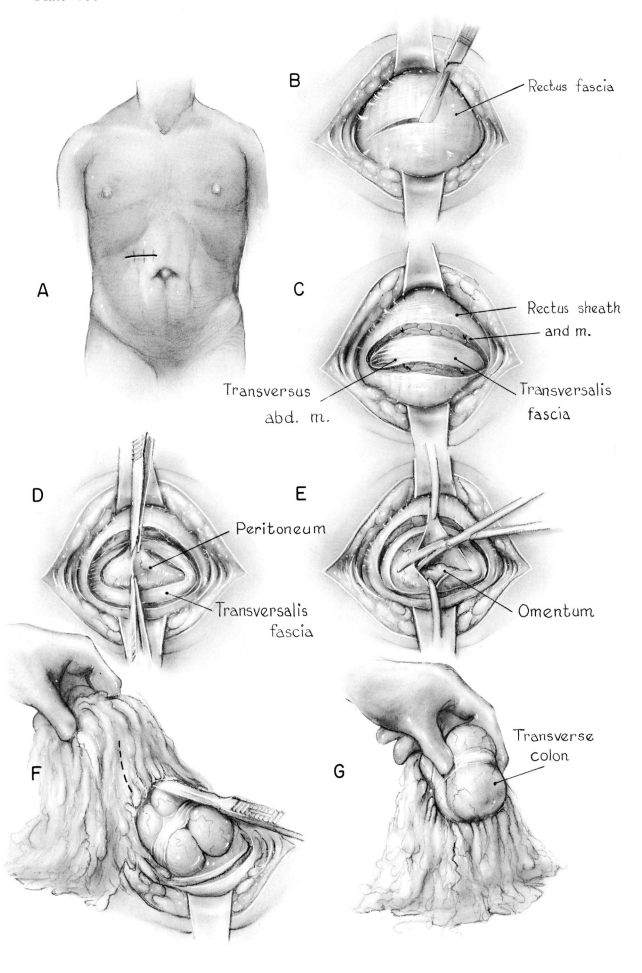

B — Rectus fascia

C — Rectus sheath and m.

Transversus abd. m.

Transversalis fascia

A

D — Peritoneum

Transversalis fascia

E — Omentum

F

G — Transverse colon

H, I. An opening is made through an avascular portion of the mesentery of the transverse mesocolon immediately subjacent to the bowel wall (H), and through this opening a solid glass rod is withdrawn (I).

J. A rubber tube is attached to either end of the solid glass rod, and the transversalis fascia and peritoneum are sutured together as a single layer using interrupted sutures of 000 silk.

K. The closure of the transversalis fascia and peritoneal layer on either side of the exteriorized loop of proximal transverse colon is completed, and the suturing of the anterior rectus sheath and rectus muscle is begun (000 silk).

L, M. The fascia (L) and skin (M) closures are completed, and, with the use of an actual cautery, an opening is made in the midportion of the anterior wall of the exteriorized loop of transverse colon (M).

N. The ends of anatomic tissue forceps (without teeth) are inserted into the lumen of the bowel to elevate the anterior wall of the colon as the incision at a right angle to its longitudinal axis is completed. The use of the forceps as demonstrated lessens the incidence of burn trauma to the mucous membrane of the posterior wall of the colon and the resulting herniation of edematous tissue through the colostomy stoma.

DISCUSSION—DR. DUNPHY (cont.)

tempt to deliver a tensely dilated obstructed colon. This brings up the question as to when cecostomy should be done rather than colostomy, and, in general, where one wishes complete diversion of the fecal stream as in inflammatory lesions of the lower colon, a colostomy is by far the better choice. On the other hand, in extremely ill, markedly distended, obese, or otherwise poor risk patients, a cecostomy is an easier operation for the patient to stand and can be performed with considerably less risk. Local anesthesia is far more suitable for a cecostomy than for a transverse colostomy.

The simple loop transverse colostomy over a glass rod, as shown in the illustrations, is an extremely valuable procedure for defunctioning the distal colon. More elaborate methods of defunctioning the bowel such as those described by Devine or Wangensteen have little to offer over this procedure, provided it is well done. The incision in the bowel, if one wishes complete diversion of the stream, should be in the transverse direction as shown in Plate 161, M, and should be sufficiently long to allow eversion of the loop and a true double-barreled colostomy. This operation has all the advantages of the more complicated procedures and yet lends itself very well, as shown later, to closure.

Plate 161

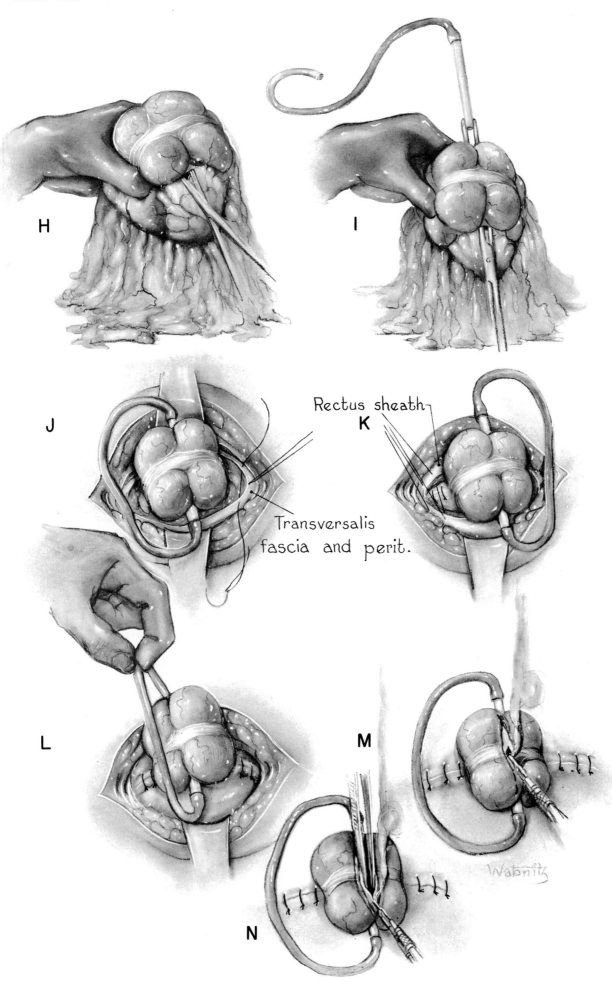

Rectus sheath

Transversalis fascia and perit.

Wabnitz

CLOSURE OF TRANSVERSE COLON COLOSTOMY

A. The longitudinal elliptical incision about the transverse colon colostomy is indicated by the dotted line. The healed lower abdominal left paramedian incision may also be seen.

B. Close-up view showing the stomas of the afferent and efferent loops of transverse colon and the elliptical incision which has been deepened into the subcutaneous tissue plane.

C, D, E. Kocher clamps for traction are applied to the skin margins immediately adjacent to the respective bowel stomas, and by scalpel dissection the afferent and efferent limbs of the transverse colon are mobilized into the wound. In this dissection the peritoneal, muscle, and fascial layers are clearly delineated.

F. The mobilization of the colonic segment is continued until the free peritoneal cavity is entered. A loop of small intestine, adherent to both the afferent and the efferent limbs of the transverse colon, is also visible.

G. By digital exploration the completeness of the mobilization of the colon intraperitoneally is determined. An intraperitoneal rather than an extraperitoneal closure of the colostomy is preferred. Furthermore, with this type of closure the incidence of postoperative incisional hernia is believed lessened.

H, I, J. The everted mucosal cuff is mobilized by scalpel dissection (H), and upon its completion the rim of skin and attached mucosa is excised (I, J).

K. The omental collar, an adherent remnant of a portion of the omentum through which the transverse colon was withdrawn in establishing the colostomy, is removed by scalpel dissection.

DISCUSSION—DR. J. ENGLEBERT DUNPHY. The time at which a transverse colostomy should be closed is always settled by a combination of factors in particular instances. However, the longer a colostomy has been present, the more it tends to contract and the easier it is to close. This is particularly true if the purpose for which the colostomy was made was of short duration and the glass rod removed early, since there is a tendency then for this type of transverse colostomy to gradually withdraw and contract into the abdominal wall. In the obese, poor risk patient this may proceed to the point where closure becomes quite simple and can be done under local anesthesia as an extraperitoneal procedure.

Intraperitoneal closure is preferable, however, particularly in younger people and those who are obliged to work, since some degree of hernia of the abdominal wall is always present in an extraperitoneal closure.

The important features of closure are well illustrated in the text. The bowel wall should be identified, and here there is always a well defined dissection plane which separates the bowel and omentum from the tissues of the abdominal wall. Once this plane is recognized, it is comparatively easy to separate the bowel successively from the fascia, muscle, and peritoneum.

Effective closure of the opening into the bowel depends on very careful freeing of the cuff of skin, subcutaneous tissue, and omentum which adhere to the serosa of the bowel. This cuff should not be dissected until the bowel is mobilized and ready for closure since the bowel becomes quite thin-walled and fragile after dissecting these tissues away from it. Sometimes, after careful freeing of the cuffs of tissue about the bowel, there is not enough bowel wall to permit the closure as shown in Plate 163, L and M. If, as the lateral cuffs of bowel are brought together, there is tension, it may be necessary to resect the area and perform an end-to-end anastomosis. One should never hesitate to do this when the closure appears insecure and an intraperitoneal closure is contemplated.

Extraperitoneal closure of a transverse colostomy is performed in much the same fashion as illustrated, except that the procedure is halted at E (Plate 162) and the bowel lumen closed. The loosely attached peritoneum often permits the bowel to be placed below the fascia and closure to be accomplished above it. This procedure has certain advantages in the very elderly and poor risk patients who may have been subjected to several difficult stage operations previously.

Fortunately, today it is rarely necessary to carry out transverse colostomy because patients are seen earlier and improved technics permit primary resection and anastomosis. On the other hand, the old adage that if there is any significant degree of obstruction, a colostomy is the wiser choice before resection is still a sound one. Despite certain opinions to the contrary, this would seem to be particularly the case in the presence of inflammatory lesions of the distal colon.

Plate 162   381

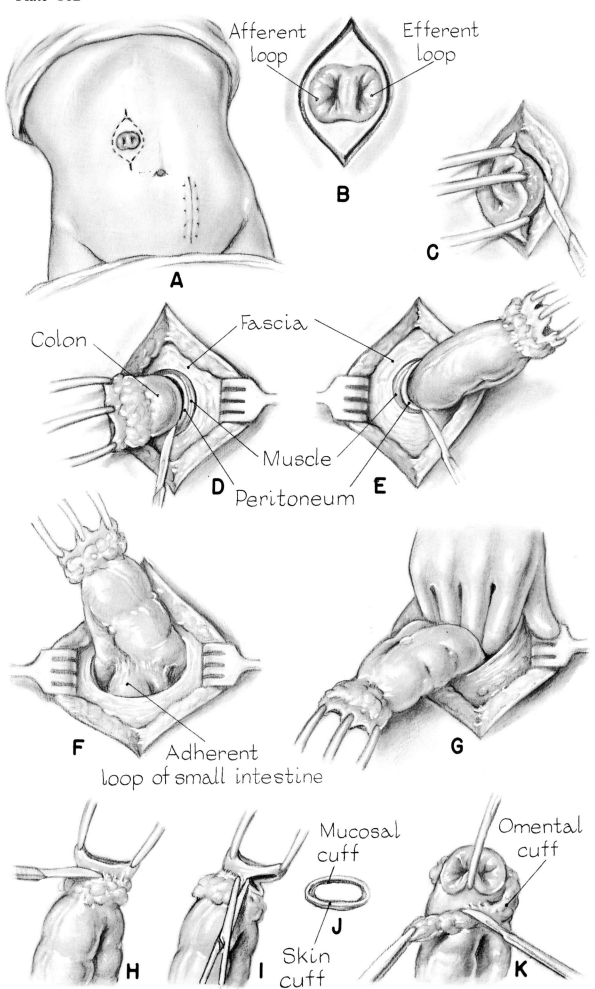

B
Afferent loop
Efferent loop

C

Colon
Fascia
Muscle
Peritoneum
D
E

F
Adherent loop of small intestine

G

H

I
Mucosal cuff
Skin cuff
J

K
Omental cuff

L. The insertion of the first anterior layer of the closure is begun. The suture (00 chromic catgut) is inserted from the "inside out" on the afferent stoma and from the "outside in" on the efferent stoma so that, when tied, the knot is on the inside of the lumen.

M. A similar suture is started from the opposite angle of the anastomosis and, when tied, it proceeds from the "inside out" on the afferent stoma. It then crosses over to the opposite side and passes from the "outside in" and from the "inside out" on the efferent stoma to place the loop of the suture on the mucosa. This inversion or Connell type of suture is continued from either angle of the anastomosis toward the center as indicated by the arrows.

N, O. Each suture, having reached the center of the anastomosis (N), is then inserted from the "inside out" in the apposing bowel lumen (O) and then tied together.

P. The second layer of the closure consists of a series of interrupted seromuscular mattress sutures (Halsted) of 000 silk. If preferred, either simple interrupted sutures or a continuous seromuscular suture (Lembert) may be used.

Q, R, S. The ends of the Halsted mattress sutures are separated, and two pieces of attached omentum are held in forceps (Q) preparatory to being placed over the line of the anastomosis (R) to which they are anchored when the long ends of the mattress sutures are tied (S).

T, U. The peritoneal, fascial, and muscle layers on each side of the incision are approximated together as one layer using the Jones type of closure. Each suture (0 silk) is inserted through the fascia, muscle, and peritoneum on one side, and through the peritoneum, muscle, and fascia on the other. The suture is then crossed over to the opposite side and is inserted through the fascial layers first on one side and then on the other (T). The complete closure is depicted in U.

V. The skin incision is closed using interrupted sutures of 000 silk. Prior to closure, the wound is irrigated with copious quantities of warm saline solution. Drainage of the wound is not employed.

Plate 163

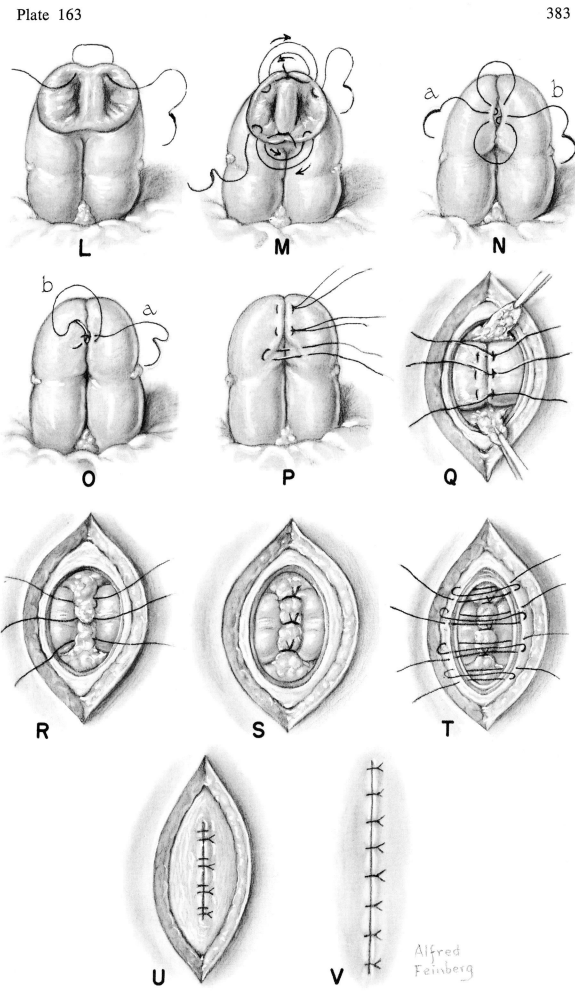

TECHNICS FOR END-TO-END ANASTOMOSIS OF THE COLON

A. Each bowel segment is stabilized by traction on the untied guy sutures at each angle of the anastomosis to facilitate the insertion of the mesenteric coapting mattress suture of Lee.

B. The guy sutures have been removed, and the insertion of the last of the horizontal mattress sutures that form the first posterior layer of the anastomosis is completed.

C. The mattress sutures are tied to approximate the bowel segments posteriorly, and the everted cut margins are being approximated with interrupted sutures of 000 silk, which form the second posterior layer of the anastomosis.

D, E. The first anterior layer is begun by the insertion of one of the angle sutures. The suture proceeds from the inside-out on the proximal segment and from the outside-in on the distal segment, so that, when tied, the knot of the suture is on the inside of the lumen (D). The sutures are inserted alternately from either angle and terminate in the center anteriorly, where the final two inversion sutures are encircled by a figure of 8 suture of 000 silk (E). This suture is tied after the previously inserted suture strands are cut, to complete the first anterior layer of the anastomosis.

Plate 164

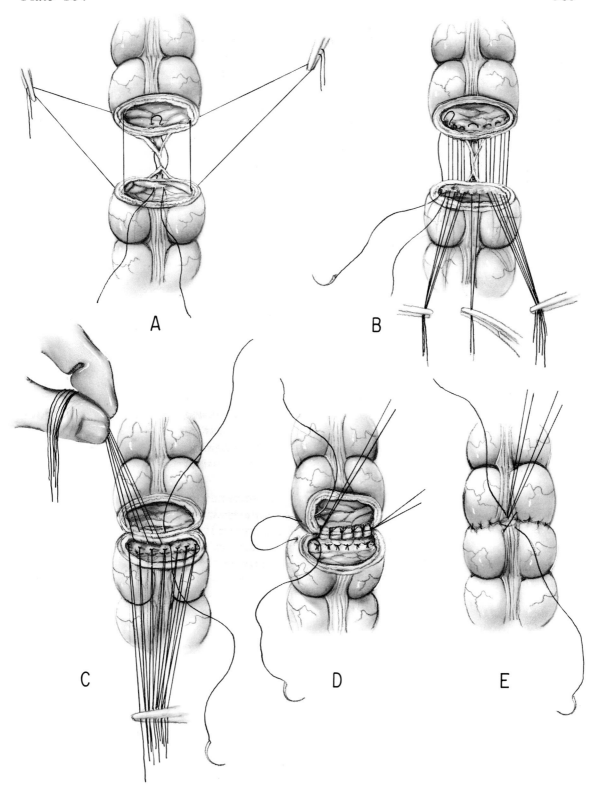

F. The second anterior layer is comprised of a series of interrupted Halsted mattress sutures, the last one having been inserted but not tied.

G, H, I, J. An alternate technic for the anastomosis is the use of a continuous interlocking suture of 00 chromic catgut for the second layer posteriorly. The suture is inserted at the angle and proceeds from the inside-out on one side and from the outside-in on the other (G). When tied, it is then continued as an interlocking suture to the opposite angle (H). At this angle it emerges from the inside-out in the lower segment and is then inserted from the outside-in to the inside-out (Connell or "loop on the mucosa" suture) in the upper segment (I) and continued as such to form the first anterior suture layer (J).

Plate 165   387

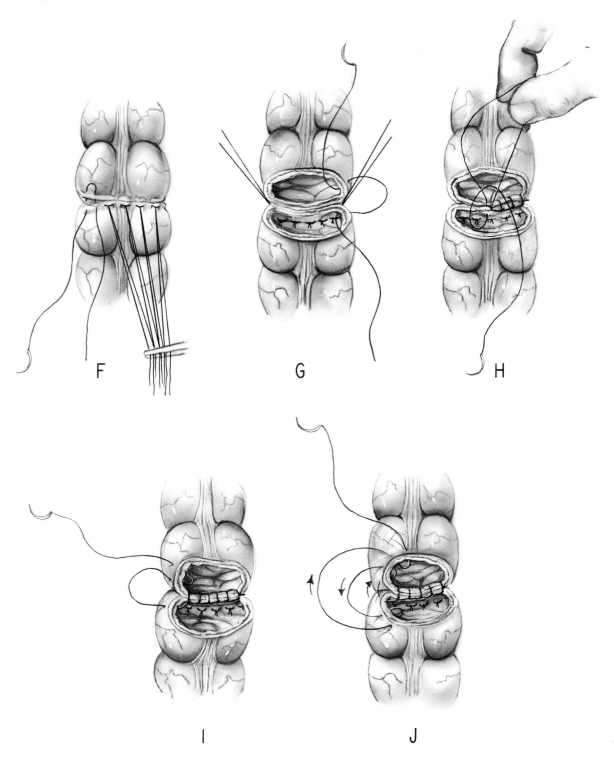

F

G

H

I

J

K, L, M. When one-half of the first anterior suture layer is completed, a second suture is inserted at the opposite angle (K) and continued toward the center as a Connell suture (L, M).

N. In the center of the anastomosis each Connell suture is terminated by being inserted from the inside-out in the lumen of the opposing segment. Each suture is inserted just beyond the exit of the opposite suture to effect a secure closure in the center of the anastomosis.

O, P. A series of interrupted Halsted mattress sutures is used for the second anterior layer. The sutures are all first inserted, the center one being the last (O), and then tied, and the sutures are cut (P) to complete the colocolostomy.

Plate 166   389

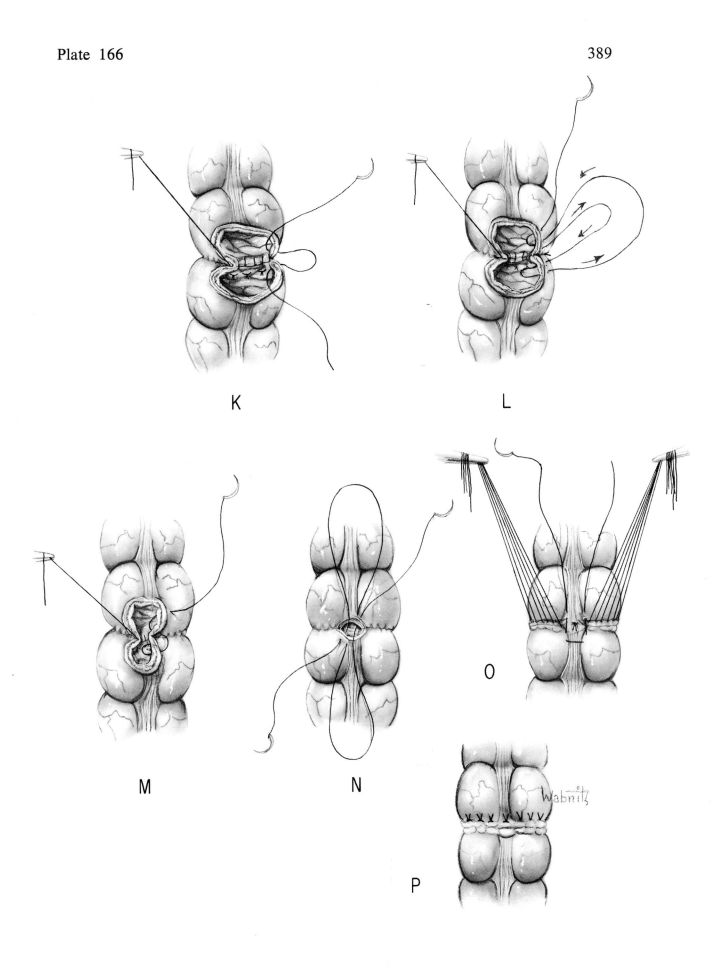

K

L

M

N

O

P

RADICAL RIGHT HEMICOLECTOMY

A. A midabdominal right paramedian muscle-retracting (lateral) incision is outlined.

B. The anterior rectus sheath is incised, the rectus muscle is retracted laterally, and the line of incision in the anterior parietal peritoneum is demonstrated.

C. The opening into the peritoneal cavity is completed, and the underlying viscera are depicted.

D. The omentum and small intestines are displaced mesially, and the mobilization of the right side of the colon is commenced by scissor dissection along the fascia fusion layer of Toldt ("white line").

E. The mobilization of the right side of the colon is continued by digital dissection in the retroperitoneal tissue plane. For purpose of clarity, the tumor mass is not covered. Routinely it is encased in a thick, moist gauze pad.

F. The hepatic flexure and the right half of the transverse colon are mobilized by clamping and dividing the right phrenocolic ligament (dotted outline) and the anterior and posterior gastric branches of the gastroepiploic arch respectively. The skeletonization of the distal half of the greater curvature of the stomach is done to include the adjacent gastrocolic ligament and greater omentum in the resected specimen. This insures the adequate removal of the lymphatic drain.

DISCUSSION—DR. HOWARD A. PATTERSON. It is in the right side of the colon that one finds many of the "bulky" neoplasms, which experience has shown to have a far better prognosis than some of the smaller types. A radical attack is often rewarded by cure, even when the abdominal wall or adjacent viscera are invaded.

Dr. Madden has outlined, compactly but thoroughly, the steps in the rather well standardized modern "right hemicolectomy," and he leaves little for the discusser to contribute by way of alteration or addition. It might be well to remind the surgeon that thorough exploration (by palpation) of the entire abdomen should *precede* local inspection of the colonic lesion, lest he become so fascinated with the excision as to forget the exploration entirely. Then, too, an abscess may be encountered alongside the lesion when least expected, which may make it unwise to proceed with exploration of the rest of the abdominal cavity.

Exposure should be adequate and reasonably quick. I prefer an incision slightly more lateral than that shown in Plate 167, A, with division of the rectus in the same line rather than retraction of the muscle outward. Retraction is tedious and limits exposure to some degree. An oblique right lower abdominal incision is an excellent alternate choice, as it affords enough exposure and is the "strongest" subsequently.

If a cecal cancer is encountered unexpectedly during surgery for appendicitis (through a Mc-Burney incision), access for a right hemicolectomy

Plate 167

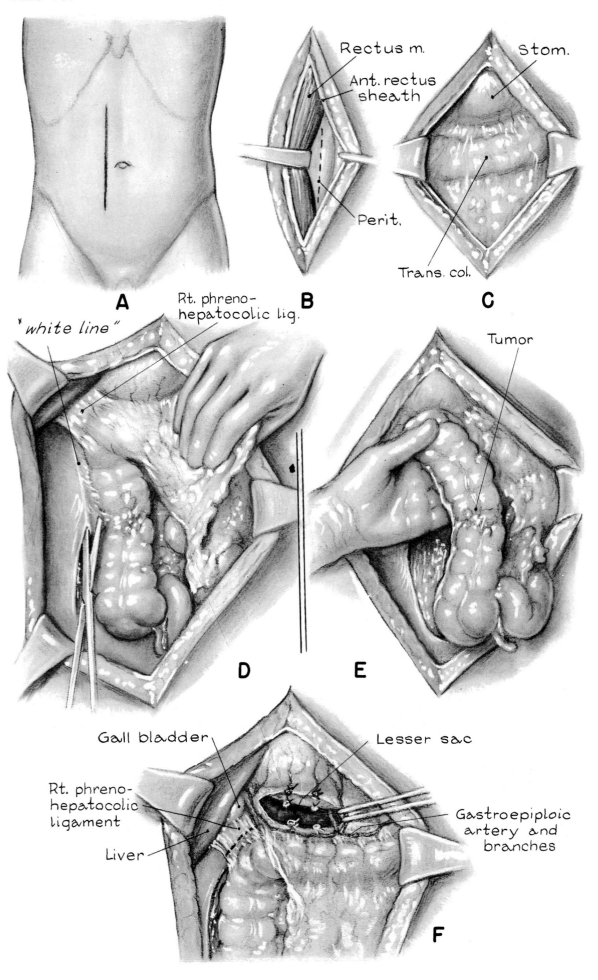

A

B

Rectus m.

Ant. rectus sheath

Perit.

C

Stom.

Trans. col.

"*white line*"

Rt. phreno-hepatocolic lig.

D

Tumor

E

Gall bladder

Lesser sac

Rt. phreno-hepatocolic ligament

Liver

Gastroepiploic artery and branches

F

G. The mobilization of the right side of the colon and the proximal half of the transverse colon is completed, and the stomach is retracted upward to expose the lesser sac and its related structures.

H. The right side of the colon is retracted toward the midline, and the retroperitoneal structures which are to be identified and protected from injury during the mobilization of the colon are depicted. These struc-tures are: (1) the internal spermatic or ovarian vessels, (2) the right ureter, (3) the inferior vena cava, and (4) the retrocolic portion of the duodenum.

I. The sites of election for transection of the ileum and transverse colon are encircled by traction tapes of rubber tissue inserted through openings in avascular segments of the mesentery in juxtaposition to the bowel wall.

DISCUSSION—DR. PATTERSON (cont.)

can be gained by extending the small incision medially and dividing the rectus sheath. The hepatic flexure is very rarely at as high a level as indicated in Plate 167, D, E, and F, and, on several occasions, I have easily removed the right colon through such an incision.

The division of the lateral peritoneum, as in D, might well be at a site further removed from the growth. If the neoplasm is adherent to the lateral wall, a row of Kocher clamps on the peritoneum and posterior sheath, rather than retractors, may be used. The surgeon may also wish to move to the left side of the table for a short while, to get a more direct look.

Warren Cole's work on the danger of implanting tumor cells in the needleholes of an anastomosis, and also on the possibility of squeezing tumor-cell emboli into the veins during operative handling of the tumor mass, surely deserves further attention and study. Ligation of the bowel (with tape) near either end of the area to be excised, *before* mobilization of the specimen, should make it less likely for the colonic wall at the site of the anastomosis to become coated with desquamated tumor cells that may be implanted by a needle. Similarly, prompt ligation of the right colic vein might theoretically prevent a tumor embolus to the liver. We may eventually know whether these refinements are really worthwhile.

The peritoneum and the thin fascia beneath it form a remarkably good barrier against direct extension, and the retroperitoneal duodenum is very rarely invaded by carcinomas of the right colon, even though they may lie side by side. When this invasion does happen, simple local excision of the obviously involved area of the duodenal wall gives extremely poor results. Hence, a more radical resection of the duodenum should be considered if a cure seems at all possible in any particular case.

Plate 168   393

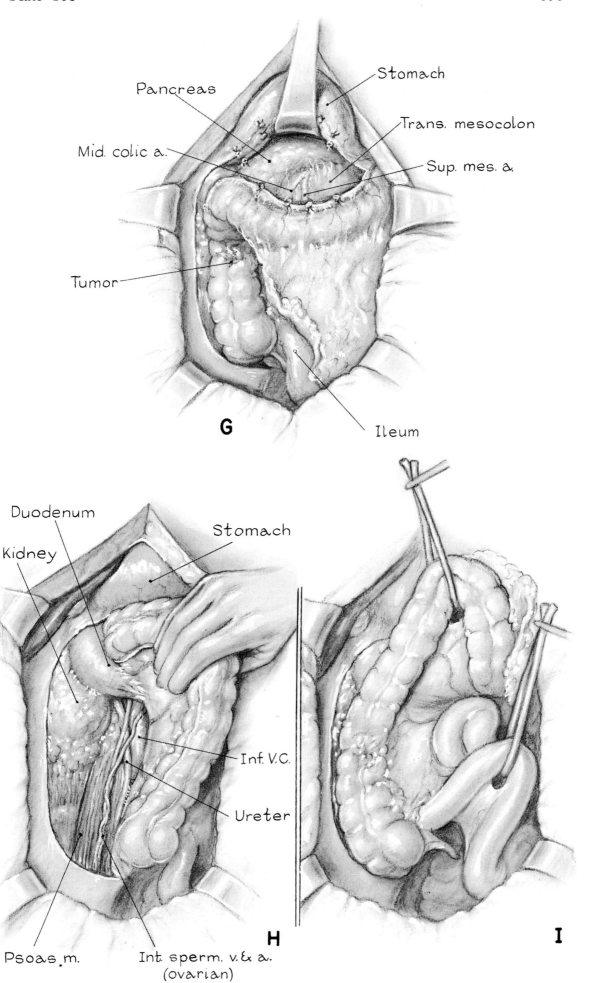

Pancreas

Stomach

Mid. colic a.

Trans. mesocolon

Sup. mes. a.

Tumor

G

Ileum

Duodenum

Stomach

Kidney

Inf. V.C.

Ureter

Psoas m.

Int. sperm. v. & a.
(ovarian)

H

I

J. Incisions, as guide tracts for division of the mesentery, are made through the serosal coverings of the transverse mesocolon and mesentery of the ileum to the respective sites of election for transection of the bowel. The apex of the incisions is at the level of origin of the right colic and/or ileocolic artery.

J'. Inset to show the grouping of the mesenteric lymph nodes about the site of origin of the ileocolic artery from the superior mesenteric artery. Accordingly, in resection of the right side of the colon for carcinoma, the necessity for ligation of the right colic and/or ileocolic artery at their respective levels of origin to include the lymphatic drain is apparent.

K. The division of the mesentery is completed to the level of origin of the right colic and/or ileocolic arteries, and hemostasis is obtained with suture ligatures of silk (000). The vascular pedicle is triply clamped prior to division between the two most distal clamps.

L, M. Insets to show method of occlusion of the vascular pedicle by a proximal ligature and a distal transfixing suture ligature of silk (00).

N. The division of the mesentery of the ileum and the colon is completed, and the isolated ileocolic segment to be resected is demonstrated. For clarity the included segments of greater omentum and gastrocolic ligament are not shown.

DISCUSSION—DR. PATTERSON (cont.)

I agree heartily with Dr. Madden's radical approach to the removal of lymph nodes and the right side of the omentum. In this connection Plate 169, J and N, and Plate 171, Z, are very helpful, though the young surgeon must be warned against too great enthusiasm. It is imperative that the superior mesenteric artery be *most* carefully safeguarded, and the pursuit of enlarged lymph nodes (Plate 169, J') may lead to damage or angulation of this artery, with subsequent thrombosis. It is well known that the majority of enlarged nodes associated with cancer of the colon turn out to be inflammatory and not neoplastic, and it would be doubly tragic to lose a patient in pursuing these nodes too far. However, this warning should not be misinterpreted as condoning half-hearted attack on the mesentery of the right colon.

There is little argument with the choice of end-to-end ileocolostomy as the quickest and best method of restoring continuity at the close of the resection.

I have never liked the end-to-side method. At times, in the very old or debilitated patient, I still close both ends and do a side-to-side anastomosis, preferring to have three suture lines that could break and do *not,* to one that could and *does.* However, the end-to-end method is usually highly satisfactory and is advisable.

Peritonization of the posterior raw surface is usually difficult. I do not attempt it and have never had any reason to regret not doing so.

The matter of establishing drainage is highly controversial. Multiple soft rubber drains may be brought out through a small flank incision and placed to the raw area. I am likely to use drainage in an obese patient, especially if the operation has been long and difficult, or there has been much inflammatory reaction in and about the tumor. This is not in anticipation of a leak at the suture line (fortunately, very rare) but to get rid of some contaminated bloody fluid. However, this is probably an unnecessarily conservative approach, now that preoperative preparation of the colon is so greatly improved.

Plate 169   395

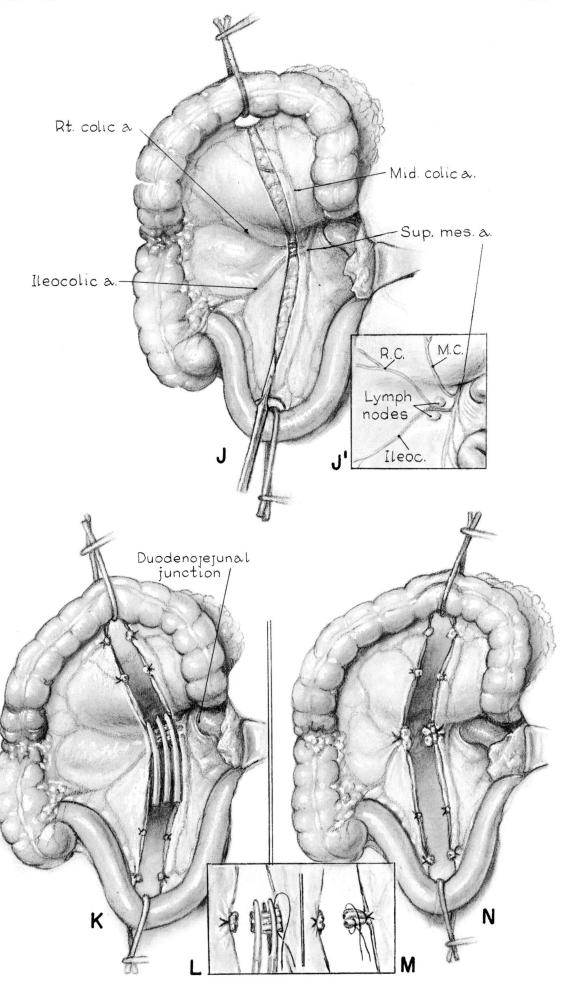

Rt. colic a.

Mid. colic a.

Sup. mes. a.

Ileocolic a.

R.C.   M.C.

Lymph
nodes

Ileoc.

J   J'

Duodenojejunal
junction

K   L   M   N

O. Noncrushing clamps (Babcock) are used to stabilize the segments of ileum and colon to be anastomosed, and crushing clamps are applied to the segments of bowel to be resected. The level of transection of the bowel is in dotted outline. The area of resection includes the terminal 8 to 10 inches of ileum and the proximal portion of the transverse colon up to the site of bifurcation of the middle colic artery into its right and left branches. Routinely the right branch, and not infrequently the whole of the middle colic artery, is included in the resection.

O′. Inset to show a close-up of the mesenteric coapting suture of Lee.

P. Guy sutures of silk are inserted through the lateral margins of the bowel wall, and the ileum is split along its antimesenteric surface to enlarge the diameter of its lumen at the site of anastomosis.

Q. The first posterior layer of the anastomosis is completed, and the first anterior layer is commenced. The central mattress suture for coaptation of the mesentery is visible. The

sutures anteriorly are inserted from the "inside out" to the "outside in" so that, when tied, the knots are on the inside of the lumen. Interrupted sutures of silk (000) are used throughout.

R. The first anterior inversion layer is completed, and the second anterior layer of seroserosal sutures (Lembert) is begun. A figure of 8 mattress suture indicates the termination of the closure in the center of the first anterior layer.

S, T. Completion of the second layer of sutures anteriorly and the rotation of the bowel on its long axis to complete the second layer posteriorly are depicted.

U, U′. The completed end-to-end ileotransverse colon colostomy and the approximation of the mesenteric borders viewed from behind and in front respectively. No attempt to reperitonize the denuded area along the right posterolateral abdominal wall is made. Closure of the opening in the mesentery, both anteriorly and posteriorly as depicted, is not required. ·

DISCUSSION—DR. EDWARD S. JUDD. The drawings are excellent and most illustrative of each step of the procedure. I agree wholeheartedly with most of the legends. The few comments I wish to make are as follows: I would prefer to cut the lateral peritoneum much more widely than is shown in D, staying well away from the tumor and stripping the posterior musculature bare. Most surgeons now ligate the bowel above and below the tumor, thinking that this might possibly reduce the incidence of recurrence at the suture line. The legend makes it clear that a pad is wrapped around the tumor and this, of course, is helpful along these same lines. The drawing (E) might have shown a great deal more omentum attached to the specimen, because the omentum is always amputated directly away from the gastric wall.

I would stress the fact that one should not be too heroic in the attack on the mesentery. The true situation is clearly shown in J, namely, that the superior mesenteric artery and vein are surprisingly close to the apex of the mesenteric incision. The inclusion of either or both of these vessels with the mesentery removed would indeed be a tragic accident. It is conceivable that, with vascular grafts available, the damage might be repaired immediately, but the caliber of these vessels is so small that the graft might be short of perfect in its result.

I prefer to divide the ileum on a slant rather than as shown in O. The slant is away from the mesenteric border. Theoretically, the blood vessels, coming as they do from the mesenteric side,

will have an easier task in supplying blood to the antimesenteric border, because the distance across the bowel is considerably shorter if the oblique method is used. Likewise, this oblique division of the bowel results in a wider stoma at this point and it is not necessary to make the additional side incision as in U, U′. I *always* close the mesenteric aperture, *not* just occasionally. I have feared small bowel obstruction and volvulus if the mesentery is left open.

In theory, the radical right hemicolectomy to include the aortocaval lymph node dissection should be a distinct advance. In practice, however, I have been struck by the eminently satisfactory long-term survival rates that can be achieved with use of the more standard right hemicolectomy, and I have not routinely added the radical lymphadenectomy. This may be pure inhibition and poor habit on my part. As the drawings clearly disclose, the chance of technical accident is considerably greater in the extended approach. Numerous vital structures are under threat, and extreme caution would be required. If the dissection always worked out as beautifully as the drawings depict, the operation would have tremendous appeal. I am concerned about this extensive dissection in the obese patient who has had numerous previous abdominal operations. I have also wondered about elderly patients and those whose surgical risk might be increased for a variety of reasons. I am not certain in my own mind just how often carcinoma of the right colon spreads into the lymph nodes lying below and behind the left renal vein.

Plate 170   397

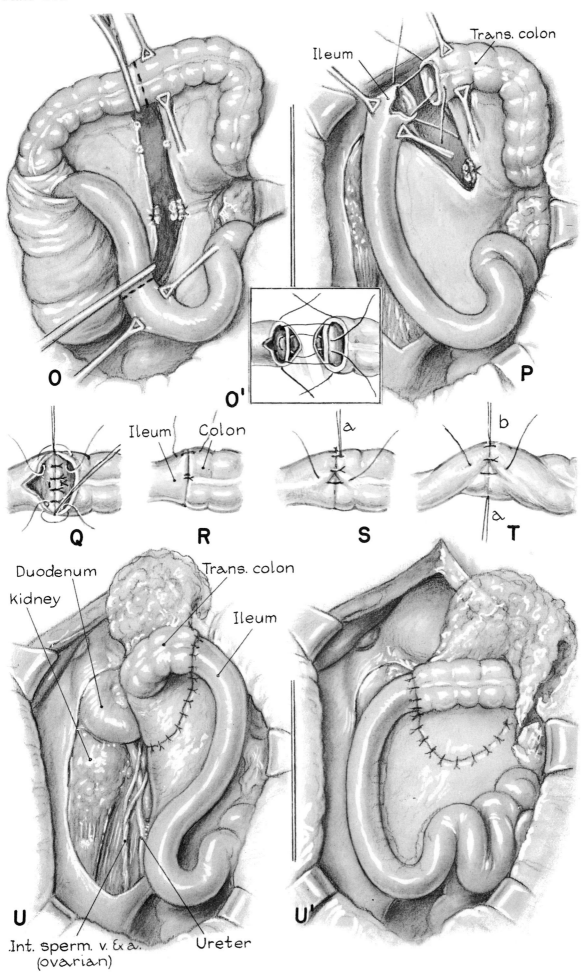

O

O'

P

Ileum

Trans. colon

Q

R

Ileum   Colon

S

a

T

b

a

U

Duodenum

kidney

Trans. colon

Ileum

Int. sperm. v. & a.
(ovarian)

Ureter

U'

V, W. The approximation of the peritoneal layer with interrupted everting mattress sutures of silk (00), alternating with simple interrupted sutures, is shown.

X, Y. The fascial layer and skin are approximated with interrupted sutures of silk (00). In the closure of the skin the needles are first inserted and individually withdrawn, then the sutures are tied.

Z. Diagrammatic representation of the extent of bowel resection in the performance of a right hemicolectomy for carcinoma involving the right side of the colon.

Plate 171   399

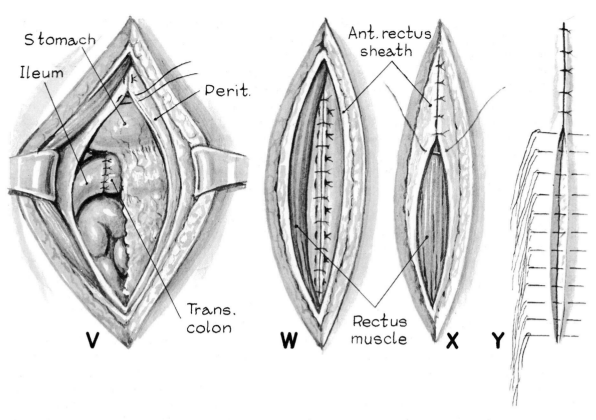

Stomach

Ileum

Perit.

Trans. colon

V

Ant. rectus sheath

Rectus muscle

W   X   Y

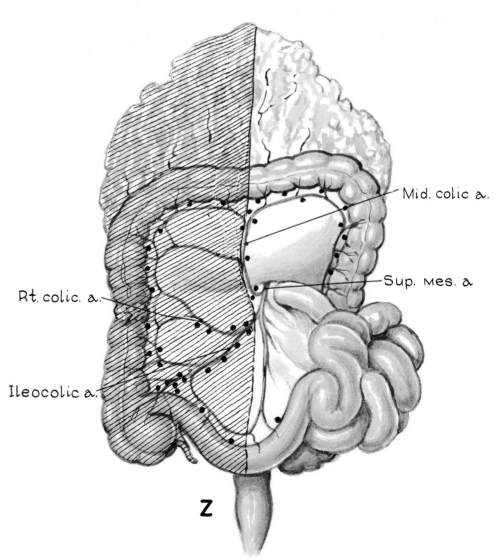

Mid. colic a.

Sup. mes. a

Rt. colic. a.

Ileocolic a.

Z

These illustrations depict the extension of the operation in the performance of a radical right hemicolectomy. In lesions of the right side of the colon, retroperitoneal aortocaval lymph node dissection is now routinely performed. This dissection is the same as illustrated in the performance of Total Gastrectomy, Splenectomy, and Partial Pancreatectomy, and Radical Left Hemicolectomy. Furthermore, there is a sound anatomic basis for this dissection, relative to the removal of the lymphatic drain, in "curative" operations for cancer of the rectosigmoid, the rectum, the testicle, the uterus, and the ovary. In one patient, exploratory laparotomy and aortocaval node dissection was performed for metastatic lymphatic disease four and one-half years after radium and roentgen therapy for a Grade III carcinoma of the cervix. In a second patient who also had a Grade III carcinoma of the cervix, necropsy was performed five and one-half years after radium and roentgen therapy, and extensive metastatic invasion of the aortocaval nodes was present. Accordingly, in the radical "curative" operation for carcinoma of the cervix one questions the logic of limiting the resection of the lymphatic drain to the pelvic nodes. In such instances, it is believed that aortocaval node dissection from the level of the renal veins downward, as illustrated, should be included.

A. The mobilization of the right side of the colon is continued, and the related retroperitoneal structures are depicted. The incision for the mobilization of the retrocolic portion of the duodenum is indicated in dotted outline.

B. The duodenum, previously mobilized by digital manipulation, is secured in a Babcock clamp and retracted upward to expose the enlarged aortocaval nodes invaded by metastases. The node constantly present behind the left renal vein, the so-called "sentinel" node, is visible.

C. The remaining attachment of the aortocaval lymph nodal mass to the left lateral margin of the aorta is severed by scalpel dissection (dotted line) to complete the radical lymphadenectomy. The uncovered aorta and vena cava and their related retroperitoneal structures may be clearly seen. The characteristic location of the terminal portion of the common bile duct between the lymph node laterally and the gastroduodenal artery medially is demonstrable.

Plate 172   401

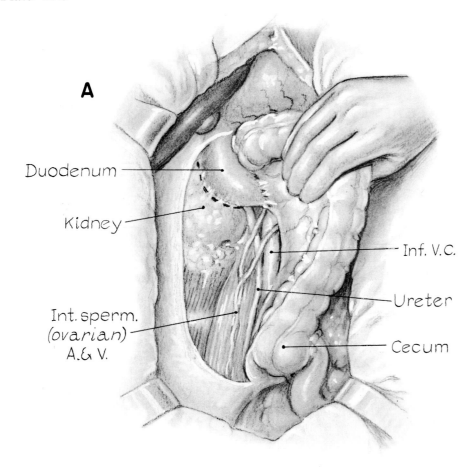

A

Duodenum

Kidney

Int. sperm.
(ovarian)
A. & V.

Inf. V.C.

Ureter

Cecum

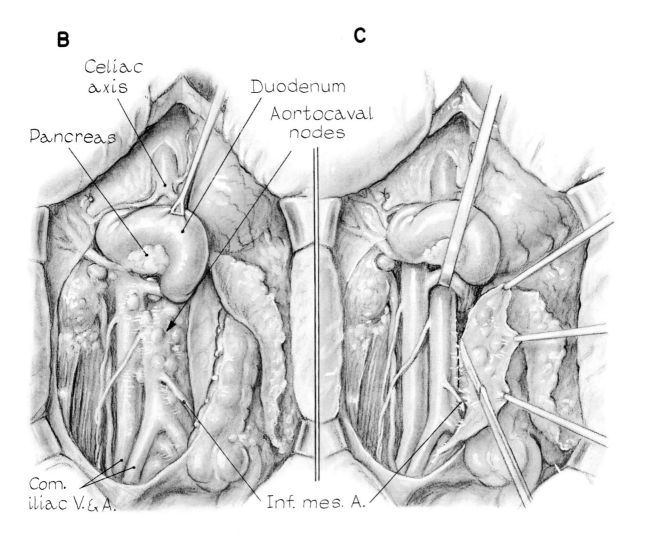

B

Celiac
axis

Pancreas

Duodenum

Aortocaval
nodes

C

Com.
iliac V. & A.

Inf. mes. A.

RESECTION FOR CARCINOMA OF THE COLON IN THE REGION OF THE SPLENIC FLEXURE

In the surgical treatment of cancer of the colon, the extent of resection of the "lymphatic drain" is widely varied, depending upon the location of the primary lesion. The operation designed for cancer of the right side of the colon, including the proximal third of the transverse colon, in general conforms with our knowledge of the lymphatic distribution. Unfortunately, however, the same does not obtain relative to the surgical treatment of tumors of the left side of the colon, including the distal third of the transverse colon. This applies in particular to carcinoma in the region of the splenic flexure, even though the inadequacy in the extent of resection in this region has been repeatedly emphasized.

In 1908, Clogg stated, "Any operation for cancer is not merely that of removal of the primary growth but also its lymphatic drain, as thoroughly as can be performed in accordance with the anatomy of the part." Clogg, and later Jamieson and Dobson, demonstrated the presence of lymphatic communications between tumors in the region of the splenic flexure and the glands in the hilum of the spleen. Moynihan was fully cognizant of this when he stated, "Any operation destined to remove the whole lymphatic area attached to the splenic flexure would, therefore, appear to be impracticable in view of the possible enlargement in it of glands in the hilum of the spleen, unless the spleen itself is excised." In addition to the hilum of the spleen, the lymphatics of the splenic flexure have drainage to nodes in the transverse mesocolon, the mesentery of the descending and proximal sigmoid colon, the omentum, the gastrocolic ligament, and the tail of the pancreas.

In the surgical treatment of carcinoma in the region of the splenic flexure, the adequate removal of its surrounding area of lymphatic drainage would embody the resection of the distal half of the transverse colon, the splenic flexure, the whole of the descending and the proximal portion of the sigmoid colon, and the whole of the attached mesentery, the distal half of the greater omentum, the proximal two thirds of the gastrocolic ligament, the spleen, and the tail of the pancreas. The technic for such an operation is shown in the following illustrations.

A, B, C. The peritoneal cavity is entered through a left rectus muscle-retracting (lateral) incision. The incision extends from the apex of the left costoxiphoid angle downward to a level approximately 3 cm. below the umbilicus.

D, E. The lesser sac is entered through an avascular area of the gastrocolic ligament above the gastroepiploic arch, and the gastrocolic ligament is serially clamped and severed to skeletonize and mobilize completely the proximal three fourths of the greater curvature of the stomach.

F. The descending colon is retracted manually toward the midline and freely mobilized by scissor dissection along the line of peritoneal fusion, the fascia fusion layer of Toldt, commonly called the "white line."

Plate 173   403

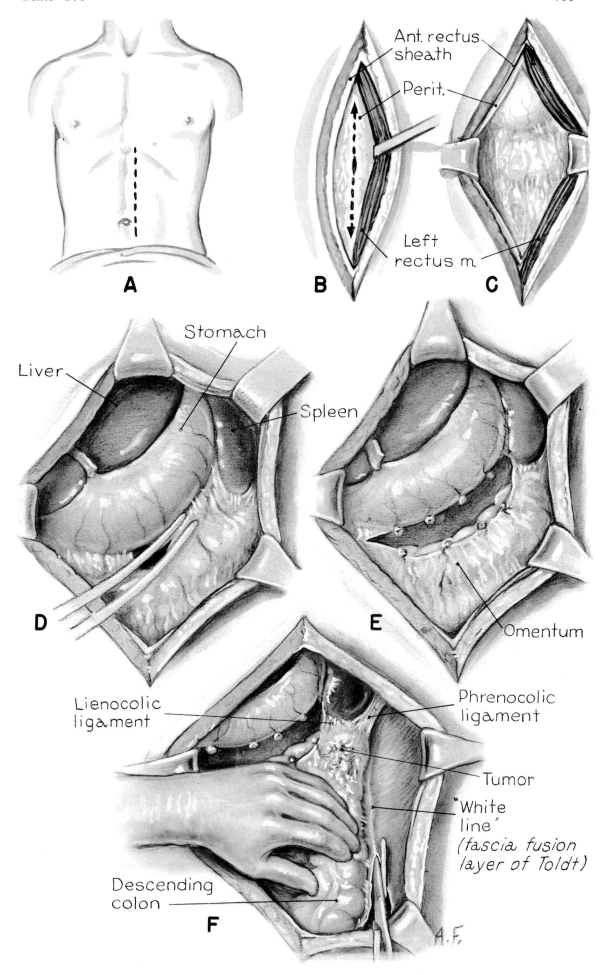

A

B   Ant. rectus sheath
    Perit.
    Left rectus m.

C

D   Liver
    Stomach
    Spleen

E   Omentum

F   Lienocolic ligament
    Phrenocolic ligament
    Tumor
    "White line" (fascia fusion layer of Toldt)
    Descending colon

A.F.

G. The mobilization of the colon is completed, first proximally to the region of the splenic flexure where the left phrenocolic ligament is severed, and then distally to the junction of the proximal and middle one third of the sigmoid.

H, I. The dissection of the colon is continued medially to expose the lower pole of the kidney, the ureter, the renal and spermatic (or ovarian) veins, the aorta, and the site of origin of the inferior mesenteric artery.

J. The duodenojejunal junction is mobilized by severance of the ligament of Treitz and the mesentery adjacent. This permits the retraction of the duodenum and proximal portion of the jejunum which, in tumors of the splenic flexure, is frequently displaced toward the site of the tumor by the foreshortened mesocolon.

K. The mobilization of the colon is completed, and the pedicle of the spleen and the tail of the pancreas are exposed anteriorly by clamping and severing the anterior layer of the gastrosplenic ligament and its contained vasa brevia.

DISCUSSION—DR. WARREN H. COLE. The illustrations and the description of technic are very concise and clear. The technic described is somewhat standard, although not all surgeons would remove the tail of the pancreas (unless it were in close proximity to the tumor). It seems probable, however, that Dr. Madden is correct in making this part of the standard technic. All surgeons would include removal of the spleen.

As soon as the tumor is palpated for mobility and operability, it should be covered with a dry laparotomy pad and kept covered throughout the operation. Many surgeons, including myself, would apply a tape ligature to the lumen of the colon a few inches proximal and distal to the tumor as soon as operability is determined and before any operative manipulation; this is done to eliminate the drifting of live cancer cells from the tumor in the lumen down to the bowel utilized in the anastomosis. Smears of luminal content made in the surgical pathology room indicate that cells desquamated before application of the tape ligatures have died and disintegrated, since none could be found outside the ligatures. Similarly, I believe that the vascular trunks should be ligated as soon as they can be isolated. The left branch of the middle colic (or the middle colic if it is to be sacrificed) can be ligated as soon as an opening is made in the lesser peritoneal sac. The left colic artery should be ligated shortly afterwards; the exposure indicated in H and I makes this readily feasible.

I agree with Dr. Madden in that a very important feature of the operation is excision of a maximum amount of mesentery and the lymph-bearing tissues, particularly that adjacent to the major vessels. Precautions must be taken to preserve vascularity of the bowel at the point where the colon is to be severed. In other words, the surgeon must be certain that the two ends of the bowel are viable because impairment of the blood supply in either end of the bowel increases the possibility of a leak at the suture line.

I favor irrigation of the two ends of the bowel just before the anastomosis is made to eliminate the possibility of local recurrence at the suture line, which has been described by numerous authors. There is no agreement as to what solution should be used for this purpose. Until an ideal drug is obtained for this purpose, distilled water might have some benefit by removing the luminal content. The crushed end of each end of the bowel should be excised to allow fresh bowel wall for approximation.

Numerous technics have been described for placement of the sutures in the anastomosis. One is probably as good as the other. I use catgut for the inside row and silk for the outside row; the posterior portion of the outside row consists of continuous 0000 silk, but the remainder (two-thirds of the circumference) is interrupted. The same ratio is used for the inside row of catgut. Interrupted sutures throughout are just as effective, but using a continuous suture for one-third the circumference posteriorly saves a little time.

I do not drain the abdominal cavity unless the viability of the ends of the bowel are in doubt or tension exists. When the tail of the pancreas is resected, however, the insertion of a drain becomes obligatory. Opinions will vary concerning closure of the mesentery. When a large opening is present, it need not be closed; when only a small opening is present, the need for closure is much greater, and in fact is obligatory.

Plate 174   405

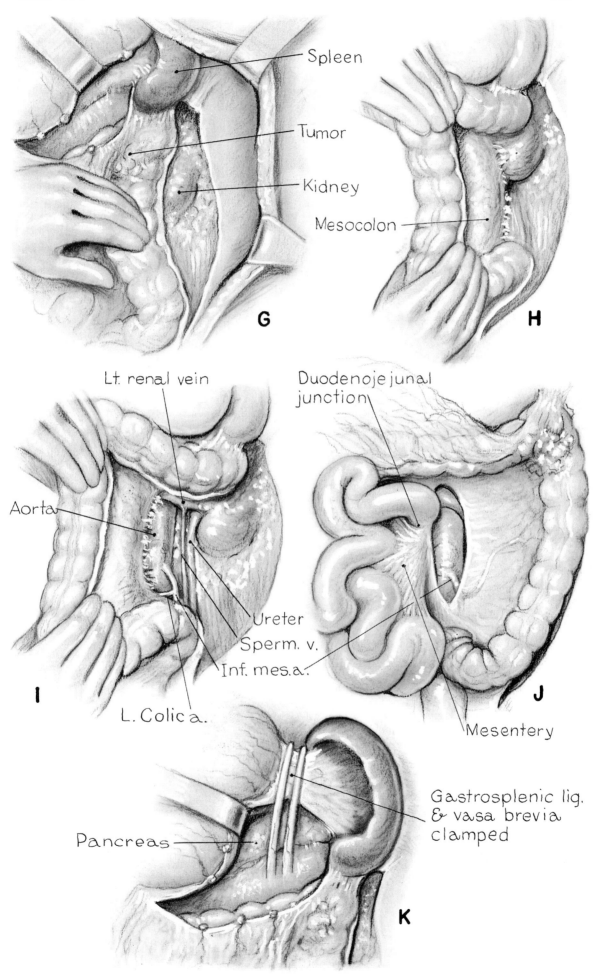

Spleen

Tumor

Kidney

Mesocolon

G

H

Lt. renal vein

Duodenojejunal
junction

Aorta

Ureter

Sperm. v.

Inf. mes. a.

I

L. Colic a.

Mesentery

J

Pancreas

Gastrosplenic lig.
& vasa brevia
clamped

K

L, M. The spleen is manually retracted toward the midline, and the posterior layer of the lienorenal ligament is severed (dotted line) to expose the posterior aspect of the vascular pedicle and the tail of the pancreas. The intimate relation between the tail of the pancreas and the pedicle of the spleen is apparent.

N. A large, warm, moist, gauze pack is placed in the "splenic bed" and the spleen is reposited laterally. The previously mobilized greater curvature of the stomach is retracted upward and medially to visualize the pancreas and the splenic vessels along its superior border. The splenic vessels are triply clamped and severed between the two distal clamps.

O, O¹. The two clamps proximally are replaced by a ligature and a suture ligature respectively of 00 silk, and the pancreas is transected subjacent to the site of severance of the splenic vessels. Hemostasis for the distal cut surface of the pancreas is obtained by the prior application of a large curved clamp and for the proximal cut surface by the serial application of Babcock clamps as the pancreas is transected. The Babcock clamps compress the pancreas adequately for hemostasis without causing undue tissue trauma.

P. The Babcock clamps have been replaced individually by mattress sutures of 00 silk, and the relation of the proximal cut end of the pancreas to the surrounding structures is depicted.

DISCUSSION—DR. J. WILLIAM HINTON. The illustrated technic for the Resection for Carcinoma of the Colon in the Region of the Splenic Flexure is most thorough for the finished surgeon. However, since the presentations in the Atlas are primarily for those in surgical training, some emphasis should be placed on certain features relative to the operation advocated.

Surgeons who have had considerable experience in the treatment of cancer of the colon are aware that the methods of surgical management of the different malignant lesions in the region of the splenic flexure are varied. Certainly, the polypoid lesion with early malignant changes does not need as extensive an operation as the ulcerated carcinoma which extends through the wall of the intestine to involve the serosa. This type of lesion will unquestionably spread more frequently through the lymphatics than the annular type of carcinoma with stenosis. The annular carcinoma with stenosis does not require the same extensive and radical operation as the type of carcinoma that has involved the entire wall of the intestine.

I believe, from my own personal observations, that the emphasis for the trainee should be more on evaluating the pathologic process encountered and on a careful consideration of the age and general physical condition of the particular patient than on a standard operative procedure for all patient. It is also believed much more difficult to teach judgment as applied to an individual patient than to teach the technic for the performance of a particular operation. I do believe, however, that the operative technic illustrated is of real value for the trained and experienced surgeon.

Plate 175

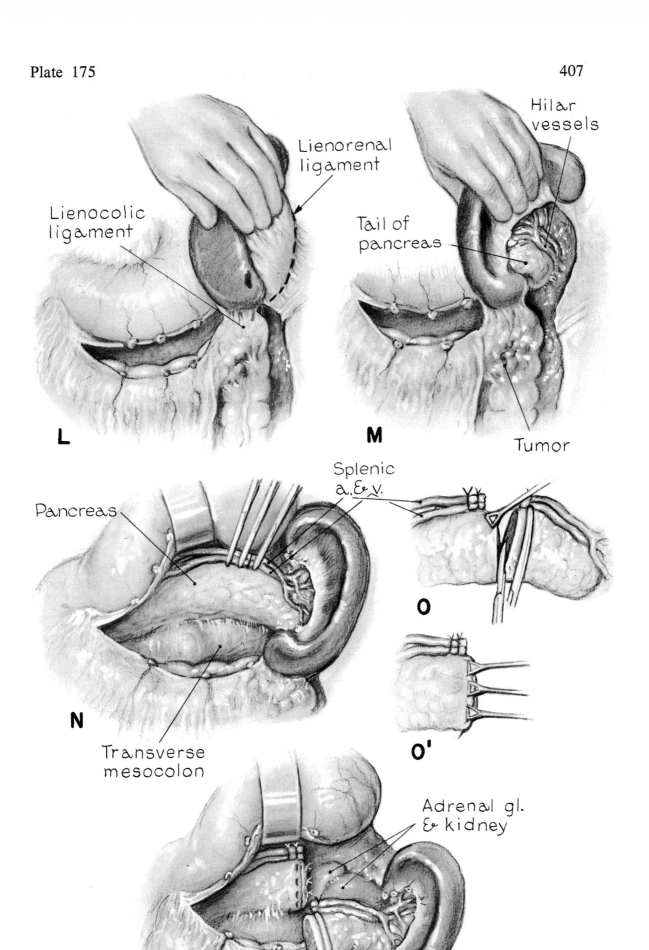

Lienorenal ligament

Lienocolic ligament

L

Hilar vessels

Tail of pancreas

Tumor

M

Splenic a. & v.

Pancreas

O

N

Transverse mesocolon

O'

Adrenal gl. & kidney

P

Q, R. The spleen and the severed distal segment of the pancreas are encased in a large, moist, gauze pad, and the mesocolon is serially clamped and cut opposite the site of election for transection of the colon. For the purpose of clarity, the apron of greater omentum and gastrocolic ligament included in the resection is not shown. In cutting the distal portion of the mesocolon, the left colic artery is doubly clamped just beyond its origin from the inferior mesenteric artery. The inferior mesenteric artery is cleanly dissected as a routine, and, if indicated, it may be sacrificed with impunity.

S, T. Prior to transgression of the continuity of the colon, the operative field is declared contaminated and is defined by the use of an appropriate red colored drape. To avoid unnecessary trauma to the tissues at the site of the anastomosis, Babcock clamps are employed to secure the proximal portion of the transverse colon and the distal segment of the sigmoid colon respectively. Medium sized crushing clamps (Payr) are applied to the colon in juxtaposition to the Babcock clamps and the colon is transected as indicated in dotted outline.

U. The operative field after the en bloc resection is shown. The divided ends of the colon are held in approximation preparatory to the performance of a two layer, end-to-end, open type of anastomosis using interrupted sutures of fine (000) silk. The open technic is preferred to the closed or so-called "aseptic" method of anastomosis.

Plate 176   409

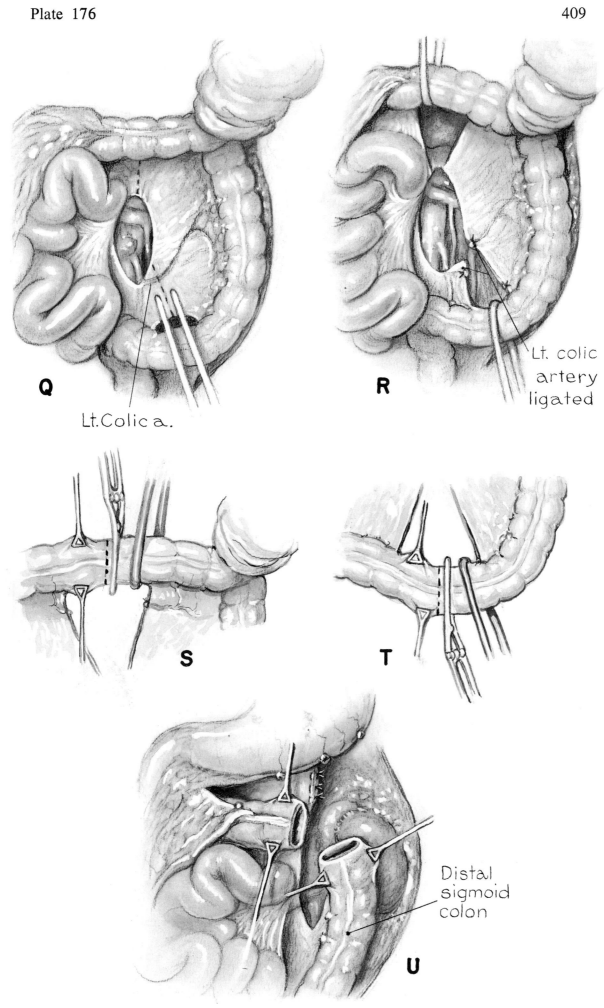

Q

Lt.Colic a.

R Lt. colic
artery
ligated

S

T

U Distal
sigmoid
colon

V, V₁. The segments of the colon are approximated with two guy sutures (000 silk), and the insertion of the first posterior layer of interrupted silk (000) sutures is completed.

V₂. The first anterior layer of sutures is inserted from the "inside out" to the "outside in" to place the knots on the inside of the lumen when the sutures are tied.

V₃, V₄. The second layer of the anastomosis is completed anteriorly using mattress sutures (Halsted) of fine (000) silk.

V₅. The two lateral mattress sutures anteriorly are left long to facilitate the rotation of the bowel on its longitudinal axis and the insertion of the mattress sutures (Halsted) posteriorly. It is technically more feasible to insert the posterior layer of seromuscular sutures at the termination rather than at the beginning of the anastomosis.

W. The relation of the completed end-to-end colocolostomy to the transected segment of the pancreas is demonstrated. The attachment of the proximal segment of the colon to the peritoneum overlying the pancreas as shown is not necessary.

X. The operation completed, the contaminated drapes, gloves, and instruments are discarded, and the operative field is again declared sterile. A Penrose (cigarette) drain is placed in the retroperitoneal area adjacent to both the anastomosis and the transected end of the pancreas, and a layer closure of the wound is performed.

Y, Z. The wound closure, using interrupted everting mattress sutures of silk (000) for the peritoneum, interrupted figure of 8 mattress sutures of silk (000) for the fascia, and simple interrupted sutures of silk (000) for the skin, is shown.

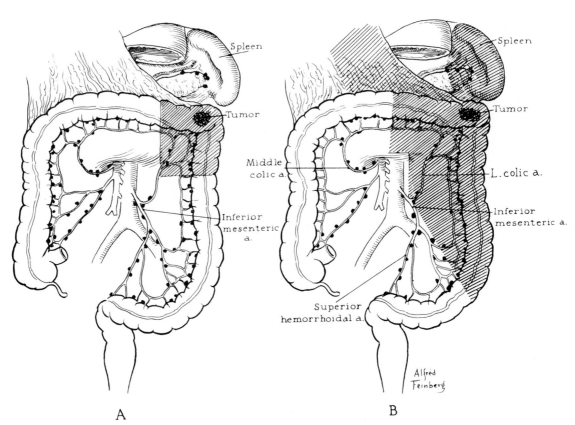

A   B

Diagrammatic illustrations of the extent of resection (shaded areas) in the surgical management of carcinoma of the colon in the region of the splenic flexure. A. The comparatively small V-shaped segment of colon that is so frequently resected. B. The extent of the resection as depicted in the preceding illustrations to include the potential zone of "lymphatic drain."

Plate 177   411

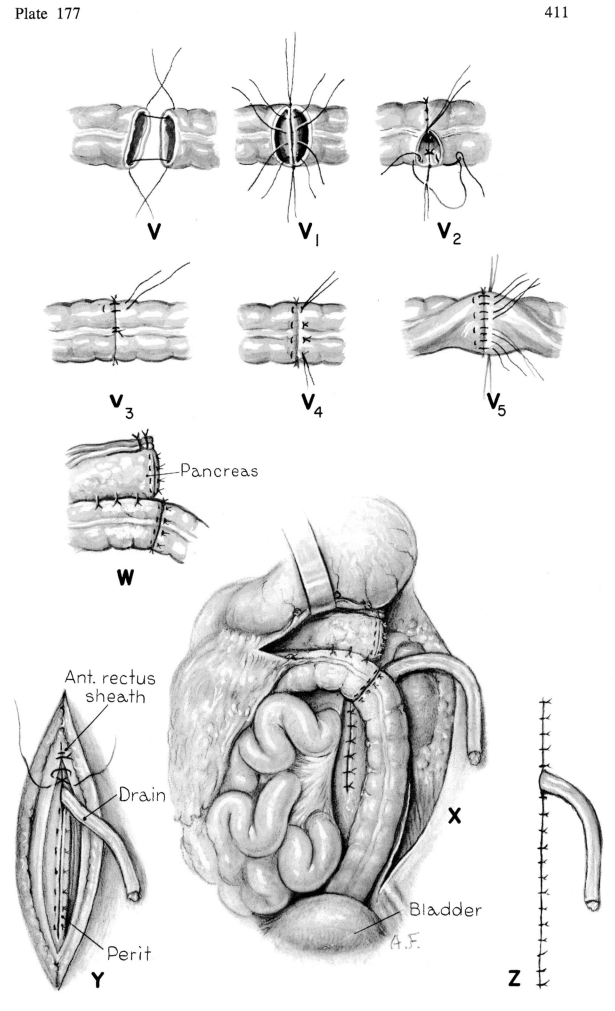

V

V₁

V₂

V₃

V₄

V₅

Pancreas

W

Ant. rectus
sheath

Drain

Perit

Y

Bladder

A.F.

X

Z

RADICAL LEFT HEMICOLECTOMY

A, B, C. The peritoneal cavity is entered through a left rectus paramedian muscle-splitting incision, and the tumor and the lower portion of the descending colon are exposed.

D. The colon, covered with a moist gauze pad and manually displaced toward the midline, is mobilized by scissor dissection along the fascia fusion layer of Toldt, commonly called the "white line."

E. To facilitate the mobilization of the splenic flexure, the lesser sac is entered through the gastrocolic ligament, and the greater curvature of the stomach is mobilized by serially clamping and severing the gastrocolic ligament cephalad to the gastroepiploic arch. This is perferred to entering the lesser sac by dissection of the omentum from the transverse colon since it permits the removal of the attached omentum and the gastrocolic ligament with the resected specimen.

F. The mobilized segments of the transverse and the descending colon are approximated, and, with downward traction maintained, the splenic flexure is mobilized by severance of the left phrenocolic and splenocolic ligaments. In some instances, because of its vascularity, it may be necessary to clamp the splenocolic ligament before it is severed.

G. The mobilization of the left side of the colon is completed to the middle third of the transverse colon, and several of the related retroperitoneal structures are depicted.

DISCUSSION—MR. J. C. GOLIGHER. The description of radical left hemicolectomy with its beautifully executed illustrations gives an admirable account of this now well-established operation, and no one studying it carefully can fail to derive a clear conception of the technic required for its performance. Consequently, little remains for a discussant to do but to reinforce or shift the emphasis in places and to suggest certain changes of technical detail, as follows.

For most surgeons the choice of incision for left hemicolectomy lies between a long left paramedian and an oblique muscle-cutting incision in the line of the external oblique fibers. The latter provides excellent access to the splenic flexure itself and leaves a very strong wound subsequently, but it is much less satisfactory in its exposure of the main vessels, particularly for a modern radical left hemicolectomy with ligation of the inferior mesenteric artery at its origin from the aorta. I have no doubt therefore that for the latter operation a left paramedian, as advised by Dr. Madden, is distinctly superior, though I myself prefer to make it as a "rectus slide" rather than a "rectus split," which inevitably sacrifices the nerve supply to the separated inner strip of the muscle. It is important however to make this incision really long—certainly longer than in A, and reaching virtually to the costal margin above and almost to the pubis below. Occasionally, in dealing with very adherent growths in the region of the splenic flexure in obese patients, it may be advisable to improve access still further by making a supplementary transverse cut extending from the main incision across the left rectus an inch or so above the umbilicus.

For the mobilization of the splenic flexure, it is an advantage for the surgeon to stand on the right of the patient and to have the table tilted 15 to 20° to that side. For the final anastomosis, which will take place in the pelvis, it is more convenient that the surgeon should take his place on the left, with the patient in a slight or moderate Trendelenburg tilt.

I should like to emphasize that the first step on opening the abdomen ought to be a careful exploration to confirm the diagnosis and determine the extent of spread of the lesion. It is a good plan to make the examination of the suspected site of the primary growth the ultimate step in this systematic palpation of the abdominal cavity, for once the primary lesion has been felt and found to be locally operable there is a not unnatural tendency for the surgeon to be carried away by the prospects of removing it and to forget to explore elsewhere. Consequently, hepatic or peritoneal metastases or a second primary growth in the colon may be overlooked. Admittedly, at the present time it is rare that a case of colonic carcinoma is turned down for excision because of the presence of secondary deposits in the liver, but under these circumstances there could be no justification for practicing a resection of the scope outlined above when a strictly limited segmental removal would suffice for all local palliative purposes.

In 1953 the late Dr. Frank Lahey recommended the use of a rubber bag to enclose the entire jejunum and ileum turned out of the abdominal cavity during colectomy and other operations. This is certainly a convenient method of controlling wayward coils of eventrated gut and is especially valuable in procedures such as the one we are now considering, during which the small intestine has to be displaced away from different areas in turn—first, the paracolic gutter and splenic flexure region; then, the front of the abdominal aorta; and, finally, the pelvis. I find it useful to enclose the small gut from just below the duodenojejunal junction almost to the ileocaecal region in a more easily sterilized disposable plastic version of this bag *as soon as the decision is made to proceed with resection,* and not to wait, as suggested in M, until a later stage of the operation.

Plate 178

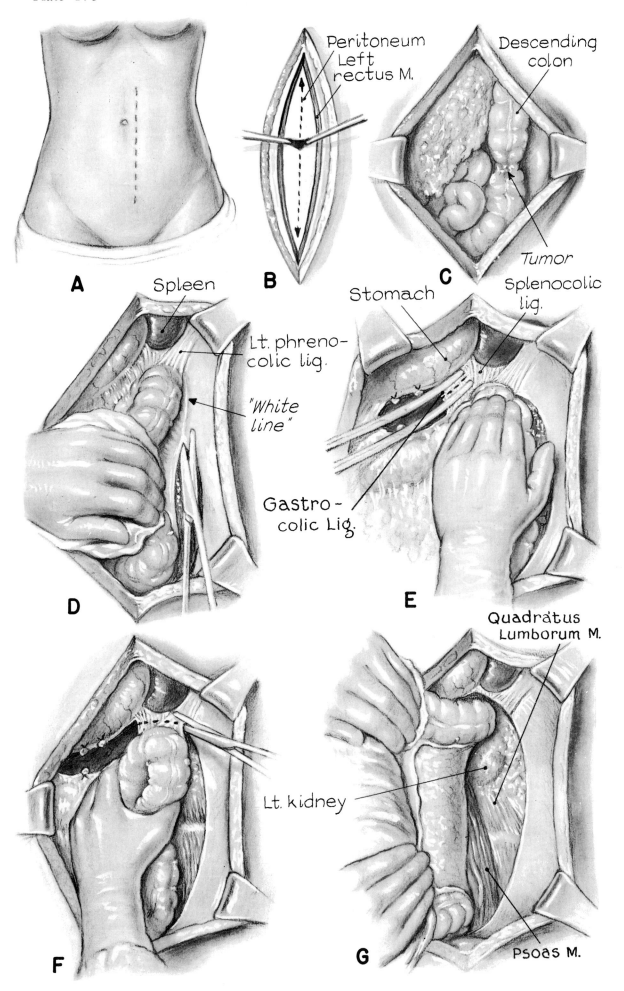

A

B
Peritoneum
Left
rectus M.

C
Descending
colon
Tumor

Spleen
Splenocolic
lig.
Stomach

D
Lt. phreno-
colic lig.
"White
line"

E
Gastro-
colic Lig.

F

G
Quadrátus
Lumborum M.
Lt. kidney
Psoas M.

H. The left side of the colon is further retracted medially to show more completely the related retroperitoneal structures. The relation of the left ureter to the bifurcation of the common iliac artery is visible. The enlarged lymph nodes overlying the anterior surface of the aorta in relation to the inferior mesenteric artery may also be seen.

I, J. The presacral space is entered by scissor dissection, and the rectosigmoid segment of the colon is mobilized by digital manipulation from the hollow of the sacrum.

K. The mobilization is completed posteriorly,

and by maintaining traction upward on the colon the recto-uterine fossa (Douglas) and the surrounding structures are shown.

L. The mobilized left side of the colon is reposited laterally, and a rubber catheter (14 F) is inserted through an avascular portion of the transverse mesocolon at the site of election for severance of the transverse colon. The transverse mesocolon is partially severed by scissor dissection along the inferior border of the pancreas where the peritoneal layers separate to cover this gland.

DISCUSSION—DR. GOLIGHER (cont.)

Readers will be familiar with the work in recent years by Warren Cole and others pointing to an increased risk during operative manipulation of carcinomata of the large intestine of exfoliation of malignant cells into the lumen of the bowel or into the venous blood draining the area. As Cole has shown, the dissemination of such cells in the lumen of the bowel can be confined largely to the vicinity of the growth by tying ligatures of tape or strong silk round the colon 2 or 3 in. proximal and distal to the primary lesion *before the manipulations leading to resection are commenced*. This may lessen the hazard of implanting malignant cells on the intestinal suture line subsequently. It is such a simple precaution that I have no doubt it ought to be adopted as a routine for what it is worth. With the object of removing or destroying any remaining cells at the site of anastomosis, it may also be a good plan to swab the open ends of colon with a soapy solution and then a cytotoxic. agent, such as nitrogen mustard, immediately prior to suture.

It is less easy to be confident about the advisability of preliminary ligation of the main vessels before mobilization of the growth to avoid a sudden gush of malignant emboli along the portal blood to the liver. The disadvantage attached to this maneuver is that it is technically a good deal more difficult—certainly in patients who are at all obese—to tie the vessels at this stage instead of after elevating the left colon with its medial leaf

of peritoneum and separating the ureter and spermatic vessels. There is, moreover, as yet no clear clinical evidence that the incidence of hepatic metastases, subsequently is reduced by this precaution. For these reasons I have not yet incorporated preliminary ligation as a routine feature of my technic for right or left hemicolectomy for malignant disease, though I do employ it in rectal excision, where it is easily practicable.

Following ligation of the inferior mesenteric artery, the only remaining source of blood for the upper rectum and distal sigmoid is the middle and inferior hemorrhoidal vessels. An important question in the conduct of radical left hemicolectomy is how far proximally this supply will suffice. My experience is that it can certainly be relied upon to maintain the viability of at least 5 or 6 in. of bowel proximal to the anterior peritoneal reflection off the rectum. A convenient level to choose for distal division of the mesosigmoid and bowel is thus about 4 in. above the reflection, or just opposite the promontory of the sacrum. This point has also the advantage that it provides a distal stump which has a peritoneal covering all round (except possibly for a short gap posteriorly) so that the anastomosis is easy and safe and it also retains sufficient bowel below to ensure excellent rectal function. Contrary to I and J, therefore, it is not necessary to open up the presacral space and mobilize the rectum from the sacral concavity.

DISCUSSION—DR. FREDERICK H. AMENDOLA. In several respects the illustrated technic for the left hemicolectomy is somewhat more radical than the operation that is generally performed. The surgical approach is well conceived, and it is quite possible that it offers, to the patient for whom it is appropriate, a better chance of cure than the less extensive procedures commonly employed. However, any added advantage which might accrue from excursion upward under the duodenum, pancreas, and left renal vein may be outweighed on certain occasions, and particularly in obese or otherwise unsuitable subjects, by the added risk that such dissection undoubtedly

creates. In extirpating regional node metastases, one must inevitably reach the point of diminishing returns and, considering the fact that mesenteric venules certainly assist in the dissemination of a considerable proportion of colon cancers, it is my feeling that this critical point is reached sooner than we think. Therefore, in deciding whether to employ a radical operation in a given patient, we must be ever mindful of the possible complications that the greater procedure entails, and we must be reasonably certain that the increased hazard is justified by improved long-term results.

The technical aspects of the radical operation are

Plate 179

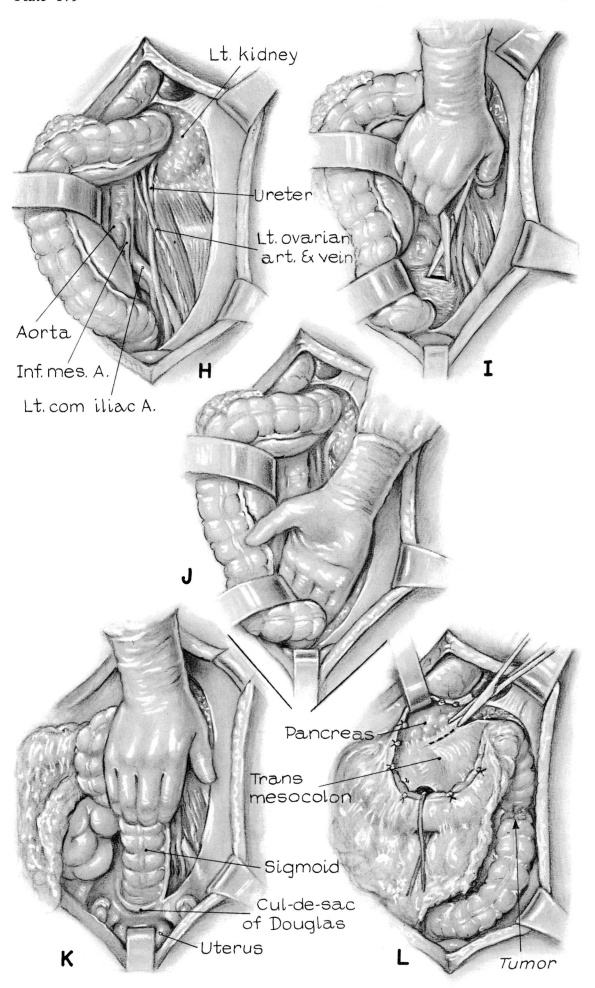

Lt. kidney

Ureter

Lt. ovarian
art. & vein

Aorta

Inf. mes. A.

Lt. com. iliac A.

H

I

J

Pancreas

Trans
mesocolon

Sigmoid

Cul-de-sac
of Douglas

Uterus

K

L

Tumor

M. The transverse colon is displaced upward by traction, and the ligament of Treitz is severed with scissors. The close relation of the inferior mesenteric vein to the duodeno-jejunal junction is visible. Exposure of both the aorta and the inferior vena cava is obtained through incisions along the attachment of the root of the mesentery of the small bowel and the peritoneal covering of the inferior border of the transverse portion of the duodenum as shown by the dotted lines. If desired the incision along the root of the small bowel mesentery may be continued around the cecum and then upward along the right side of the colon to mobilize completely this segment of the large bowel. The mobilized small and large bowel is then inserted into a Lahey type rubber bag and placed on top of the upper portion of the abdomen. This type of mobilization has been performed when indicated to improve the surgical exposure. If used, one must be certain that hemostasis is complete relative to the mobilized segment of the right side of the colon. Otherwise excessive blood loss (800 to 1000 ml.) into the bag may occur. Occult hemorrhage of this nature was observed on two occasions.

N. The mobilized small intestine is covered, first with a large piece of rubber tissue dam and then with a moist gauze pad before it is retracted from the operative field. The aorta and the enlarged lymph nodes on its anterior surface are now more clearly seen. The transverse mesocolon, subjacent to the site of election for severance of the transverse colon, is serially clamped and severed, and the inferior mesenteric vein is doubly clamped at the apex of the paraduodenal fossa prior to its severance.

O, P. The operative field is more widely exposed by further retraction of the small bowel and its mesentery in conjunction with the mobilization of the whole of the duodenal loop and the head of the pancreas. The mass of matted nodes and lymphatic tissue about the aorta and inferior vena cava is completely exposed. A node that is constantly present and referred to as the "sentinel" node is located on the front of the aorta just behind the junction of the left renal vein with the inferior vena cava. Elevation of the left renal vein (P) is required for the exposure and removal of this node. In its removal caution should be observed to prevent injury to the adjacent right renal artery.

The surgical importance of the mobilization of the duodenum and the head of the pancreas in the performance of the retroperitoneal node dissection should be emphasized. Normally the inferior border of the duodenum overlies the aorta at the level of origin of the inferior mesenteric artery. In fact, in some instances the origin of this artery may be seen only after the duodenum is mobilized and elevated. Accordingly, if the cephalad portion of the retroperitoneal dissection is limited to the level of the inferior border of the duodenum, the lymphatic tissue and nodes overlying a long segment (7 to 8 cm.) of the aorta and inferior vena cava, which may be either invaded or potentially invaded by metastatic disease, are not included in the dissection. This is obviated by mobilizing and retracting upward the duodenum and the head of the pancreas. The illustrations depict clearly the extent of the exposure of both the aorta and the vena cava proximal to the level of origin of the inferior mesenteric artery when this is done.

Q. The removal of the group of aortacaval lymph nodes is commenced by sharp dissection. A short segment of the inferior mesenteric artery and its origin from the aorta may also be seen.

DISCUSSION—DR. AMENDOLA (cont.)

shown clearly and accurately in the illustrations. The incision (Plate 178, A) might usefully be extended a few inches higher toward the costal margin. Mobilization of a deeply placed splenic flexure can be difficult and time consuming, and if exposure is inadequate, the serosa of the lower pole of the spleen may be stripped inadvertently and necessitate splenectomy for control of obstinate oozing. Before the descending colon is too extensively mobilized, it might be well to place ligatures around the bowel immediately above and below the lesion, as suggested by Warren Cole. Exfoli-ated tumor cells will thus be trapped within this segment and the likelihood of their implantation in the anastomotic suture line will be appreciably reduced.

Excision of the portion of the greater omentum (Plate 178, E) that is attached to the segment of transverse colon to be removed is sound. The alternative method, leaving the omentum behind after dissecting it away from the transverse colon, is acceptable only in the excision of benign or inflammatory lesions.

For tumors of the descending colon or high sig-

Plate 180   417

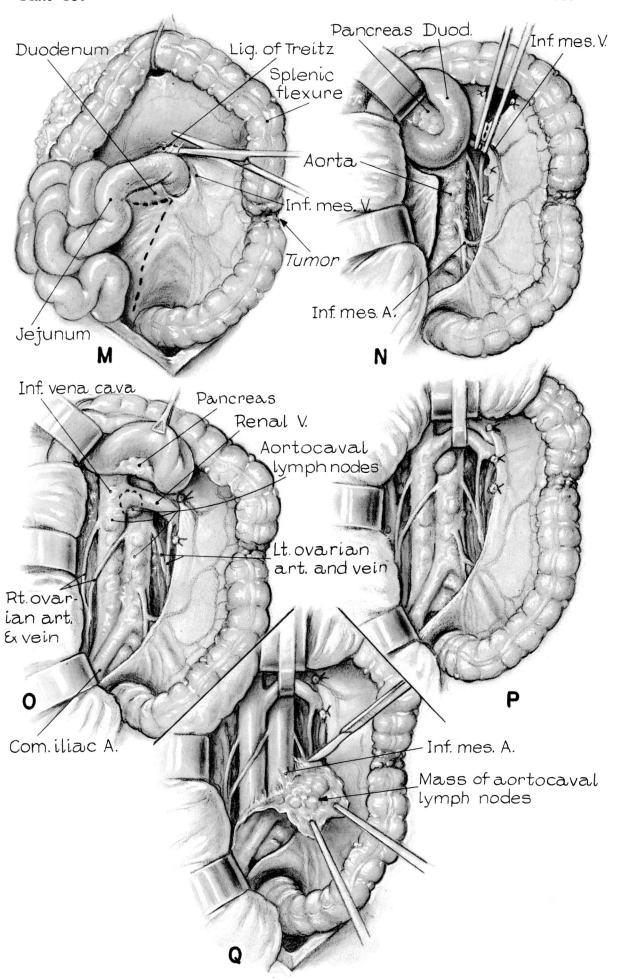

M — Duodenum, Lig. of Treitz, Splenic flexure, Aorta, Inf. mes. V., Tumor, Jejunum

N — Pancreas, Duod., Inf. mes. V., Inf. mes. A.

O — Inf. vena cava, Pancreas, Renal V., Aortocaval lymph nodes, Lt. ovarian art. and vein, Rt. ovarian art. & vein, Com. iliac A.

P — Inf. mes. A., Mass of aortocaval lymph nodes

Q

R, S. The retroperitoneal dissection is continued, and the mass of lymphatic tissue and contained lymph nodes is peeled down off of the inferior mesenteric artery. This artery is first ligated proximally (silk, 00) at its origin and then doubly clamped as shown prior to its severance. To secure hemostasis a suture ligature of silk (00) is inserted through the proximal stump of the severed artery immediately distal to the first occluding ligature (S). In utilizing this technic of exposure of the inferior mesenteric artery by tissue dissection from above downward, that is from behind, the likelihood of cutting across lymphatics laden with cancer cells is lessened. On the contrary, this likelihood is increased when the inferior mesenteric artery is exposed by tissue dissection from in front at the level of its origin from the aorta.

T. Following the completion of the ligation and division of the inferior mesenteric artery, scalpel dissection is continued and the aortacaval lymphatic mass is removed from the common iliac vessels.

U. The mobilized lymphatic mass is reposited temporarily onto the aorta and the vena cava, and preparations are made for the resection of the left side of the colon. The proximal segment of the transverse colon is secured with two Babcock clamps, and the distal segment is occluded with a straight crushing type clamp (Kocher). The site of division of the colon is indicated by the oblique dotted line. The mesosigmoid subjacent to the site of election for transection of the bowel distally is doubly clamped prior to its severance.

V. The operative field is declared contaminated, and it is walled off with a red colored laparotomy sheet. The transverse colon is severed and the distal cut end is covered with a moist gauze pad. For clarity the temporary covering of the proximal open end of the colon is omitted. The lower portion of the sigmoid colon is occluded proximally with a straight crushing clamp (Kocher) and secured by two Babcock clamps distally preparatory to its transection as indicated by the dotted line. Following the resection of the colon, the dissection of the lymphatic mass is continued along the external iliac vessels to the inguinal ligament and removed en bloc.

DISCUSSION—DR. AMENDOLA (cont.)

moid it should not often be necessary to mobilize the rectosigmoid segment as indicated in Plate 179, I and J. For lesions in the lower sigmoid this maneuver is, of course, indispensable and very useful in affording needed length in the distal limb.

In Plate 180, the steps suggested for excision of proximally placed pre-aortic nodes are illustrated. These steps must be executed with great care if troublesome bleeding is to be avoided. In a patient who is overweight a thick deposit of retroperitoneal fat in this strategic area may make dissection difficult. In the average subject I have usually been content to divide the inferior mesenteric artery as close to its origin at the aorta as good ligation permits. This frequently requires mobilization upward of the inferior border of the duodenum. I have not pursued the chain of pre-aortic nodes as high up under the left renal vein as the illustrations indicate. Involvement of the nodes at that level would be very ominous, but I see no reason why extirpation of such nodes should not be attempted under *suitable* conditions. Removal of all nodes and areolar tissue situated around the origin of the inferior mesenteric artery and distally from the aorta and vena cava (Plate 181, S and T) is essential and, in some respects, more important than the excision of tremendous lengths of bowel above and below the lesion. I have always felt that the really significant step in the performance of an adequate resection for carcinoma of the colon is accomplished by removing the *central areas* of lymphatic spread—that is, the node-bearing tissue about the origin of the vessel which is to be sacrificed—and a generous but reasonable segment of mesentery and bowel above and below the growth.

The illustrations U and V, Plate 181, show the tumor bearing segment being excised. It might be a helpful suggestion to the operator that the transverse colon be divided at a point that permits its easy approximation to the sigmoid loop without tension. This point may be selected by testing before actual transection is done. An additional few inches of length will often facilitate the approximation immeasurably. When I have resected a long segment of transverse colon, I have found it necessary on a number of occasions to mobilize the hepatic flexure to avoid tension on the suture line. Because of the frequency of multiple tumors in the colon, it might be wise to introduce a sterile sigmoidoscope into the open limbs of bowel before the anastomosis is performed. The presence of a small unsuspected carcinoma or polyp may be disclosed by this simple maneuver.

Plate 181   419

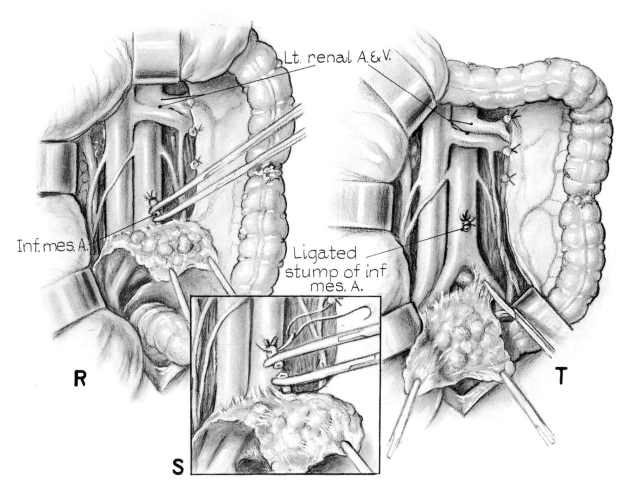

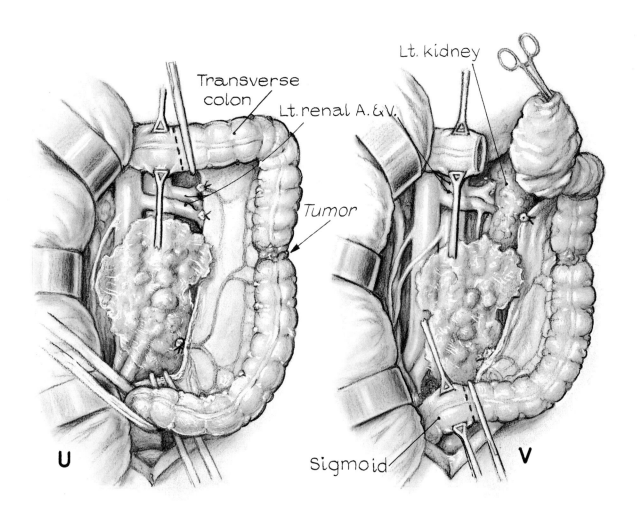

W. The operative field following the completion of the radical left hemicolectomy and retroperitoneal lymph node dissection is shown. The proximal end of the transverse colon will be united with the distal segment of the sigmoid colon by an open type end-to-end anastomosis.

X, X^1. Guy sutures of silk (000) are inserted through the lateral margins of each segment of large bowel, and the first posterior layer of the anastomosis, using interrupted sutures of silk (0000), is completed.

X^2, X^3, X^4. The second posterior suture layer, a continuous interlocking suture of chromic catgut (00), is inserted and continued anteriorly as a Connell ("loop on the mucosa") type of suture (*a*). This suture *a* which forms the first anterior layer of the anastomosis is inserted from the "outside in" to the "inside out" and "over" to invert the bowel wall and obtain a serosa-to-serosa approximation. A second chromic catgut suture *b* is commenced at the opposite angle of the anastomosis and is continued as

the first suture layer anteriorly similar to *a* to avoid an angle closure of the suture line.

X^5, X^6. The two inversion sutures forming the first anterior layer are terminated in the midline opposite each other. Each of these sutures is in turn inserted through the bowel wall on the opposite side from the "inside out" (X^5) and then tied together (X^6) to complete the first layer of the closure anteriorly.

X^7, X^8. The second layer anteriorly (*a'*) consists of a series of interrupted mattress sutures of the Halsted type which, if warranted, may be continued as an additional reinforcing suture layer posteriorly (X^8).

Y. The operative field and the related structures after the completion of the end-to-end colocolostomy are demonstrated. The drain in the retroperitoneal space, in close approximation to the anastomosis, is brought out through the abdominal incision rather than through a stab wound toward the flank.

Discussion—Dr. Amendola (cont.)

The illustrations in Plate 182 show in detail the technic of the anastomotic suture. Dr. Madden employs two layers of sutures. I have always preferred a single layer of carefully placed Halsted sutures of 0000 silk. However, whichever method one does employ, it is important to remember that excessive inversion of the line of closure may produce dangerous narrowing of the lumen at the stoma. At the conclusion of the anastomosis, the patency and adequacy of the stoma should be tested carefully with the thumb and forefinger.

The operator should be reminded of the importance of closing the mesenteric defect following any form of intestinal resection in order that internal herniation of the small bowel be avoided.

The need of placing a drain routinely at the site of the anastomosis is, in my opinion, open to question. There can be no reasonable objection to drainage of a widely denuded retroperitoneal area although I believe that even this is unnecessary. On the other hand, I have always introduced a drain down to the anastomosis in the pelvis when I have united a proximal loop of bowel covered by serosa to a distal loop that was not so protected. That there is always some insecurity about an anastomosis done at so low a level is amply demonstrated by the appreciable incidence of local leakage and fistula formation following so-called anterior resection for a very low sigmoid lesion.

I am in complete agreement with Dr. Madden that our resections for carcinoma of the colon must be planned to encompass, at the first procedure, those regional nodes that might harbor cancer cells. This must be done, however, within reasonable limits of safety. In the final analysis the estimation of risk involved in an extended procedure in a specific patient must be left to the judgment of the responsible surgeon.

Plate 182   421

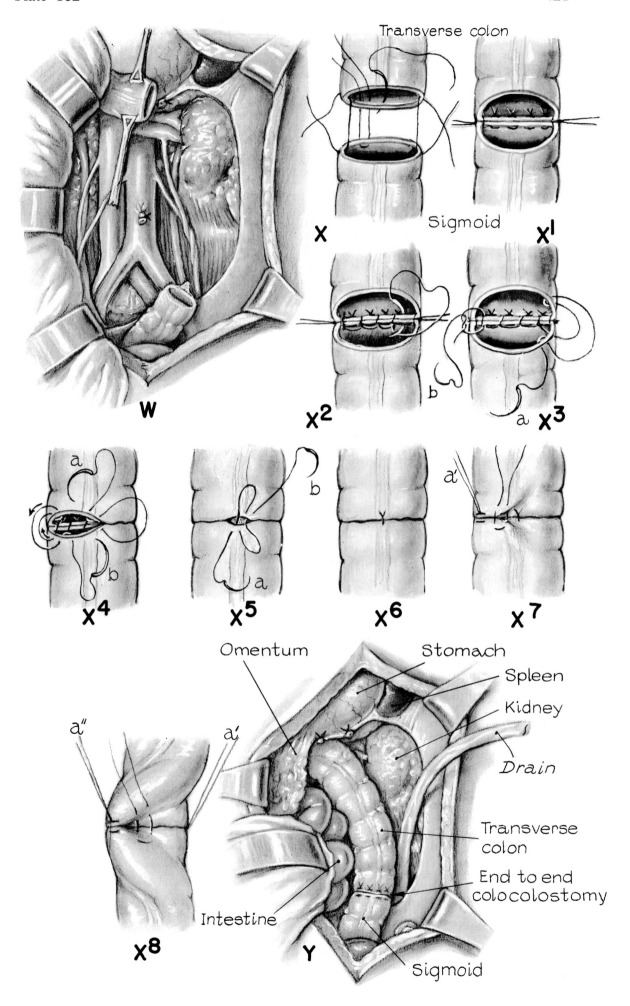

Transverse colon

Sigmoid

X

X¹

W

b

X²

a X³

a

b

X⁴

b

a

X⁵

X⁶

a′

X⁷

Omentum   Stomach

Spleen

Kidney

Drain

a″   a′

Transverse
colon

End to end
colocolostomy

Intestine

X⁸   Y

Sigmoid

ANTERIOR RESECTION OF THE RECTOSIGMOID COLON

In the performance of an anterior resection of the rectosigmoid colon the preliminary phases of the operation are the same as those used in the abdominal phase of the one-stage combined abdominoperineal resection of the rectum and are depicted in the illustrations of that operation, A through S.

A. Traction is maintained upward on the sigmoid colon, and traction sutures of silk and a right angle clamp respectively are applied to the rectal wall below the level of the tumor. The site for the transection of the rectum is shown by the dotted line. For clarity the tumor mass is uncovered.

B. The transection of the rectum is completed, and the site for severance of the sigmoid colon proximally is shown. Crushing clamps are not applied to either segment of the bowel that is used for the anastomosis. The open type of anastomosis, using interrupted sutures of silk (00), is preferred.

C. Lateral angle approximation sutures are inserted, and the lumen of each bowel segment is irrigated with copious quantities of warm (112° F.) isotonic saline solution, which is immediately removed by suction siphonage. This is done for the purpose of washing away any desquamated tumor cells that may be present and thereby tends to lessen the incidence of tumor recurrence at the anastomotic site.

D. The first suture layer posteriorly is completed. This layer consists of interrupted through and through sutures of silk (000) which are first all inserted, tied individually, and then cut.

D′. Inset to show an alternate and frequently preferred method for the closure posteriorly. A series of interrupted horizontal mattress sutures are inserted as the first posterior layer. This causes an eversion of the cut margins of the bowel which are approximated by a continuous suture of fine chromic (00) catgut, either as a simple over and over suture as shown, or one of the interlocking type. This suture, the second layer posteriorly, is then continued anteriorly as an over and over or an inverting Connell type of suture and tied to its starting point. This completes the first anterior layer. The second anterior layer is completed by the insertion of a series of interrupted horizontal seroserosal mattress sutures of fine silk (000).

E, F. The first layer of the closure anteriorly consists of interrupted sutures of silk (000) which are inserted from the "inside out" to the "outside in," so that, when tied, the knots are on the inside of the lumen. The closure terminates in the midline using a figure of 8 mattress suture of silk (000). This method of closure is believed to lessen the hazard of leakage of the anastomosis by the avoidance of an "angle" closure.

G, H. The completion of the second layer anteriorly, using interrupted mattress sutures of silk (000), is depicted.

I. Either lateral suture of the second layer anteriorly is left long to permit axial rotation of the bowel and to facilitate the insertion of the second layer of interrupted silk (000) mattress sutures posteriorly.

J. The anterior resection and the infraperitoneal anastomosis are completed. A drain is inserted into the hollow of the sacrum alongside of the anastomosis, and the reconstruction of the new pelvic floor is commenced. In all infraperitoneal anastomoses between serosal and aserosal segments of the large bowel, a complementary transverse colon colostomy is routinely performed.

DISCUSSION—DR. MICHAEL R. DEDDISH. This operation has essentially supplanted the Miles' type of resection where it is possible to obtain 6 cm. of normal rectal wall below a carcinoma. This measurement is determined only upon completion of the surgeon's dissection within the pelvic cavity and should be of the same extensive scope as described for the abdominal phase of the abdominoperineal resection. In the markedly obese patient, or where a very small male pelvis is encountered, this operation may not be feasible.

In my experience the use of 0 chromic catgut suture material to effect the anastomosis is preferred. The use of silk sutures has made postoperative evaluations difficult and in some instances has resulted in stricture at the anastomosis. Infection may be present about a silk suture for many months, and it is most difficult to determine whether one is dealing with an abscess or residual disease at the anastomosis. Reperitonealization is not necessary, and the use of a suprapubic drain brought out through the lower angle of the abdominal wound is used routinely. A complementary transverse colostomy should be used where there is any question about the security of the anastomosis and especially in elderly patients.

Plate 183

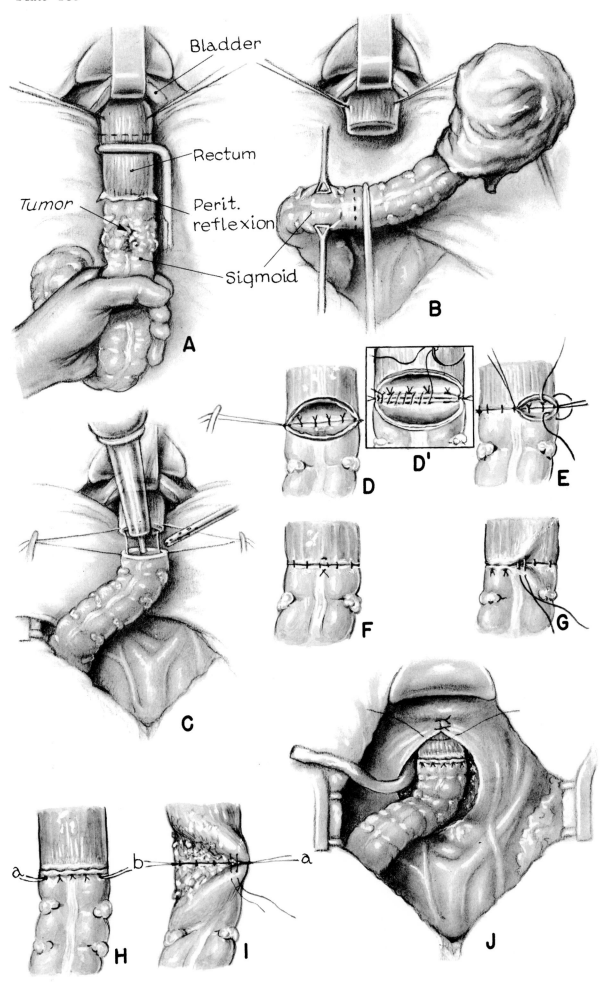

Bladder

Rectum

Tumor

Perit.
reflexion

Sigmoid

A

B

C

D

D'

E

F

G

H

I

J

a

b

a

ONE–STAGE COMBINED ABDOMINOPERINEAL RESECTION OF THE RECTUM (MILES)

A, B, C, D, E. The peritoneal cavity is entered through a left paramedian longitudinal muscle-splitting incision which extends from the symphysis to a level just above the umbilicus. The fibers of the rectus muscle are separated along the line of junction of the inner and middle thirds.

F. The patient is placed in the Trendelenburg position, and with the aid of moist gauze protective pads or preferably a large sheet or rubber tissue dam, the small bowel is displaced upward out of the operative field.

Not infrequently, a low attachment of the terminal ileum to the posterior parietal peritoneum is present and will require scissor dissection for its mobilization. In this dissection one should be careful to avoid injury to the subjacent right ureter.

G. The sigmoid colon is manually retracted toward the midline by the first assistant, and its mobilization laterally is commenced by scissor dissection along the fascia fusion layer of Toldt ("white line") down to the rectovesical or recto-uterine fossa.

Plate 184

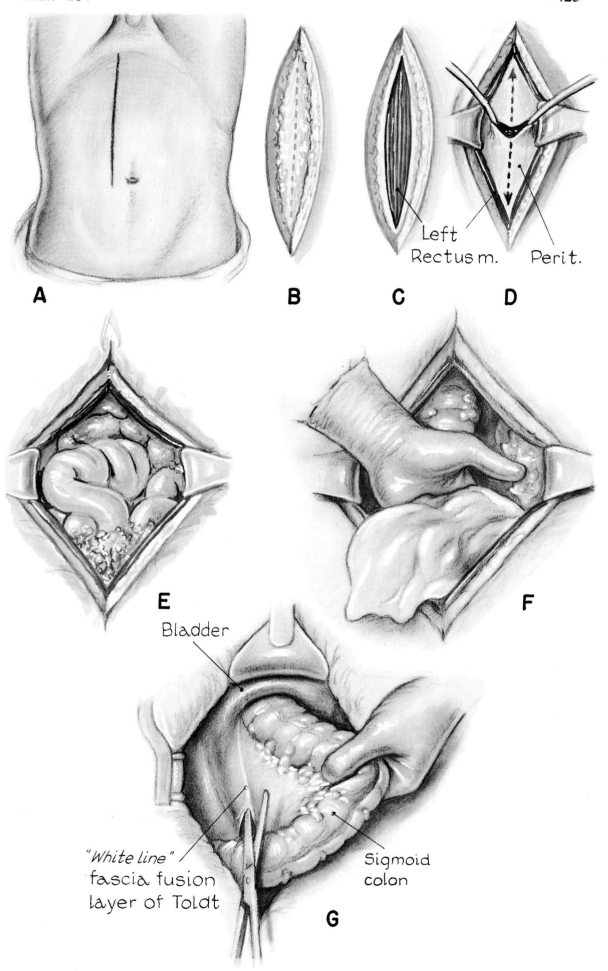

A

B

C Left
Rectus m.

D Perit.

E

F

Bladder

G

"White line"
fascia fusion
layer of Toldt

Sigmoid
colon

H. The mobilization of the sigmoid colon laterally is completed, and the three main anatomic landmarks are identified. These are the spermatic (or ovarian) vessels, the left ureter, and the superior hemorrhoidal artery.

I. The sigmoid colon is retracted to the left, and the peritoneum at the base of the mesosigmoid is incised. This incision extends from the level of the origin of the left colic artery downward to the rectovesical or recto-uterine fossa and terminates opposite the incision on the lateral side. An opening through a relatively avascular segment of the mesosigmoid for the insertion of clamps is made adjacent to the superior hemorrhoidal vessels just below the bifurcation of the aorta.

J. The location of the superior hemorrhoidal artery in the base of the mesosigmoid is determined by visualization and/or palpation. Through the openings previously made in the mesosigmoid, the artery and its accompanying veins are triply clamped and severed between the two distal clamps. This is the site of election for severance of the vessels in the classic one stage abdominoperineal resection originally described by Miles. However, in recent years, the "curative" operation has been extended to include not only ligation and division of the inferior mesenteric artery but also the mobilization and elevation of the duodenum and the head of the pancreas and the skeletonization of the aorta and vena cava by dissection of the lymphatic tissues from the level of the left renal vein downward into the pelvis along the iliac vessels. The technic for this procedure which is advocated in all "curative" operations performed for cancer of the rectum, rectosigmoid, and left side of the colon is shown in the illustrations depicting the technic for Radical Left Hemicolectomy.

K. The colon is encircled by a traction tape of rubber tissue at the site of election for subsequent transection. From this site an incision is made through the serosal layer of the mesosigmoid as a direction line for its severance and extends to the level of the division of the superior hemorrhoidal vessel.

Plate 185

427

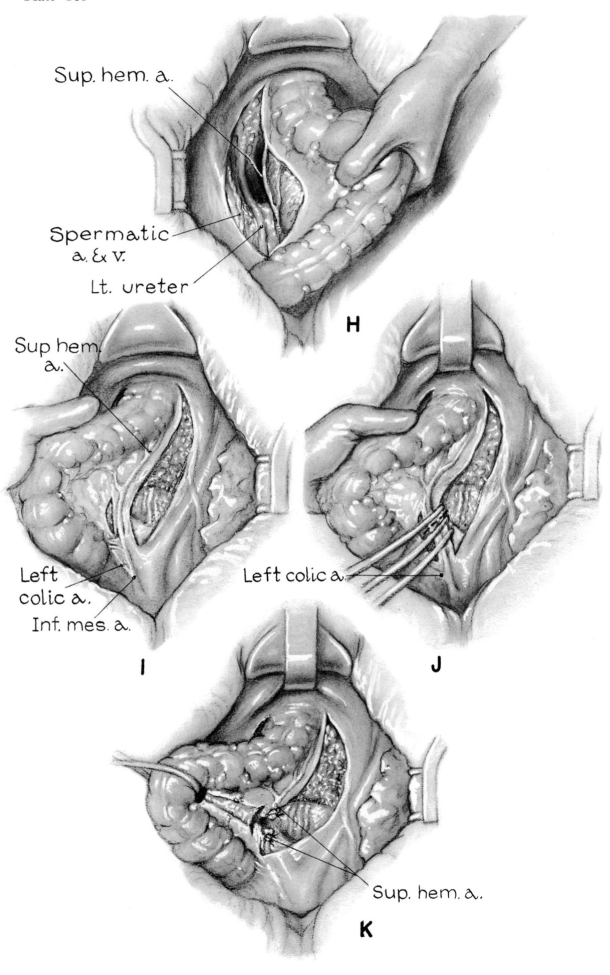

Sup. hem. a.

Spermatic
a. & v.

Lt. ureter

H

Sup hem.
a.

Left
colic a.

Inf. mes. a.

I

Left colic a.

J

Sup. hem. a.

K

L. The mesosigmoid is serially clamped and severed as indicated in dotted outline. Hemostasis is obtained with suture ligatures of 000 silk.

M. By scissor dissection, an opening is made in the fatty areolar tissue of the retrorectal and presacral space.

N. Traction is maintained upward on the sigmoid colon, and by manual dissection in the presacral space the rectosigmoid and rectum are freed from the hollow of the sacrum downward to the level of the tip of the coccyx.

O. A warm, moist gauze pad is placed in the hollow of the sacrum, and with traction on the sigmoid colon maintained, the lateral peritoneal incisions are united by division of the rectovesical or recto-uterine layer of peritoneum anteriorly. This is facilitated by preliminary digital dissection beneath the peritoneal floor as demonstrated.

P. A clamp for traction is placed on the distal cut margin of the rectovesical layer of peritoneum, and by digital dissection the avascular areolar tissue space posterior to the rectovesical fascia (Denonvilliers') is entered. The dissection of this space is continued down to the level of the tip of the prostate or the cervix uteri. Care should be taken to enter the proper plane of cleavage; otherwise troublesome bleeding may occur.

Plate 186

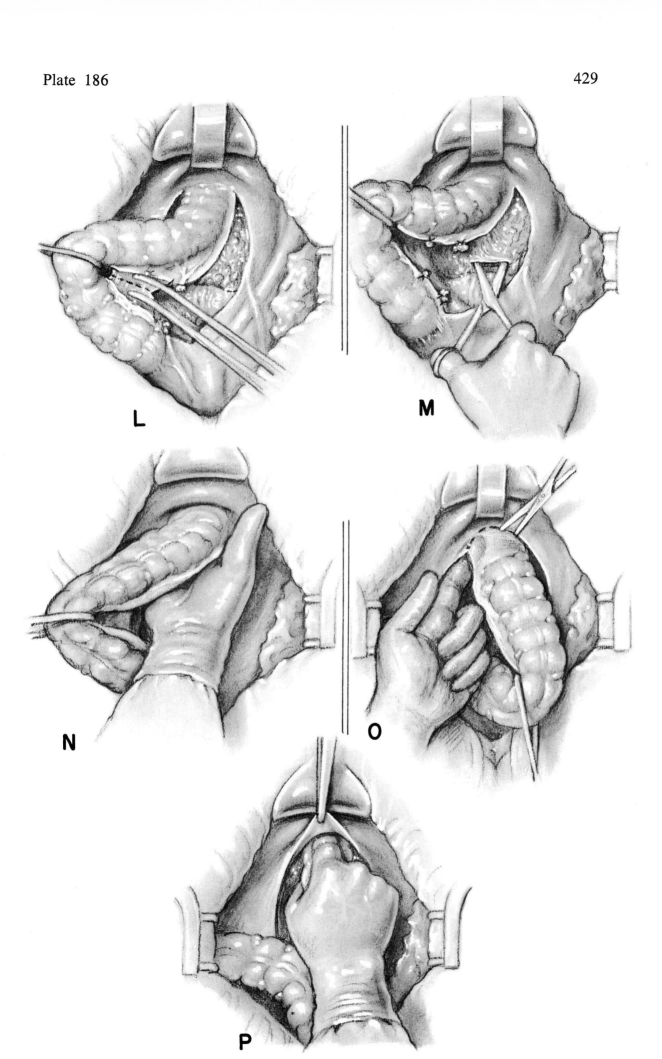

L

M

N

O

P

Q. The dissection is completed anteriorly, and the prostate gland, seminal vesicles, and portions of the lateral ligaments are visible.

R. The colon is retracted laterally to the left, and the severance of the taut right lateral ligament with long scissors is commenced. In this dissection, ligation of the middle hemorrhoidal artery contained within the lateral ligament is seldom required.

S. The sigmoid colon is retracted toward the midline, and the left lateral ligament is similarly severed as depicted by the dotted line.

T. After the severance of the lateral ligaments the dissection of the rectum is continued down to the level of the levator floor, and the distal bowel segment is divided between clamps.

Plate 187

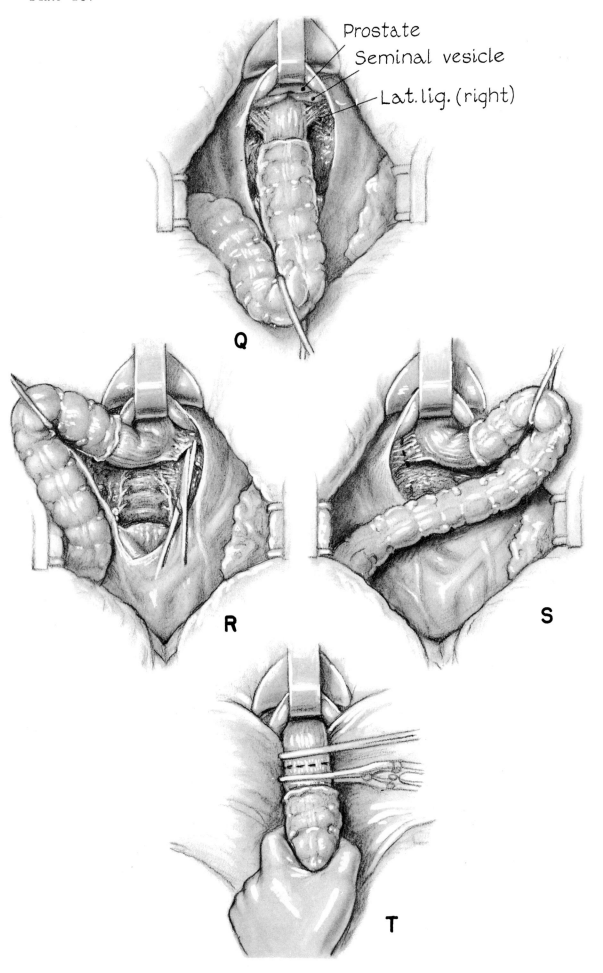

Prostate

Seminal vesicle

Lat. lig. (right)

Q

R

S

T

U, U′, U″. The proximal end of the rectum is occluded with a ligature of heavy silk (No. 1) and coverd with a small sheet of rubber tissue.

V, V′. To facilitate both the displacement of the distal segment of the bowel into the hollow of the sacrum and the reperitoniza-

tion of the pelvic floor, a low division of the bowel and resection of the redundant segment ("nuisance loop") may be required. However, this should be avoided whenever possible because of the potential danger of transecting lymphatic vessels that may be either grossly or microscopically infiltrated by cancer cells.

DISCUSSION—DR. MICHAEL R. DEDDISH. This operation is indicated for cancer of the rectum at the level of the levator muscles, or just above, and for most cancers of the anal canal.

A left paramedian longitudinal muscle-retracting lower abdominal incision seems preferable to the muscle-splitting incision as illustrated. This incision leaves the left rectus muscle intact with its blood and nerve supply and gives better support to a midline colostomy. Predisposition to a ventral or paracolostomy hernia should be avoided when possible. Such a complication usually interferes with the proper function of the colostomy.

The medial and lateral leaves of the sigmoid mesentery should be developed with a wide margin about the tumor as might be indicated by the extent of visceral peritoneal involvement. Miles originally described incising the peritoneum at the pelvic brim. Too frequently, cancer-invaded peritoneum is left in the pelvis in the effort to allow adequate peritoneum with which to construct a new pelvic floor.

Extending the Miles' type of resection to include the ligation of the inferior mesenteric artery at the aorta has quite naturally led to the dissection of the lymphatic-bearing tissues about the great vessels of the lower abdomen. Better mobilization of the distal

Plate 188

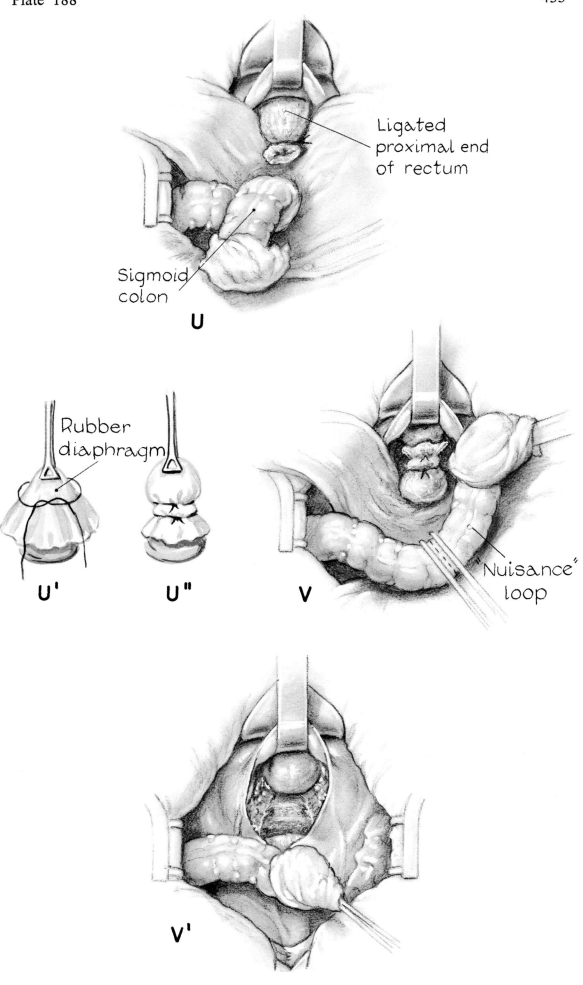

Ligated
proximal end
of rectum

Sigmoid
colon

U

Rubber
diaphragm

U'   U"

'Nuisance'
loop

V

V'

W. Sagittal section to show the completed abdominal phase of the operation. The reperitonization of the pelvic floor, the "turn-in" of the distal cut end of the sigmoid and proximal segment of the rectum into the hollow of the sacrum, and the location of the tumor are demonstrable.

X. The reperitonization of the pelvic floor when viewed through the abdominal incision.

Y. The operation table is levelled, and the closure of the abdominal incision is commenced. The small bowel is replaced into the pelvis and the proximal cut end of the sigmoid colon is exteriorized through the abdominal incision at a site where it is without either undue angulation or tension. This is usually at the junction of the upper and middle one third of the incision. To prevent herniation of the small bowel the sigmoid colon is anchored to the lateral parietal peritoneum with interrupted sutures of fine (000) silk. However, many surgeons of experience do not think that this is necessary. In the closure of the incision the modification of the Jones technic, using interrupted sutures of silk (00) rather than stainless steel wire is preferred. In this closure the sutures

are inserted through the fascia, muscle, and peritoneal layers on one side, and through the peritoneal muscle, and fascia layers on the other. The suture is then crossed over the incision and reinserted through the fascia layers only, on either side.

Z. The completed modified "Jones closure" of the fascia, muscle, and peritoneal layers is demonstrated.

Z'. The closure of the skin layer using interrupted sutures of silk (000) is completed. No sutures are used to anchor the exteriorized segment of the sigmoid colon to any part of the abdominal wall during the wound closure. The clamp on the colon is removed within 12 hours, and following the separation of the agglutinated ends of the bowel, its lumen is digitally explored. If desired, the clamp on the colon may be removed immediately upon the completion of the wound closure and the cut end of the bowel sutured to the skin margins either at the site of its exteriorization in the incision or to the margins of a lateral "stab" wound. The technic for its performance is the same as illustrated for the establishment of an ileostomy stoma as advocated by Brooke and depicted in Plate 156 of the illustrations for Ileostomy and Subtotal Colectomy.

DISCUSSION—DR. DEDDISH (cont.)

descending colon is so effected. The inferior mesenteric vein and the sigmoid branches of the inferior mesenteric artery should be isolated and ligated individually near their junction with the marginal vessel. Conservatism in our treatment of this portion of the mesentery has resulted in leaving residual disease.

Definite emphasis might be made on the extent of the abdominal phase of the pelvic dissection. This should include a clean dissection of the node-bearing tissues about the iliac and hypogastric vessels. The pelvic fascia with its extensions should be excised at the most lateral attachments and should include

the supralevator fascia. This latter step greatly facilitates the perineal resection of the rectum and should eliminate the possibility of rupturing the operative specimen from below and the resultant "seeding" of tumor within the pelvic cavity. A comment on the extent of the abdominal phase of this operation would not be complete without stating that any adjacent organs intimately associated with a rectal tumor, including the omentum and ovaries, should also be resected. It has been my experience that closure of the abdominal incision by the Jones technic, using No. 32 stainless steel wire, has resulted in much fewer wound infections and foreign body reactions.

Plate 189

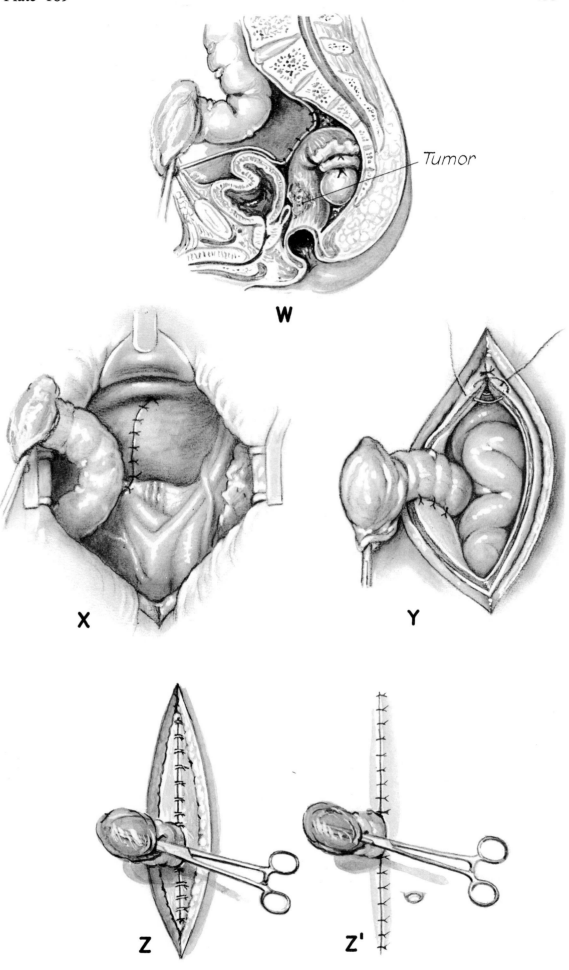

W

X

Y

Z

Z'

Tumor

A. The patient is placed in the left lateral prone (Sims') position with the left buttock over the edge of the operation table. If preferred, the lithotomy position may be used. A purse-string suture of heavy silk (No. 1) is inserted to occlude the anal orifice, and the elliptical incision employed is outlined. For clarity the draping of the operating field is eliminated.

B, C, D. The purse string suture is tied, and first the lowermost and then the uppermost portion of the perianal elliptical incision is deepened into the subcutaneous fatty tissue plane. The severed branches of the external hemorrhoidal artery are clamped and ligated with fine silk (0000).

E. The tip of the coccyx is identified by palpation and the anococcygeal raphe is divided transversely to expose the fascia propria. This is similarly cut transversely and the presacral space is entered.

F. The left index finger is used to tent the levator sling above, and the muscle is widely excised out to the ischial tuberosity.

DISCUSSION—DR. DEDDISH (cont.)

At the perineal resection of the rectum, the distance of the skin incision from the anal margin is determined by the proximity of the tumor to the anal canal. In other words, for a low-lying tumor there should be wide excision of the perineal skin, removal of the ischiorectal space fat, and transection of the levator ani muscles at their most lateral extent. Control of the pudendal vessels is best secured by suture ligatures. The use of plain catgut ligatures for the smaller vessels will eliminate many troublesome sinuses due to foreign body reaction. In patients whose work requires heavy manual labor, a gauze pack in a rubber sheet or a size eight surgeon's glove is placed in the lower pelvic cavity. This is secured by interrupted skin edge sutures and is kept in place until the patient has recovered from postoperative ileus and is on a full diet. After removal of the pack, the outlet of the pelvis fills with granulation tissue, dense scarring, and subsequent better support. In my experience, primary suture of the subcutaneous fat and skin has resulted in a greater incidence of perineal herniae. There is also a psychologic advantage to the patient when the gluteal cleft is preserved.

Plate 190 437

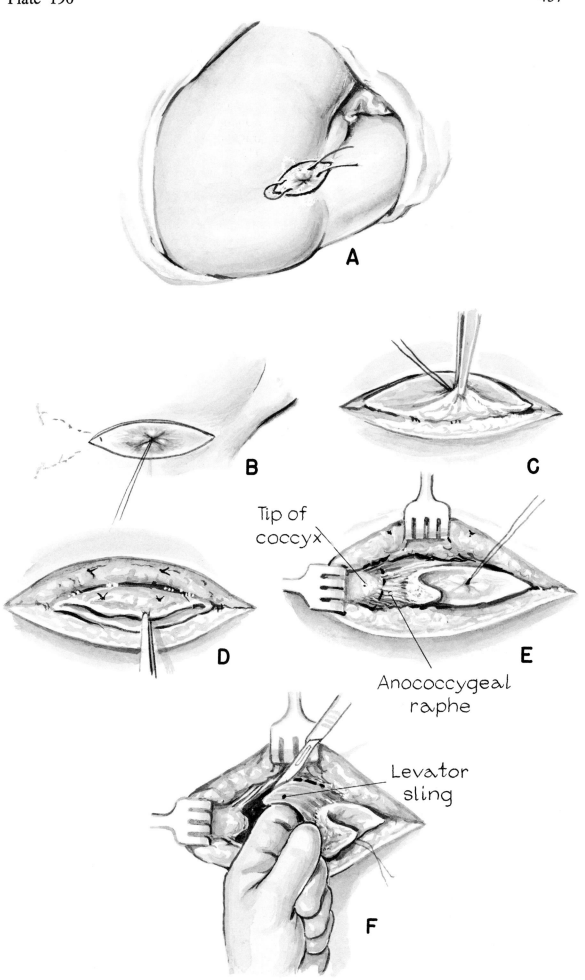

Tip of
coccyx

Anococcygeal
raphe

Levator
sling

G, H. The levator sling below is similarly widely excised, and the rubber covered distal cut end of the rectosigmoid segment is easily withdrawn from the hollow of the sacrum.

I. The division of the levator muscles anteriorly is completed, and the cut margin of the central tendon of the perineum is demonstrable. Traction is maintained anteriorly, and the rectum is separated by sharp dissection from the prostate gland and the adjacent tissue. In this dissection one must be careful to avoid injury to the underlying membranous portion of the urethra.

J, K. The perineal portion of the operation is completed, and a rubber tissue cigarette drain is inserted to the level of the base of the prostate gland. A drain is preferred to the use of a diaphragm pack because of the more rapid and more satisfactory wound healing that is obtained.

L, M. The closure of the perineal wound is completed using both simple interrupted and vertical "on-end" mattress sutures of silk (000). The application of a soft absorbent perineal dressing and T-binder support completes the operation. The drain is removed routinely on the fourth day postoperatively. Daily thereafter a soft rubber catheter (12 F) is inserted through the drain site and the depths of the wound are gently irrigated with a solution containing equal parts of hydrogen peroxide and isotonic saline. The patient is allowed out of bed on the fourth to sixth day postoperatively, and the skin sutures are removed on the eighth to tenth postoperative day.

Plate 191

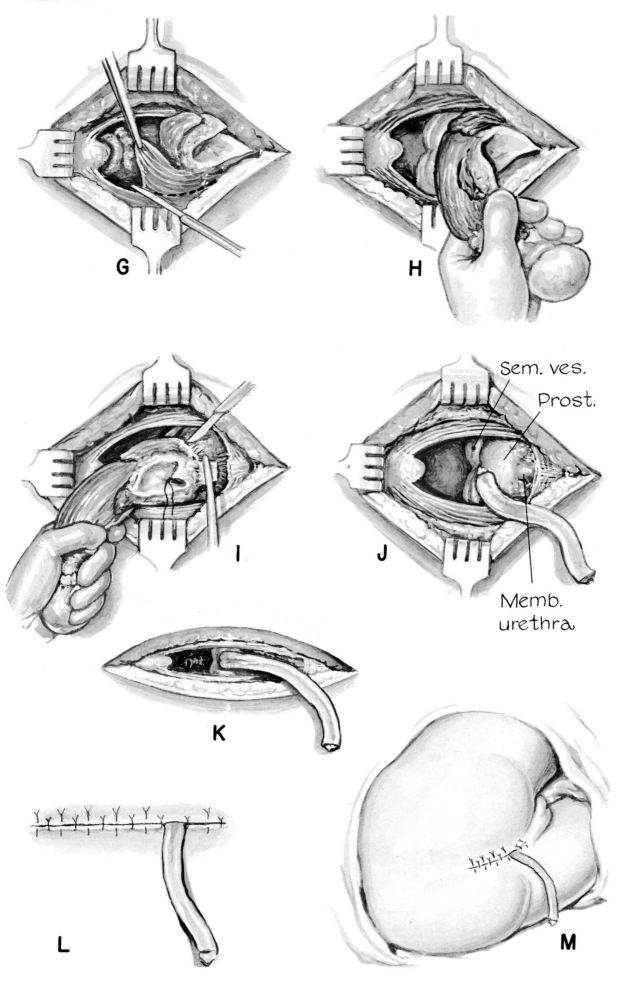

G

H

I

J

Sem. ves.

Prost.

Memb.
urethra

K

L

M

END-TO-SIDE URETEROSIGMOIDOSTOMY

The patient, a 74-year-old white man, was operated upon for an obstructive lesion of the sigmoid colon. The left ureter was markedly dilated, and when traced distally, it was found incorporated in a large infiltrative tumor mass. Because of the ureteral obstruction, the tumor mass was presumed malignant. However, when the resected surgical specimen was opened, it proved to be a benign diverticulitis of the sigmoid colon with extensive inflammatory induration and edema.

A. The patient is in the supine position, and the left lower paramedian muscle-splitting incision is indicated by the solid black line.

B. This is a view of the pelvic portion of the peritoneal cavity following the resection of the benign obstructive inflammatory lesion (diverticulitis) of the sigmoid colon and the incorporated distal segment of the left ureter. The ligated proximal end of the left ureter is behind the colon, the continuity of which has been restored by an end-to-end anastomosis, using the "open" technic. The broken line on the ureter indicates the site of election for its transection preparatory to anastomosis with the proximal segment of the sigmoid colon.

C. Guy sutures of silk (0000) are inserted on either side of the ureter, just distal to which the ureter is transected with scissors. The short ureteral segment distally, the lower end having been previously ligated, is now removed.

D. A longitudinal opening is made into the lumen of the colon corresponding in size to the transverse diameter of the severed end of the ureter. Sutures of 00000 arterial silk have been inserted in each angle of the anastomosis but not tied. The first of a series of through-and-through sutures of arterial silk (00000), which include the whole thickness of the wall of the ureter and the colon, is similarly inserted but not tied.

E. All of the sutures have been inserted and, when tied, will form the posterior layer of the anastomosis. One suture layer only is used posteriorly.

Plate 192

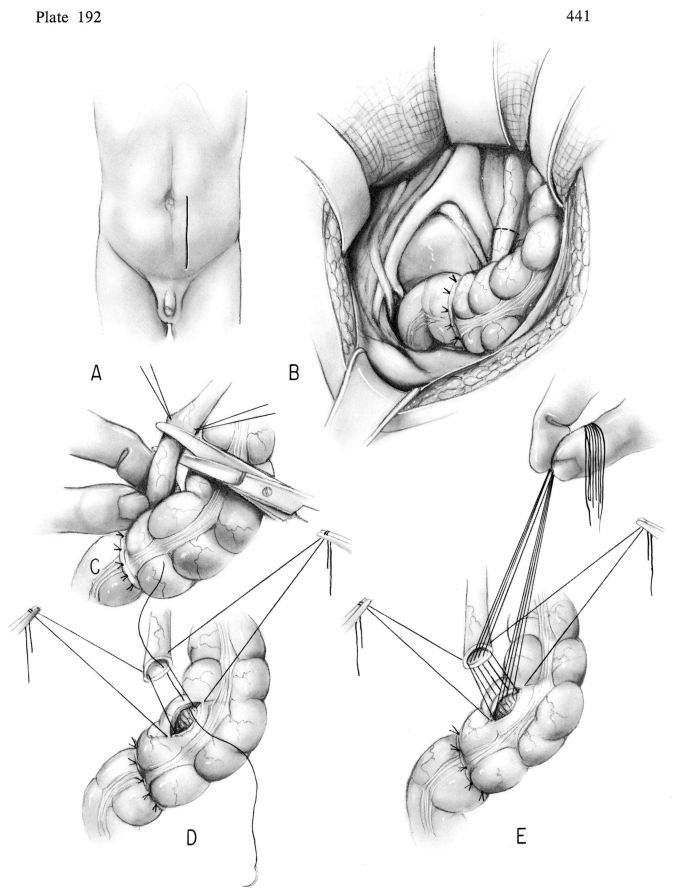

A

B

C

D

E

F, G. The posterior suture layer is completed, and the first layer anteriorly is begun by the insertion of interrupted sutures (00000 silk) at each angle of the anastomosis. Each of the "angle" sutures is inserted from the inside-out on one side to the outside-in on the other, so that, when tied, the knot of the suture is on the inside of the lumen. Inward traction on the previously inserted "angle" suture posteriorly facilitates inversion of the tissues (F). The remainder of the sutures that will comprise the first anterior layer of the anastomosis are simple interrupted through-and-through sutures that include all the layers of the ureter and colon (G).

H. The first anterior layer of the anastomosis is completed, and the second of a series of Lembert-Cushing mattress sutures (00000 silk), which comprise the second anterior layer, is being inserted.

I. The mattress sutures have been inserted and tied to complete the mucosa-to-mucosa end-to-side ureterosigmoidostomy.

The technic illustrated for the performance of a ureterosigmoidostomy is based on the principle of mucosa-to-mucosa union previously stressed by Cordonnier. This principle, long accepted in gastrointestinal surgery, has only relatively recently been established as of basic importance in the union of the ureter with the intestines.

In reviewing the development of surgery of the esophagus, the earlier technics were based on the "pull through" principle. The open transected end of the esophagus was left "dangling" in the lumen of the stomach, the anterior wall of which was anchored to the muscular wall of the esophagus about its circumference. This technic was subsequently discarded because esophageal stenosis inevitably occurred. It was only when the principle of mucosa-to-mucosa union was practiced that uniformly good results were obtained.

Similarly, in the development of uretero-intestinal anastomoses, the early technics, such as those established by Coffey, were on a modified "pull through" principle and did not effect an accurate mucosa-to-mucosa approximation. This is believed the basic cause for the failures that occurred. The same reasoning applies to the failures in the anastomoses of the common duct to the intestinal tract, an operation that is generally held, I believe unjustly, in bad repute.

It is a time honored observation that intestinal fistulas will not close spontaneously when the intestinal mucosa is adherent to the skin surface. In the anastomosis of a conduit to the intestinal tract, whether it be ureter, common duct, or pancreatic duct, an accurate mucosa-to-mucosa union precludes spontaneous closure of the stoma. Accordingly, this type of union is considered the best prophylaxis for stenosis of the stoma.

Finally, it cannot be overemphasized that regurgitation of intestinal contents through the anastomotic stoma is in itself of no consequence. It is the stenosis of the stoma and not the regurgitation through it that is the basic factor in the production of symptoms.

Plate 193

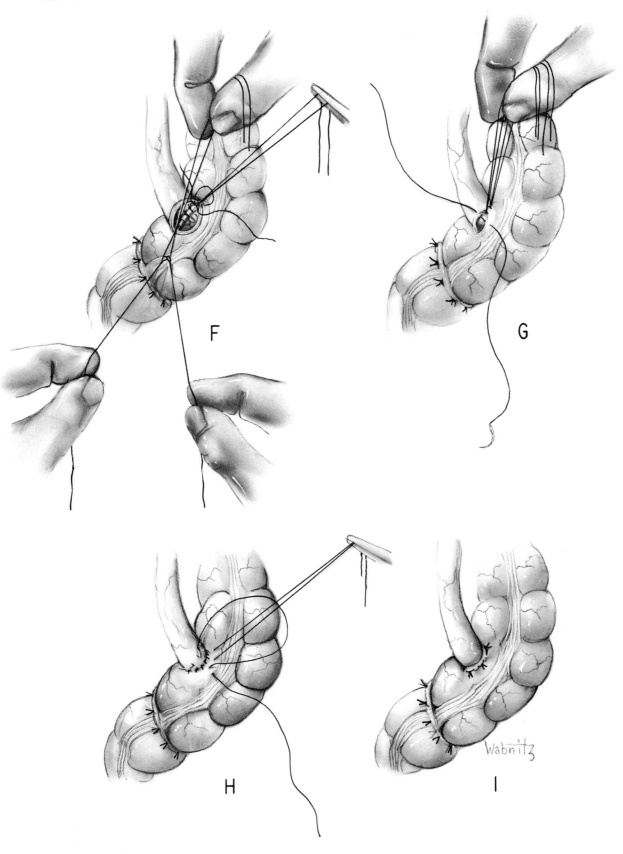

F

G

H

I

Wabnitz

CONGENITAL MEGACOLON (HIRSCHSPRUNG'S DISEASE)

A. The patient is placed in the supine position with the buttocks overhanging the edge of the operation table and the hips and knees maintained in a flexed position by suitable strapping. In this position the perineum and the lower abdomen are accessible surgically without moving the patient. The left rectus paramedian muscle-retracting (lateral) incision is indicated by the solid black line.

B. The peritoneal cavity is entered, and the dilated, redundant loop of sigmoid colon is exteriorized. The narrow segment of the colon distally in comparison with the dilated segment proximally is visible.

C, D. The mobilization of the sigmoid colon is begun by severance of the lateral parietal peritoneal reflection using scissor dissection (C). When this is completed, the three anatomic landmarks routinely demonstrated are the left ureter, the ovarian or spermatic vessels, and the superior hemorrhoidal artery (D).

E, F. The superior hemorrhoidal vessels are triply clamped and severed (dotted line) between the two most distal clamps (E). The two most proximal clamps are replaced by a ligature and a suture ligature respectively of 00 silk. Subsequently the mesentery of the sigmoid colon and its contained vessels are serially clamped, severed, and ligated, and the freed mesenteric border of the bowel wall is encircled by a tape of rubber tissue (F). The presacral areolar tissue space is entered by scissor dissection (F) prior to the mobilization of the rectum from the hollow of the sacrum.

DISCUSSION—DR. ROBERT B. HIATT. The positioning of the patient for a pull-through procedure is most easily done by lowering the foot of the operation table and placing the buttocks near the edge with the legs placed on arm boards and separated as far as possible. This allows easy access to the anus when the time comes to intussuscept the rectum and lower sigmoid through the anus.

While the incision depicted (Plate 194, A) is adequate for this procedure, I prefer the lower transverse incision with a cephalad curve above the left anterior superior spine. I find it easier to detach the splenic flexure through this incision if the aganglionic segment is unusually long, and the cosmetic result is much better.

If there is any doubt about the length of the aganglionic segment, one should take a button of muscularis from the anterior taenia for frozen section. It is not necessary to enter the lumen since one is primarily interested in the ganglion cells between the two muscle coats only. In freeing the rectum from its surrounding structure, the surgeon should keep in mind the importance of preserving the autonomic enervation of the bladder and seminal vesicles. To do this, the hypogastric plexus must be avoided by dividing the superior hemorrhoidal vessels as near to the rectum as possible. The presacral space can then be entered in the midline and the rectum separated from the sacrum, coccyx, and posterior levators. The lateral ligaments of the rectum (Plate 195, J) can then be stripped anteriorly to their attachments in each anterolateral angle of the rectum and subsequently divided between clamps adjacent to the rectum itself without compromising the sympathetic trunks as they swing from the hypogastric plexus around the lateral pelvic wall to enervate the bladder and seminal vesicles.

Plate 195, I, is most misleading because, in the male, this phase of the rectal dissection is of utmost importance and cannot be properly done by blunt dissection until Denonvillier's fascia is identified and separated from the rectum by sharp dissection. Once this is done and the bare muscularis of the anterior wall of the lower rectum visualized, the dissection can be easily completed to the anal level by blunt finger dissection.

If the surgeon uses the proper sequence in the rectal dissection, it is possible to accomplish all of the maneuvers under direct vision with controlled hemostasis. In principle it simply means performing all of the posterior maneuvers before attempting to dissect anything anteriorly. I will outline this sequence as follows: (1) Divide the superior hemorrhoidal ves-

Plate 194   445

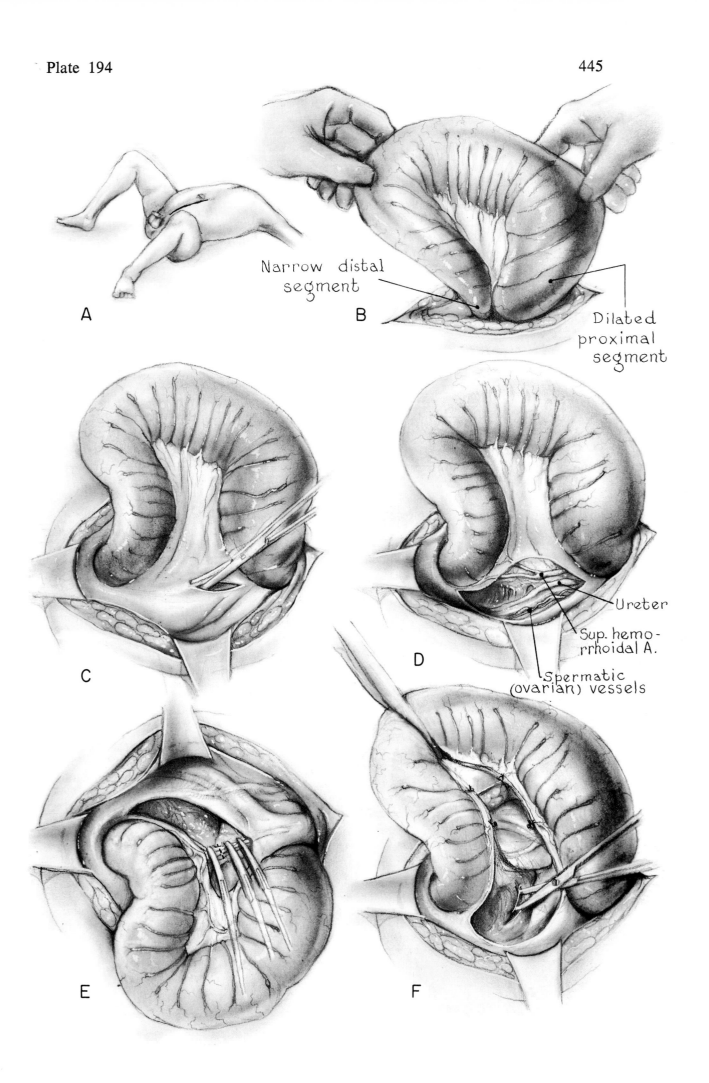

A

B   Narrow distal segment

Dilated proximal segment

C

D   Ureter

Sup. hemorrhoidal A.

Spermatic (ovarian) vessels

E

F

G. By blunt digital dissection in the presacral space, the rectum is mobilized from the hollow of the sacrum down to the tip of the coccyx.

H. The rectovesical fold of peritoneum is freed by blunt digital dissection and severed with scissors as depicted.

I. The lower cut margin of the rectovesical fold of peritoneum is retracted downward in a clamp (Babcock), and blunt digital dissection in the rectovesical space behind Denonvilliers' fascia is performed. In this dissection it is most important to enter the proper tissue plane to avoid injury to the prostate or seminal vesicles, as well as troublesome bleeding.

J. The right lateral ligament is being cut by scissor dissection. The severance of the left lateral ligament is indicated by the dotted line. In this dissection the middle hemorrhoidal vessels are severed, and if bleeding is excessive, the severed ends are clamped and ligated. Generally no untoward bleeding is observed.

K. The lateral ligaments are cut, and the mobilization of the rectum down to the levator floor is completed.

L. The anterior wall of the distal sigmoid colon is indented by the index finger, and the inverted wall is grasped in a ring clamp which is inserted through the rectum. By a combination of traction from below and digital inversion from above, the sigmoid colon is telescoped into the lower sigmoid segment and protruded inside-out through the anus. This is the technic advocated by Hiatt. If preferred, the recommendation of Swenson—transection of the sigmoid colon distally and closure of the proximal transected end—may be followed. The cut margins of the distal transected end are secured in two guy sutures of silk (00) which are withdrawn through the anus to turn the lower segment inside-out. The closed proximal transected end is then withdrawn through the anus with the distal segment encircling it as an everted sleeves. The proximal transected end is then opened, and a two-layer anastomosis between the everted (inside-out) lower segment and the pull-through proximal segment is performed.

DISCUSSION—DR. HIATT (cont.)

sels away from the hypogastric plexus just before the artery branches. (2) Enter the presacral space in the midline and separate the rectum from the sacrum, coccyx, and posterior perineum. To do this, it is usually necessary to divide the posterior attachments of the lateral ligaments of the rectum. (3) Strip the lateral ligaments of the rectum anteriorly to their ultimate attachments to the rectum in the anterolateral quadrants. (4) Divide these ligaments and the contained middle hemorrhoidal arteries between clamps close to the rectum. (5) Carefully separate Denonvillier's fascia from the anterior wall of the rectum by sharp dissection, and complete the distal dissection to the anus under direct vision.

Before everting the rectum through the anus, the distal dissection should be checked by having an assistant gently place his finger in the anal canal from below. The operating surgeon should then be able, from within the pelvis, to palpate the assistant's finger with ease around the entire circumference of the anorectal junction.

When the eversion of the rectum is being done by the assistant, the surgeon must be certain that the area of the sigmoid he has chosen to anastomose to the anus reaches the anal level accurately and without torsion. This is most easily accomplished by placing a stay suture in the anterior taenia at the point of election for anastomosis and holding the free end in one hand while checking its descent with the other hand until it lies accurately in the anterior anus. This can be checked by the assistant's palpating through the anterior portion of the everted anus.

It must be remembered that the levator ani muscle has its attachments to the external sphincter and not to the rectum. The dissection should be carried to the sphincter level so that, when the rectum is everted through the anus, the anus itself should also be everted. For this reason the illustrations M, N, O, P, and Q (Plate 196) are inaccurate. The circumferential incision in the anorectal junction should be made in the columnar epithelium of the everted anus within 0.5 to 1 cm. of the stratified squamous epithelium of the anus. It is an inadequate resection to leave any of the distal rectum in place. The technic as portrayed here is for congenital megacolon of the classic variety in which the aganglionic segment extends proximally to a point between the midrectum and midsigmoid. The megarectum (short aganglionic segment type) and the extremely long aganglionic segment, which extends to any point in the colon proximal to the sigmoid, require slightly altered technics for proper handling.

Plate 195

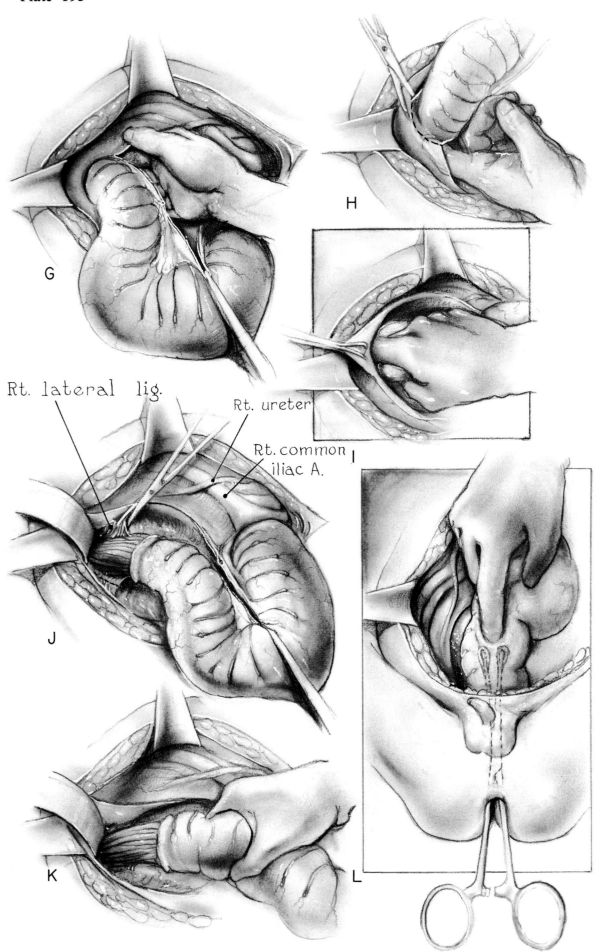

G

H

I

Rt. lateral lig.

Rt. ureter

Rt. common
iliac A.

J

K

L

M. Through guy sutures of silk (000), traction is maintained on the protruded segment of the colon, and a circular incision is made through the mucosa, muscularis, and serosa of the outer bowel wall.

N. This illustration shows the first or sero-serosal layer of silk sutures (000) being inserted.

O. The circular incision about the whole of the circumference of the outer wall of the telescoped segment of bowel and the first or seroserosal anastomotic layer are completed.

P. The distal cut margin of the outer bowel wall is pulled downward, and the length of the telescoped segment of bowel to be amputated is visible. An incision through the whole of the thickness of the "inner" bowel segment, serosa, muscularis, and mucosa is being made by scalpel dissection.

Q. The interrupted sutures (000 silk) which form the second layer of the anastomosis are inserted through the whole thickness of each segment of the bowel wall.

R. The insertion of two of the four quadrants of sutures (000 silk) which form the second layer of the anastomosis is completed, and the remaining attachment of the protruded bowel segment is being severed by scissor dissection.

S. The remaining two quadrants of sutures are inserted to complete the second layer of the anastomosis. The view is magnified for clarity.

T, U. By digital manipulation (T), the anastomotic ring is inverted into the anal canal to complete the operation. The appearance of the anus following this maneuver is normal (U).

DISCUSSION—DR. ORVAR SWENSON. Experience has proved that a more adequate suspension of the patient's legs than indicated in A is needed for this long operation. In order to prevent nerve damage, I have found it necessary to suspend the legs of infants and small children from a crossbar at the foot of the operation table with the use of adhesive tape. In older children, I prefer to tape the feet to a board and then tape the knees to a crossbar. In either position there is no damage to any of the peripheral nerves. I have found a vertical incision such as is shown in the drawings to be satisfactory. Providing a muscle-retracting incision is used, postoperative dehiscence is eliminated.

Beginning with E, my technic differs radically from that presented. In E, I do not ligate both the superior hemorrhoidal artery and vein. Rather, I ligate only the superior hemorrhoidal artery to reduce bleeding as the pelvic dissection progresses, and I leave the vein untouched so that there will be no venous obstruction which would actually increase bleeding in the pelvis. Blunt dissection in the pelvis, as shown in F, may be dangerous. Patients with associated defects in ennervation of the bladder who have been subjected to this type of dissection have suffered loss of their ability to initiate micturition. The dissection illustrated is actually the type used in cancer surgery, and it has no place in the treatment of megacolon. The dissection in a patient with Hirschsprung's disease should be carried out right on the bowel wall so that *the superior hemorrhoidal vessels and all adjacent soft tissues are left in place in the pelvis.* If care is taken to do this, there is no disturbance in ejaculation. In G the lateral ligaments are shown being divided some distance from the bowel. Here again, it is extremely dangerous to allow the dissection to wander away from the bowel surface. None of the drawings suggest how one may determine when the dissection should be terminated. There is, in fact, no landmark that will demonstrate absolutely, in every case, when this point is reached. I believe the only way to determine this is to divide and resect the bowel in the abdominal portion of the operation. First of all, this insures adequate material for biopsy to be sure ganglion cells are present at the proximal margin. In the second place, it leaves a short rectosigmoid and rectal stump that can be prolapsed readily and returned to the pelvic cavity if the dissection has not progressed far enough. The dissection is sufficient if one can observe continuity from the bowel wall to the skin when the prolapsed rectum is placed under traction and the perianal skin is given countertraction. If the telescoping technique is used, as depicted in the drawing, it is impossible to observe this because the anal canal is extremely full of prolapsed bowel and one cannot determine the extent of the pelvic dissection. Furthermore, in the event the surgeon feels the dissection has not been carried far enough, it is extremely difficult to replace all this into the pelvic cavity. A third advantage of the abdominal resection technic is that one can clean the area much more carefully, simply because there is not a great length of prolapsed bowel protruding from the anal canal.

The actual construction of the anastomosis is satisfactory. My only comment is that there is no indication as to just where the rectum should be cut across in relation to the mucocutaneous margin. I find that by actual measurement one should be within 2 or 3 cm. of the mucocutaneous margin anteriorly and 1 cm. posteriorly, which results in an oblique cut across the rectum that in its posterior aspect actually removes some of the internal sphincter.

In recent days there has been considerable discussion about the results of resection of the aganglionic segment in Hirschsprung's disease. The difference in reported results in all probability is related to technical differences in the way the operation is performed. In Europe the operation is performed as outlined in these illustrations. By and large, the results reported have not been as good as those obtained when there has been strict adherence to the principles set forth in this discussion.

Plate 196

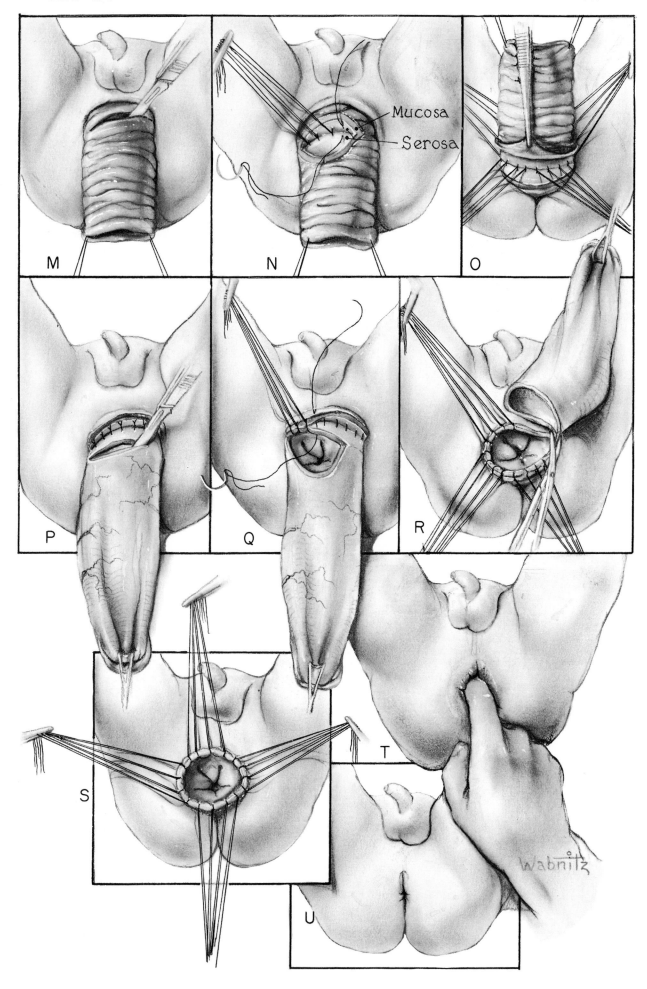

Mucosa

Serosa

M

N

O

P

Q

R

S

T

U

Wabnitz

IMPERFORATE ANUS

A. A sound is inserted into the rectal lumen through the ectopic anal opening in the fourchette. The vertical incision extending posterior from the fourchette through the dimple indicative of the normal site of the anus is depicted by the dotted line. This incision bisects the sphincter ani musculature.

B. The vertical incision is partially completed into the underlying subcutaneous tissue, and the circumscribed incision about the ectopic anus in the fourchette is shown in dotted outline.

C, D, E. Dissection is continued deeper into the underlying tissues, and the rectum is mobilized by scissor dissection.

F, G, H. The mobilization of the rectum is completed, and its relation to the transected perineal body and to the margins of the levator ani muscles is shown. A suture (00 silk) is being inserted (H) to approximate the fibers of the levator ani muscles in front of the mobilized rectum.

Plate 197   451

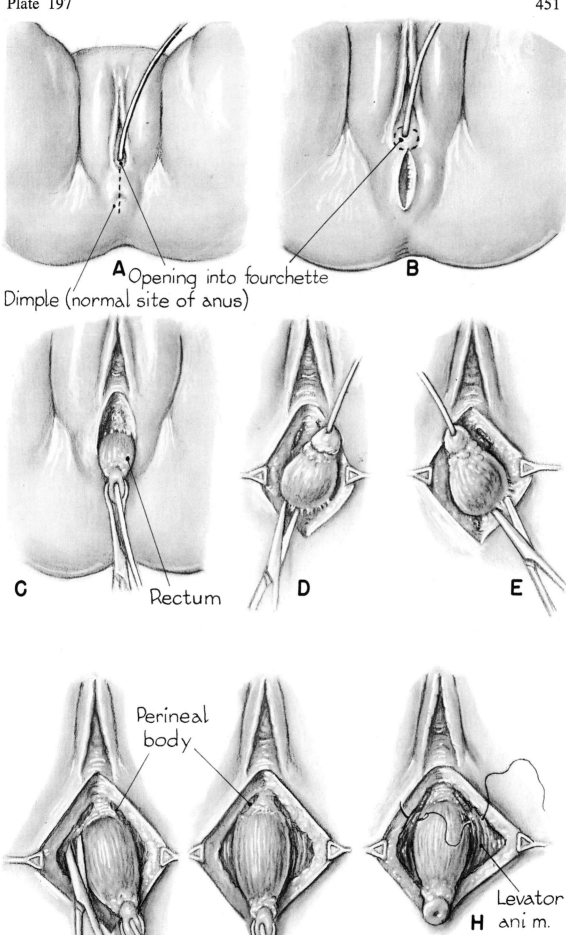

A Opening into fourchette

Dimple (normal site of anus)

B

C Rectum

D

E

Perineal body

F

G

H Levator ani m.

I, J, K. A second suture (00 silk) is inserted in the levator ani muscles (I) and tied (J) to complete the approximation of these structures anterior to the rectum. The first of two sutures is inserted in the transected ends of the perineal body (J), which are approximated when the sutures are tied (K). The skin closure of the perineum is begun by the insertion of a suture of 000 silk (K).

L. The last perineal skin suture anterior and the first one posterior to the rectum include a "bite" of its muscle layer.

M. The anchoring perineal skin sutures just inserted (L) are tied, and the site of transection of the rectum proximal to the contracted segment of the ectopic anal canal is indicated by the dotted line.

N. The transection of the rectum is being completed by scissor dissection.

O. The cut margins of the rectum are approximated to the surrounding skin margins by four cardinal guy sutures of silk (000).

P, Q. The four cardinal guy sutures are tied, and the intervening approximation sutures are all first inserted (P) and then tied (Q) to complete the construction of the new anus.

R. By digital manipulation, the perianal suture line is inverted into the rectal canal, and the relation of the patulous anal opening to the other structures in the perineum is visible.

This patient, a white infant girl, delivered spontaneously at full term, was perfectly normal with the exception of the ectopic anal orifice within the fourchette. The operation as illustrated was performed the day after birth, and the postoperative convalescence was uneventful. The follow-up period to date is 28 months. Except for occasional bouts of constipation, bowel function and control are completely satisfactory.

Plate 198

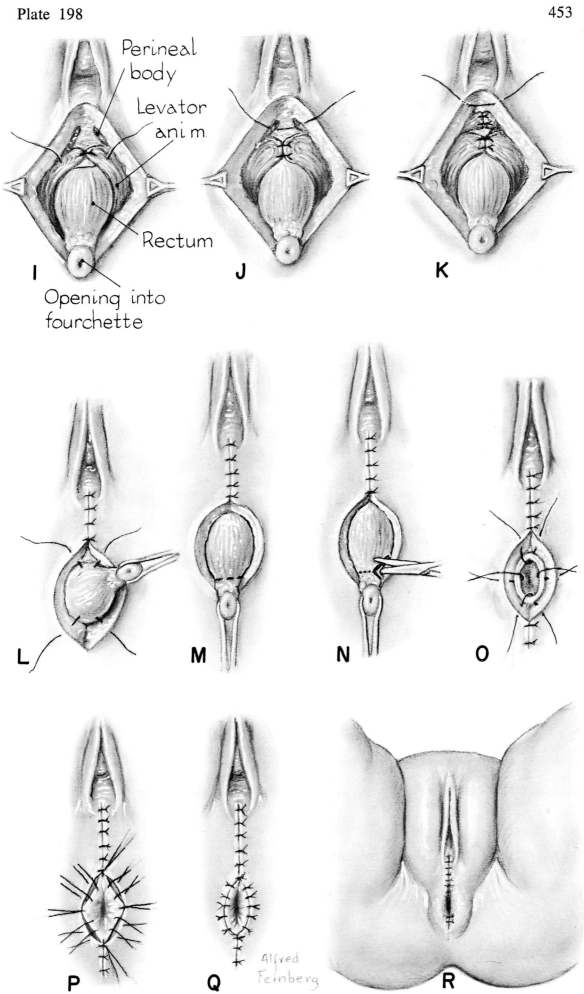

Perineal body

Levator ani m.

Rectum

I

Opening into fourchette

J

K

L

M

N

O

P

Q

Alfred Feinberg

R

EXCISION OF FISSURE IN ANO

A, B. The patient is placed in the prone modified "jackknife" position (Buie), and the buttocks are separated by adhesive tapes. The "sentinel pile" (Brodie) that is visible (A) is shown in a close-up view (B).

C. An anoscopic view within the anal canal shows the anatomic pathologic characteristics of a fissure in ano—(1) the "sentinel pile" of Brodie, (2) the fissure, (3) the hypertrophied anal papilla.

D. The mucocutaneous junction of the anus is retracted by triangular (Pennington) clamps placed at equidistant points about the anal orifice.

E. A curved probe is inserted to show the depth of the sinus beneath the lower margin of the fissure and leading into the base of the "sentinel pile."

F. The tip of the "sentinel pile" is grasped in a clamp, and, with downward traction maintained, a wide excision of the fissure is begun.

G. Traction on the "sentinel pile" is then directed upward, and the incision is continued on either side of the fissure into the mucosa of the anal canal to include the site of the hypertrophied anal papilla.

H. The wide excision of the fissure is completed, and a partial severance of the superficial fibers of the subcutaneous external sphincter muscle is being performed.

I, J. Upon completion of the partial sphincterotomy (I), the operative area is inspected for bleeding, and a narrow strip of sterile gauze impregnated with petrolatum is inserted into the anal canal (J).

K. A sterile gauze dressing is applied and subsequently secured by the use of a T-binder.

DISCUSSION—DR. CON AMORE V. BURT. It is rare that I do a simple excision of a fissure. Almost invariably, in my experience, there are associated hemorrhoids or large crypts. It seems desirable to remove these along with the fissure. It is most important to remove any associated anal papillae and to excise the mucocutaneous line above the fissure. Usually there is an enlarged papilla above the fissure.

It is important to have an adequate drainage area in the skin of the verge, as shown in H. If the external wound heals before that of the anal canal, the fissure persists.

The old fibrous tissue at the base of the fissure should be carefully removed. Usually this means excising the superficial surface of the underlying sphincter.

It is only in the old recurrent fissure that I feel it is necessary to incise the sphincter. I rarely do a sphincterotomy, and when I do, I make a much deeper cut into the sphincter than that shown in H and I. The proper use of local anesthesia in oil generally leaves the sphincter relaxed. In older people there is sometimes, around the entire anal canal, a rather marked degree of fibrosis, which must be broken down during the anal dilatation. In these cases a sphincterotomy is particularly desirable.

Since the passing of hard stools is the cause of most fissures, proper instructions as to bowel hygiene is an important consideration postoperatively. The use of zinc peroxide, local anesthesia in oil, antibiotics, mineral oil, and so forth is the same as prescribed for hemorrhoidectomy.

Plate 199   455

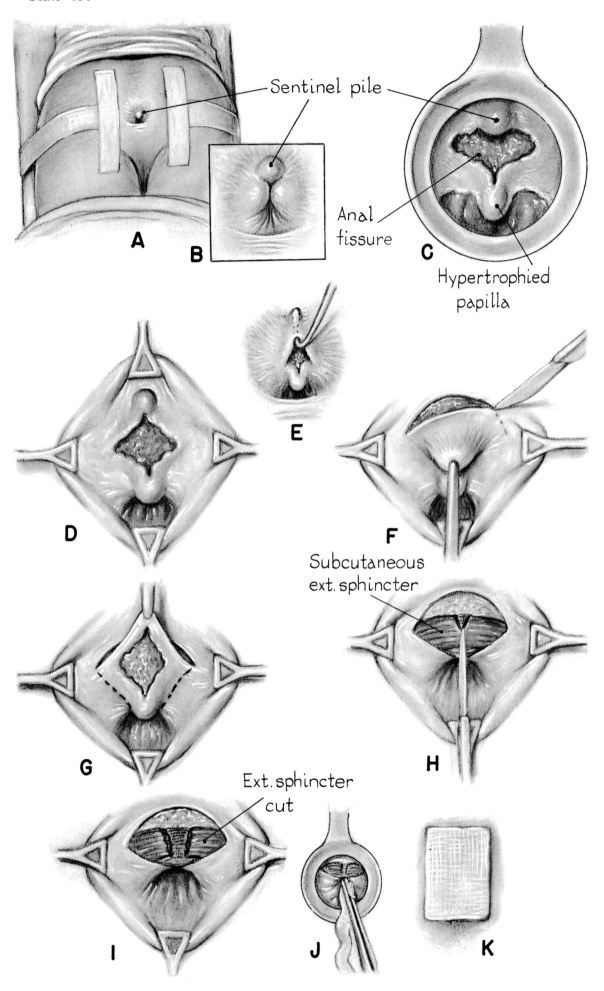

Sentinel pile

Anal
fissure

Hypertrophied
papilla

A

B

C

D

E

F

Subcutaneous
ext. sphincter

G

H

Ext. sphincter
cut

I

J

K

EXCISION OF FISTULA IN ANO

A. The patient is placed in the prone modified "jackknife" position (Buie), and the buttocks are separated by adhesive straps to expose the external opening of the fistula (seven o'clock) in relation to the anal orifice.

B, C. With the index finger in the anal canal for palpation, a probe is inserted through the external orifice of the fistula into the fistulous tract (B) and then through the internal opening into the anal canal (C).

D. The terminal portion of the probe, bent on itself, is extruded through the anal orifice, and the overlying tissue along the length of the fistulous tract is incised as indicated by the dotted line.

E, F. The chronically infected fibrous tissue base of the fistula and the surrounding indurated tissues are elliptically excised as demonstrated.

G, H. The new bed formed by healthy subcutaneous fatty tissue is loosely packed with a dry sterile gauze packing and subsequently covered with a compression gauze dressing to complete the operation. Excision of the fistula and primary closure of the defect is neither practiced nor recommended.

DISCUSSION—DR. CON AMORE V. BURT. Fistulas in ano may vary widely in degree and extent. I agree in general with the procedure of Dr. Madden in the very simple fistula. Most of mine, however, do not seem to be so simple. Again, there are usually associated internal hemorrhoids and generally many enlarged anal crypts from which most anal abscesses and subsequent fistulas result. It is my practice to always remove these hemorrhoids and crypts rather than subject the patient to another operation. Also, I think the wound heals better if these are removed at the same time.

In many instances in the more extensive fistulas, it is my usual practice to excise completely the fistulous process and repair the internal and external sphincters at the same time. This has saved many patients from some degree of incontinence and further operations. To promote proper drainage it is important to leave the skin and subcutaneous tissue open without suturing.

It is desirable to prepare the bowel with antibiotics and proper cleansing preoperatively. It seems to make little difference postoperatively whether the patient is kept without a bowel movement for 8 or 10 days or is given mineral oil and cathartics to promote normal function.

Many of these repaired sphincters become infected, and it is necessary to cut through the repair within 8 to 10 days postoperatively. However, the retraction of the sphincter ends is minimal, and usually incontinence is either minimal or absent. In the extensive fistulas, if the sphincters are not repaired, considerable incontinence is frequently observed.

If the fistula extends up along or close to the vaginal wall, it is extremely important to keep one finger in the vagina during the dissection. It is easy to buttonhole the vaginal wall and produce a rectovaginal complication.

Where previous operations have destroyed much of the sphincters, it is sometimes necessary to do a preliminary colostomy. Otherwise the repair of the fibrous-tissue-laden structures will not be successful.

The use of zinc peroxide, antibiotics, mineral oil, cathartics, and postoperative dilation once or twice a week to prevent adhesions and to relax the sphincters is similar to the postoperative care after hemorrhoidectomy.

Plate 200   457

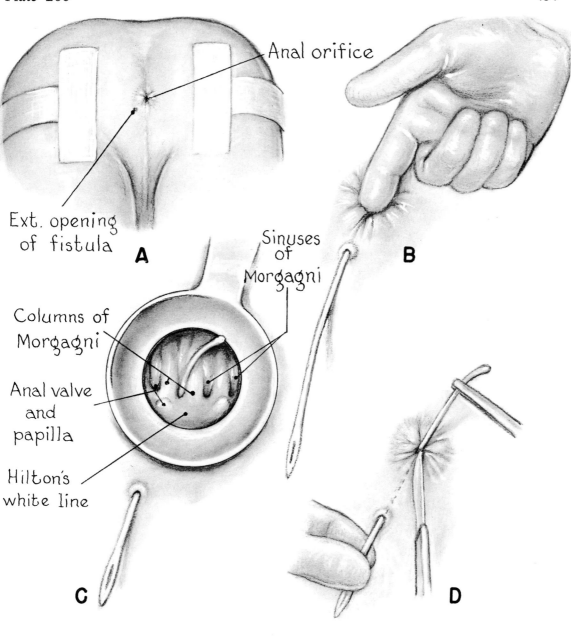

Anal orifice

Ext. opening
of fistula

A

B

Sinuses
of
Morgagni

Columns of
Morgagni

Anal valve
and
papilla

Hilton's
white line

C

D

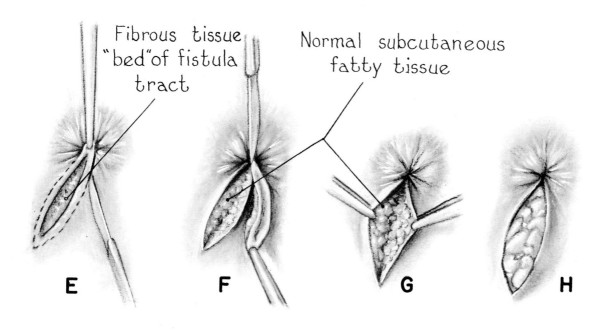

Fibrous tissue
"bed" of fistula
tract

Normal subcutaneous
fatty tissue

E   **F**   **G**   **H**

HEMORRHOIDECTOMY

A, B. The muscle structures of the perianal region (A) and the relation of the external and internal hemorrhoidal plexuses to the intermuscular septum and the adjacent muscles (B) are visible.

C. The patient is placed in the prone, modified "jackknife" position (Buie), and the ends of two gauze strips are protruded through the lumen of the anoscope previously inserted into the anal canal and lower rectum.

D, E. The anoscope is withdrawn over the gauze strips (D) which are subsequently withdrawn to evert the hemorrhoidal masses (E). With the patient in the prone position, the location of each primary hemorrhoid is shown. The subsequent steps in the illustrated technic are based on the principles set forth by Milligan of England.

F. Four Pennington clamps are placed equidistant from each other about the anal orifice, and a curved clamp is applied to the dentate line in relation to the primary hemorrhoid at one o'clock.

G. The Pennington clamp laterally is removed, and, with medial traction on the hemorrhoid through the curved clamp, an angular incision extending well on to the cutaneous margin is made laterally (dotted lines).

H. The tip of the cut margin of the angular incision is grasped in a clamp, and by a combination of traction and scalpel dissection the hemorrhoid is mobilized. In this mobilization the dissection is behind the hemorrhoidal mass and continued well beyond the subcutaneous external sphincter muscle which is an important anatomic landmark to be identified. Bleeding is usually minimal when this technic is used.

DISCUSSION—DR. CON AMORE V. BURT. It is my practice to place the patient in the lithotomy position, mainly because of the greater ease of administration of gas–oxygen anesthesia which I use as a supplement to local anesthesia–analgesia (eucupin in oil). Local anesthesia is fraught with some danger of abscess formation, but this has proved an infrequent complication. However, if the local anesthesia is not pooled and is evenly distributed there is diminution of postoperative pain and relaxation of the sphincters.

It is important to dilate the sphincters but not divulse or tear them. The sphincters are completely relaxed after the local in oil is placed subcutaneously and submucosally in the anal canal. Caution is observed to avoid injection into the muscles. The use of gauze for eversion of the hemorrhoids has not been necessary in my experience. I place Allis clamps anteriorly and bilaterally on the skin at the anal verge or over the subcutaneous sphincter. With gentle traction on these clamps, the hemorrhoids are completely exposed.

My primary incision is the same as shown in Plate 201, G and H, so as to include all of the redundant external tags. It is our objective to leave the perianal area streamlined. The patients object to tags postoperatively, and they are interpreted to be persistence of the hemorrhoids. In the excision, it is important to include the smaller or secondary hemorrhoids. One should be careful not to excise too high and too wide both in the internal and external hemorrhoidal zones, as this contributes to postoperative anal stenosis.

It is my practice to ligate the pedicle as shown in Plate 202, K and L, and then close the skin margins with the same suture running out to the anal verge. It is very important to leave open one area of excision, usually posteriorly, so that good drainage is provided. This reduces postoperative edema and discomfort. The drainage tract should extend outside the verge so that the external wound does not heal earlier than the wounds in the anal canal.

To reduce postoperative pain further, I usually instruct patients to eat lightly the day before operation and to take achromycin tablets (250 mg.) three times a day for three days preoperatively to sterilize the colon contents. An enema is given the day before operation and a sedative at bedtime. Postoperatively, antibiotics for four or five days, hot sitz baths and mineral oil (1 ounce) twice daily, and a cathartic the evening of the first postoperative day are prescribed. The mineral oil is continued until the wound is healed, which is about one month after operation.

At the completion of the operation, I place in the anal canal about six wicks of 1-inch gauze (folded) soaked in a zinc peroxide suspension. This is bacteriostatic for the anaerobic organisms, comes away easily, and reduces the odor.

Plate 201

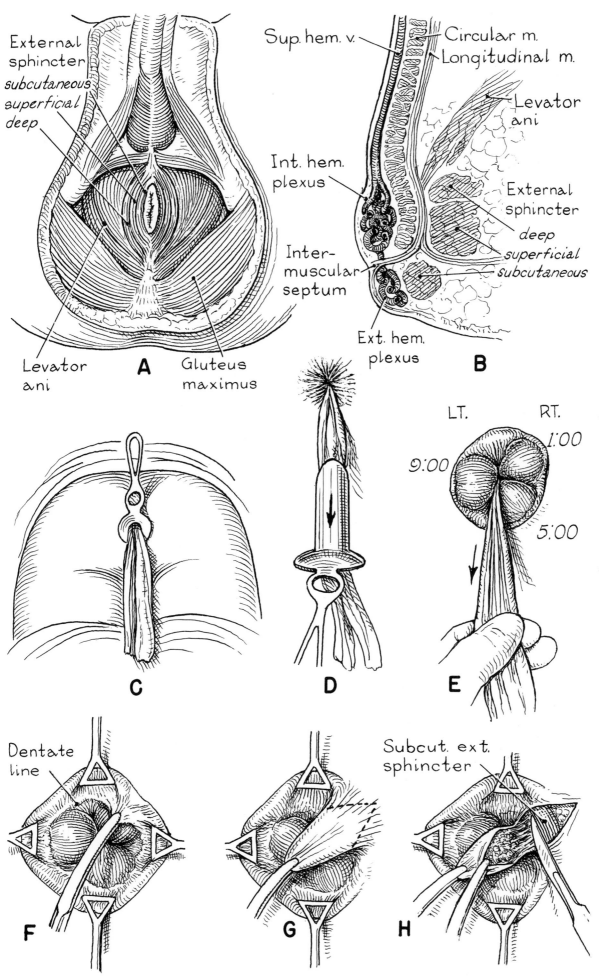

A

External sphincter *subcutaneous superficial deep*

Levator ani

Gluteus maximus

B

Sup. hem. v.

Circular m.

Longitudinal m.

Levator ani

Int. hem. plexus

External sphincter *deep superficial subcutaneous*

Intermuscular septum

Ext. hem. plexus

C

D

E

LT.

RT.

9:00

1:00

5:00

F

Dentate line

G

H

Subcut. ext. sphincter

I. Following completion of the dissection posteriorly the hemorrhoidal mass is displaced laterally, and the angular incision to be made in the mucous membrane is shown (dotted lines).

J. The mobilized hemorrhoidal mass is again displaced medially, and a ligature of 00 chromic catgut is being applied to the base of its pedicle.

K, L. The pedicle is doubly clamped and severed (dotted line) distal to the ligature (K), and a suture ligature of 00 chromic catgut is inserted in the pedicle between the remaining clamp and ligature (L).

M. The location of the ligature on the hemorrhoidal pedicle in relation to the external and internal hemorrhoids and the subcutaneous external sphincter is shown.

N. The mobilization of the primary hemorrhoid at five o'clock is being completed as previously described.

O. Upon completion of the hemorrhoidectomy the anoscope is reinserted, and the ligated pedicle of each primary hemorrhoid and the adjacent raw surfaces are carefully inspected for bleeding. If bleeding is present, hemostasis is obtained with suture ligatures of 00 chromic catgut. The stellate appearance formed by the raw surfaces after excision of the three primary hemorrhoids is visible. The extension of the incisions well onto the cutaneous margins minimizes postoperative tissue edema and pain. The insertion of a thin petrolatum gauze wick and the application of a sterile compression dressing complete the operation. Postoperative sedation is prescribed as required. The day after operation the vaseline gauze strip is removed and sitz baths twice daily are prescribed. Mineral oil (1 ounce) twice daily for four days is also prescribed. Subsequently, mineral oil (1 ounce) is ingested once a day every other day for the next seven days.

A, B, C, D. The technic for removal of a thrombotic external hemorrhoid is depicted. Using 0.5 ml. of procaine (1 per cent), a weal is raised in the mucous membrane overlying the thrombus (A). The mucous membrane is incised, and a portion of the overlying thrombus is visible (B). By blunt tissue dissection with a clamp the thrombus is evacuated (C, D). Bleeding is usually minimal and readily controlled by momentary pressure with a dry gauze sponge.

Plate 202   461

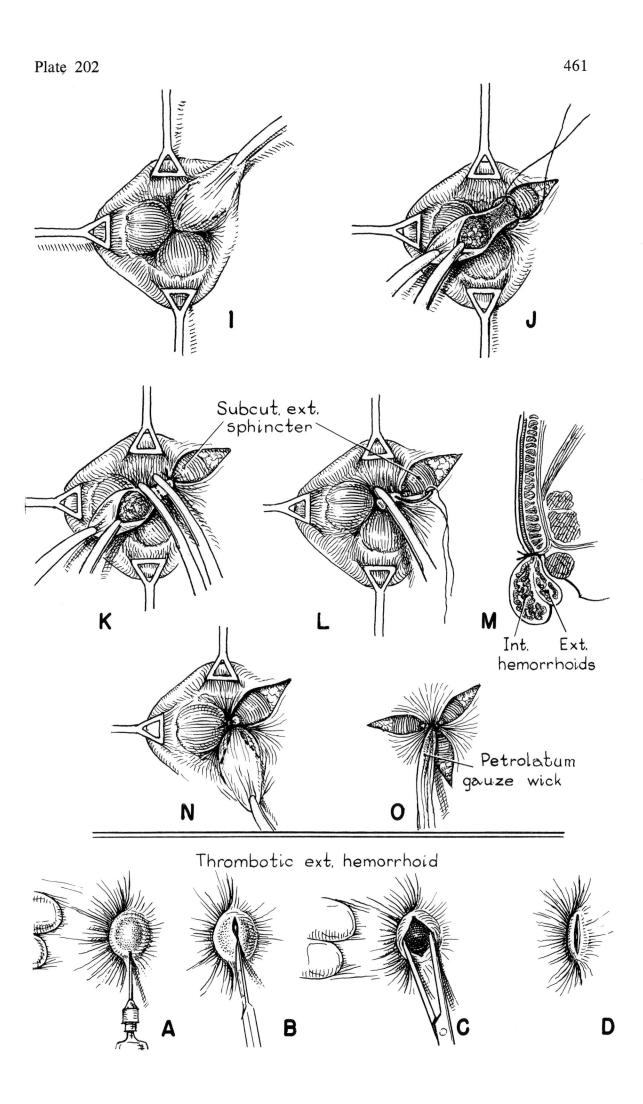

Subcut. ext.
sphincter

Int.   Ext.
hemorrhoids

Petrolatum
gauze wick

Thrombotic ext. hemorrhoid

I

J

K

L

M

N

O

A

B

C

D

LEFT HEPATIC LOBECTOMY

A. The longitudinal left upper quadrant par-amedian muscle-retracting (lateral) incision employed and the horizontal T-shaped extension to the right, which was required subsequent to exploration, are indicated in dotted outline.

B. The peritoneal cavity is entered, and the large protuberant tumor mass in the left lobe of the liver may be seen. The horizontal extension of the incision in the peritoneum is indicated by the dotted line.

C. The tumor mass, soft in consistency, is displaced digitally to the left as its fibrous tissue attachments are severed by scissor dissection.

D, E. The mobilization of the tumor mass is continued, and its deeper attachments to the anterior wall of the stomach and the left lobe of the liver are exposed and severed as indicated (E).

DISCUSSION—DR. ALEXANDER BRUNSCHWIG. The incision as illustrated in Plate 203, A, is unusual for exposure of the left lobe. I employ the high midline or left paramedian incision with horizontal component extending to the left. Under certain circumstances, I use a left high paramedian incision, with the upper end curving toward the left over the costal arch and transecting the arch without necessarily entering the left thoracic cavity (or pericardium). Division of the costal arch adds to retractability of the exposure incision.

Usually the left lobe does not have numerous adhesions about it. In some instances the left lobe may be quite adherent to a carcinoma of the stomach; this lobe is then excised en masse with the stomach.

Detachment of the falciform ligament may or may not be necessary, but, when carried out, it certainly adds mobility to the left lobe.

In this case, the tumor in the left lobe was removed separately, but usually the tumor and the left lobe are excised en masse. Benign or even malignant neoplasms sometimes are easily "cored out" of the liver, and there is surprisingly little bleeding from the bed. This is not often done intentionally.

Plate 203

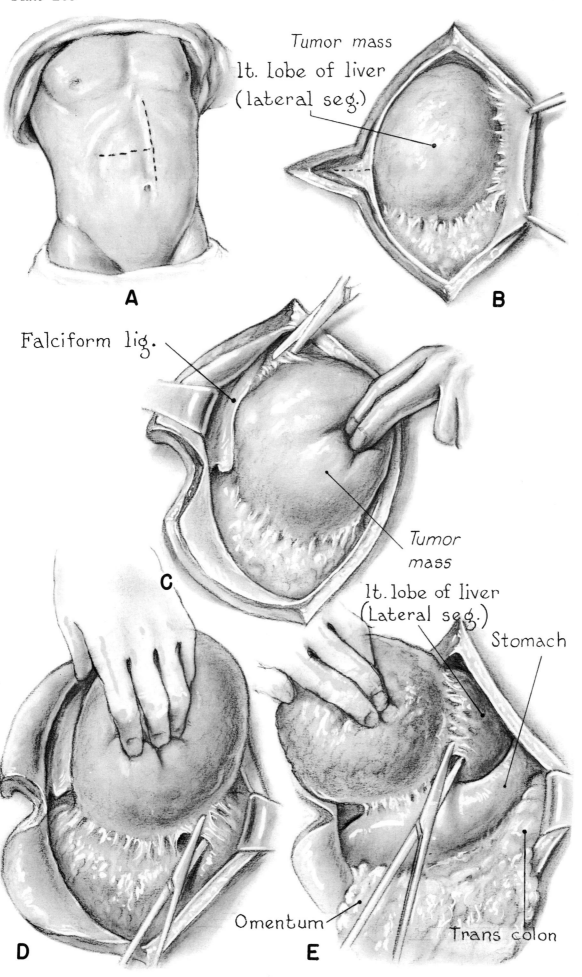

Tumor mass
lt. lobe of liver
(lateral seg.)

A

B

Falciform lig.

*Tumor
mass*

C

lt. lobe of liver
(Lateral seg.)

Stomach

Omentum

Trans colon

D

E

F. The dissection of the soft friable tumor mass from its bed in the lateral segment of the left lobe of the liver is completed. The tumor, a primary hepatoma, felt like a large incompletely organized hematoma. The removal of the protuberant portion of the tumor mass was not associated with undue hemorrhage and permitted the exposure of the underlying lateral segment of the left lobe of the liver and its contained residual tumor.

G. The left and right lobes of the liver are retracted upward to expose the site of the incision (dotted line) to be made in the gastrohepatic ligament.

H. The incision in the gastrohepatic and the hepatoduodenal ligaments is completed, and the underlying vascular and ductal structures are depicted. The large lymph node, uniformly present overlying the hepatic artery just distal to its bifurcation into hepatic propria and gastroduodenal branches, and the node characteristically found lateral to the terminal portion of the common bile duct are visible.

I. The left lobe of the liver is manually depressed downward, and its mobilization is begun by severance (dotted line) of the avascular left triangular ligament by scissor dissection.

DISCUSSION—DR. BRUNSCHWIG (cont.)

The approach to the porta hepatis is well illustrated in Plate 204, G and H, and, in the absence of fat and edema in the gastrohepatic ligament, the structures depicted may be fairly well visualized and palpated before any dissection is begun. During the identification and isolation of the left branch of the hepatic artery and left branch of the portal vein, it is very important to be on the alert for anomalies in the distribution of these vessels. As a matter of principle, they should be transected as near the liver as feasible. The right and left hepatic ducts join at varying levels, and the actual confluence may be partially or entirely within the hepatic parenchyma. The left hepatic artery and the left branch of the portal vein are the important structures to divide before the left hepatic duct is secured, although, for exposure, early transection of the left hepatic duct may be necessary. When the left hepatic artery and the left portal vein branch are divided, almost all of the left lobe will assume a dark bluish hue.

In dividing the left triangular ligament over the dome of the left lobe, care must be exercised as the transection is carried toward the midline, because an anomalous left hepatic vein within the mesial portion of the ligament may be inadvertently opened, with consequent severe hemorrhage.

The transection of the base of the left lobe is depicted in Plate 205, J, as beginning above and progressing downward. Personally, I begin this transection below and proceed upward—separating parenchyma by a somewhat teasing motion with the scalpel or by using the scalpel handle for such blunt dissection. In this manner the left lobe becomes finally detached except for the left hepatic vein, which is then doubly clamped and transected.

The inset Plate 205, J[1], depicts the true anatomic lobar division of the liver. Thus, if left hepatic lobectomy is defined as resection of the tissue to the left of the falciform ligament, it really represents resection of the left lateral segment of the liver.

The method, depicted in Plate 205, M, of covering the transected stump of the left lobe by turning the falciform ligament downward is one of several methods followed as a final step in this operation. Any method that a surgeon uses and that is found to give satisfaction may be employed. Personally, I leave perhaps a little more stump to the left of the falciform ligament and, as a final step, insert an over and over parenchymal compressing suture of No. 2 chromic catgut on a blunt-tipped large curved needle. The bites are taken through each margin of the base —anteriorly and posteriorly. If oozing is a little more marked, I tamponade the cut surface with long 4-inch wide gauze pack, allowing the end to protrude from the upper end of the wound. The pack is removed in toto in three or four days under pentothal anesthesia. One or two large soft rubber drains are inserted to the region of the lesser curvature of the stomach and brought out through a stab wound to the left of the midline incision.

Plate 204   465

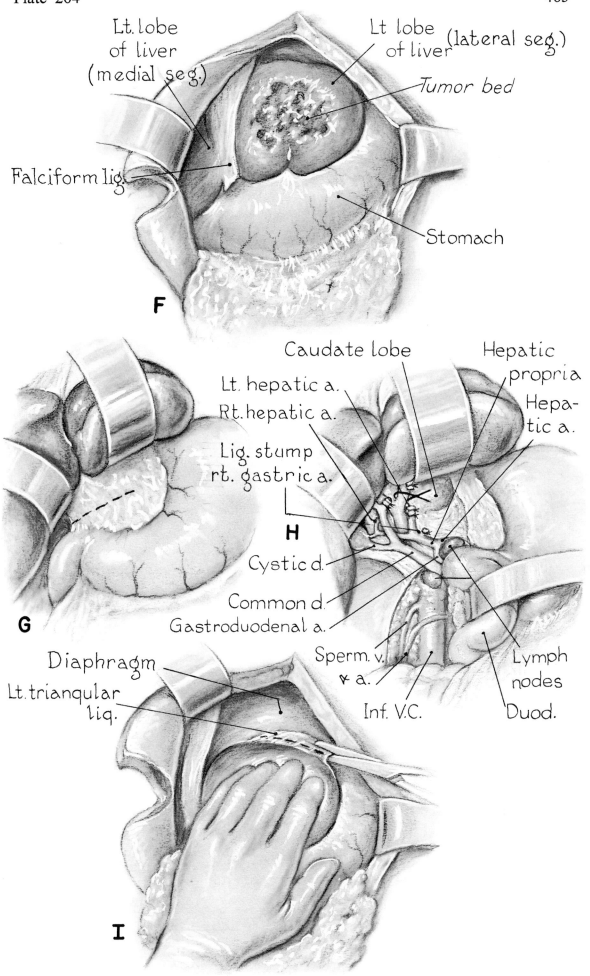

Lt. lobe of liver (medial seg.)

Lt lobe of liver (lateral seg.)

Tumor bed

Falciform lig.

Stomach

F

G

Caudate lobe

Hepatic propria

Lt. hepatic a.

Rt. hepatic a.

Hepa- tic a.

Lig. stump rt. gastric a.

H

Cystic d.

Common d.

Gastroduodenal a.

Sperm. v. & a.

Inf. V.C.

Lymph nodes

Duod.

Diaphragm

Lt. triangular lig.

I

J. The ligation and transection of the left hepatic duct, the left hepatic artery, and the left hepatic tributary of the portal vein are completed, and the resection of the lateral segment of the left lobe of the liver is begun by severance (scalpel) of the liver parenchyma in the intersegmental tissue plane between the medial and lateral segments of the left lobe of the liver. This plane is frequently and incorrectly referred to as the interlobar tissue plane. However, the true interlobar plane bisects the fossa of the gallbladder and the fossa of the inferior vena cava respectively (J¹). Accordingly, the left lobe of the liver is anatomically separated into two segments: (1) a medial segment located between the true interlobar plane previously mentioned and the falciform ligament; (2) a lateral segment between the falciform and left triangular ligaments which is commonly and incorrectly referred to as the left lobe of the liver (J¹). A portion of the left hepatic vein tributary is visible. This vein drains the entire lateral segment of the left lobe and the superior area of the medial segment of the left lobe of the liver. It normally unites with the middle hepatic vein to form a common hepatic venous trunk, as first stressed by Rex, which empties into the inferior vena cava. The middle hepatic vein drains the inferior area of the anterior segment of the right lobe and the inferior area of the medial segment of the left lobe of the liver. In the performance of a resection of the whole of the lateral segment of the left lobe of the liver, the potential danger of inadvertently ligating the common venous channel formed by the left hepatic and middle hepatic veins is decidedly less when compared to the performance of a right hepatic lobectomy, as is subsequently shown.

J¹. This inset shows schematically the plane of the true lobar division of the liver into right and left lobes. This plane bisects the gallbladder and inferior vena cava respectively. The separation of the left lobe into medial and lateral segments is also depicted. Accordingly, it is an error in anatomy to speak of the lateral segment of the left lobe as if it were the whole left lobe of the liver.

K, L. The left hepatic vein tributary is severed and ligated, and the incision in the liver parenchyma is deepened to the plane of the tributaries of the left portal vein between the medial and lateral segments of the left lobe of the liver. This is accomplished with negligible bleeding because of the preliminary extrahepatic ligation of the vascular supply to the left lobe of the liver. The intersegmental tributaries of the left portal vein are individually doubly clamped, severed (dotted line) (K), and ligated (L) to complete the total resection of the lateral segment of the left lobe of the liver (L). The ligated stumps of the vascular and duct structures to the left lobe of the liver are visible.

M. The resection of the whole of the lateral segment of the left lobe of the liver is completed, and the raw surface of the medial segment of the left lobe is covered by the falciform ligament which is anchored to the subjacent tissues with sutures of 000 silk.

N. The operative field, upon completion of the operation and the insertion of two cigarette drains (Penrose), is shown.

O. The wound closure is in layers, using a continuous interlocking double strand suture of 00 chromic catgut for the peritoneum, as shown, interrupted sutures of 00 silk for the fascia, and 000 silk for the skin. The drains have their exit through the incision rather than through adjacent stab wounds.

Plate 205

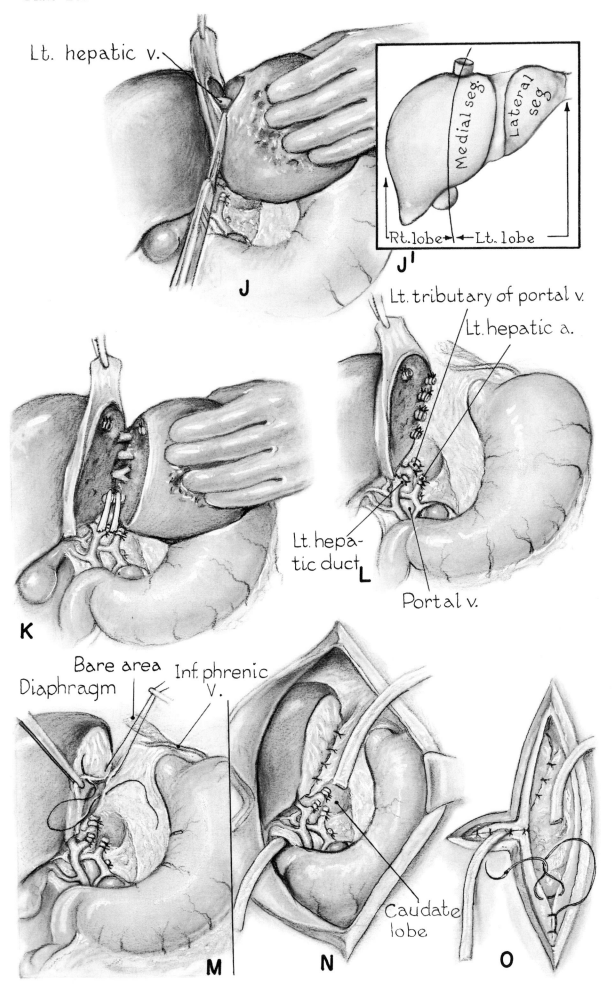

Lt. hepatic v.

Medial seg.

Lateral seg.

Rt. lobe — Lt. lobe

J¹

J

Lt. tributary of portal v.

Lt. hepatic a.

Lt. hepatic duct

L

Portal v.

K

Bare area

Diaphragm

Inf. phrenic v.

Caudate lobe

M

N

O

RIGHT HEPATIC LOBECTOMY

A. The right side of the patient is elevated on a pillow support, somewhat higher than that indicated in the illustration, and the thoraco-abdominal incision (ninth interspace) routinely employed is shown by the solid black line.

B. The incision is completed to convert the peritoneal and right pleural cavities into one common cavity. The resultant exposure of the underlying viscera is shown.

C. The right lobe of the liver is manually displaced toward the midline preparatory to severance of the right triangular ligament by scissor dissection.

D, E. The undersurface of the liver is exposed, and the gastrohepatic and hepatoduodenal ligaments are incised to demonstrate the structures within the hepatic trinity. In E, these structures are more clearly defined,

and the retrocolic portion of the duodenum is mobilized and retracted toward the midline to show the subjacent retroperitoneal structures. The right adrenal gland, in relation to the superior pole of the kidney, and the entrance of the right adrenal vein into the inferior vena cava are also visible. The characteristic locations of the lymph nodes, in relation to the hepatic artery, and the distal portion of the common duct are depicted.

F. This is a schematic illustration to show the completion of the ligation and severance of the right hepatic artery, the cystic duct, the right hepatic duct, and the right hepatic tributary of the portal vein. The passage of the portal vein beneath the arch formed by the gastroduodenal branch of the hepatic artery is also visible. This is an important anatomic landmark surgically for the identification of the portal vein.

DISCUSSION—DR. ALEXANDER BRUNSCHWIG. The incision as depicted in Plate 206, A, indicates more of a thoracic than an abdominal component. In making thoracoabdominal exposure for the right hepatic lobectomy, I usually perform a high right rectus incision with extension of the upper end obliquely upward to the right and over the costal arch in the eighth interspace for not more than 4 inches. The right cartilaginous costal arch is severed, and the diaphragm is split down to the inferior vena cava. After transection of the right triangular ligament and division of the falciform ligament, the whole liver is rotated upward. The incision described permits free access to the porta hepatis as indicated in Plate 206, E. I usually do not mobilize duodenum and head of pancreas as shown, nor do I particularly visualize the right suprarenal gland. The first step that I carry out is isolation and transection of the cystic duct. The right branch of the hepatic artery, the right branch of the portal vein, and the right branch of the hepatic duct are identified, isolated, and transected well out to the right in the porta hepatis rather than in the midportion of this region. After the right hepatic artery and the right branch of the portal vein are divided, most of the right lobe turns a bluish color, with a 2 to 3 cm. wide zone of the right lobe to the right of the falciform ligament retaining its normal color. In Plate 207, G, H, and I, the rotation of the right lobe to the left to expose the hepatic veins going into the vena cava is well demonstrated. As soon as they are identified, they are doubly clamped with small

hemostats and ligated, using silk for all the ligatures. There may be considerable variation in the anatomy of the principal hepatic vein draining the right lobe and emptying into the inferior vena cava; also, in the large central hepatic vein, which may enter the inferior vena cava directly or join with the right hepatic vein to form a common trunk or even join with the left hepatic vein to form a large single hepatic vein emptying into the vena cava. Not infrequently I search for the terminations of the right hepatic vein and the central hepatic vein by permitting the right lobe to fall back into normal position and inserting a retractor over the upper surface of the liver just to the right of the falciform ligament. When this retractor is pulled downward, the large trunks mentioned above can sometimes be visualized as they go into the inferior vena cava. Thus, they can be traced backward into the liver where they may be secured and divided. Some blunt dissection with the scalpel handle may greatly facilitate the exposure.

Too much emphasis cannot be placed upon the importance of isolation of the large right and middle hepatic veins with sparing of the left hepatic veins during right hepatic lobectomy. It is in carrying out these steps that very severe hemorrhage might arise, and, of course, in clamping bleeding areas, great care must be exercised not to clamp too much. Likewise, in clamping and dividing the shorter and smaller hepatic veins coming from the lower portions of the right lobe directly into the vena cava, great care must be taken to avoid tearing the inferior vena cava itself, since such tearing may lead to disaster. The dis-

Plate 206

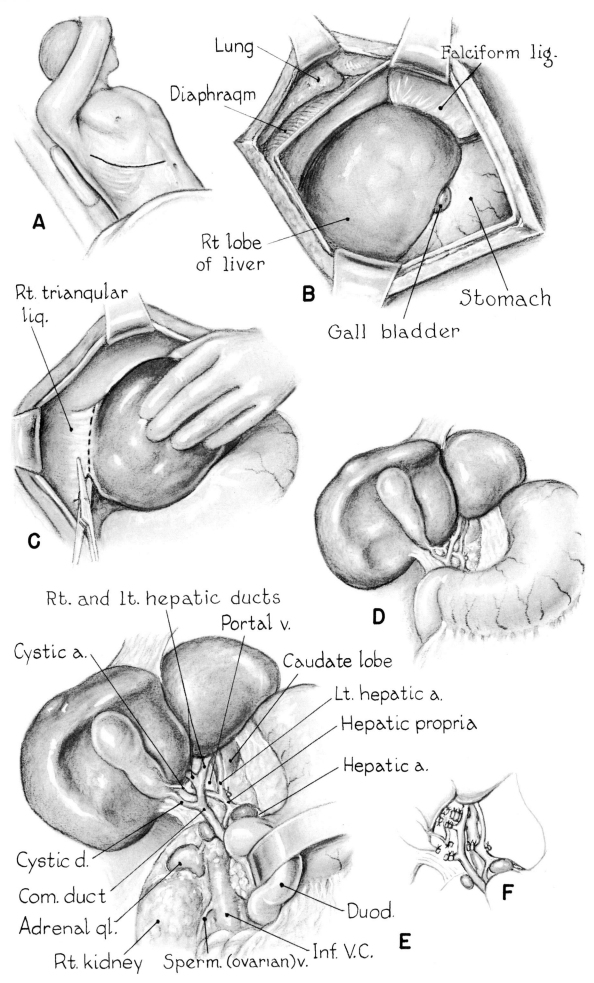

A

Lung

Diaphragm

Falciform lig.

Rt lobe
of liver

B

Stomach

Gall bladder

Rt. triangular
lig.

C

D

Rt. and lt. hepatic ducts

Portal v.

Cystic a.

Caudate lobe

Lt. hepatic a.

Hepatic propria

Hepatic a.

Cystic d.

Com. duct

Adrenal gl.

Rt. kidney   Sperm. (ovarian) v.

Duod.

Inf. V.C.

E

F

G, H. The right lobe of the liver is manually retracted toward the midline as dissection of the "bare" area (G), enclosed by the attachments of the right triangular ligament, is continued to expose the inferior vena cava and its two major right hepatic vein tributaries, two minor right hepatic vein tributaries, and right adrenal vein tributary (H).

I. The ligation and severance of the first plane of hepatic veins which drain the right lobe of the liver is completed, and the second plane of smaller hepatic veins draining the posterior surface of the right lobe of the liver is visible.

J. The ligation and severance of the first and second planes of hepatic veins which drain the right lobe of the liver are completed, and the formation of a common hepatic vein tributary of the inferior vena cava by the union of the middle and left hepatic veins, as previously mentioned in the description of left hepatic lobectomy, may be seen. Accordingly, in the performance of a right hepatic lobectomy, it is most important that the middle hepatic vein be ligated proximal to this common channel of communication to prevent obstruction of the venous drainage of the lateral segment of the left lobe of the liver through the left hepatic vein.

K. The right lobe of the liver is replaced into its normal position, and the hepatic parenchyma is incised (scalpel) to the plane of the intersegmental tributaries of the left portal vein. The union, within the liver substance, of the middle and left hepatic veins, draining the medial and lateral segments respectively of the left lobe of the liver, to form a common hepatic vein tributary of the inferior vena cava is again visible. The danger of compromise of the venous outflow of the lateral segment of the left lobe of the liver by inadvertent ligation of the common channel of communication rather than selective ligation of the middle hepatic vein is apparent.

L. The hepatic parenchyma is incised in the intersegmental plane to the right of the falciform ligament to expose the intersegmental tributaries of the left portal vein, which are doubly clamped and severed (dotted line) prior to ligation (00 silk). As previously stated in reference to left hepatic lobectomy, if preliminary extrahepatic selective ligation of the vascular supply to the right lobe of the liver is performed, there is minimum bleeding from the incised liver tissue.

DISCUSSION—DR. BRUNSCHWIG (cont.)

tribution of hepatic veins, their size, and the ease with which they are isolated and clamped may be seriously altered by the presence of large bulky tumor masses in the right lobe. Such tumor-bearing right lobes are extremely friable, and, even with the most gentle manipulation, the right lobe may suddenly fissure or splinter causing severe hemorrhage. Another point to emphasize in regard to the shorter hepatic veins entering the vena cava below the entrance of the one or two large hepatic veins mentioned above is the fact that the shorter veins might be draining both lobes of the liver even though they appear to enter the vena cava entirely from the right lobe.

It is my own practice to transect the base of the right lobe 1½ to 2½ cm. to the right of the falciform ligament within the narrow zone of unchanged color of parenchymal tissue and accept what bleeding may occur. Such bleeding can be controlled by clamping the individual bleeding points.

The statements which I have made relative to the treatment of the stump of the left lobe apply equally well to the treatment of the stump of the right lobe.

In connection with hepatic lobectomies, I always use silk for all vessel and bile duct ligations.

I agree with the method described in terminating the operation as shown in Plate 208, O, P, and Q, but in some instances I leave a hard rubber drain connected to a negative suction apparatus in the upper right portions of the abdomen for 48 or 72 hours. In some instances, although the right costal arch may be divided, actual entry into the right pleural cavity is not necessary and is not carried out. The advantages of this are obvious in that complications relative to right thoracotomy are avoided. Where the right diaphragm has been split throughout most of its length, i.e., down to the inferior vena cava, repair is made by carefully placed and tied interrupted silk or linen sutures.

An alternate method for amputation of the right lobe consists of insertion of two rows of compressing sutures 2 cm. apart and incision downward between these two rows to a depth of about 2 cm. where two more rows of compressing sutures are inserted. This procedure is continued until the whole thickness of the base of the right lobe is transected. The surgeon must be constantly on the lookout for large vessels and bile ducts. When these are seen, they are bluntly dissected, doubly clamped, ligated, and transected. This type of guillotine amputation of the right lobe may be carried out in combination with a preliminary transection of the large vessels and ducts as shown in Plate 206, E and F.

Plate 207 471

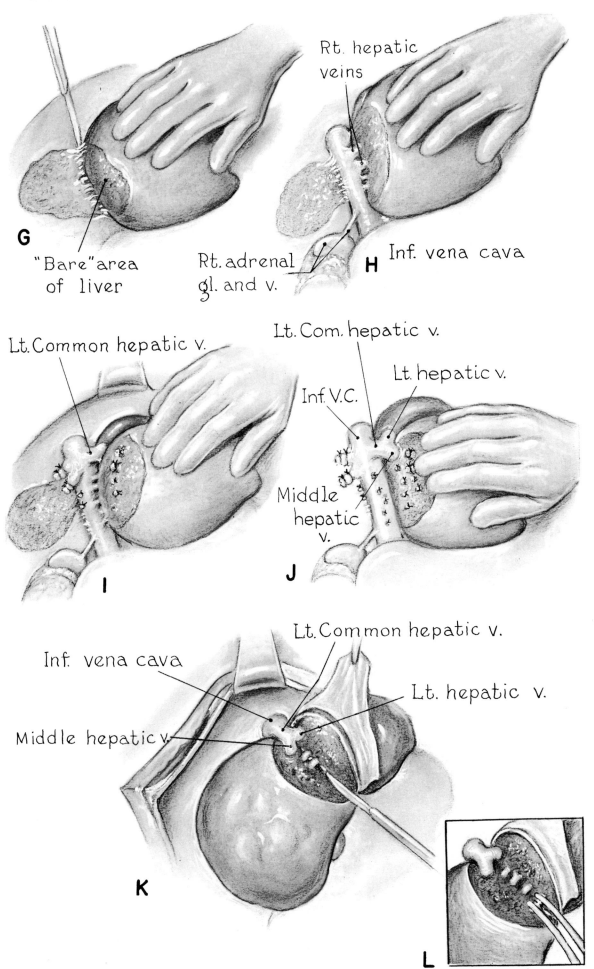

G "Bare" area of liver

Rt. hepatic veins

Rt. adrenal gl. and v.

H Inf. vena cava

Lt. Common hepatic v.

I

Lt. Com. hepatic v.

Inf. V.C.

Lt. hepatic v.

Middle hepatic v.

J

Inf. vena cava

Lt. Common hepatic v.

Lt. hepatic v.

Middle hepatic v.

K

L

M. The middle hepatic vein, which drains the inferior area of the anterior segment of the right lobe and the inferior area of the medial segment of the left lobe of the liver, is clamped and severed, and its cephalad end is occluded with a ligature and a suture ligature respectively of 00 silk.

N, O. The right hepatic lobectomy is completed (N), and the raw surface of the lateral segment of the left lobe of the liver is covered by suture (000 silk) of the falciform ligament to the subjacent structures (O).

P. The operative field, upon completion of the operation and the insertion of a cigarette drain (Penrose), is shown.

Q. The wound is closed in layers. Water-seal drainage (Foley catheter No. 16 F) of the right pleural cavity through a stab wound site subjacent to the incision is routinely practiced. The intraperitoneal drain has its exit through the abdominal incision rather than through a separate stab wound drainage site.

Plate 208   473

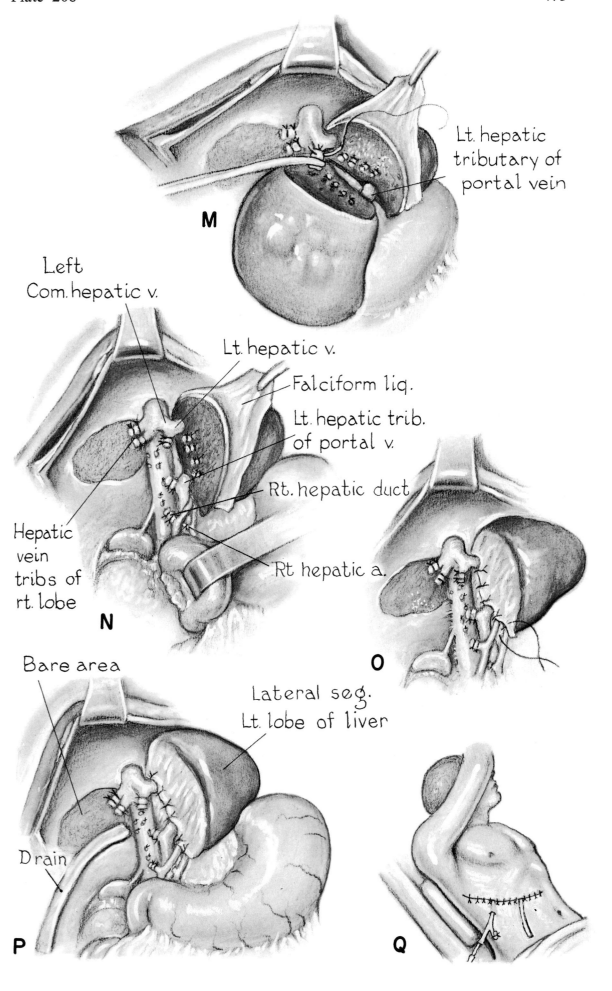

M

Lt. hepatic
tributary of
portal vein

Left
Com. hepatic v.

Lt. hepatic v.

Falciform lig.

Lt. hepatic trib.
of portal v.

Rt. hepatic duct

Hepatic
vein
tribs of
rt. lobe

Rt hepatic a.

N

O

Bare area

Lateral seg.
Lt. lobe of liver

Drain

P

Q

CHOLECYSTECTOMY

A. An oblique right paramedian muscle-retracting (lateral) incision, depicted by the solid black line, is the one of choice. If preferred, either a subcostal or transverse incision, as shown in dotted outline, may be used.

B, C. The anterior rectus sheath is incised, and the medial border of the right rectus muscle is mobilized by a combination of sharp and blunt dissection from its midline attachment and retracted laterally. Accordingly, the nerve supply to the muscle is not interrupted.

D, E. Upon entrance into the peritoneal cavity, the intraperitoneal and the adjacent retroperitoneal viscera are carefully explored, and a record of the findings is made. A curved (Kelly) clamp is placed upon the fundus of the gallbladder, and the right hand is inserted over the dome of the right lobe of the liver into the subphrenic space. The clamp on the gallbladder is held in the left hand, and, while traction is maintained

upward, the right hand is used to rotate manually both the inferior surface of the liver and the gallbladder into the operative field (E).

F. To isolate the operative field, three medium-sized moist gauze pads are used. One is placed over the anterior surface of the stomach, another is inserted into the hepatorenal (Morison) space, and a third is placed over the transverse colon and the first portion of the duodenum. A second curved (Kelly) clamp is placed upon the gallbladder in the region of its ampulla, and, with traction maintained upward, the cholecystoduodenal ligament is made taut prior to its division by scissor dissection.

G. The dissection of the cholecystoduodenal ligament is completed to expose both the cystic duct and artery and their related structures. The long cystic duct and the origin of the cystic artery from the convex arch formed by the right hepatic artery are clearly visible.

DISCUSSION—DR. FRANK GLENN. The abdominal incision that promises the best exposure of the biliary fossae should be determined by the surgeon for each patient. Over the years it seems to me that the subcostal approach (Plate 209, A) has been the one most often used. However, muscle-reflecting incisions (Plate 209, B, C) are much more comfortable for the patient. Dislocation of the liver (Plate 209, D) is a useful maneuver but is not always needed if the exposure is good. Linear incisions parallel to the common duct and made just through the peritoneum after dividing any cholecystoduodenal adhesions enable one to ⸱ visualize the cystic duct with minimal effort.

Identification of the cystic duct and the placing of a ligature about it enable one to place traction upon it so that the next step of identification and dissection of the cystic artery as it enters the gallbladder can be done with safety under clear vision. It is here that mistaken identity of strictures may result in common duct injury. Even where these structures are satisfactorily identified and when retrograde removal of the gallbladder is planned, it is recommended that the cystic artery be divided just proximal to its bifurcation as it enters the gallbladder wall and before the cystic duct is transected.

In retrograde removal of the gallbladder (Plate 211, P, P'), sharp dissection, keeping close to the

Plate 209

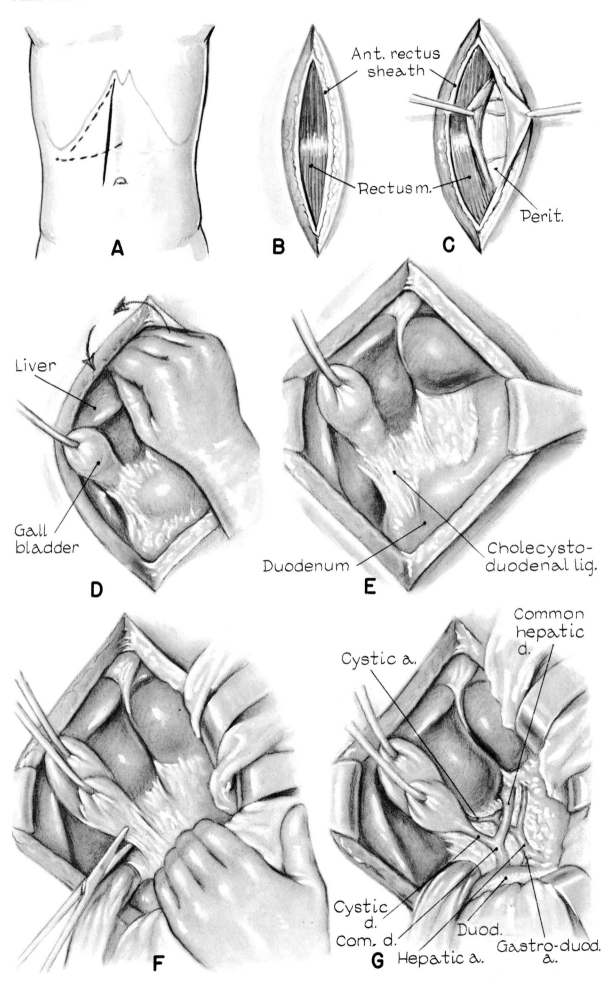

A

B

Ant. rectus
sheath

Rectus m.

C

Perit.

Liver

Gall
bladder

D

Duodenum

Cholecysto-
duodenal lig.

E

F

Cystic a.

Common
hepatic
d.

Cystic
d.

Com. d.

Duod.

Hepatic a.

Gastro-duod.
a.

G

H, H¹, I. The cystic duct and the cystic artery are individually doubly clamped and severed, and the proximal ends are occluded with both ligatures and transfixion suture ligatures of silk (000). To facilitate the division of the cystic duct and artery, a curved (Kelly) clamp is applied distally and a right angled (Mixter) clamp is applied proximally.

J. If preferred, the proximal ligatures may be applied prior to the application of clamps to either the cystic duct or artery.

K, L. The cystic duct and cystic artery are in turn doubly clamped and severed, and transfixion sutures of silk (000) are inserted as previously described.

M. An unusually short cystic artery is demonstrated which permitted the application of only one clamp distal to which the artery was divided.

N. The right hepatic artery courses anterior to the common hepatic duct, and from its convex arch a short cystic artery arises. This anatomic finding demonstrates the absolute necessity for careful tissue dissection and the individual isolation of structures to lessen the chance of injury to the right hepatic artery. Whenever the cystic artery is either shorter than the cystic duct (M) or anterior to the common hepatic duct (N), it is clamped and severed first. If this precaution is not observed, there is danger of an avulsion tear of the artery with resultant hemorrhage.

O. Upon completion of the severance and ligation of both the cystic duct and cystic artery, traction is maintained upward on the gallbladder and an incision is made through its peritoneal covering in juxtaposition to the inferior surface of the liver.

DISCUSSION—DR. GLENN (cont.)

gallbladder wall particularly in the proximal one third, enables one to visualize more readily accessory bile ducts extending from the liver into it. It also affords protection to biliary channels within the liver adjacent to the gallbladder bed. Scarring and distortion of these is frequent in longstanding and recurrent cholecystitis. Every effort should be made not to cut into liver tissue. It is preferable to open into the gallbladder rather than into a bile channel in the liver. Finger dissection (Plate 211, Q) may result in dividing the liver with subsequent oozing of blood and bile. Again sharp dissection enables one to avoid this. Approximation of the margins of the peritoneum from which the gallbladder was dissected (Plate 211, T, U, R) should be done only when it can be accomplished without tension. Meticulous attention to hemostasis and recognition of injured bile channels should precede this step if it is carried out.

DISCUSSION—DR. ROBERT S. SPARKMAN. It is my opinion that in all instances cholecystectomy can be performed more safely by removing the gallbladder from above downward rather than from below upward. This allows one to straighten out the mobilized gallbladder and cystic duct and to demonstrate more clearly the junction between the cystic duct and common duct before clamping or dividing the cystic duct. Moreover, it is easier to see and ligate all structures in the bed of the gallbladder and in the serosal cuff if the dissection is carried out from above downward.

Two preliminary steps are accomplished, as follows: (1) division and ligation of the cystic artery and (2) provisional ligation of the cystic duct at or near its junction with the gallbladder. This ligature serves to prevent displacement of stones from the gallbladder into the common duct during surgical manipulation of the gallbladder.

If the cystic artery cannot be seen readily, it usually can be located by identifying any arterial branch on the wall of the gallbladder and tracing it proximally until it moves away from the gallbladder. The single lymph node found in this area is a reliable guide to the location of the main cystic artery or its anterior branch.

After complete mobilization of the gallbladder, the surgeon proceeds finally to the division and ligation of the cystic duct. It is better to leave every cystic duct too long than to cut a single one too short.

Plate 210

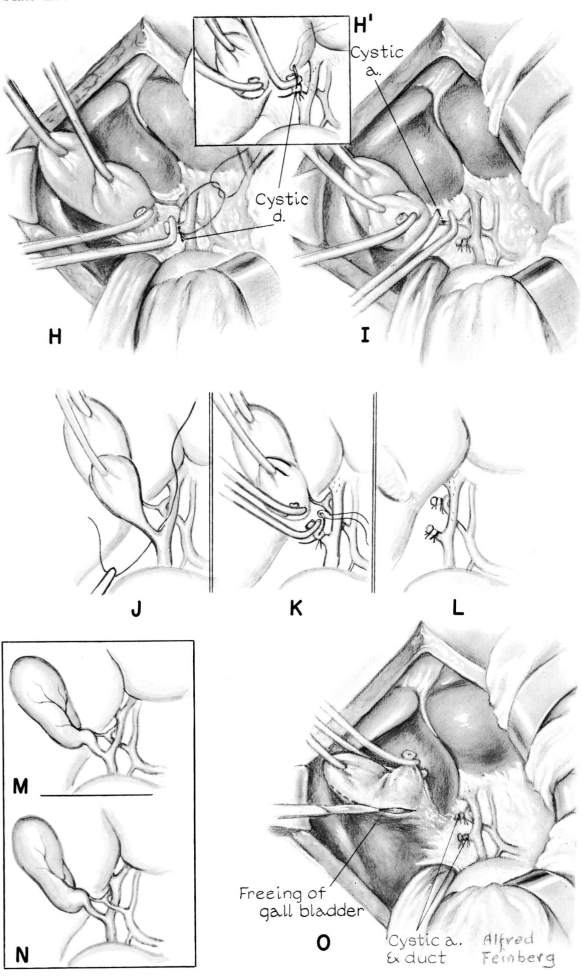

H'

Cystic
a.

Cystic
d.

Cystic
d.

H

I

J

K

L

M

N

O

Freeing of
gall bladder

Cystic a.
& duct

Alfred
Feinberg

P. Similarly, as in O, the peritoneal covering on the opposite side of the gallbladder is incised.

P¹, Q. The mobilization of the gallbladder from its bed is commenced by scissor and continued by blunt digital dissection.

R. Scissors are again used to complete the dissection of the gallbladder from the liver bed. An aberrant duct arising from the right hepatic duct at the porta hepatis may be seen passing across the lower portion of the gallbladder bed. A branch of the duct which entered the liver bed was inadvertently divided and required the application of a ligature as depicted.

S. After its mobilization, the gallbladder is allowed to lay on the surface of the abdomen for purpose of traction, and the liver bed is inspected for bleeding areas. The use of transfixion sutures of silk (000) for hemostasis is preferred to the various nonsuture methods.

T, U, V. The gallbladder bed of the liver is peritonized, and the vascular peritoneal attachment of the gallbladder to the liver is clamped, severed, and occluded with a suture ligature of silk (000).

W. A portion of a Penrose (cigarette) drain is inserted into the foramen of Winslow, and a layer closure of the wound completes the operation. The exit of the drain through the incision is preferred to the use of a stab wound.

DISCUSSION—DR. E. LEE STROHL. The incision for cholecystectomy is determined by the choice of the surgeon, the physical characteristics of the patient, and the anticipated findings at the time of operation. In the obese patient, I prefer the Kocher or subcostal incision (A). Furthermore, I feel that the respiratory exchange is more comfortable for the patient when this incision is used.

The right paramedian muscle-reflecting incision (B and C) is the incision that I use more frequently in the patient who is not obese. Downward dislocation of the liver, which permits the entrance of air between the liver and the diaphragm, is helpful in adding to the exposure, irrespective of the type of incision used (D).

Adhesions between the duodenum and the gallbladder should be separated with care, and the cystic duct identified (E and F). Tension on the gallbladder using curved 8-in. hemostats is helpful in this identification.

No attempt at removal of the gallbladder is made until all structures in the biliary triad are identified (G). It is my policy to identify the cystic duct, the cystic artery, the common bile duct, and the common hepatic duct before proceeding further with the operation. In my experience, "anybody can remove it, if they can see it." Therefore, proper exposure is one of the most important factors in any operation.

In most instances common duct stricture and hepatic artery injuries are the result of inadequate exposure and other technical errors. First, the cystic artery is clamped, cut, and doubly ligated with 00 silk, just beyond its bifurcation, as it enters the gallbladder. Similarly, the cystic duct is then clamped, cut and doubly ligated. It is not my policy to transfix the cystic duct stump, because on one or two occasions I have had leakage of bile from a transfixion suture, even though in my opinion the ligation was distal to the area in the cystic duct through which the needle was inserted (K).

The clamp applied to the cystic duct should not encroach upon the common bile duct; otherwise, stricture may result. I prefer to identify these structures and deliver the gallbladder from below upward, leaving a peritoneal cuff to be used as a cover for the gallbladder notch (O). When the gallbladder is removed in a retrograde manner, (P, P'), I keep close to the gallbladder wall so that all necessary ducts emerging from the liver may be identified separately. At this stage of the operation, I exchange positions with my first assistant and carry out the remainder of the dissection of the gallbladder from his position rather than from my normal position on the right side of the patient. Injury to the liver tissues should be avoided at all costs to prevent bile leakage. The peritoneal edges are then closed, without undue tension over the notch in which the gallbladder was lying (T, U, V, W). Complete hemostasis and recognition of any necessary bile duct channels must be secured before the closure of the peritoneum (S).

Plate 211

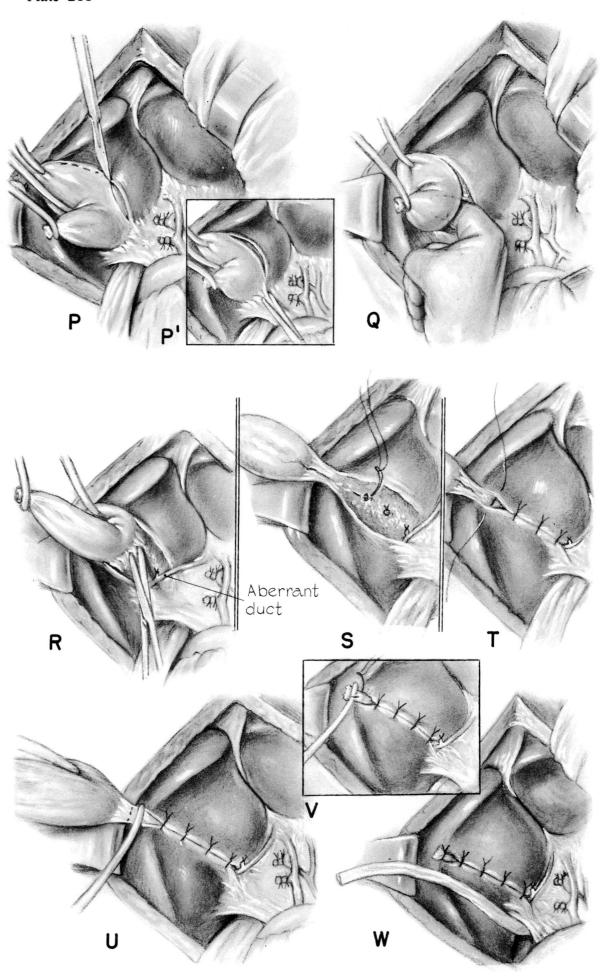

P

P'

Q

R

Aberrant
duct

S

T

V

U

W

CHOLECYSTECTOMY FOR ACUTE CHOLECYSTITIS

In the surgical management of patients with acute cholecystitis, rigid individualization is practiced. Consequently in some patients the gallbladder is removed in the acute stage, whereas in others cholecystectomy is performed as an elective procedure in a quiescent period at some later date.

A. Acute cholecystitis with distention of the gallbladder and surrounding inflammatory edema.

B. The operative field is "walled off" with protective moist gauze pads, and the gallbladder is decompressed, using a trocar and canula.

C. The opening in the fundus of the gallbladder is occluded with a curved (Kelly) clamp, and the mobilization of the gallbladder from

above downward by sharp dissection is commenced.

D, E. The detachment of the gallbladder from its bed is continued by blunt digital and scissor dissection.

F. The scissor dissection is continued anteriorly in the edematous cholecystoduodenal ligament to expose the underlying cystic duct and artery.

DISCUSSION—DR. ROBERT S. SPARKMAN. It is implied by the author that preliminary evacuation of the acutely inflamed gallbladder is practiced routinely. I do not believe that it is always necessary or desirable to empty the acute gallbladder prior to its removal. Indeed, in many instances subserous dissection will be facilitated if the tense gallbladder is left intact.

The key to successful hemostasis in retrograde removal of the acutely inflamed gallbladder lies in the delineation of a broad serosal cuff and the establishment of the proper subserous plane of dissection. If this is done, it is usually possible to grasp and ligate every bleeding point as it is encountered.

At times the acutely inflamed gallbladder is grossly infected with highly pathogenic organisms. Coliform bacteria are the most common. These, in conjunction with salmonella and clostridia, are the most dangerous. Positive cultures are more likely to be obtained from the wall of the gallbladder than from its contents. In acute cholecystitis cultures should always be taken both from the bile and from the gallbladder wall and should be grown under both aerobic and anaerobic conditions.

DISCUSSION—DR. FRANK GLENN. Cholecystectomy for acute cholecystitis (Plates 212, 213) may be embarked upon with safety if after decompression of the distended inflamed viscus one can identify the cystic duct and cystic artery. If one removes a gallbladder from the fundus downward without temporarily occluding the cystic artery, bleeding may be considerable. If the cystic duct is not identified, cholecystectomy is hazardous because of the danger of injury to the common duct. These factors, together with others, require evaluation in arriving at a decision as to whether to do a cholecystectomy or a cholecystostomy for acute cholecystitis.

Drainage following cholecystectomy (Plate 213, J) has been demonstrated to be an essential step in making it a safer procedure. Drains should be placed so that they provide the most direct route. A generous stab wound that permits the drain to reach the exterior and not pass through the abdominal wound is desirable. The incidence of postoperative hernia is greater in abdominal wounds through which drains are placed. Care is to be exercised to see that a drain from the operative area does not protrude into the lesser peritoneal sac through the foramen of Winslow. This may result in a lesser sac abscess.

Plate 212

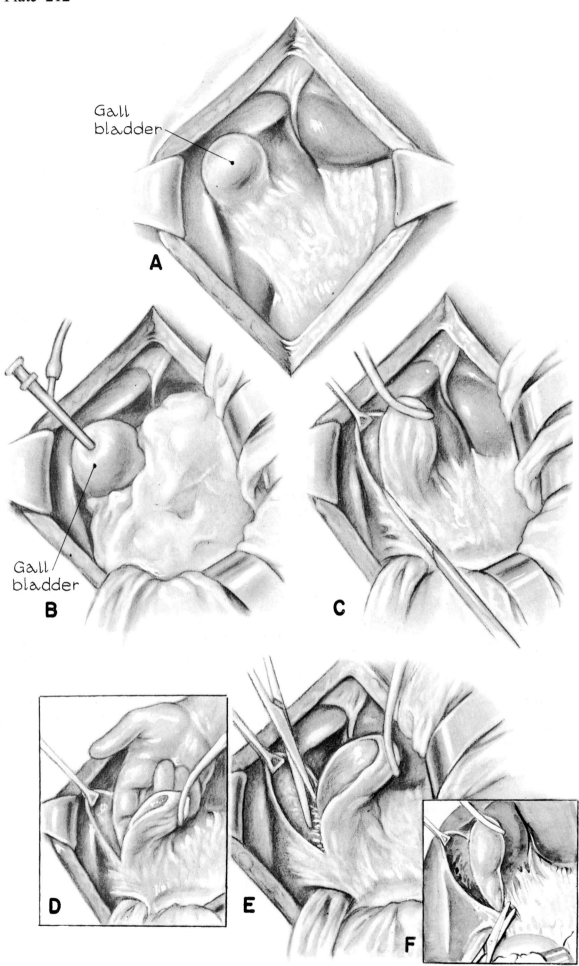

Gall bladder

A

Gall bladder

B

C

D

E

F

G. The mobilization of the gallbladder from its liver bed is completed. The only attachments remaining are the cystic duct and cystic artery.

H. The cystic artery, because of its shorter length, is the first to be doubly clamped, severed, and occluded proximally with a ligature and a transfixion suture of silk (000).

I. In like manner the cystic duct is clamped, divided, and ligated, and the gallbladder is removed.

J. A drain is inserted routinely into the foramen of Winslow and has its exit through the wound. The open liver bed is preferred to the peritonization method previously illustrated.

K. Layer closure of the wound, using interrupted sutures of silk (00) for both the peritoneum and fascia. In the closure of a paramedian incision, the rectus muscle serves as a protective barrier between the lines of closure in the peritoneal and fascial layers.

DISCUSSION—DR. E. LEE STROHL. During the early phase of acute cholecystitis, in most instances removal of the gallbladder can be done with safety. In my earlier writings, I recommended that the operation be performed within the first 72 hours. Recently, I have extended this interval to any time within the first week following an acute attack, and have had no reason to regret this change.

Acute cholecystitis is basically a sterile inflammatory disease due to blockage of the cystic duct with stones. Infection is a secondary phenomenon, with bacteria invading the obstructed gallbladder by way of the lymphatics, the blood stream, or the biliary tree.

Up to one week following the acute onset of symptoms, the gallbladder can be removed more easily than at a later interval of two or three weeks, at which time fibrosis and fibroplasia make surgical dissection more difficult.

The distended gallbladder is immediately decompressed to aid in the identification of the structures in the biliary triad. In the presence of excessive edema and inflammation, and when bleeding is a disturbing feature, cholecystectomy and choledochostomy are hazardous. In my opinion, under these conditions cholecystostomy is a safer procedure (A-F). Cholecystostomy under local anesthesia or regional block is the procedure of choice in the "poor risk" patient or in one seen in an advanced stage of the disease.

When the biliary triad is obscured so that accurate anatomic delineation is impossible, cholecystectomy should be abandoned, and either cholecystostomy or partial cholecystectomy performed. When a partial cholecystectomy is done, the fundus is removed, leaving the neck intact, but well drained, using a catheter and Penrose tube. Definitive surgery with removal of the gallbladder remnant can be carried out at a more propitious time, if and when indicated. When the indications exist, exploration of the common duct may be done in the "good risk" patient in the early stages of acute cholecystitis. However, in the aged or "poor risk" patient in an advanced stage of acute cholecystitis, cholecystostomy done as a life-saving measure will release the obstruction and provide adequate drainage. If it is necessary, the gallbladder can be removed at a later date.

In a recent collective review, I found that in 7,708 patients with acute cholecystitis the incidence of gangrene and perforation of the gallbladder was 8.3 per cent. The mortality rate in those patients who had perforation of the gallbladder was 19.0 per cent. In a recent 10-year study of the autopsy material from Cook County Hospital, there were 20 cases of gangrene of the gallbladder with perforation. It is because of the complications of acute cholecystitis that early operation is recommended. It should be performed as soon as the patient is in optimum condition.

In my opinion, whenever the biliary tract is approached surgically, the serious consequences of bile peritonitis can be avoided by the use of drains. The drains are brought out of the abdominal wall through a counterincision, never through the abdominal wound. The reason for preferring the counterincision is that postoperative hernias occur more frequently when drains are brought out of the abdominal cavity through the incision. I use a small rubber tube drain, as well as a Penrose tube. The rubber drain may also be used to inject an opaque media for roentgenographic survey, should leakage of bile continue for an undue period of time.

Plate 213   483

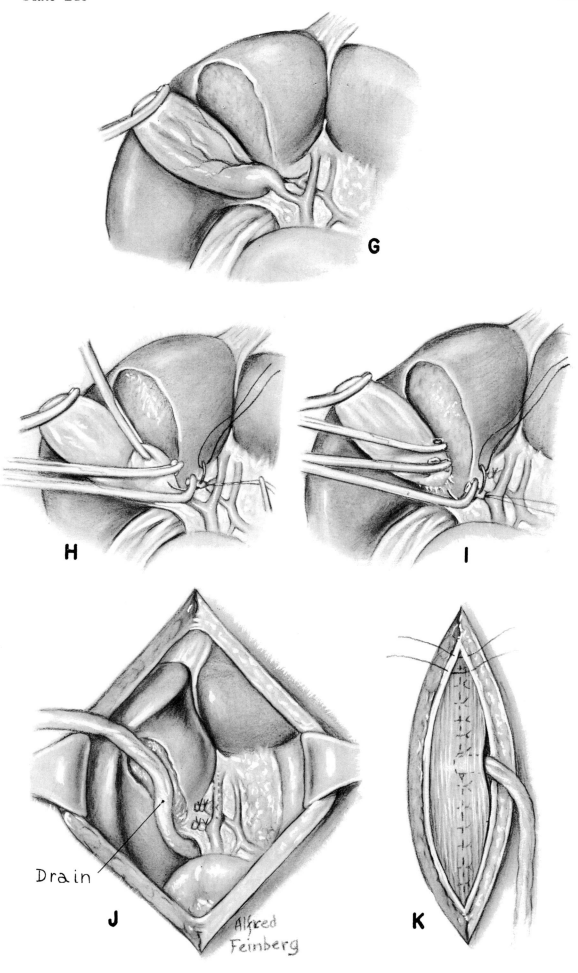

G

H   I

Drain

J   K

Alfred
Feinberg

COMMON DUCT EXPLORATION

The indications for exploration of the common duct are: (1) palpable stone; (2) roentgeno-graphic visualization of a stone; (3) jaundice either recent or present; (4) dilatation of the duct and/or thickening of its wall; (5) multiple small stones in the gallbladder in conjunction with a large cystic duct; (6) the aspiration of murky bile; (7) when in doubt.

A. In all secondary explorations, and frequently in primary explorations of the common duct, the hepatic flexure is mobilized by severance of the right phrenocolic ligament, as depicted in dotted outline.

B. The mobilized hepatic flexure and the proximal portion of the transverse colon are displaced downward, and scissor dissection of the cholecystoduodenal ligament is commenced. The curved dotted line indicates the line of incision (Kocher) in the posterior parietal peritoneum for the mobilization of the retrocolic portion of the duodenum.

C. By blunt digital dissection in the retroperitoneal tissue plane, the duodenum and the head of the pancreas are mobilized and rotated toward the midline.

D. The mobilization of the second portion of the duodenum is completed to expose the retroduodenal portion of the common duct and its related structures. The lymph node laterally and the gastroduodenal artery medially are excellent landmarks for the identification of the distal portion of the common duct.

DISCUSSION—DR. FRANK GLENN. In exploration of the common duct (Plates 214, 215), mobilization of the duodenum (Plate 214, B, C, D) enables one to examine the course of the common duct from the cystic duct to its entrance into the duodenal wall. There is considerable variation in the anatomic relationship of the duodenum, ascending colon, and subhepatic structures. Thus it is sometimes of advantage to make an incision through the peritoneum from the area of the junction of the duodenum and common duct laterally and downward to enable one to reflect the colon and duodenum. It is a very useful maneuver in secondary operations where identification of the common duct, portal vein, and hepatic artery may be difficult. This approach requires a very generous abdominal incision.

An adequate common duct exploration is one that leaves no stones behind and demonstrates any cause of obstruction, if present. Linear incisions in the common duct equal or greater than its diameter afford the needed portal of exploration. Instruments that are used to detect stones including bougies, probes, catheters, and pituitary spoons have special merit according to the dexterity and experience of those who use them. A conviction that the ductal system being explored contains a stone or stones is a great stimulus and determines to a considerable degree the care and thoroughness with which the procedure is accomplished.

Following choledochotomy the common duct may be drained by one of two ways. The first is to place a catheter through the cystic duct remnant and close the wall of the common duct. The second is to employ a T-tube and bring it out through the proximal end of the choledochotomy wound. In either event a water-tight closure of the common duct is to be done. Leakage results in periductal accumulations. Interrupted sutures of 00000 silk or 000 catgut enable one to attain such a closure. Careful testing of the integrity of the closure by injection of saline into the tube while temporarily compressing the duct above and below is an important step.

Plate 214   485

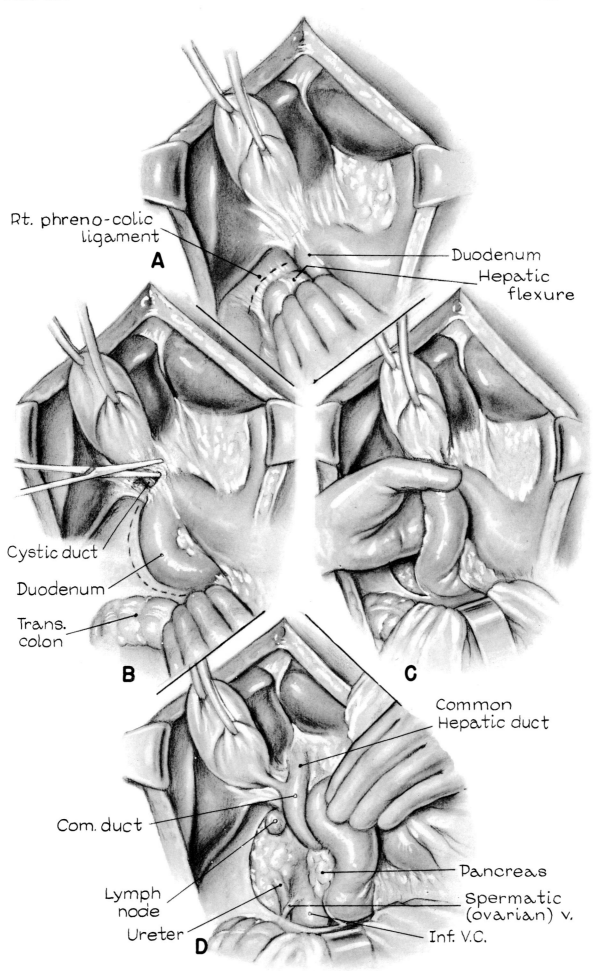

Rt. phreno-colic
ligament

A

Duodenum

Hepatic
flexure

Cystic duct

Duodenum

Trans.
colon

B

C

Common
Hepatic duct

Com. duct

Lymph
node

Ureter

D

Pancreas

Spermatic
(ovarian) v.

Inf. V.C.

E. In explorations of the common duct, the gallbladder, because it serves as a technical expediency, is not removed until the exploration is completed. However, prior to exploration, the terminal portion of the cystic duct is occluded with a ligature of silk to prevent egress of stones from the gallbladder into the common duct. The incision in the anterior wall of the duct between guy sutures of silk (00000) is shown in dotted outline. The location of the terminal portion of the common duct, between the lymph node laterally and the gastroduodenal artery medially, is visible.

E'. A new set of guy sutures is inserted through the incised margins of the common duct, and the guy sutures in the wall of the duct are removed.

F. The lumen of the dilated common duct is explored distally with a small scoop, and a stone present is removed.

G. Digital palpation along the outside wall of the common duct against an indwelling probe is performed. This maneuver is a technical aid in the detection of small stones which may be felt to grate against the probe.

H. The exploration of the common duct is continued with the use of a Bâkes dilator (4 mm.). If possible, the dilator is inserted through the papilla of Vater into the duodenum. If successful, progressively larger dilators are used up to one of 8 mm. in size. In using the dilators, one must avoid undue trauma and the establishment of false passages.

I. A soft rubber catheter (No. 12 F) is inserted into the duct and irrigation of its lumen with copious quantities of warm saline solution is performed. This procedure is considered one of the best methods for the removal of occult stones.

J. A two-holed rubber catheter (No. 12 F) is inserted into the lumen of the common duct and directed toward the liver. This size catheter is used regardless of the degree of dilatation of the common duct and is removed routinely on the fourth postoperative day if the cholangiogram taken at this time is negative. Catheter drainage of the common duct is preferred to the use of a T-tube.

K. The operative field after the completion of the exploration of the common duct, the establishment of a catheter choledochostomy, and cholecystectomy.

Plate 215   487

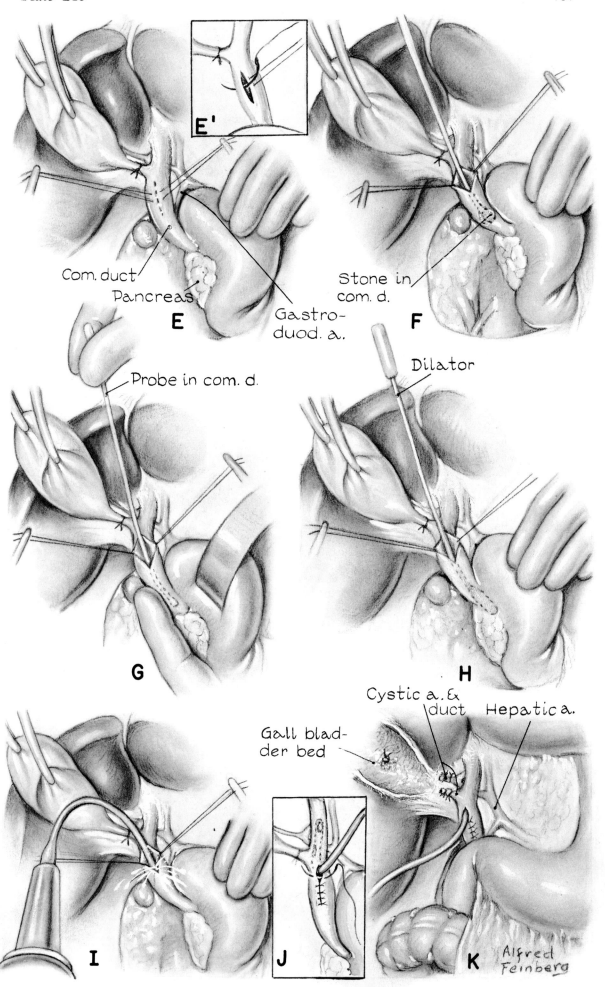

Com. duct

Pancreas

Gastro-
duod. a.

E'

E

Stone in
com. d.

F

Probe in com. d.

Dilator

G

H

Cystic a. &
duct   Hepatic a.

Gall blad-
der bed

I

J

K

Alfred
Feinberg

DISCUSSION—DR. E. LEE STROHL. In exploration of the common duct, the duodenum must first be mobilized (B, C, D), in order to examine the route of the common duct from the cystic duct to its entrance into the duodenal wall. The "Kocher maneuver" may be helpful in mobilizing both the duodenum and the ascending colon. The paramedian incision is usually the one of choice, and must be adequate in length.

Changes in the biliary tree occur when obstruction is produced by stones. The changes vary with the frequency, degree, and duration of the obstruction. Dilatation of the common duct and other segments of the biliary tree as well as secondary infection, with cholangitis and hepatitis, are frequent sequelas of an obstructed duct. In many of the patients a varying degree of pancreatitis is also found.

The common duct may be difficult to locate, particularly in secondary operations. Aspiration with a needle is frequently helpful in making positive identification of the common duct. Exploration of the duct, if indicated, is done before the gallbladder is removed. A 1.5 to 2 cm. incision is made in the anterior wall of the duct, cephalad to the site where the duct passes beneath or into the pancreas (E, E'). This site is 2 or 3 cm. distal to the junction of the cystic and common ducts. It is preferable to use two traction sutures (E', F) of fine silk to hold the walls of the incised duct apart, rather than risk injury to the duct with the use of instruments. The bile, as it escapes, is removed by suction. This flow of bile may also wash out stones present in the common duct.

If an attempt is made to probe the ducts before biliary decompression is completed, stones may be impacted in the tributaries of the bile ducts. After decompression is complete, the proximal and distal portions of the duct are flushed with saline, through a small catheter. Exploration is then carried out with a malleable scoop, bougies, probes, or a small pituitary spoon (F, G, H). Every effort should be made to remove the stones intact; if they are fragmented, all the fragments must be removed (I). It should be emphasized that occasionally a probe or catheter may be passed through the sphincter of Oddi into the duodenum, even though a stone is present in the distal portion of the common duct. Palpation of the duct along a metallic instrument or catheter may be helpful in the identification of a stone (F, G, H). This maneuver may be more easily accomplished by the surgeon when it is carried out from the left side of the operation table.

After exploration the common duct is drained with a T-tube. The Mayo Robson catheter type of drainage is an alternate procedure (J, K). I do not like to drain a common duct through the remnant of a cystic duct. A T-tube is preferred because it remains in place and will not be dislodged when inadvertently tugged or pulled. After exploration of a common duct, drainage is always carried out. I am not a proponent of primary closure of the common duct after it is explored. The T-tube should always be tested for patency. I have found a T-tube with a complete diaphragm which blocked the lumen. A notch should be made in the tube, opposite the T-crossarm, to facilitate its removal. The limbs of the T-tube are trimmed to suitable length and the upper limb should not impinge on the bifurcation of the right and left hepatic ducts. I do not use a long-arm T-tube because of the possibility of inciting the highly lethal postoperative complication of acute hemorrhagic pancreatitis. A water-tight closure of the common duct is then done using 0000 chromic catgut sutures, both above and below the exit of the T-tube. The forceful injection of saline into the T-tube is used to test the water-tight closure of the duct.

In a collective review previously reported, I found the average incidence of common duct exploration in 25,807 operations for chronic cholecystitis to be 23 per cent. The incidence of common duct stones was 11.3 per cent. Accordingly, approximately two common ducts were explored for each duct in which stones were found.

In a recent study at Presbyterian-St. Luke's Hospital, Chicago, it was found that in the performance of cholecystectomy concomitant exploration of the common duct was done in 22 per cent of the patients and in 53 per cent of these, the exploration yielded one or more stones. Furthermore, in patients over 60 years of age, the incidence of stones in the common duct was proportionately higher.

DISCUSSION—DR. ROBERT S. SPARKMAN. In exploration of the common duct, nothing has been quite so helpful to me as the Randall stone forceps. This set of four instruments, devised for removal of stones from the renal pelvis, is ideally constructed for manipulation within the bile ducts. In addition to their function as grasping instruments, they are of great value for manipulation of the duodenal ampulla. When conventional dilators, probes, or catheters are employed, the sphincter tends to evert into the duodenum in advance of the instrument and often will not yield to it. The appropriate Randall clamp is passed distally until the tip everts the ampulla into the duodenum; the jaws of the instrument are then opened and closed several times, while a gentle everting force is still applied. This seems to overcome spasm of the ampulla, and the tip of the instrument will usually pop suddenly into the duodenum. Thereafter, the various probes, dilators, and catheters may be introduced with ease.

I prefer a T-tube to the straight catheter. The caliber of the tube should be distinctly smaller than the lumen of the bile duct. The T-limb should be notched and trimmed so that it may be withdrawn easily. Some slack should be provided in the tube between the point of its emergence from the duct and the site of its fixation to the abdominal skin; otherwise, coughing or abdominal distention may drag the tube out of the duct.

T-tubes have been pulled out inadvertently by irrational patients. This mishap may be prevented if the tube is properly anchored. At the point of exit of the tube on the abdominal wall, a deep bite is taken in the skin with a suture of #28 or 30 stainless steel wire. This is tied down loosely. The two ends of the wire are wrapped around and around the tube in opposing spirals for 4 or 5 in. The wire ends are then twisted together several times and cut. It is almost impossible to dislodge a tube that has been secured in this manner.

CHOLECYSTOJEJUNOSTOMY

A. The peritoneal cavity is entered, and the distended gallbladder, in relation to its surrounding structures, is visible.

B, C. A trocar and canula are inserted into the lumen of the gallbladder (B) and the trocar is withdrawn to decompress the gallbladder by suction siphonage (C). Only after the gallbladder is decompressed (C) are the clamps (Babcock) applied.

D, E. The transverse colon is elevated, and an opening is made by blunt dissection in a relatively avascular plane of the transverse mesocolon (D). Through this opening a loop of jejunum secured by traction guy sutures of silk (000) is withdrawn (E).

E$_1$. If preferred, the jejunum may be brought in front (antecolic) of rather than behind (retrocolic) the colon.

DISCUSSION—DR. RALPH COLP. Patients with severe obstructive jaundice in whom palliative procedures are indicated are those with inoperable carcinomatous infiltration either of the head of the pancreas, of the duodenum, or of the terminal portion of the common duct, and occasionally those with advanced chronic pancreatitis. In these pathologic conditions, the distal area of the choledochus is either infiltrated by tumor or compressed by scar tissue formation or neoplasm. Regardless of the preoperative diagnosis, exploration is indicated unless hepatic metastases are definitely palpable, ascites is present, or rectal examination reveals the presence of a Blumer's shelf.

Preoperatively, these patients should be prepared by a high carbohydrate and protein diet, vitamin K, blood transfusions, and the correction of electrolytic imbalances. In the performance of the operation, spinal anesthesia is preferred. An upper oblique right rectus muscle-splitting incision usually provides adequate exposure. Exploration in most cases reveals a dilated gallbladder and a dilatation of the common bile duct. If the cause of the obstruction cannot be removed, the jaundice may be relieved by a side-tracking biliary-intestinal anastomosis.

The choice of operation depends upon the surgeon's preference and his judgment. Prior to any type of anastomosis, the large gallbladder is carefully isolated by abdominal pads. A 1-inch incision is made through the serosa of the gallbladder parallel to, and at least 1 inch from the liver margin. A trocar is introduced into its lumen and the thick viscid bile is aspirated. The original serosal incision is now deepened through all the walls of the gallbladder and its interior is palpated for the presence of biliary cal-

culi. The thin gallbladder should be handled with care. Any type of grasping clamp used should be loosely applied. This may be dispensed with if guy sutures of silk are used for traction. The gallbladder may now be anastomosed either to the stomach, duodenum, or jejunum. The basic technics illustrated by the author are applicable, with minor variations, to all types of anastomoses.

Our own preference is a cholecystogastrostomy. This not only presents fewer technical difficulties, but is followed by a negligible mortality and an insignificant morbidity. If the jejunum is used, many prefer the Roux-en-Y method of cholecystojejunostomy. This procedure is time consuming and entails certain operative hazards. In its performance the mesentery of the jejunum is partially divided about 24 inches from the ligament of Treitz. The bowel is then transected between Von Petz clips or rubber-covered intestinal clamps. The distal end of the jejunum is anastomosed to the gallbladder, and intestinal continuity is restored by implanting its proximal end into the distal limb either by an end-to-side or a side-to-side jejunojejunostomy. This anastomosis is made about 18 inches below the site of the cholecystojejunostomy. Following a side-to-side cholecystojejunostomy, some surgeons elect to perform a complementary jejunojejunostomy about 12 inches from the anastomosis.

There are theoretic reasons for the Roux-en-Y anastomosis or the addition of a complementary jejunojejunostomy. It is believed that the danger of an ascending infection from a reflux of jejunal contents into the ducts of the liver via the gallbladder is minimized by either one of these two methods.

Plate 216   491

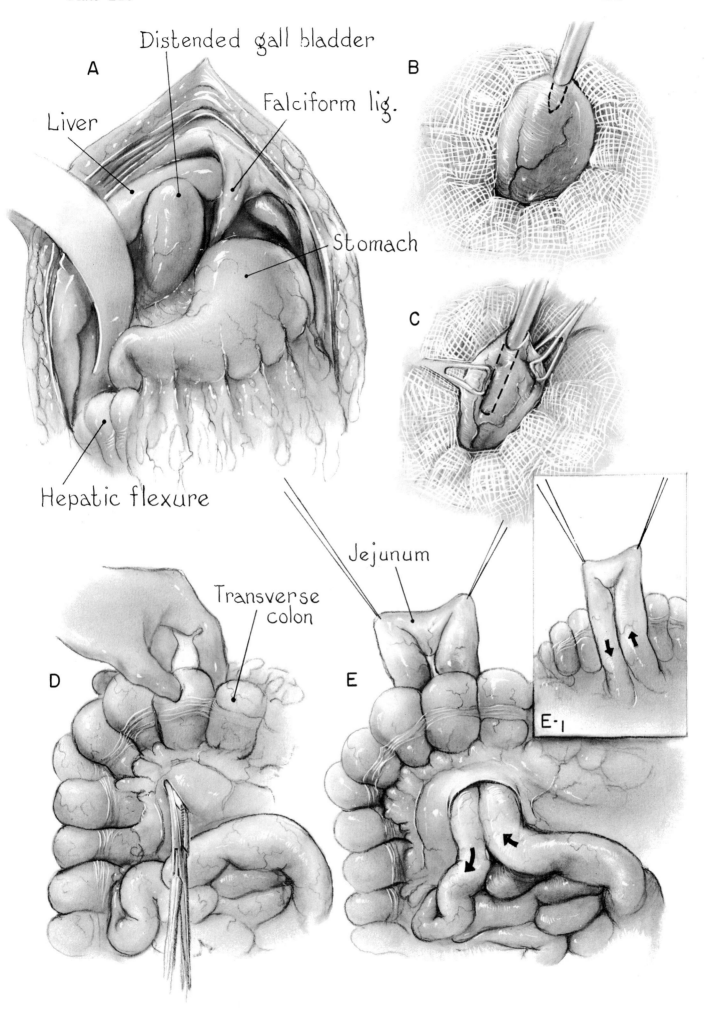

A

Liver

Distended gall bladder

Falciform lig.

Stomach

B

C

Hepatic flexure

Jejunum

Transverse colon

D

E

E-1

F. Guy sutures of silk (000) are inserted at either angle of the enlarged opening in the gallbladder, and the first posterior layer of sutures (000 silk) to approximate the gallbladder and jejunum is inserted, but the sutures are not tied.

G, H. An incision is made through the seromuscular layer of the jejunum (G) to expose the vessels in the submucosa. These vessels are undersewn with hemostatic suture ligatures of 000 silk (H).

I, J. An opening is made into the lumen of the jejunum between the two rows of hemostatic suture ligatures (I) and then enlarged by scissor dissection (J).

K. Upon completion of the opening in the jejunum, the sutures of the first posterior layer are tied, and the insertion of the second posterior layer, a series of interrupted sutures (0000 silk) which includes all of the layers of the jejunum and gallbladder, is begun.

DISCUSSION—DR. COLP (cont.)

Ascending infection is a potential hazard in any type of biliary intestinal anastomosis. However, it is not dependent upon the reflux alone. It is more dependent upon biliary stasis with infection secondary to a stenosis of the anastomotic stoma. This unfortunate complication may be lessened by making the primary anastomosis sufficiently large and approximating the mucosa of the gallbladder most carefully to the mucosa of the stomach, duodenum, or jejunum. These precautions will result in an adequate stoma with a minimum of scar tissue formation. However, most patients die from metastatic carcinoma before ascending infection ever becomes a serious threat to life. Minor episodes of concurrent infection usually can be controlled by the use of appropriate antibiotics.

In some instances, the gallbladder is either contracted because of disease or absent because of previous cholecystectomy. Under such circumstances, the dilated common duct must be carefully explored. If necessary, an anterior duodenotomy is indicated to eliminate the possibility of an impacted ampullary calculus. If exploration discloses that the obstruction is due to an inoperable carcinoma, the dilated duct may be anastomosed either to the duodenum or the jejunum. The duodenum is mobilized by incising the peritoneum along its lateral border, and the side of the dilated duct is anastomosed to the lateral wall of the duodenum. If mobilization of the duodenum is impractical, a transverse incision is made into its first portion in close proximity to the common duct, and an end-to-side choledochoduodenostomy is performed. If the duodenum, because of carcinomatous infiltration, is unsuitable for an anastomosis, the choledochus and the jejunum may be joined by a Roux-en-Y choledochojejunostomy. If either of these operations is performed, it may be safer to do a complementary biliary intestinal intubation. The technic is simple. After the posterior double row of sutures has been placed, a fenestrated rubber tube is introduced into the proximal choledochus so that it fits rather snugly. The distal end of the tube is then inserted into the duodenum or jejunum for about 8 inches. The two anterior layers of the anastomosis are now completed. The tube not only insures the immediate flow of bile from the liver to the intestines, but it acts as a supporting scaffold and prevents obstructive edema of the stoma. Before discharge, patients should always be apprized of the fact that a rubber tube has been left in situ, but that it will eventually be passed per rectum.

Following any type of palliative diverting procedure, intraabdominal drainage of the abdomen is unnecessary. The anterior abdominal wall should be closed in layers and reinforced with through and through sutures. In jaundiced patients with carcinoma the tissues heal slowly and poorly. Accordingly wound dehiscence and evisceration are not infrequent complications. Postoperatively, gastric suction should be maintained until normal gastrointestinal peristalsis occurs. During this period, the electrolyte and fluid balances should be maintained by intravenous solutions.

Plate 217

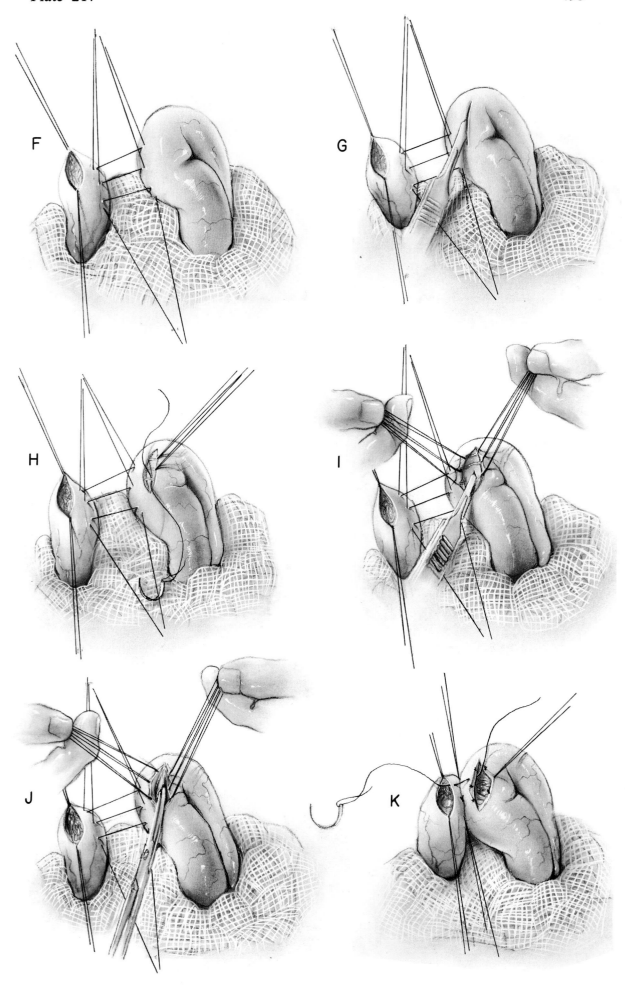

L, M, N, O. The sutures of the second posterior layer are inserted and tied (L). The long strands of the sutures are cut, and the insertion of the first anterior inverting layer of sutures (000 silk) is begun (M). These sutures are inserted from the "inside out" on one side and from the "outside in" on the other so that, when tied, the knots of the sutures are on the inside of the lumen. To facilitate the inversion of the tissue layers, traction on the previously inserted suture is maintained in the long axis of the anastomosis as each succeeding suture is tied. The sutures are inserted alternately from either angle (M, N) toward the center where the termination of the last two sutures is encircled by a figure of 8 mattress suture before the long strands are cut (O).

P, Q. The figure of 8 mattress suture is tied and cut, and the second anterior layer of sutures (Lembert) is first inserted (P) and then tied and cut (Q).

R, S. Following completion of the cholecystojejunostomy, the margins of the opening on the inferior surface of the transverse mesocolon are anchored to the afferent and efferent loops of the jejunum (R). On the superior aspect of the transverse colon a similar anchoring suture of the mattress type is inserted (S). These sutures serve to obliterate any opening through which herniation of additional small bowel loops may occur. If desired, an enteroenterostomy may be performed between the afferent and efferent loops proximal to the site of the cholecystojejunostomy.

Plate 218   495

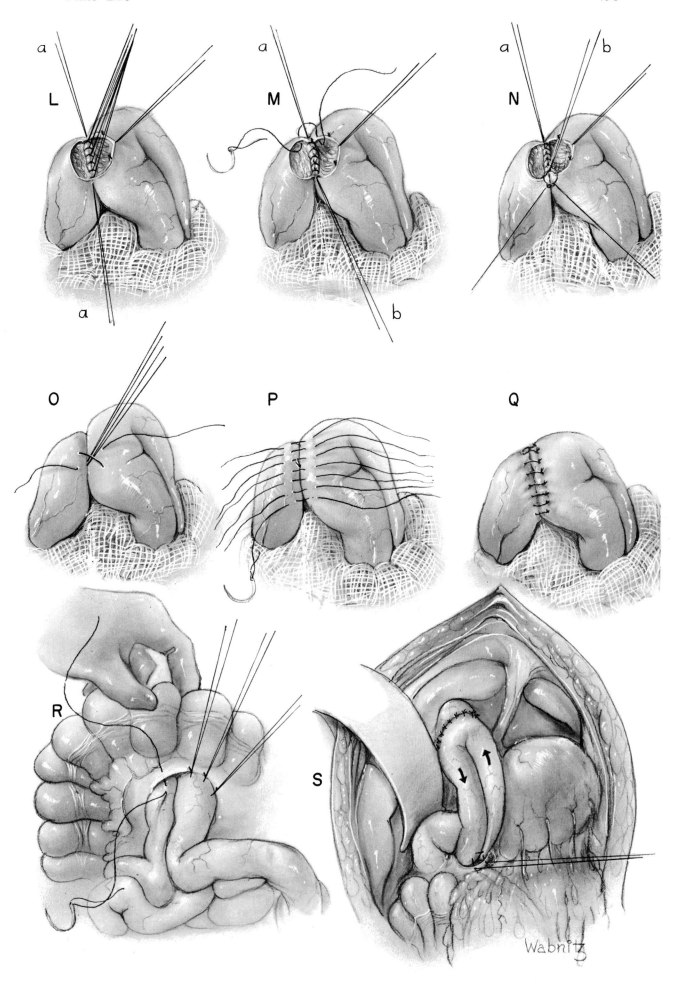

SPHINCTEROTOMY

A, B, C. The scar of the previous operation (cholecystectomy) is elliptically excised (dotted lines) (A), and the peritoneal cavity is entered through a muscle-splitting incision (B). The postoperative intraperitoneal adhesions between the liver and colon are readily visible (C).

D. The colon is freed from the liver, and the hepatic flexure is mobilized by the severance of the right phrenocolic ligament as indicated by the dotted line.

E. The hepatic flexure is displaced downward toward the left lower quadrant of the abdomen, and the lateral incision for the mobilization of the duodenum (Kocher) is shown in dotted outline.

F. The mobilized duodenum is rotated and displaced toward the midline (Moynihan rotation maneuver), and the site of the transverse incision in the common duct (dotted line) and the adjacent related structures are visible.

G. If desired, a longitudinal incision in the common duct which is elongated transversely by traction guy sutures of silk (00000) may be used in preference to the transverse incision.

DISCUSSION—DRS. I. S. RAVDIN AND GERALD W. PESKIN. Sphincterotomy is practiced for the removal of stones impacted in the distal common bile duct and to relieve recurrent attacks of pancreatitis. Although the incision for this operation may be made through the scar of a previous rectus incision, a new subcostal approach is often used to obtain better exposure and wound healing, particularly in the patient with a wide costal angle. When the rectus incision is elected, it is wise to attempt lateral retraction rather than splitting of this muscle in order to conserve nervous innervation. When the posterior rectus sheath and peritoneum are incised, elevating the anterior rectus fascia with a series of Kocher hemostats decreases the likelihood of entering a viscus rather than the free peritoneal cavity.

Once inside the abdomen, the first step is to clear the subhepatic area of organs adherent to the liver. By staying close to the liver edge and using sharp dissection, the attached hepatic flexure of the colon and displaced duodenum are quickly freed. Mobilization of the lateral aspect of the duodenum is completed by the Kocher maneuver as depicted in Plate 219, E, and the pancreas is manually examined for pseudocysts and abscesses. The common duct is approached from the lateral free edge of tissue representing the duodenohepatic ligament, using the pulsation of the hepatic artery as the medial guide. The blue-green color of the duct is invaluable in its identification. When doubt exists as to the exact location of the duct, a hypodermic needle attached to a small syringe is used to probe the general area in search of bile. This maneuver is of great help in avoiding accidental injury to the portal vein or hepatic artery. It is unnecessary and even hazardous to attempt the wide clearing of structures depicted in Plate 219, F.

Following the placement of two guide sutures of 000 chromic catgut (atraumatic), a longitudinal incision is made in the common duct about 1 inch above the superior edge of the duodenum or, if the gallbladder is present, just distal to the junction of the cystic duct with the common duct. Again it is a wise practice to aspirate the structure thought to be the common duct before incising it. The common duct is then probed and irrigated to remove any residual debris.

When a Bâkes dilator cannot be made to traverse the sphincter or when the primary intent of operation is sphincterotomy, the area around the duodenal loop is carefully walled off with sponges to minimize soilage upon opening the duodenum. With the dilator in the distal common duct as a guide, a 2-inch vertical incision is made in the anterolateral wall of the duodenum and centered over the tip of the probe. After ligating small subserosal bleeding points, Babcock clamps are placed to retract the cut margins of the duodenum. A small, tagged tape is then inserted into the proximal duodenal lumen to prevent gastric and duodenal secretions from obscuring the area of the papilla. The papilla is thrown into prominence by gentle pressure on the dilator within the common duct. If the ductal orifice is still not apparent with this maneuver, 1 or 2 ml. of methylene blue can be instilled into the common duct, and its appearance in the duodenum within a few moments will pinpoint the papillary ostium. Incision of the papilla is performed in a manner similar to that depicted in Plate 220, L, employing 1 cm. as the safe distance for obtaining an adequate aperture without risking perforation of the duodenum. Dilators are passed upward and downward through the enlarged sphincter until adequate patency is assured. Because of occasional hemorrhage from this site in the past, we have found it valuable to tack the cut

Plate 219

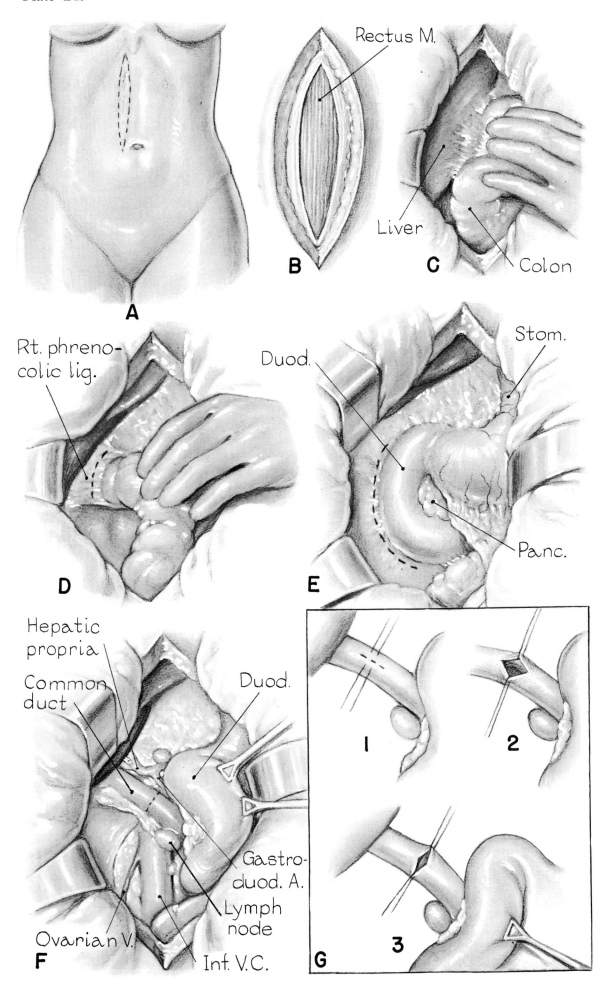

A

B Rectus M.

C Liver — Colon

D Rt. phreno-colic lig.

E Duod. — Stom. — Panc.

F Hepatic propria — Common duct — Duod. — Gastro-duod. A. — Lymph node — Ovarian V. — Inf. V.C.

G 1 2 3

H. A probe is inserted through the incision in the common duct into its lumen. However, the probe could not be passed through the papilla of Vater into the duodenum. When this occurs, it is imperative for the surgeon to determine the presence or absence of an obstruction in the region of the papilla of Vater. Accordingly, a duodenotomy is advised, and, in the absence of a tumor or calculus as a cause of the obstruction, either a sphincterotomy or a choledochoduodenostomy is recommended. Under such circumstances a choledochoduodenostomy is frequently preferred.

I. The lumen of the common duct is irrigated thoroughly, and frequently occult calculi will be flushed out.

J. An incision is made through the seromus-

cular coat of the posterior wall of the duodenum overlying the region of the papilla, and the vessels in the submucosal layer are undersewn with hemostatic suture ligatures.

J^1. Inset showing the incision into the lumen of the duodenum being made by scissor dissection between the two rows of hemostatic sutures.

K. The cut margins of the duodenum are retracted in Babcock clamps, and the probe in the common duct is held firmly against the papilla to project it more prominently into the lumen of the duodenum.

L, L^1. The mucosa of the duodenum overlying the probe is incised with a scalpel (L), and the probe is then readily passed into the lumen of the duodenum (L^1).

DISCUSSION—DRS. RAVDIN AND PESKIN (cont.)

edge of the common duct wall to the cut edge of the duodenal wall with several sutures of 00000 atraumatic chromic catgut. Not only does this provide hemostasis, but it serves to prevent stricture of the sphincterotomy site. Care must be taken, in placing these sutures, not to encroach upon the pancreatic duct opening. This may be probed if serious doubt exists as to its location. A roentgenographic evaluation of the pancreatic duct may be obtained at this point by placing a fine polyethylene catheter into the duct of Wirsung through the sphincterotomy opening and injecting a radiopaque material. If the pancreatic duct appears obstructed on the roentgenograms, distal pancreaticojejunostomy must be seriously considered.

Transverse closure of the duodenotomy is accomplished after removal of the pack within the duodenal lumen employing O chromic catgut (atraumatic) for the first layer and beginning at each lateral margin of the incision. A running, inverting, Connell-type stitch is utilized, catching a minimal amount of tissue with each bite. The sutures are tied at the center of the incision. Interrupted seromuscular Lembert sutures of 000 silk are used to complete the closure

after gloves and drapes have been changed. A tag of omentum may be fastened over the duodenal wound when available.

In contrast to the technic employed in Plate 221, O, we prefer to employ the largest rubber T-tube which will comfortably fit within the common duct (usually No. 18 or No. 16 French). Water-tight closure of the duct is accomplished in a longitudinal fashion with interrupted sutures of 000 chromic catgut (atraumatic).

A sump drain is routinely placed just lateral to the junction of the duodenum and common duct, and it and the T-tube are led out of the peritoneal cavity through separate stab wounds in the flank. This provides more dependent drainage, does not weaken the wound, and makes accidental removal of the drain or T-tube during dressing changes less likely. Abdominal wound closure is performed in layers using interrupted No. 28 stainless steel wire for the anterior rectus fascia.

It is extremely important to remove the gallbladder, if present, at the time of sphincterotomy to avoid the serious sequelae which may result from malfunction of this organ.

Plate 220

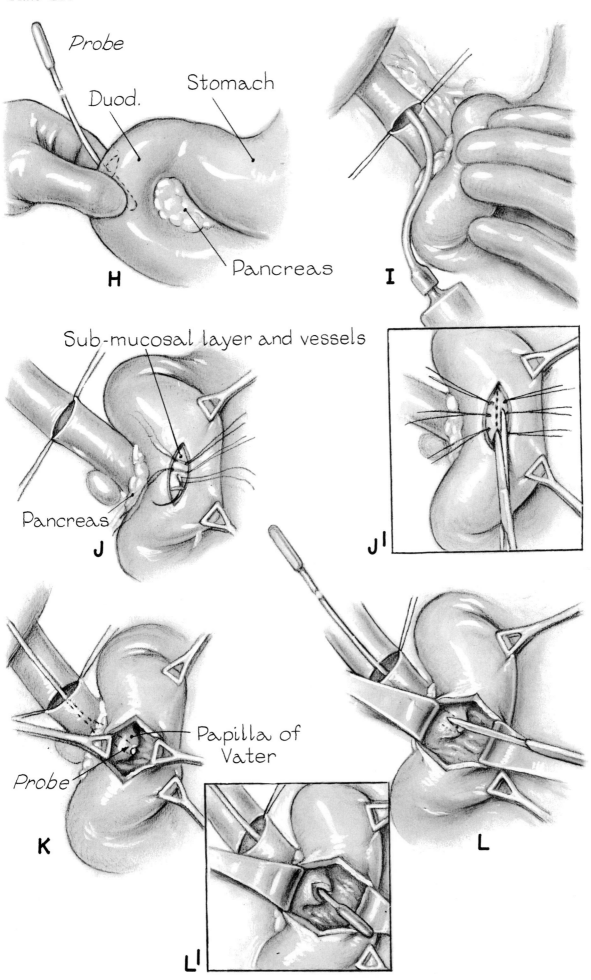

Probe

Duod.

Stomach

Pancreas

H

I

Sub-mucosal layer and vessels

Pancreas

J

J¹

Papilla of Vater

Probe

K

L

L¹

M. The probe is easily inserted in a retrograde manner through the incised sphincter into the lumen of the common duct and out through an opening in its anterior wall.

N, N¹, N², N³, N⁴. The longitudinal opening in the duodenum is closed transversely in two layers using interrupted sutures of silk (000). The sutures forming the first layer are inserted alternately from either end and from the "inside out" to the "outside in", (N, N¹) so that, when tied, the knots of the sutures are on the inside of the lumen. The site of the termination of the first layer of sutures in the center of the anastomosis is

reinforced by an encircling figure of 8 suture (N²) and the second layer of interrupted seromuscular sutures is inserted (N³, N⁴).

O. The completed closure of the incisions in the common bile duct and the duodenum and their relation to the surrounding structures are visible.

P, Q. The peritoneal (P) and fascial (Q) layers are closed about the peritoneal drain and the common duct catheter (No. 12 F). Drainage through the incision is preferred to the use of stab wound drainage sites in the flank.

DISCUSSION—DR. ROBERT J. COFFEY. In recent years this operative procedure has been most commonly employed for the relief of chronic pancreatitis. However, other indications for division of the sphincter of Oddi do exist. In several patients I have found it necessary to divide this structure, exposing the terminus of the common duct, in order to remove a solidly impacted common duct stone. In removal of calculi from the duct of Wirsung, division of the sphincter is necessary to obtain exposure of the terminus of the major pancreatic duct. Sphincteritis is a poorly understood but very real entity in which fibrotic changes involve the sphincter, division of which affords surgical relief.

In addition to these indications for sphincterotomy, it is not infrequently necessary to surgically expose the major papilla and to palpate the region of the sphincter of Oddi. Such a procedure is indicated if a tumor of the ampulla is suspected or if the surgeon is unable to successfully introduce a probe through the common duct into the duodenum.

The primary step in carrying out a sphincterotomy is mobilization of the descending duodenum by division of its lateral peritoneal reflection. This permits one to more accurately palpate the entire duodenal wall, as well as to identify the major papilla transduodenally. One's ability to feel this structure through the unopened duodenal wall is directly related to the frequency with which he attempts to palpate the structure. In chronic pancreatitis the major papilla is abnormally conspicuous and therefore is easily palpable. In most instances, a tumor of the ampulla can be readily felt as an abnormal structure prior to opening the duodenal wall.

To either divide the sphincter or explore the major papilla, I incise the anterior wall of the

duodenum in a vertical direction opposite the palpated major papilla. This incision is usually 2 to 3 in. in length. Once the duodenum is opened and bleeding of the incised edges controlled, exposure of the major papilla may be effected by employing infant-size Dever retractors. Very often ejection of a spurt of bile will identify the major papilla. In addition, the minor papilla, situated approximately 1 in. above and medial to the major papilla, should be palpated. If division of the sphincter is to be carried out, fine silk guide sutures are placed on either side of the upper edge of the papilla; after appropriate dilatation, a small scissors can be readily introduced, and the terminus of the common duct, sphincter, and duodenal mucosa can be divided for a distance of 0.5 to 1 cm. Attempts to suture the corners marked by the silk guy sutures in a retracted position are, in my opinion, unnecessary. If sphincteritis is suspected, a wedge excision of the sphincter and adjacent mucosa should be secured for pathologic examination. On division of the sphincter, the ampulla is immediately exposed. One should attempt to identify the stoma of the major pancreatic duct as it empties into the ampulla posteriorly. If stones exist in this ductal system, removal via the ampulla can be carried out after appropriate dilatation of the terminus of the duct of Wirsung.

It is not always necessary to open the common duct prior to carrying out a sphincterotomy. This is true if the indication is chronic pancreatitis or removal of stones from the pancreatic ducts. It is quite generally agreed that cholecystectomy should supplement sphincterotomy, inasmuch as the function of the gallbladder is seriously impaired following division of the sphincter. If it is felt that removal of the gallbladder will result in an undue extension of the operative procedure, however, its removal is not essential.

Plate 221   501

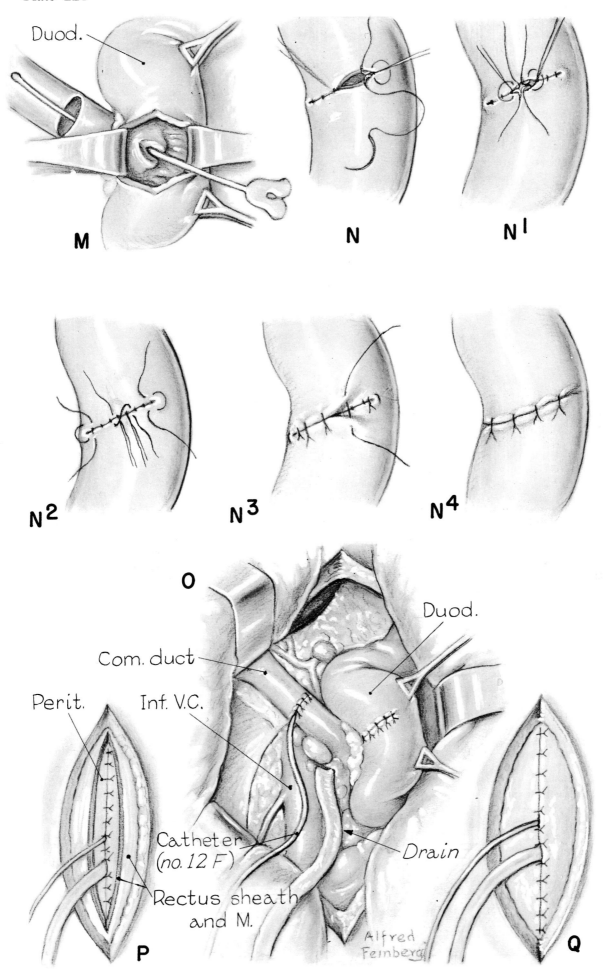

Duod.

M

N

N¹

N²

N³

N⁴

O

Com. duct

Duod.

Perit.

Inf. V.C.

Catheter
(no. 12 F)

Drain

Rectus sheath
and M.

P

Q

Alfred
Feinberg

CHOLEDOCHODUODENOSTOMY

The technic for exposure of the operative area is the same as that shown in the first plate of the illustrations for sphincterotomy and, accordingly, is deleted here.

A. The first posterior layer of interrupted silk (0000) sutures, which approximates the posterior aspect of the first portion of the duodenum to the side of the common bile duct, is shown being inserted. The dotted line indicates the site of the incision to be made in the duodenum.

B. The insertion of the first posterior layer of sutures which are not tied is completed. An incision has been made through the seromuscular layer of the duodenum, and the vessels in the submucosa are undersewn with hemostatic sutures of 0000 silk.

B¹. The first posterior layer of sutures is tied, and the second posterior layer of interrupted through and through silk (0000) sutures is being inserted.

B², B³, B⁴. The insertion of the second posterior layer of sutures is completed, and the first anterior layer is begun. This layer consists of interrupted silk sutures which are inserted from the "inside out" to the "outside in" so that when tied the knots are on the inside of the lumen (B², B³). These sutures meet in the center of the anastomosis anteriorly where a reinforcing figure of 8 suture ligature is inserted (B⁴).

C. The insertion of the second anterior layer, a series of interrupted mattress sutures of silk (0000), completes the operation.

DISCUSSION—DRS. I. S. RAVDIN AND GERALD W. PESKIN. While our experience with choledochoduodenostomy is limited because of a preference for sphincterotomy in the treatment of chronic pancreatitis, we have had some success with this procedure. Since the common channel theory of the etiology of pancreatitis provides the rationale for this operation, we believe that complete division of the duct with end-to-side anastomosis of the proximal segment to the duodenum is important. This affords absolute protection against the reflux of bile into the pancreatic ducts, whereas only partial division is accomplished by the technic illustrated in the plates.

After exposure of the area as described under sphincterotomy, the common duct is freed from surrounding structures just above the superior edge of the duodenum. A lubricated hernia tape is placed around it, and, with the aid of gentle traction on the tape, the duct is cleared for a distance of 2 cm. A site for transection of the duct which should be as far distally as possible is selected, allowing just enough space to close the distal stump without passing sutures through the pancreas or duodenum. Before transection of the duct, a longitudinal choledochostomy incision is made about one-half inch above the anticipated line of resection for subsequent insertion of a T-tube. The duct is then divided with fine, straight scissors (such as right angle vascular scissors), and the distal stump is closed with a running over and over suture of 0000 or 00000 silk (atraumatic). The duodenal area selected for the anastomosis shown in Plate 222, A and B, is posterior and distal to the site which we ordinarily use. The

duodenal incision is usually placed just beyond the junction of the first and second portions at the anterolateral margin. This site allows for an anastomosis which is free of kinks. Guide sutures of 00000 silk (atraumatic) are placed at the lateral angles of the common duct opening, and the duct is gently lifted to approximate the duodenum to it. The posterior row of interrupted 00000 silk (atraumatic) sutures is placed, taking care not to go completely through all layers of the common duct. In this manner, nonabsorbable material is not placed within the duct lumen. When these sutures have been tied, an opening is created in the duodenum, approximating the size of the common duct. After hemostatis is obtained, a posterior row of interrupted 00000 chromic catgut (atraumatic) mucosal sutures is placed. A large caliber (No. 16 to No. 18) T-tube is then inserted through the longitudinal choledochostomy incision, and its distal limb is led through the anastomotic area and into the duodenal lumen for about 1 inch. The interrupted mucosal suturing is completed anteriorly, with the T-tube splint affording absolute assurance of a patent lumen. The final step is a serosal closure anteriorly with interrupted 00000 silk (atraumatic). In this manner a splinted, patent, unkinked anastomosis is created. The choledochostomy is closed around the T-tube in the fashion described under sphincterotomy, and the T-tube is led from the peritoneal cavity through a separate stab wound. Drainage is again by a sump drain placed near the anastomosis and led from the peritoneal cavity through a stab wound.

Plate 222

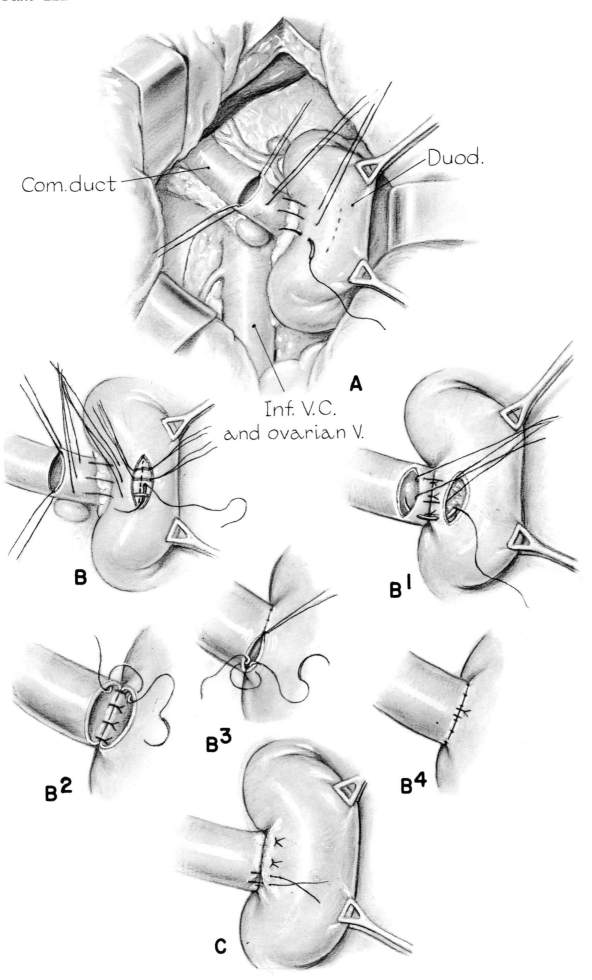

Com.duct

Duod.

Inf. V.C.
and ovarian V.

A

B

B¹

B²

B³

B⁴

C

SIDE-TO-SIDE CHOLEDOCHODUODENOSTOMY

A. Through a right paramedian muscle-splitting incision, the operative field is exposed. The gallbladder has been removed and the hepatic flexure of the colon mobilized and retracted downward and medially. The broken lines indicate the sites of the incisions to be made in the common duct and duodenum, respectively.

A₁. In this close-up view, the incision in the duodenal wall is deepened through the seromuscular layer. The blood vessels in the submucosal layer are undersewn on each side of the incision with interrupted sutures of 0000 silk for hemostasis. The last of these sutures is inserted but not tied. The incision to be made into the lumen of the duodenum is indicated by the broken line.

B. An opening is made into the lumen of the common duct between guy sutures of 00000 silk and the opening into the lumen of the duodenum is completed. One of the hemostatic sutures in the anterior layer of the duodenal incision is left long for traction to facilitate the insertion of the posterior layer of sutures. The first suture in the posterior layer is the center one, which is inserted from the inside-out on the duodenum and from the outside-in at the caudad angle of the choledochotomy.

C. Upward traction through a clamp is maintained on the untied strands of the center suture, and sutures of 00000 silk are inserted from the inside-out in each angle of the incision in the duodenum to the outside-in in the center of each wall of the incised common duct.

D. The "angle" sutures are tied, and a series of interrupted sutures of 00000 silk that incorporate the full thickness of the wall of the duodenum and the common duct are inserted. These sutures form the single posterior layer of the anastomosis.

In surgery of the biliary tract, the operation of side-to-side choledochoduodenostomy is in general held in bad repute in the United States. On the continent of Europe and in the British Isles, however, it enjoys much favor. Basically it is believed a sound surgical procedure, and its use is enthusiastically recommended.

The prime indication for side-to-side choledochoduodenostomy is the presence of a primary or stasis type of stone in the common duct. This type of stone is characterized by its friability, which permits it to be easily crushed between the fingers. It is usually solitary and associated with an enlargement of the common bile duct that is out of proportion to the extent of the associated disease process in the biliary tract.

The presence of an unusually dilated common bile duct in conjunction with either minimal or no evidence of concomitant biliary tract disease should make one suspicious of the presence of a primary or stasis type of stone in the common duct secondary to stenosis of the sphincter of Oddi. In such circumstances the simple removal of the stone is not believed sufficient. To prevent recurrence of the stone, a sphincterotomy or biliary-intestinal bypass operation is required. The bypass operation, a side-to-side choledochoduodenostomy is preferred. A transduodenal sphincterotomy (internal choledochoduodenostomy) is used only for the removal of a stone impacted in the intramural portion of the common duct.

A more frequent indication for side-to-side choledochoduodenostomy is the presence of a single or multiple secondary (gallbladder origin) stones in the common duct. The basic reason for its use as a primary operation is that, regardless of the experience and skill of the surgeon and the thoroughness of the exploration of the common duct, one or more stones may remain. Accordingly, the old adage states, "When the last stone is removed from the common duct, go back and remove the remaining stone." Admittedly under such circumstances an operative cholangiogram may prove useful. No matter how skillfully performed and expertly interpreted, however, this ancillary diagnostic aid still has a disturbingly high incidence of both false positive and false negative reports.

Side-to-side choledochoduodenostomy, advocated and performed by Riedel in 1888 and Sprengel in 1891, was first suggested and practiced by Sasse in 1913 as a primary method of treatment for common duct stones. In later years it received enthusiastic support from Flörcken in Frankfurt, Pribram in Berlin, and Jurasz in Posnan, while more recently Sou-

Plate 223   505

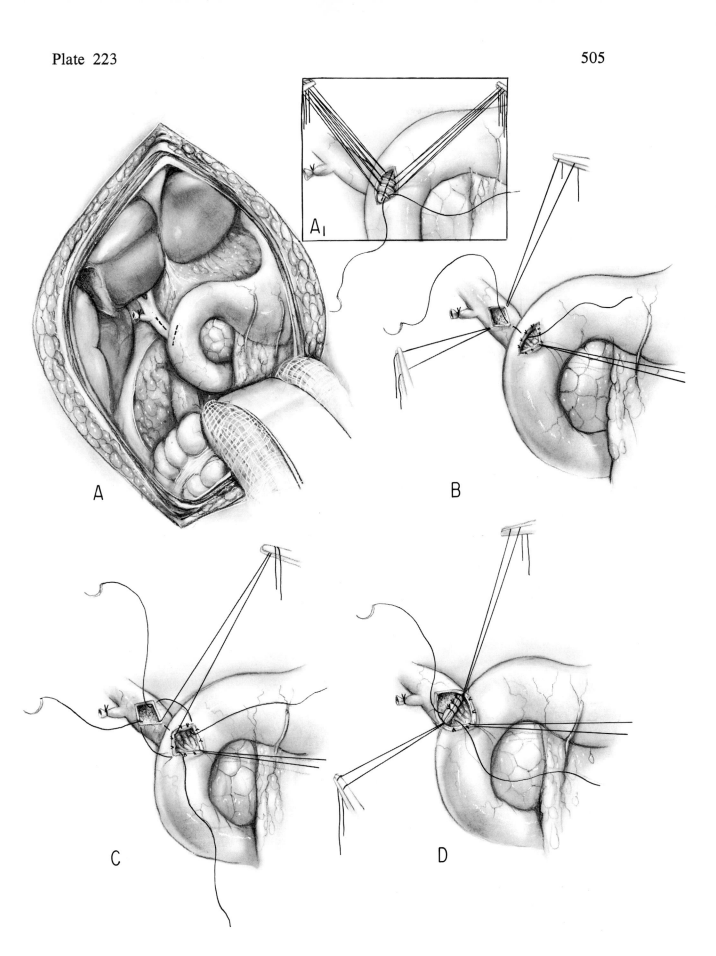

A

A₁

B

C

D

E. The first anterior layer of the anastomosis is begun by the insertion of inversion sutures in each angle of the anastomosis. Each of these sutures is inserted from the inside-out on the duodenum and from the outside-in on the common duct, so that, when tied, the knot is on the inside of the lumen. Traction on each of the previously inserted "angle" sutures posteriorly facilitates the inversion of the tissues.

F. The remainder of the sutures comprising the posterior layer are simple interrupted sutures that include the whole thickness of the wall

of the duodenum and the common bile duct, respectively.

G. The insertion of the first anterior layer of sutures is completed, and the last of a series of Lembert-Cushing mattress sutures is being inserted to complete the second anterior layer of the anastomosis.

H. The mattress sutures (00000 silk) are tied, and the seromuscular layer of the duodenum is enfolded onto the common duct to effect a cap-like serosal covering of the suture line.

palt in Paris, Valdoni in Rome and Pi-Figueras in Barcelona have strongly recommended its use. Pi-Figueras performed this operation in a consecutive series of 128 patients, the one indication being stone or stones in the common duct. The follow-up period varied between a minimum of one year and a maximum of 13 years. There were unfavorable results in only eight patients, an incidence of 6.7 per cent.

In the United States side-to-side choledochoduodenostomy as a primary operation for choledocholithiasis is uniformly condemned. The main objection to its use is the fear of cholangitis as a complication. In a personal experience with 85 patients in each of whom a side-to-side choledochoduodenostomy was performed, this complication has not occurred. It cannot be overemphasized that it is not the reflux of the intestinal contents through the anastomosis that causes difficulty, but the stenosis at the site of the anastomosis. The stenosis is prevented by meticulous care in the performance of the operation.

The indications for a side-to-side choledochoduodenostomy are generally associated with an enlargement of the common bile duct, which facilitates the performance of the anastomosis. The vertical incision in the common duct should be 2.0 to 2.5 cm. in length, and the horizontal incision in the duodenum should be comparable in size. Interrupted sutures of 00000 arterial silk are used for the anastomosis, which is clearly depicted in the artist illustrations. The necessity for a careful mucosa-to-mucosa apposition is particularly stressed. Posteriorly, the knots of the sutures are on the inside of the lumen. This is frequently objected to on the theoretical basis that it provides a nidus for the deposition of bile pigments. However, in my own experience this objection has not been substantiated.

In the posterior and first anterior layers, the whole thickness of the walls of the duodenum and common bile duct are united together. The second anterior layer is comprised of a series of interrupted mattress sutures that coapt the seromuscular layer of the duodenum to the anterior surface of the common duct. A Penrose ("cigarette") drain is inserted to the region of the anastomosis and has its exit through the incision rather than through a stab wound.

It is firmly believed that side-to-side choledochoduodenostomy is an operation that is deserving of more popular appeal in the United States. Its use as a primary procedure in the treatment of primary or stasis stones and multiple secondary (gallbladder origin) stones is unreseruedly recommended and routinely practiced.

DISCUSSION—DR. ROBERT J. COFFEY. When this operative procedure is indicated, the technic demonstrated in the illustrations is the one to employ. However, I utilize this operative procedure almost exclusively as a palliative procedure in carcinoma of the head of the pancreas. In such cases, the expectancy of survival averages six to nine months, and for this reason complications resulting from anastomosis of the common duct of the duodenum are not important. In an individual whose prospects for longevity are good, however, I do not

consider this operative procedure a sound one. Ascending cholangitis is inevitable and over a period of years may lead to serious hepatic impairment. In those situations in which choledochoduodenostomy might be carried out for benign disease, such as sphincteritis or obstruction of the lower end of the common duct as a result of chronic pancreatitis, anastomosis of the common duct to an isolated loop of jejunum, as suggested by Bowers, is a preferable procedure.

Plate 224

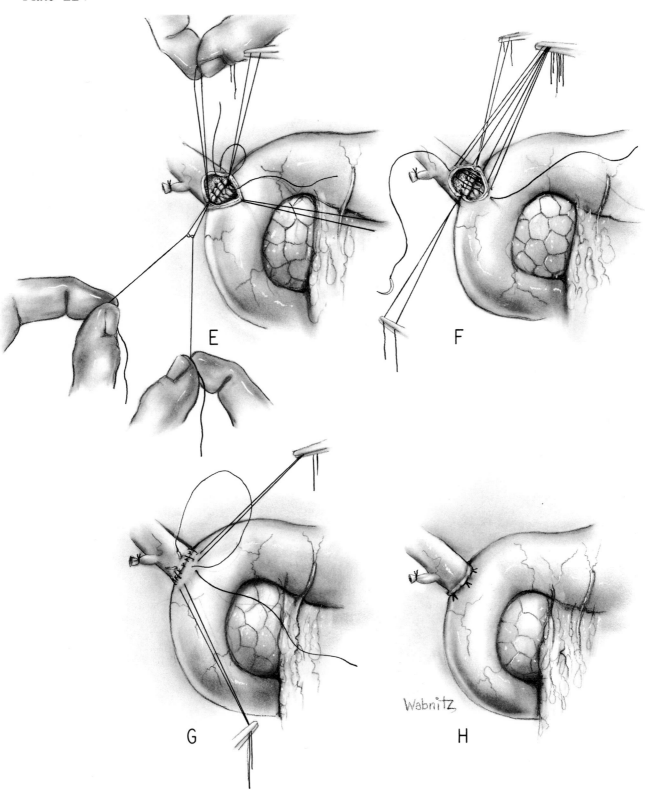

E

F

G

H

Wabnitz

RECONSTRUCTION OF THE COMMON BILE DUCT

A. The site of the benign traumatic (postoperative) stricture and the related anatomic structures are visible. Exposure of this operative field is obtained as demonstrated in the first plate of illustrations depicting the technic for sphincterotomy.

B. The strictured segment is encircled by a guy ligature of silk (0) through which traction is maintained as the duct structures proximally and distally are mobilized by scissor dissection.

B¹. Inset showing the mobilized segment of the common duct distal to the stricture being transected with scissors. The level for the transection of the common duct proximally is indicated by the dotted line.

C, D. The transected ends of the common hepatic and common bile ducts are approximated by lateral "angle" sutures of 00000 silk (C), and the insertion of the posterior layer of interrupted through and through sutures of silk (00000) is completed (D).

D¹. The sutures forming the posterior layer are tied and the insertion of the anterior layer of sutures is begun.

E. The completed end-to-end anastomosis

without an internal splint or stent support is shown. The relation of the distal end of the common duct to the gastroduodenal artery medially and the lymph node laterally is visible.

F. Inset showing an alternate method of performing an end-to-end anastomosis of the common duct. Three cardinal guy sutures of silk (00000) are inserted at equidistant points through the transected ends of the ducts (1) and tied (2). The ends of the guy sutures are left long to facilitate the axial rotation of the duct ends, and the insertion of interrupted silk (00000) sutures completes the anastomosis (3, 4). This technic is preferred to the previous one illustrated because the knots of the sutures are on the outside of the lumen, and the foreign body tissue reaction is thereby lessened. Suture knots on the inside of the lumen may be the nidus for the formation of secondary common duct calculi. However, in the patient on whom the technic as illustrated (C–E) was used, no untoward clinical manifestations were observed as late as 30 months postoperatively. If preferred, interrupted sutures of 00000 chromic catgut on a swedged-on minimum trauma needle may be used.

The technic for reconstruction of the common duct by end-to-end anastomosis without the use of an internal splint or stent is illustrated. Admittedly this is contrary to the generally accepted practice. Most commonly, a tube or stent about which the common duct is reconstructed is used and allowed to remain three months, six months, and even a year or longer. The necessity for this practice is questioned because a stent, regardless of its type, is a foreign body and, as such, may cause a foreign body tissue reaction. This is believed to be nature's attempt to eject the "intruder," which indeed may become an actuality. Furthermore, the tissue reaction may be accompanied by a deposition of varying quantities of fibrous connective tissue. Under such circumstances it is logical to assume that one may be causing that which he is trying to prevent—cicatricial stenosis of the anastomotic stoma. If a stent is used, the necessity for its presence beyond 21 days is dubious.

From our own experience, both clinically and experimentally, reconstruction of the common bile duct without the use of internal splints or stent supports has proved satisfactory. This technic was employed clinically for the first time in October, 1950; the patient has remained asymptomatic. Subsequently three other patients were similarly operated upon and have remained asymptomatic for periods of 57 months, 32 months, and 22 months, respectively. Experimentally, primary and secondary reconstructions of the common duct without the use of stents or internal splint supports have been performed in 84 animals, and, except in one animal, postoperative strictures of the common duct did not occur.

In the illustrated technic, the anatomic pathologic findings at operation were ideal for the resection of a strictured segment of the common duct and the performance of a primary end-to-end anastomosis. Plastic reconstruction of common duct strictures by a

Plate 225

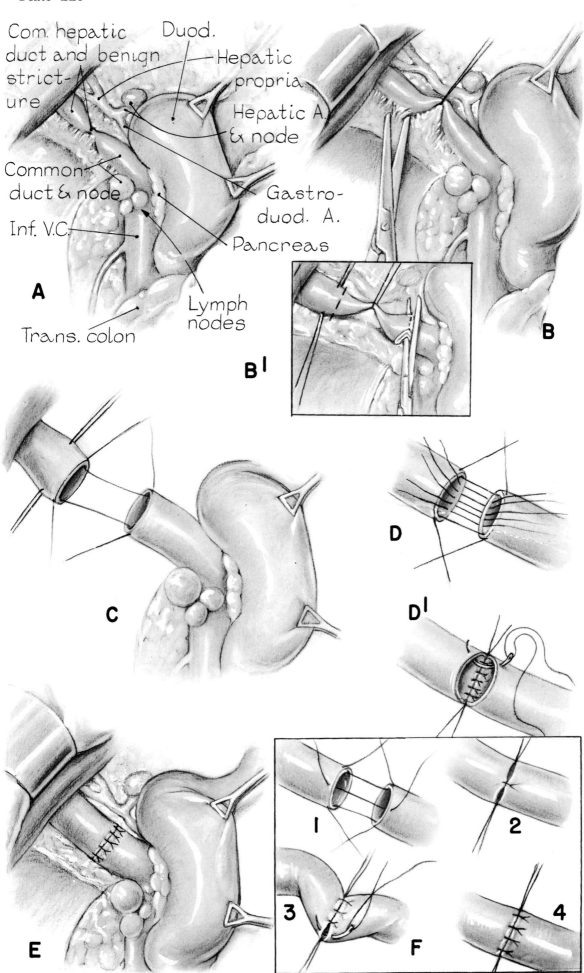

Com. hepatic duct and benign stricture

Duod.

Hepatic propria

Hepatic A. & node

Common duct & node

Inf. V.C.

Gastro-duod. A.

Pancreas

Lymph nodes

Trans. colon

A

B

B¹

C

D

D¹

E

F

1

2

3

4

longitudinal incision of the stricture and closure transversely, the Heineke–Mikulicz principle, is believed basically unsound and is neither practiced nor recommended. Frequently, the distal segment of the severed common duct is retracted into the region of the pancreas and, accordingly, is not visible. In this regard, the anatomic landmarks stressed by Cattell for the location of this segment of the common duct, namely, the lymph node laterally and the gastroduodenal artery medially (E), are a distinct aid. However, many surgeons are of the opinion that the distal segment, even if isolated, is too fibrotic for use. This has not been the experience of the author. In fact, the apparent normalcy of the tissue is most surprising. Commonly the epithelial lining is glistening in appearance and the lumen is readily distensible, which facilitates the performance of the anastomosis to the dilated duct segment proximally. Accordingly, an attempt is always made to reconstruct the common duct by an end-to-end anastomosis. If this does not prove feasible, an end-to-side choledochoduodenostomy without either proximal bile duct drainage or internal splint support is preferred.

DISCUSSION—DRS. I. S. RAVDIN AND GERALD W. PESKIN. Reconstruction of the common bile duct is one of the most difficult of all surgical procedures demanding experience, knowledge of anatomy, gentle surgical technic, and patience. This is not a procedure for the occasional operator. Wide exposure is necessary, preferably through a long subcostal incision. Good illumination is of inestimable aid. Dissection is started at the superolateral side of the adhesive mass beneath the liver, staying as close to the liver capsule as possible. Once the hepatic flexure of the colon has been freed and rotated to the patient's left, the duodenum is found adherent to the liver hilum. During the dissection necessary to release the duodenum, special attention must be paid to observation for fistulous openings between the bile ducts and the duodenum, and any opening into the duodenum must be carefully closed in layers. All of this dissection is sharp, and the moderate ooze which usually ensues can be readily controlled by firm pressure with a warm, moist sponge. The region of the common duct is then approached from the lateral side, using the palpated pulsation of the hepatic artery as a medial landmark. Aspiration with a hypodermic needle is valuable in locating the proximal duct at the liver hilum. If the duct does not protrude below the liver edge, it may be necessary to cut out a segment of liver to free it after bile has been obtained by aspiration. The proximal duct is usually large, with a rounded end and a somewhat shiny appearance. Once it is cleaned, the Kocher maneuver is performed, and the duodenum is rotated medially to aid in locating the distal segment of duct. It may be necessary to split the pancreatic head or to expose the papilla of Vater through the duodenum in order to find the distal duct. Plate 225, B, represents a stage of the operation reached only after considerable time has been consumed in careful, slow dissection. One should not be misled by the clean appearance of the tissues in this plate as this is not the usual situation in our experience. Rather, all of the structures of the portal triad are covered with a dense layer of scar.

It is important to isolate enough of the duct to perform a good anastomosis, but no more than this should be mobilized lest the vascular supply be damaged to a point of causing poor healing. The use of a hernia tape or silk suture encircling the strictured area is helpful in the mobilization of the duct.

Before cutting away the strictured segment, a longitudinal choledochostomy incision is made about one-half inch proximal or distal to the anticipated line of transection of the duct (usually in the distal duct). The duct is then cut using fine, straight scissors, and angle guide sutures of 00000 silk (atraumatic) are placed. The ends of the segments should be inspected and any frayed areas with doubtful blood supply removed. If there is a question as to the presence of mucosa, a frozen section may be obtained to be certain one is not suturing scar tissue.

The anastomosis is begun posteriorly with interrupted sutures of 00000 silk (atraumatic), utilizing the guide sutures for rotating the two ductal segments. The sutures are started from "outside in" rather than from "inside out" as shown in Plate 225, D, so that the knots are tied on the serosal rather than the mucosal side. In addition, an attempt should be made not to include the full thickness of common duct wall since foreign material within the lumen may serve as a nidus for infection or stone formation. Upon tying the posterior row of sutures, the T-tube is inserted through the vertical choledochostomy incision with one limb traversing the anastomosis. The anterior stitches are then placed and tied with the assurance that the T-tube has maintained the patency of the lumen. It is often surprising how few sutures are necessary to effect a good anastomosis. It is extremely important that the site at which the T-tube leaves the common duct be away from the line of anastomosis, since leading the tube out through the suture line usually is followed by recurrence of the stricture.

Closure of the longitudinal choledochostomy incision, drainage, and abdominal wall closure are similar to the technic described under sphincterotomy. Before closing, however, saline solution should be injected through the long limb of the T-tube to test the water tightness of the anastomosis. The T-tube is usually left indwelling for from three to six months.

DISCUSSION—DR. ROBERT J. COFFEY. In the vast majority of cases, the prime indication for reconstruction of the common bile duct is the stricture that results from the surgical trauma incident to a previous cholecystectomy. It should be emphasized that the ideal time to repair such an injury is at the time it is inflicted. The surgeon who recognizes the fact that he has damaged the common duct after having removed a gallbladder and who then calmly and carefully carries out a reconstructive procedure on the common duct has demonstrated his mettle in a most impressive way. In the illustrations, the stricture is quite apparent and the method of repair is the classic and acceptable one. However, I do feel that more evidence must accumulate before one can confidently claim that use of a stent does more harm than good. I personally insert a T-tube either above or below but not at the point of repair. This, of course, can be taken out after whatever interval the surgeon pre-

fers. It should be mentioned that not all strictures are localized or lend themselves to excision with approximation of healthy edges of common duct above and below. Cattell has quite appropriately stressed the fact that, by careful dissection of the retropancreatic portion of the common duct, considerable added length may be obtained in these trying circumstances. In several of my patients, this stricture has involved most of the visible common duct, extending into the hepatic ducts. In these patients, it was necessary to anastomose the two hepatic ducts to an isolated loop of jejunum, fashioned by the Roux "en-Y" method.

It has for many years been a cherished hope of surgeons that in those patients in whom lengthy strictures of the common duct are present, some prosthesis or graft would be found that would effectively provide a conduit for the bile. However, no such device is available.

SPLENECTOMY

A. A left rectus paramedian muscle-splitting incision, the one preferred, is depicted. In this patient the spleen was huge and produced a visible bulge on the left side of the anterior abdominal wall.

B. Alternate incisions which may be used: a′, combined abdominothoracic, b′, transverse and subcostal incisions; the dotted line shows the possible extension of the subcostal incision.

C, D, E. The dotted lines indicate the incisions through the anterior rectus sheath, the left rectus muscle, and the peritoneum respectively.

F. The peritoneal cavity is entered, and the wound margins are retracted to show the notched border of the enlarged spleen and its related structures.

G. By careful manual manipulation the spleen is displaced medially, and the incision in the layer of peritoneum which forms the posterior layer of the lienorenal ligament is shown in dotted outline. Ordinarily this layer is avascular. However, in some instances of hypersplenism, particularly the so-called Banti's syndrome, its marked vascularity necessitates the application of clamps prior to division.

H. By digital manipulation in the retroperitoneal tissue plane, the mobilization of the spleen is continued. The lienocolic ligament is shown doubly clamped before it is severed.

DISCUSSION—DR. WILLIAM D. HOLDEN. The principal hazard encountered in performing a splenectomy is hemorrhage. The operative procedure may be relatively simple, or it may tax the patience and ingenuity of the surgeon to the utmost.

The type of incision is of great importance in facilitating technical maneuvers during the operation. The left paramedian incision (Plate 226, A) extending upward to the vicinity of the xiphoid process provides better exposure than either a transverse or subcostal incision (Plate 226, B). This extension is especially worthwhile because the densest peritoneal attachments of the spleen to the posterior parietal peritoneum are frequently at the upper pole. The gastrosplenic ligament can also be exposed and clamped most easily when the incision is extended upward as far as possible. When a splenorenal anastomosis is anticipated and considerable portacaval collateral channels exist, a combined thoracoabdominal incision (Plate 226, B) provides better exposure and minimizes the danger of bleeding. A combined incision is not ordinarily necessary, however, even when splenic venous hypertension exists, if care is taken and the surgeon has had experience with this type of surgery.

With a paramedian incision the muscle preferably should be retraced laterally rather than split (Plate 226, D). Fewer anatomic relationships are disturbed, and trauma to the motor branches of the intercostal nerves supplying the rectus is reduced.

When a splenectomy is being performed for thrombocytopenia, the subcutaneous tissue in the incision oozes blood diffusely and continuously while the remainder of the incision through the abdominal wall is being made. This is apt to occur to a variable degree whether or not fresh whole blood or platelet suspensions are given just prior to the operation. This oozing ordinarily stops during the course of the operation and should not disconcert the operator.

After incising the peritoneum, the surgeon should not explore manually the peritoneal cavity of thrombocytopenic patients because of the likelihood of producing retroperitoneal ecchymoses which can assume significant proportions.

Because of difficult exposure, it is not always possible to incise the lienorenal ligament, which, in essence, is the posterior parietal peritoneum as it comes medially and anteriorly over the spleen (Plate 226, G). With experience the retroperitoneal space may be entered with the tip of a finger and the peritoneum separated bluntly. It is important not to place this peritoneal opening too close to the spleen, in order to avoid stripping the peritoneum from the splenic tissue, with resulting bleeding.

The gradual and gentle separation (Plate 226, H) of the splenic pedicle from other retroperitoneal tissues is perhaps the most important maneuver in the operation. A few extra minutes here may save considerable blood loss and many minutes of frustrating effort to control the bleeding. After completion of this manipulation, the spleen will ordinarily be sufficiently mobile to enable the remainder of the operation to be done under direct vision. Occasionally however, the spleen cannot be completely mobilized because of insufficient length and elasticity of the splenic vessels. In these circumstances, it is worthwhile to place a sponge or hernial tape loosely about the pedicle so that any sudden hemorrhage can be controlled promptly. If it becomes necessary to tighten this hemostatic

Plate 226

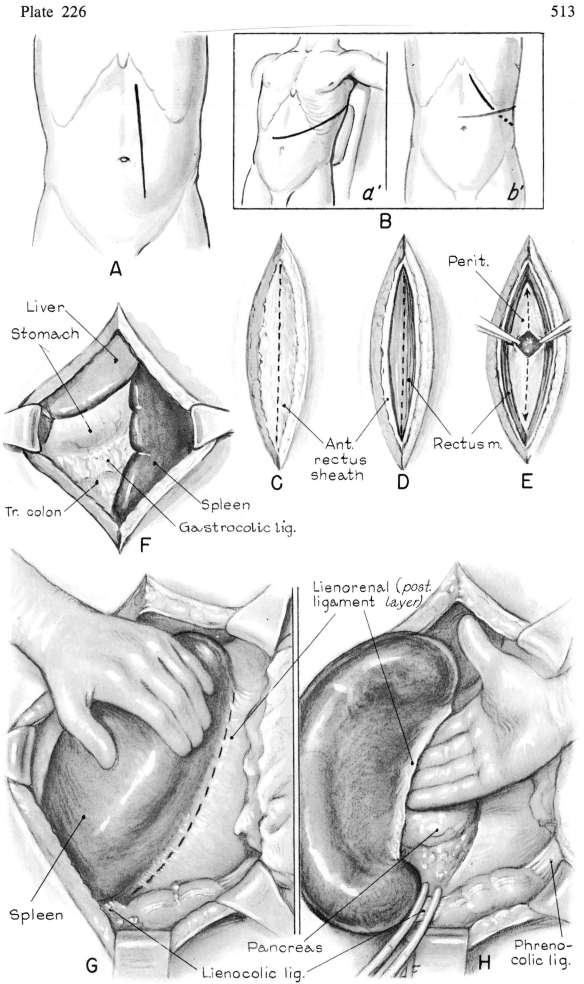

A

B

a'

b'

Liver

Stomach

Perit.

Tr. colon

Spleen

Gastrocolic lig.

F

Ant.
rectus
sheath

C

Rectus m.

D

E

Lienorenal (*post.*
ligament *layer*)

Spleen

Pancreas

Lienocolic lig.

G

Phreno-
colic lig.

H

I. The mobilization posteriorly is completed, and the spleen is easily displaced upward into the abdominal incision. The posterior aspect of the splenic pedicle and its relation to the tail of the pancreas is demonstrated. In the dissection posteriorly, particular precaution should be taken to avoid injury to the tail of the pancreas which is frequently in close approximation to the hilum of the spleen and its vascular pedicle.

J. The spleen is withdrawn through the incision and rotated laterally onto the anterior abdominal wall, and traction upward on the greater curvature of the stomach is maintained. The line of division of the anterior layer of the gastrosplenic ligament and its contained vasa brevia is shown in dotted outline.

K. The division of the gastrosplenic ligament is almost completed, and the anterior aspect of the splenic pedicle is visible. The uppermost part of the anterior layer of the gastrosplenic ligament is relatively short. Accordingly, in the application of clamps to this ligament one must be careful to avoid injury to the greater curvature of the stomach and the superior pole of the spleen. Furthermore, the uppermost part of the gastrosplenic ligament contains one of the vasa brevia. An avulsion tear of this vessel may be a frequent cause of troublesome hemorrhage during the performance of a splenectomy.

L. The spleen is completely mobilized and its vascular pedicle, which is contained within the posterior layer of the gastrosplenic ligament and the anterior layer of the lienorenal ligament, is triply clamped prior to its division between the two distal clamps. In the application of the clamps to the splenic pedicle, injury to the tail of the pancreas should be avoided. If preferred, triple ligation in continuity without the use of clamps may be performed. The center ligature is of the transfixion type distal to which the pedicle is severed. The artery and vein may be ligated either separately or as a unit structure. This method is used frequently because of the friability of the vessels. In every splenectomy performed for hypersplenism, a diligent search is always made for accessory splenic nodules, one of which is depicted in juxtaposition to the hilum. Removal of all such nodules is mandatory.

M, N. The application of a proximal ligature and a distal transfixion suture ligature of silk (00) to the vascular pedicle following the removal of the spleen is depicted.

DISCUSSION—DR. HOLDEN (cont.)

tourniquet, the tail of the pancreas may be included in it. Temporary constriction of the pancreas, however, does no permanent damage.

The splenic artery and vein may be brittle or friable, especially in elderly patients. In these circumstances, no effort should be made to separate the vein from the artery for individual ligation. Because of the danger of tearing the vessels, the application of clamps (Plate 227, L) prior to ligation is not always desirable. Two 00 silk ligatures passed around the main vessels create less trauma and are less hazardous.

Fortunately, most accessory spleens (Plate 227, L) will be encountered around the hilus of the spleen. Throughout the operation, however, the surgeon must be aware of the possibility of finding them elsewhere, such as along the course of the splenic vessels, in the gastrocolic omentum, or even in the tail of the pancreas.

Preliminary double ligation in continuity of the

Plate 227   515

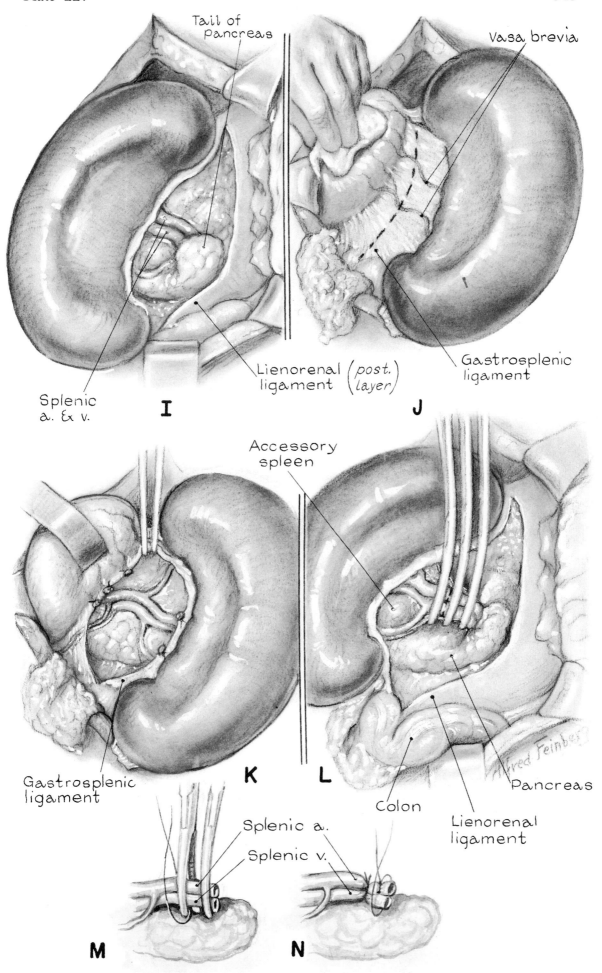

Tail of
pancreas

Vasa brevia

Splenic
a. & v.

Lienorenal (*post.
layer*)
ligament

Gastrosplenic
ligament

I   **J**

Accessory
spleen

Gastrosplenic
ligament

K   **L**

Colon

Lienorenal
ligament

Pancreas

Splenic a.

Splenic v.

M   **N**

O. The operation is completed, and the occluded vascular pedicle of the spleen and its related structures are demonstrated.

P. The anatomic relations of the intraperitoneal viscera prior to wound closure.

Q, R, S. Layer closure of the abdominal incision using interrupted mattress sutures of 00 silk for the peritoneum, interrupted sutures of 00 silk for the fascia, and interrupted sutures of 000 silk for the skin.

T. This insert depicts the preliminary double ligation in continuity of the splenic artery as advocated by the late A. O. Singleton as a technical aid in the removal of a large or densely adherent spleen. The lesser sac is entered through an opening in the gastrocolic ligament, and the splenic artery is identified by inspection and palpation as it courses along the superior border of the pancreas. The peritoneum of the posterior wall of the lesser sac overlying the pancreas is divided, and the artery is ligated in continuity with two ligatures of silk (00).

DISCUSSION—DR. HOLDEN (cont.)

splenic vessels (Plate 228, T) to facilitate the removal of a densely adherent spleen can be of value. When a previous inflammatory process has been present along the upper border of the pancreas, it is not always easy to dissect the vessels out. Ligation must be done distal to the origin of the left gastroepiploic artery; otherwise, little is gained.

An essential feature of this operation is careful inspection for bleeding of the splenic pedicle and the denuded retroperitoneal space after the spleen has been removed. It is much easier to find a small bleeding vessel, and to either ligate or suture it, at this time than several hours later.

Plate 228   517

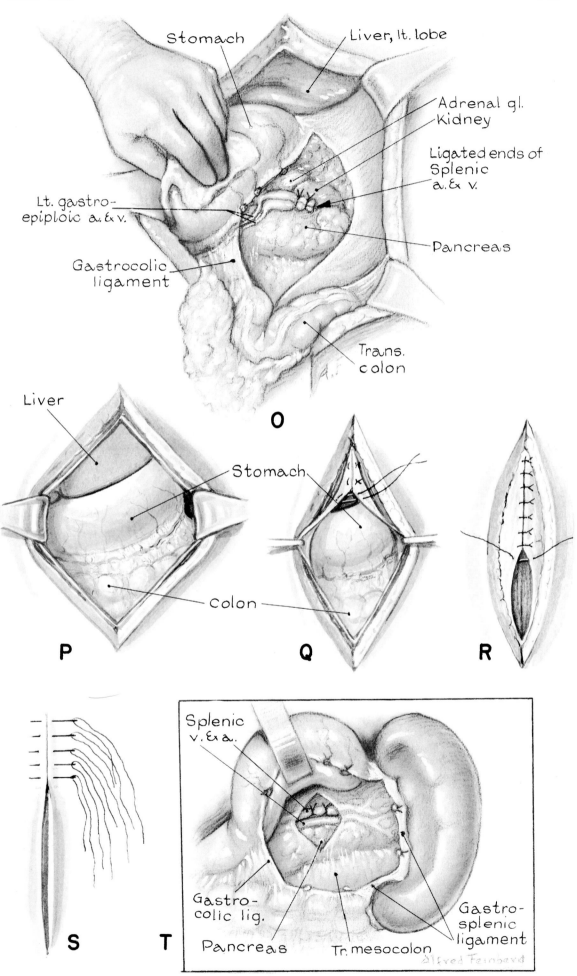

Stomach

Liver, lt. lobe

Adrenal gl.
Kidney

Ligated ends of
Splenic
a. & v.

Lt. gastro-
epiploic a. & v.

Pancreas

Gastrocolic
ligament

Trans.
colon

O

Liver

Stomach

Colon

P

Q

R

S

T

Splenic
v. & a.

Gastro-
colic lig.

Pancreas

Tr. mesocolon

Gastro-
splenic
ligament

ANNULAR PANCREAS

A. The right paramedian upper abdominal incision is shown by the solid line.

B. The peritoneal cavity is entered, and the right side of the transverse colon is displaced downward to show the middle of the second portion of the duodenum, the perivaterian segment, encircled by a constriction ring of pancreatic tissue.

C, D. The annular constriction ring of pancreas is mobilized by blunt dissection on a curved (Kelly) clamp (C) preparatory to being doubly clamped and severed (D).

E. The severed ends of the constriction ring are occluded with suture ligatures of silk (00). One of the suture ligatures is inserted and the other is being inserted prior to removal of the clamp. Even though the annular island of pancreas was severed, the constriction effect on the lumen of the duodenum was noted to persist. Furthermore, the circulation of the bowel wall appeared impoverished and was a potential site for spontaneous perforation to occur.

F. Because of the persistence of the constriction effect on the lumen of the duodenum and the potential danger of spontaneous perforation, a duodenoduodenostomy was deemed advisable. Accordingly the area was covered by the insertion of an overlying layer of interrupted seromuscular sutures (000 silk) which also formed the first posterior layer of the duodenoduodenostomy.

G. The insertion of the first posterior layer of sutures is completed. An incision is being made through the seromuscular layer of the distal segment of the duodenum to expose the vessels in the underlying submucosa. A similar incision was previously made in the proximal segment of the duodenum, and the vessels in the submucosa were undersewn with hemostatic suture ligatures of 0000 silk.

H. Traction is applied to the hemostatic suture ligatures in the distal segment of the duodenum, and the initial scalpel opening into the lumen of the duodenum is extended by scissor dissection. In like manner the lumen of the duodenum proximally was entered prior to cutting the long strands of the hemostatic ligatures.

The operation illustrated was performed in a 46-year-old white man who had intermittent digestive symptoms of 10 years duration. These symptoms were characterized by recurrent attacks of abdominal pain, nausea, and vomiting. Roentgenograms demonstrated a partial blockage in the second portion of the duodenum, the cause of which was not determined preoperatively. Diabetes mellitus controlled by dietary management was also present.

In this patient the annular constriction ring was doubly clamped, severed, and ligated as illustrated. A logical objection to this method is the potential danger of a complicating postoperative pancreatitis secondary to leakage from the severed duct which is usually contained within the constriction ring of pancreatic tissue. Although this complication did not occur in the patient operated upon, the severance of the ring did not affect a release of the constriction of the lumen of the duodenum. In fact, the segment of the duodenum uncovered after severance of the annular pancreas was exceedingly thin walled and perforation appeared imminent. Accordingly, the area was covered by the insertion of an overlying layer of seromuscular sutures (F, G) preparatory to doing a duodenoduodenostomy.

In the surgical treatment of annular pancreas, however, severance or resection of the constriction ring of pancreatic tissue about the duodenum should not be done. Either a duodenoduodenostomy (preferred) or a duodenojejunostomy (antecolic or retrocolic) is recommended. The performance of a gastrojejunostomy is not a satisfactory operation because it does not prevent the cyclic attacks of vomiting due to regurgitation of the obstructed duodenal contents into the stomach.

Plate 229

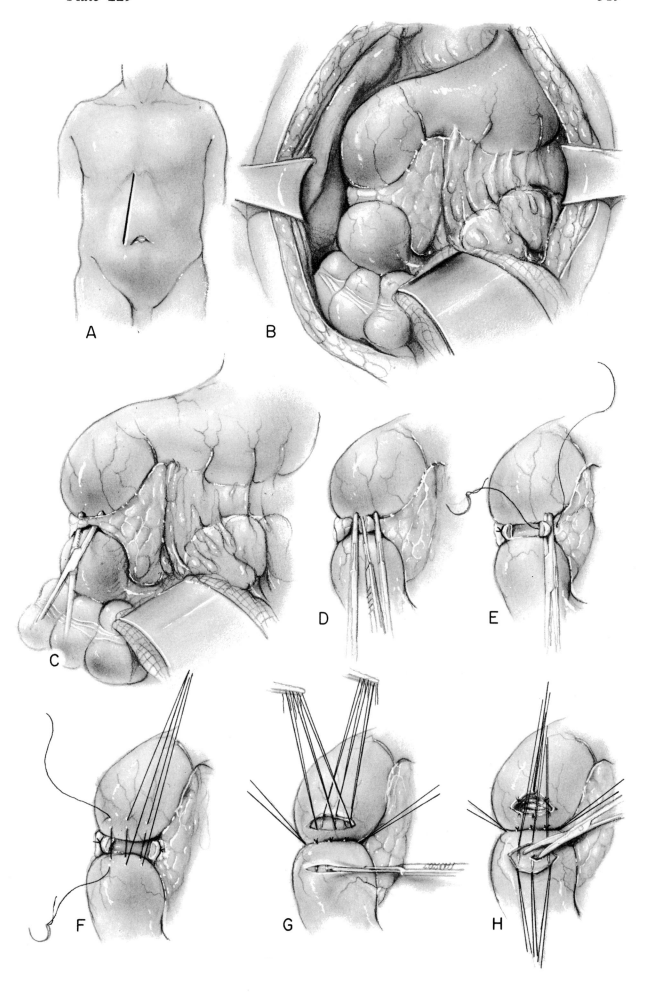

I, J, K. The insertion of the second layer of sutures (000 silk) posteriorly is begun (I). These sutures are first all inserted, tied individually (J), and then cut (K). If preferred, fine chromic catgut (000–0000) sutures may be used for the approximation of the mucosal layers. However, no complications have been observed with the use of silk sutures as depicted. The insertion of the first layer of sutures anteriorly is begun at either "angle" of the anastomosis (K). Each suture is inserted from the "inside out" to the "outside in" so that, when tied, the knots are on the inside of the lumen and inversion of the tissue layers is obtained.

L. The last two sutures of the first anterior layer of the anastomosis are encircled by an untied figure of 8 mattress suture.

M, N. The long strands of the terminal two sutures are cut, and the figure of 8 mattress suture is tied to reinforce the site of termination of the first anterior layer of the anastomosis. The interrupted seromuscular (Lembert) sutures (000 silk) which form the second anterior layer are all first inserted (M), tied individually, and then cut (N), to complete the duodenoduodenostomy.

O, P. An operation performed by many in the treatment of annular pancreas (O) is the use of a simple bypass, side-to-side anastomosis between the proximal portion of the duodenum and the jejunum. The anastomosis may be performed either anterior (antecolic) as depicted or posterior (retrocolic) to the colon.

DISCUSSION—DR. THOMAS V. SANTULLI. In this rare condition, the severity of the symptoms depends on the degree of duodenal obstruction resulting from the constricting ring of pancreas. The obstruction is almost always incomplete, but it may be severe enough to present symptoms in early life. Many of the patients do not come to surgery until late in life because of a relatively mild degree of duodenal obstruction.

The legends accompanying the illustrations state that the division of the constricting pancreatic tissue may be dangerous. It would be more prudent not to disturb the pancreas but simply to perform the anastomosis illustrated in F through N. Duodenoduodenostomy seems preferable to the duodenojejunostomy illustrated in P.

However, in infancy, the anastomosis of choice is duodenojejunostomy because of the anatomic findings and technical considerations. In all instances, it is preferable to avoid gastrojejunostomy.

In infancy, one of the important considerations is the high incidence of serious associated anomalies, i.e., malrotation, Mongolism, duodenal atresia, and so forth. The prognosis usually depends on these associated anomalies.

DISCUSSION—DR. W. H. SNYDER, JR. In infancy, any attempt to sever the pancreatic ring has been shown to be hazardous (1). Furthermore, it is my opinion that, because the duodenum beyond the annulus is so tiny and immobile, a duodenoduodenostomy should not be attempted. A duodenojejunostomy, as shown in P, or a retrocolic type, which is my preference, is indicated.

I prefer a single layer of interrupted 00000 silk suture anastomosis. The sutures are placed about 1 mm. apart and include all layers. In the posterior layer the knots are tied within the lumen, and in the anterior layer, on the surface of the bowel. Air within the stomach is then forced through the anastomosis while a little saline is dropped over it. If any bubbles are seen, an additional suture is taken. I feel that interrupted sutures are important, because a running suture may tend to constrict an already very small opening.

REFERENCE

1. Hays, Daniel M., Greaney, E. M., Jr., and Hill, James T. Annular pancreas as a cause of acute neonatal duodenal obstruction, Ann. Surg., 153, Jan., 1961.

Plate 230

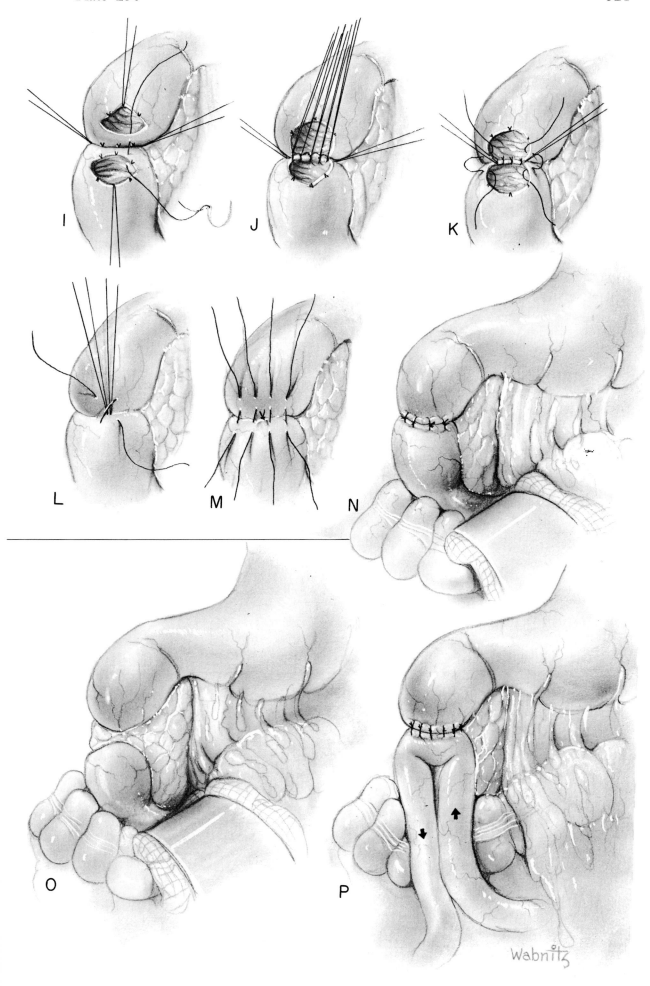

PSEUDOCYSTS OF THE PANCREAS

In this patient two pseudocysts of the pancreas, one in the head and one in the tail, were present. In addition multiple calculi both in the gallbladder and in the common duct were found. Accordingly, drainage of the cysts, cholecystectomy, and choledochostomy were performed.

A. The right paramedian muscle-retracting (lateral) incision and the extension from its midpoint transversely to the left are shown by the solid lines.

B. The peritoneal cavity is widely exposed, and the relation of the pseudocysts of the pancreas to the surrounding structures is visible.

C. The right hepatic flexure of the colon is mobilized and displaced downward toward the left lower quadrant, and the mobilization of the duodenum by scissor dissection of the posterior parietal peritoneum is indicated by the dotted line. The widened duodenal sweep is clearly shown.

D. The mobilized duodenum is secured by Babcock clamps while an incision is being made through its seromuscular layer.

Plate 231   523

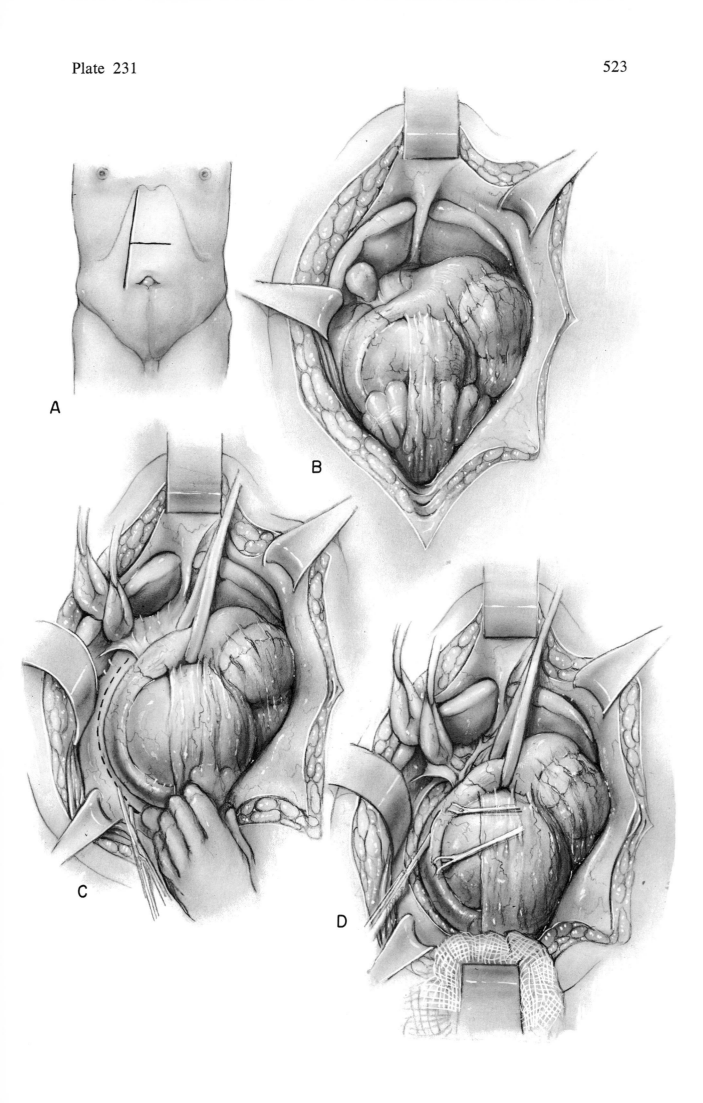

A

B

C

D

E, F. The common duct is opened, and a Bâkes dilator is inserted distally toward the papilla of Vater. Multiple stones were removed from the common duct, subsequent to which the dilator readily entered the lumen of the duodenum (E). The vessels in the submucosal layer of the duodenum are undersewn with hemostatic suture ligatures of 0000 silk (E) preparatory to incision into its lumen with a scalpel (F).

G, H. The opening into the lumen of the duodenum is enlarged by scissor dissection (G), and the cut margins are retracted to show the incision being made through the mucosal layer of the posterior wall of the duodenum (H).

Plate 232

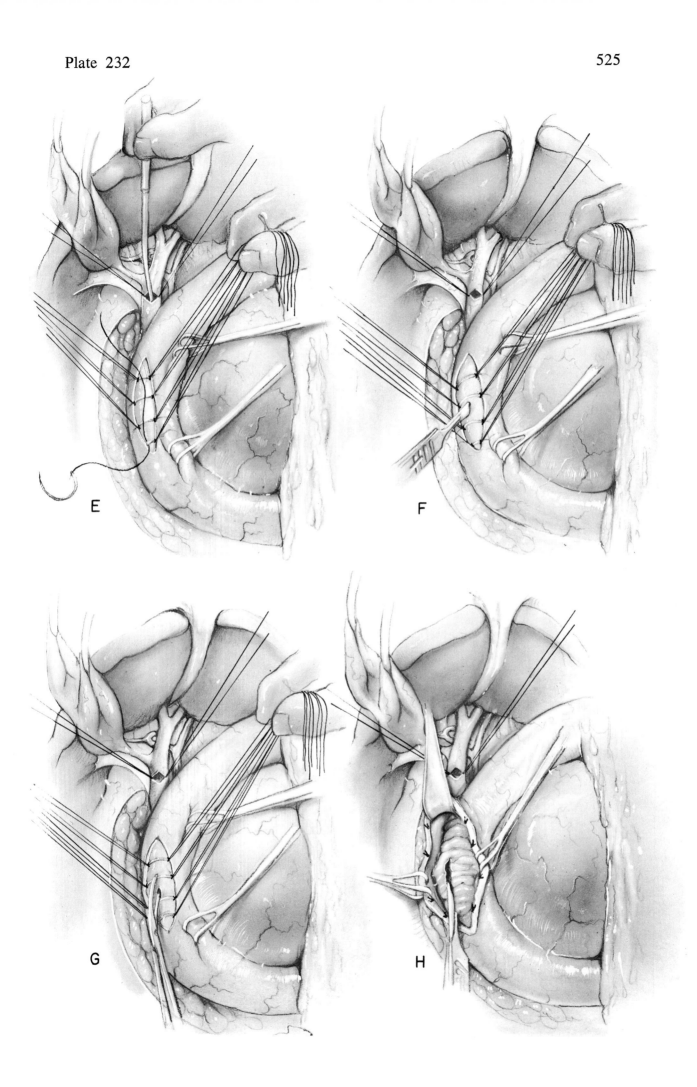

E

F

G

H

I. A trocar and canula are inserted into the cyst cavity through the partially incised posterior wall of the duodenum, and, on withdrawal of the trocar, suction decompression of the cyst within the head of the pancreas is performed.

J. The opening into the cyst cavity is enlarged by scissor dissection, and the incised margins are oversewn with a continuous hemostatic suture of chromic catgut (00).

K. The anterior wall of the cyst may be seen elevated on the tip of a clamp inserted through the opening in the posterior wall of the duodenum.

L, M, N, O. The longitudinal opening in the anterior wall of the duodenum is closed in a transverse plane by a continuous interlocking suture of 000 silk (L). A second layer of inverting Halsted mattress sutures are inserted (M, N) and tied (O) to complete the closure of the duodenotomy incision.

Plate 233

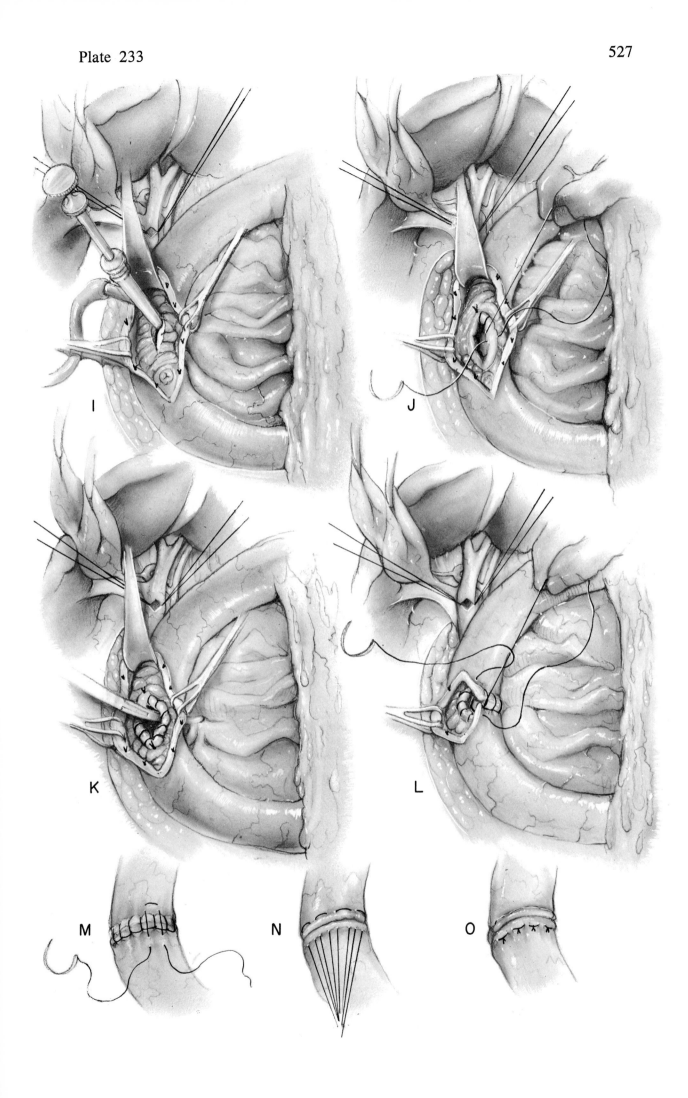

P. The pancreatocystoduodenostomy is completed, and the incision for the transgastric drainage of the cyst in the tail of the pancreas is shown by the solid line. Prior to making this incision, the lesser sac was entered and the spleen was mobilized in anticipation of performing a combined splenectomy and excision of the cyst-bearing area of the tail of the pancreas. However, the extent of the inflammatory induration of the tissues precluded the completion of the contemplated operation.

Q. The longitudinal incision through the sero-

muscular layer of the anterior wall of the stomach is completed, and the vessels in the submucosal layer are undersewn with suture ligatures of silk (000).

R, S. A scalpel is used to make an opening into the gastric lumen (R) which is enlarged by scissor dissection (S).

T. The incised margins of the anterior wall of the stomach, grasped in Babcock clamps, are retracted to show the incision being made through the mucosa of the posterior gastric wall.

Although in the past trauma has been considered a frequent etiologic factor in the formation of pseudocysts of the pancreas, it is believed that the basic cause is an acute pancreatitis either with or without associated biliary tract disease.

Pseudocysts differ from true cysts of the pancreas in that they have no epithelial lining. However, the same may obtain in true cysts of long standing because of pressure atrophy of the lining membrane.

In the surgical management of pseudocysts, excision is frequently mentioned as the ideal in treatment. However, based on the most probable pathogenesis of the formation of pseudocysts, namely, acute pancreatitis with the escape of pancreatic fluid usually into the lesser sac wherein it is encysted, this is not believed a feasible operation. The operation most commonly used is marsupialization. This is technically simple and was performed for the first time in 1881 by Gussenbauer. The objections to this operation are: (1) persistent fistula, (2) skin excoriation, and (3) recurrent cyst formation.

In the treatment of cysts located in the tail of the pancreas, resection of this segment of the gland with splenectomy may be performed in selected instances. Rarely, proximal pancreatoduodenectomy may be required as a curative procedure in instances of severe pancreatic fibrosis of the head of the pancreas complicated by pseudocyst formation.

In recent years internal drainage of pseudocysts into the proximal gastrointestinal tract has become increasingly popular. Cystogastrostomy was employed first by Jedlicka in 1923. In 1929, Jurasz performed a transgastric cystogastrostomy, and, in the same year, Kerschner drained a cyst of the head of the pancreas by the transduodenal route. The tech-

nic for each of these procedures is depicted in detail in the illustrations. They are the preferred methods for internal drainage of pseudocysts either in the head or tail of the pancreas. The theoretic objection that the stomach or duodenal contents may pass into the cyst rather than the reverse is not substantiated in fact.

Hahn, in 1926, first employed the jejunum for the drainage of pseudocysts. Chesterman of England reported its use in 1943 and was under the mistaken impression that this was the first time that pancreatocystojejunostomy was performed. Technics for its performance are illustrated in Plate 237. At present the use of the jejunum, particularly the Roux-en-Y type of anastomosis (Plate 237, A and A[1]), is believed the method most generally employed. However, the simplicity and the therapeutic effectiveness of transgastric and transduodenal drainage, either alone or combined as in the case illustrated, are factors which are believed to make either of these methods preferable to others for internal drainage of pseudocysts of the pancreas.

Finally, sphincterotomy, stressed particularly by Doubilet, may be employed. Although not used by the author in the treatment of pseudocysts of the pancreas, it is considered sound in principle, and it may prove an effective and preferred method of treatment. However, if it is used, there must be demonstrated a free communication between the cyst contents and the pancreatic duct to allow free drainage into the duodenum following the sphincterotomy. The presence of an obstruction between the duodenum and the pseudocyst precludes its use unless the obstructive factor is concomitantly relieved.

Plate 234

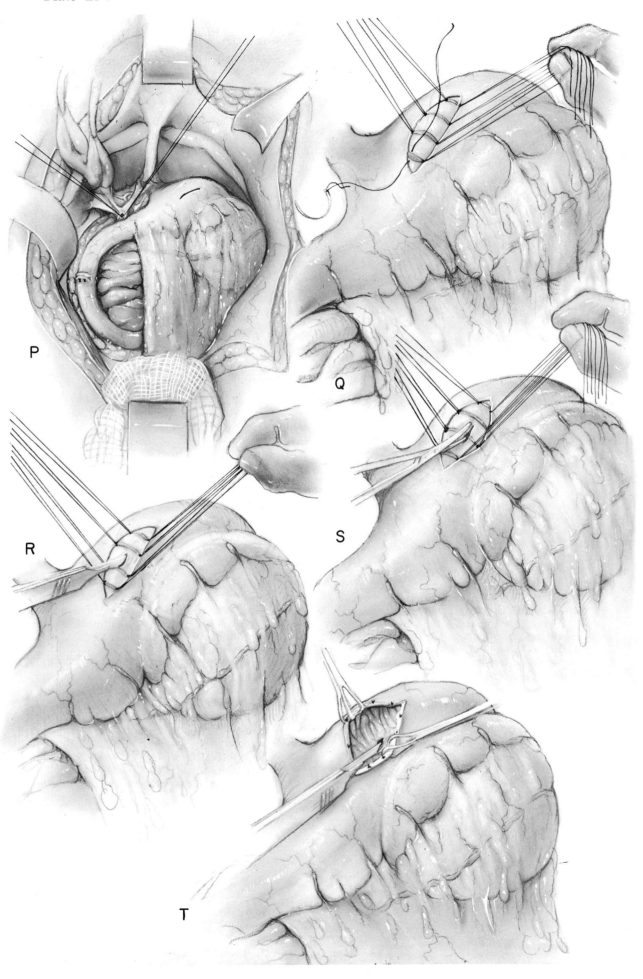

U. A trocar and canula are inserted through the incised mucosa into the lumen of the cyst which is drained by suction siphonage.

V. Following the decompression of the cyst, the opening into its cavity is enlarged (3 to 4 cm.) by scissor dissection, and the incised margins are oversewn with a continuous hemostatic ligature of 00 chromic catgut.

W, X. The longitudinal incision in the anterior wall of the stomach is closed transversely to its longitudinal axis with interrupted through and through sutures of silk (W). This line of closure is then reinforced with a series of interrupted seromuscular inversion mattress sutures (000 silk) of the Halsted type (X).

DISCUSSION—DR. HENRY DOUBILET. Since pseudocyst formation is one of the complications of an attack of acute pancreatitis, it is important to consider the etiology of the acute attack. In my opinion, the disease is caused by reflux of bile into the pancreatic duct as a result of spasm of the sphincter of Oddi. If the necrotizing process opens one or more of the smaller ducts, pancreatic juice passes into the retroperitoneal space in which the pancreas lies. Since resistance to flow into this space is less than through the spastic sphincter, the pseudocyst enlarges and extends. It will not become stabilized until the resistance of surrounding structures is equal to the resistance of the sphincter of Oddi. It is not necessary to excise, drain, or anastomose pseudocysts. Section of the sphincter of Oddi reduces the pancreatic intraductal pressure, and the pseudocyst will empty through the pancreatic duct into the duodenum. At the same time, sphincterotomy will cure the underlying disease of pancreatitis and prevent further formation of pseudocysts, a not unusual event following procedures such as marsupialization or anastomosis.

The case presented here might serve to illustrate this principle. After cholecystectomy and removal of the common duct stones, the sphincter might have been sectioned. Following this, a plastic tube could have been inserted into the duct of Wirsung and a pancreatogram performed. In the absence of any obstruction in the pancreatic duct, no further procedure would have been necessary. The two pseudocysts would have collapsed and disappeared. This has been our experience in 26 cases.

If pancreatographic study reveals obstruction in the duct, I prefer to perform a split pancreaticojejunostomy. The body of the pancreas is transected, and the ends of the sectioned duct are anastomosed to each side of a loop of jejunum (Roux-en-Y). This procedure permits drainage of the pancreatic duct from the tail, the body, and the head, and at the same time conserves all the pancreatic tissue. As a result of reduction of intraductal pressure, the pseudocyst disappears. The operations depicted by the author are unnecessary. They are anatomically unsound, since essentially each of these procedures produces an anastomosis between the gastrointestinal tract and the retroperitoneal space.

Several other points may be worth noting. The lesser omental sac is not part of the retroperitoneal space, and pseudocysts do not form there but behind it. Inflammatory adhesion of the posterior parietal peritoneum to the posterior wall of the stomach merely gives this impression. The posterior parietal peritoneum overlying the pancreas is firmly adherent and, in our experience, is not seen lifted off the surface of the organ as illustrated in Plate 238. The exudate often spreads behind the pancreas and pushes it anteriorly. The incision depicted in Plate 231, A, gives an adequate approach to the biliary tract and pancreas, but, in the experience of this commentator, a transverse incision is superior in terms of exposure, ease of closure, and resulting firmness of the wound.

A final point that might be stressed is that, on physiologic grounds, it is preferable to close the duodenal incision (Plate 231, D) in a longitudinal direction instead of transversely (Plate 233, L, M, N, O). I believe that this produces less interference with the very important peristaltic activity of the duodenum. Closure is made in two layers, a running everting chromic suture (000) to the mucosa for hemostasis, and interrupted fine silk sutures to draw the muscle and serosa together.

Plate 235

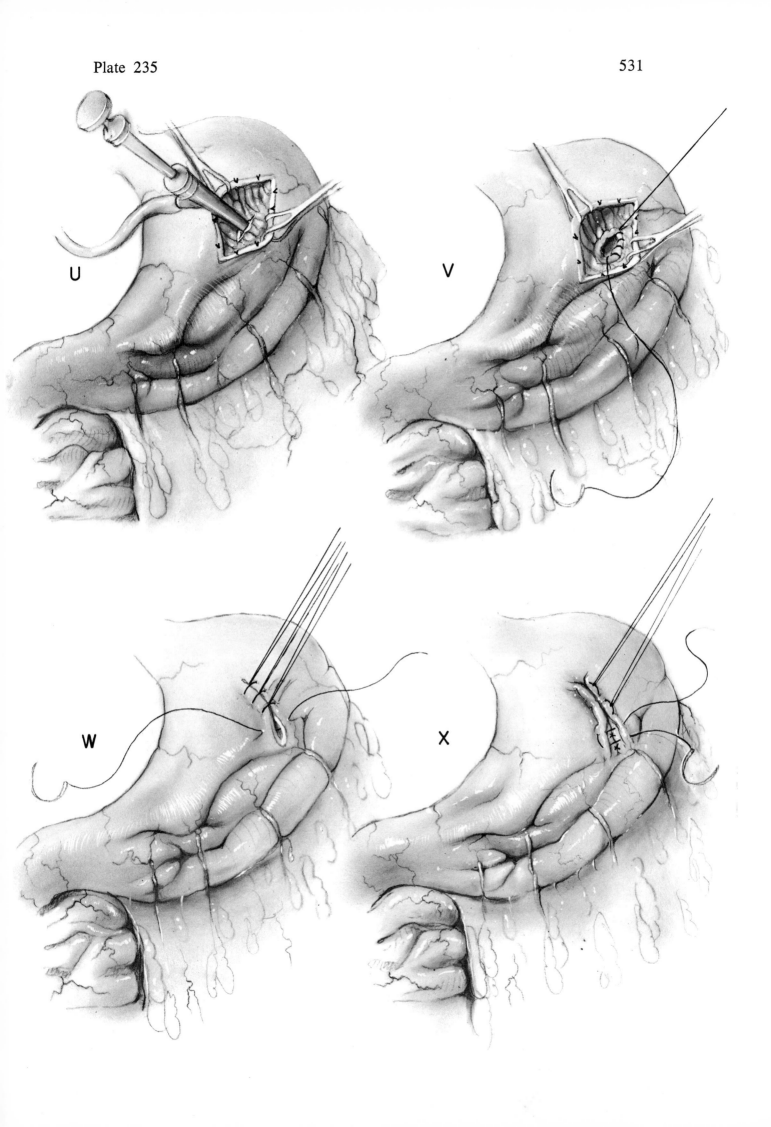

U

V

W

X

Y. Upon completion of the transgastric pancreatocystogastrostomy, the stones present in the common duct are removed preparatory to excision of the gallbladder. Prior to the exploration of the common duct the cystic duct is ligated (00 silk) to prevent the possibility of egress of stones from the gallbladder into the common duct. Subsequently the cystic duct is doubly clamped proximal to the ligature previously applied and is severed between the clamps.

Y[1]. A transfixion suture ligature of silk (000) is inserted between the clamp and the ligature on the distal severed segment of the cystic duct to reinforce its closure.

Y[2]. The proximal severed end of the cystic artery, which arises from the convex arch formed by the right hepatic artery, is similarly ligated, and the gallbladder is being mobilized from its liver bed by incision of its peritoneal attachments.

Y[3]. The cholecystectomy is completed, and the incision in the common bile duct is being closed with 00000 arterial silk sutures about a catheter (12 F) which is preferred to a T-tube for drainage of the common duct.

Z. This illustration shows the whole of the operative field upon the completion of the transduodenal and transgastric drainage of the pancreatic cysts, the cholecystectomy, and the common duct exploration. A Penrose cigarette drain, which is routinely used, is inserted into the foramen of Winslow prior to closure of the abdominal incision. The catheter and the drain have separate exits through the abdominal incision rather than through stab wounds in the flank.

DISCUSSION—DR. MAURICE MERCADIER. Pseudocysts of the pancreas are collections that represent the evolution of a more or less important form of pancreatic necrosis. Their cause is usually acute hemorrhagic pancreatitis, but as this varies from patient to patient, it is really difficult to always determine the cause. The pseudocysts may be the result of an autodestruction of the pancreas, however, which may be due to (1) circulatory insufficiency (vascular spasm, obstruction of an artery, or venous thrombosis), (2) acute retention of pancreatic secretions associated with hypersecretion of the pancreas, or (3) the activation of the pancreatic secretions by the reflux of bile from the choledocus into the duct of Wirsung. This reflux may be due to the presence of a functional (spastic) or an organic (sclerotic) block of the sphincter of Oddi.

Pseudocysts of the pancreas differ from true cysts in that they have no epithelial lining and contain pancreatic secretions, hemolyzed blood, and necrotic material. There are two types of pseudocysts: (1) the small intrapancreatic collections, which occur within a pancreatic parenchyma altered by sclerosis, and (2) the peripancreatic collections, which form in the omental bursa or at the level of the detachable cellular spaces in contact with a relatively normal or minimally altered gland. As a rule, when the cystic collections are large and expansive, they have no connection with the excretory system of the pancreas, whereas they do when they are either small or resolving. In any event, it is believed important to determine whether or not there is a communication between the pseudocyst and the pancreatic excretory system. Accordingly, operative roentgenograms are obtained routinely after the injection of a contrast medium into both the lumen of the cyst (cystography) and the duct of Wirsung (ductography).

An operative cholangiogram and determination of the intraductal (common duct) pressure are also obtained routinely.

The intraparenchymatous pseudocysts are moderate in size and occur frequently in a parenchyma altered by sclerosis (chronic pancreatitis). They are encircled by an area of chronic pancreatic fibrosis, in which the ducts and acini are distorted and filled with mucoprotein debris and calcium precipitates. The treatment of intraparenchymatous pseudocysts depends on their location and whether or not a communication with the duct of Wirsung or one of its accessory ducts is present. Pseudocysts located in the tail of the pancreas are well suited for combined distal pancreatectomy and splenectomy, provided the peripancreatic inflammatory reaction does not make the involved surgical procedure a hazardous one. Pseudocysts of the proximal portion of the pancreas sometimes have been treated by pancreaticoduodenectomy. This operation is indicated only when the pancreas is extensively diseased. Otherwise, one of the following simpler operations is preferred: (1) sphincterotomy and drainage of the duct of Wirsung (if the cyst communicates with the pancreatic duct), (2) cystoduodenostomy with drainage of the cyst into the second or third portions of the duodenum (when the lowermost part of the cyst is in close proximity with the duodenum), or (3) cystojejunostomy using the Roux "en-Y" principle (when the cyst is some distance away from the duodenal cadre but level with the anterior surface of the pancreas).

The extraparenchymatous pseudocysts often are extremely large and may arise either anterior or posterior to the pancreas. They are surrounded by a fibrous tissue reaction, which causes an adherence to the surrounding structures. In the majority of cases these pseudocysts present anterior

Plate 236

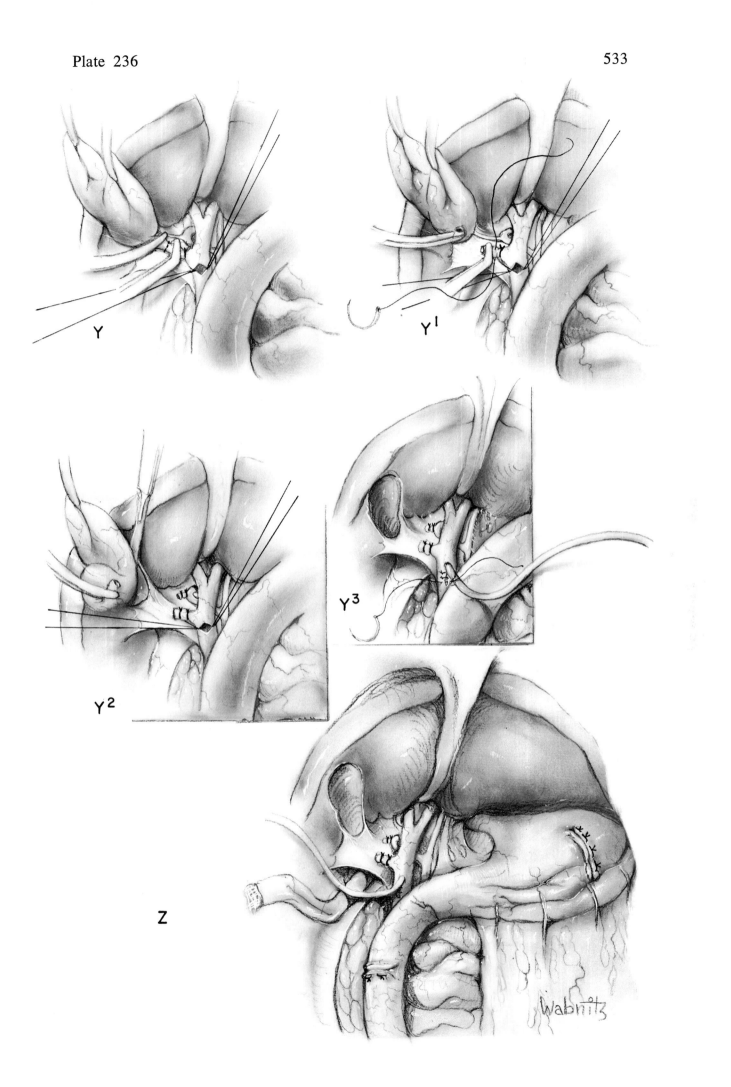

Y

Y¹

Y²

Y³

Z

A. The internal dependent drainage of a pseudocyst of the head of the pancreas by a Roux-en-Y type of anastomosis using an isolated limb of jejunum is demonstrated. The jejunum is transected 15 to 20 cm. from the ligament of Treitz, and the length of the isolated segment of jejunum cephalad to the end-to-side jejunojejunostomy varies between 30 and 35 cm.

A[1]. If preferred, a side-to-end rather than a side-to-side cystojejunostomy may be used.

B, B[1]. A pancreatocystojejunostomy may also be employed as a simple side-to-side anastomosis either without (B) or with (B[1]) a concomitant proximal enteroenterostomy (Braun anastomosis).

DISCUSSION—DR. MERCADIER (cont.)

to the pancreas and within the omental bursa. They may fill the whole cavity or be limited to one portion. Also, they may occur posterior to the pancreas in the retroperitoneal cellular tissue and project in various directions toward the left lumbar "gutter," the celiac region, the inferior portion of the posterior mediastinum, the retro-duodenopancreatic free space, and the right iliac fossa.

Sometimes the cysts are in direct communication with the pancreatic ducts, as Doubilet has demonstrated. In such cases an attempt may be made to collapse them by sphincterotomy, complemented by drainage of the duct of Wirsung. Most frequently, as demonstrated by operative cystography and ductography, these cysts do not communicate with the excretory system. Under such circumstances, sphincterotomy and drainage of the duct of Wirsung are inadequate. To insure proper drainage, external or internal drainage of the cyst is required.

Marsupialization or simple drainage of the pseudocysts has been and is still frequently used. However, these methods predispose to pancreatic fistulas, excoriation of the abdominal wall, hemorrhage, and recurrences of the pseudocysts. To prevent some of these complications, continuous suction drainage through a catheter inserted into the cystic cavity is advised. However, this method is not curative and does not prevent certain of the complications previously mentioned. Mallet-Guy recommends, as a curative procedure, reoperation three to four weeks after simple drainage of the cyst and the removal of the necrotic focus. This method is technically difficult, however, and increases the surgical risk to the patient.

Internal drainage of the collection into some nearby segment of the digestive tract eliminates these risks. Cystodigestive tract anastomosis has been objected to because it permits the reflux of intestinal contents into the cystic cavity and thereby creates a source of infection with its secondary complications of suppuration and hemorrhage. In reality, such complications are not due to reflux but to stasis, which can be avoided by placing the anastomosis in the most dependent part of the cyst. This to me is a fundamental principle. As for the role attributed to the corrosive action of the pancreatic secretions in contact with the mucous membrane of the digestive tract, this notion in my opinion has been overemphasized. It is well known that this contact is a normal physiologic occurrence within the digestive tract. Internal drainage of the contents of the pseudocyst can be assured by anastomosis of the pseudocyst to the stomach, duodenum, or jejunum.

Historically, the first cystogastrostomy was performed in 1923 by Jedlicka. It was achieved by a direct anastomosis between the pseudocyst and the lesser curvature of the stomach. Unfortunately, the anastomosis was located too high to provide adequate drainage of the cyst, and, accordingly, the operation was a failure.

Jurasz, in 1931, reported for the first time transgastric drainage of a pseudocyst of the pancreas, the technic for which is clearly illustrated. It should be mentioned that this technic is applicable only when the pseudocyst is located high behind the lesser curvature or the body of the stomach. It is not applicable when the fundus of the pseudocyst is located lower than the greater curvature of the stomach. Under such circum-

Plate 237

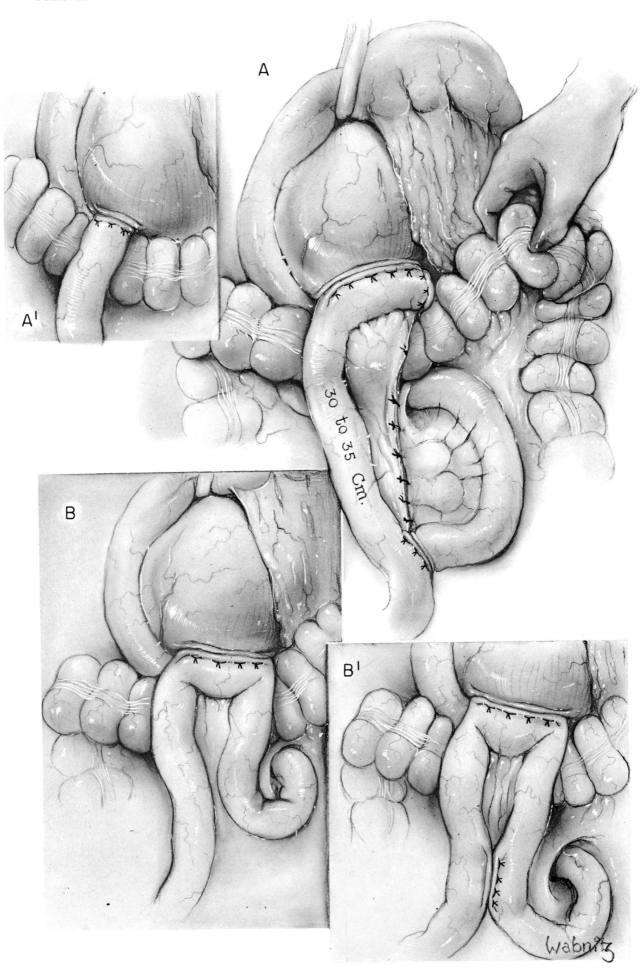

A

A'

B

B'

30 to 35 Cm.

Wabnitz

This plate (after Judd, Mattson, and Mahorner) depicts the common pathways of extension of pseudocysts of the pancreas. In addition to those illustrated, extension of a pseudocyst into the posterior mediastinum may also occur.

A. Projection of the cyst between the inferior surface of the liver and the anterior wall of the stomach is shown. This is the second most common pathway of enlargement. Access to cysts in this area is best obtained through an opening in the gastrohepatic ligament.

B. This is the most common location for pseudocysts of the pancreas, namely, between the stomach above and the transverse colon below. Access to cysts in this area is readily obtained through the gastrocolic ligament.

C, D. Pseudocysts of the pancreas may project between the leaves of the transverse mesocolon and enlarge downward toward the pelvis (C) or ventrally toward the anterior abdominal wall (D).

E. In some instances pseudocysts may extend retroperitoneally either upward into the posterior mediastinum or downward into the pelvis as depicted. When a retroperitoneal extension into the pelvis occurs, there may be difficulty in differentiating it from a large ovarian cyst. In fact, in the case reported by Bozeman (1882), which was the first successful excision of a pseudocyst of the pancreas reported, the preoperative diagnosis was an ovarian cyst.

DISCUSSION—DR. MERCADIER (cont.)

stances, the anastomosis does not insure complete drainage of the cyst.

The first cystoduodenostomy was done in 1911, by Ombredanne. The anastomosis was done between the cyst and the second portion of the duodenum. The operation failed because of tension on the suture line and a disruption of the anastomosis.

Kerschner, in 1929, introduced transduodenal cystoduodenostomy. This operation is also clearly demonstrated, and I have nothing to add to the technic of its performance. It must be emphasized, however, that it is essential to place the anastomosis in the most dependent portion of the cyst. This operation is indicated only for the high-lying pseudocyst in the head of the pancreas. Low-lying collections should be drained into the third portion of the duodenum, not into the second or descending portion.

Cystojejunostomy is considered the best method for internal drainage, provided it is done by means of the Roux "en-Y" type of anastomosis using an isolated limb of jejunum. The technic for this operation is adequately illustrated. The antiperistaltic type of anastomosis minimizes reflux of intestinal contents, and stasis is prevented by placing the anastomosis in the most dependent part of the cyst. It should be mentioned, however, that the operation is more difficult and longer than the preceding ones described. To be successful, it is necessary that the walls of the cyst be well organized, firm, and able to hold the sutures. I use it only for the drainage of pseudocysts located below the greater curvature of the stomach and behind the gastrocolic ligament and for the pseudocysts of the head of the pancreas that are not in apposition with the medial wall of the duodenum.

In summary, the preferred methods of surgical management for the various types of pancreatic pseudocysts are as outlined: (1) for pseudocysts communicating with the main pancreatic ducts, sphincterotomy associated with or without drainage of the duct of Wirsung using a polyethylene tube; (2) for pseudocysts not communicating with the main pancreatic duct and not expansive, external drainage by continuous catheter suction aspiration, followed in three to four weeks by secondary surgical removal of the necrotic debris; and (3) for pseudocysts not communicating with the main pancreatic duct and expansive, internal drainage through one of the various methods illustrated for internal drainage into the gastrointestinal tract.

In the selection of the type of internal drainage, the following recommendations are made: (1) transgastric cystogastrostomy (Jurasz) for pseudocysts lying above and behind the stomach; (2) transduodenal cystoduodenostomy (Kerschner) when the pseudocyst is located in the head of the pancreas in juxtaposition to the duodenum; and (3) cystojejunostomy, on the Roux "en-Y" principle, for the large expansive pseudocysts located in the omental bursa and below the greater curvature of the stomach and for the pseudocysts in the head of the pancreas that are not in apposition with the medial wall of the duodenum.

Plate 238

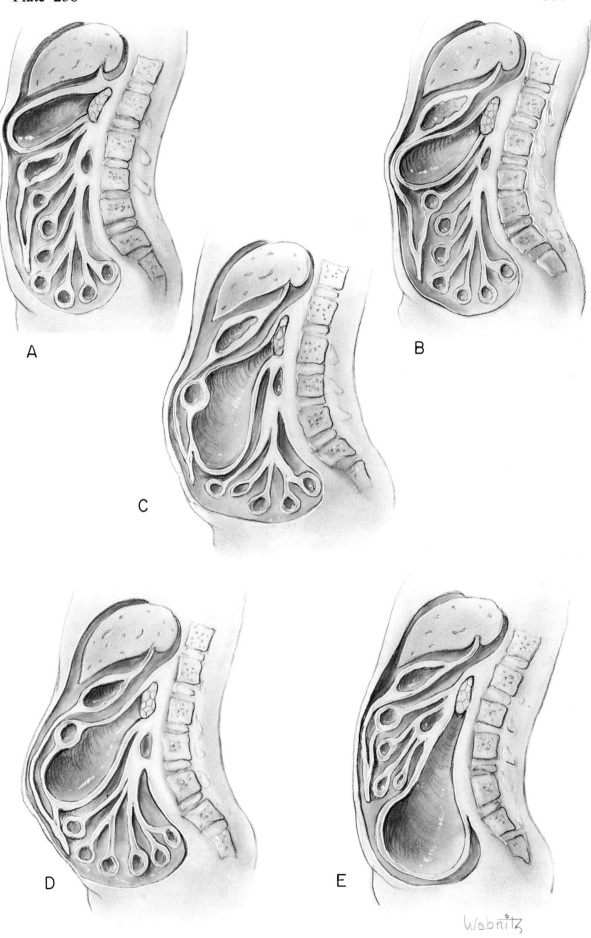

A

B

C

D

E

Wabnitz

TRANSDUODENAL EXCISION OF TUMOR ABOUT THE PAPILLA OF VATER

A. The right upper quadrant oblique paramedian muscle-retracting (lateral) incision employed is shown by the solid black line.

B. The peritoneal cavity is entered. After a thorough exploration of its contents in this patient, it was deemed advisable to explore the common duct. On exploration of the duct, a probe could not be passed into the lumen of the duodenum. Accordingly, preliminary to mobilization of the retrocolic portion of the duodenum, the right phrenocolic ligament was incised (dotted line).

C. The hepatic flexure is displaced downward and to the left, and the posterior parietal peritoneum is incised by scissor dissection preparatory to mobilization of the duodenum (Kocher).

D, E. By blunt digital dissection in the retroperitoneal tissue plane, the duodenum and the head of the pancreas are mobilized and rotated toward the midline (Moynihan rotation maneuver) (D). Palpation of the duodenum at this time revealed a tumor mass in the region of the papilla of Vater, and, accordingly, a duodenotomy was performed (E).

The patient, a seventy-year-old white woman, was admitted to the hospital with the history that, during the preceding four months, recurrent attacks of chills and fever of increasing severity were noted. Anemia and a weight loss of 13 pounds were associated clinical manifestations. Jaundice was never a symptom.

During the three-week hospital period prior to operation, a battery of diagnostic blood tests, stool examinations, and roentgenographic studies of the stomach, small bowel, colon, and kidneys were done. These were all normal. The only positive roentgenographic finding was a faint visualization of the gallbladder following ingestion of the dye. In view of this finding and in conjunction with the remittent fever and the persistence and progressive severity of the recurrent bouts of chills and fever, operation was advised. The operative findings and the surgical procedure performed are illustrated. The postoperative course of the patient was entirely satisfactory. A cholangiogram obtained on the seventh postoperative day was normal. Both catheters were removed two days later, and the Penrose drain was removed on the tenth day after operation. The temperature returned to normal within 48 hours after operation and remained normal throughout the remainder of the hospital stay. Follow-up examination at the end of 10 weeks showed the patient to be in excellent condition, and there were no subjective complaints. The pathologic diagnosis was benign sessile papillomatosis with early atypical changes and secondary inflammatory reaction.

DISCUSSION—DR. ALEXANDER BRUNSCHWIG. Every surgeon has his own particular method in connection with the minutiae of procedures such as this one. The fact that there are so many variations indicates that there is probably no one method superior to all others. In the main, I would concur with the procedure as depicted but will comment as follows.

In most instances simple firm retraction downward and mesially of the hepatic flexure will expose the first and second portions of the duodenum. A few extra "wipes" with a gauze sponge will further mobilize the hepatic flexure downward away from the duodenum.

In exploring the common duct, I would make a longitudinal incision to pass the probes and dilator.

In mobilizing the duodenum, I would grasp the upper and lower portions with Babcock clamps and incise the posterior parietal peritoneum along the greater curvature of the duodenum. Occasionally small vessels are fairly numerous, and after incising the peritoneum, the surgeon must pause to secure hemostasis by ligating all clamped vessels. The duodenum is then mobilized mesially by digital dissection, as is well shown in D. I have always known this as the "Kocher maneuver."

In opening the duodenum (E), I have usually extended the incision lower or made it lower than at first thought necessary, because in my experience the papilla of Vater is visualized lower than expected on the posterior wall of the duodenum.

As pointed out by Dr. Madden, benign lesions of the papilla of Vater are surprisingly mobile

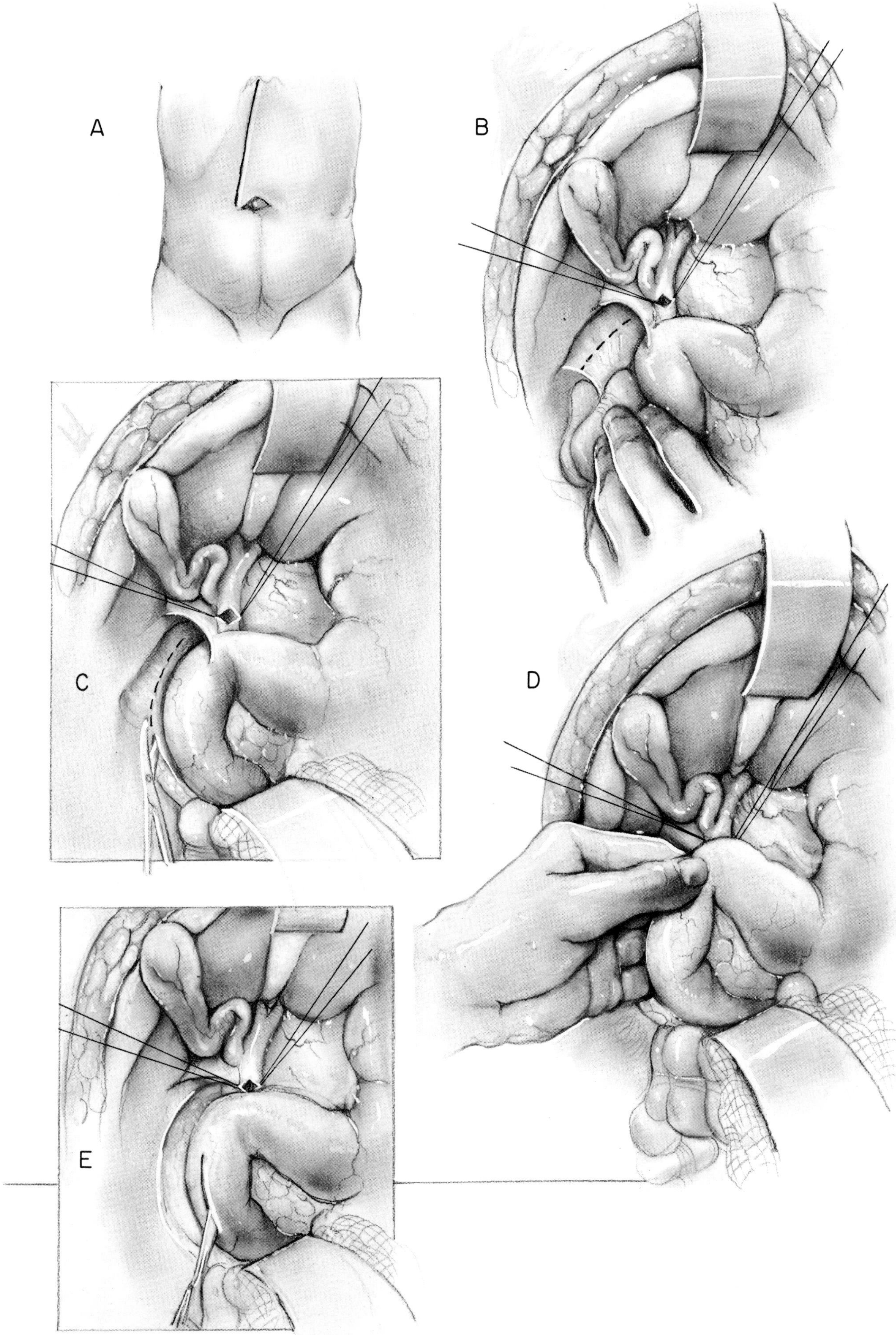

Plate 239

F. On retraction of the incised margins of the duodenum, a sessile, cauliflowerlike mass in the region of the papilla of Vater was observed. Beneath this mass a second firm, oval tumor was palpated. The head of the pancreas and the liver were normal. A Bâkes dilator (4 mm.) was inserted into the common duct and protruded through the center of the sessile tumor mass into the lumen of the duodenum.

G. The Bâkes dilator was replaced by a catheter (14 F), and a second catheter (14 F) was readily inserted into the adjacent orifice of the pancreatic duct. In view of the local characteristics of the lesion and the age and general condition of the patient, a total excisional biopsy was the operation of choice. It was surprising how readily both the common and pancreatic duct orifices were catheterized through the center of the tumor mass.

H, I. A transverse elliptical incision is made first through the mucosa of the posterior wall of the duodenum beyond the border of the tumor (H) and then deepened through its underlying layers to expose the terminal portions of the common and pancreatic ducts (I). The oval tumor mass previously palpated beneath the sessile tumor was subsequently proved to be an impacted stone in the intramural portion of the common duct.

J. Traction guy sutures of silk (00000) are placed in the walls of the pancreatic and common ducts proximally, prior to their severance distally as indicated.

K. The transection of the duct structures is completed and the repositioning of the proximal transected ends into the lumen of the duodenum is begun. The cut margins of the elliptical opening in the duodenum posteriorly are approximated with interrupted mattress sutures of silk (000), which include all of the layers of the bowel wall and separate the duct structures from each other.

L, M. The mattress sutures are tied, and the transected ends of the pancreatic (L) and common (M) ducts are sutured to the cut margins of the mucosa of the posterior wall of the duodenum using 00000 arterial silk.

DISCUSSION—DR. BRUNSCHWIG (cont.)

and can be readily elevated by probes inserted downward through the common duct. A wide excision, as depicted, entails transection of both the terminal common duct and the pancreatic duct and these are immediately identified. In the few cases I have operated upon, these ducts were first sutured together by two interrupted sutures of 000 silk passing through the entire thickness of the walls. The posterior duodenal wall was brought snugly about the united ducts by one layer of interrupted sutures, also of 000 silk. A T-tube is then inserted into the incision in the dilated common duct proximally. The proximal segment of the tube is cut short, and the distal segment is preserved long enough to pass into the duodenum through the open sutured-in common duct. Interrupted sutures of catgut (00) close the common duct about the T-tube. I have not cannulated the pancreatic duct and encountered no difficulties because of this.

In general, the incision into the duodenum is closed transversely in two layers. If it is unusually long, it is closed longitudinally. By not cannulating the pancreatic duct, no tube passes out of the duodenum through the anterior abdominal wall. I make a point of placing the soft rubber drain in the right kidney fossa which is the lowest point in this area, when the patient is in the reclining position.

Plate 240

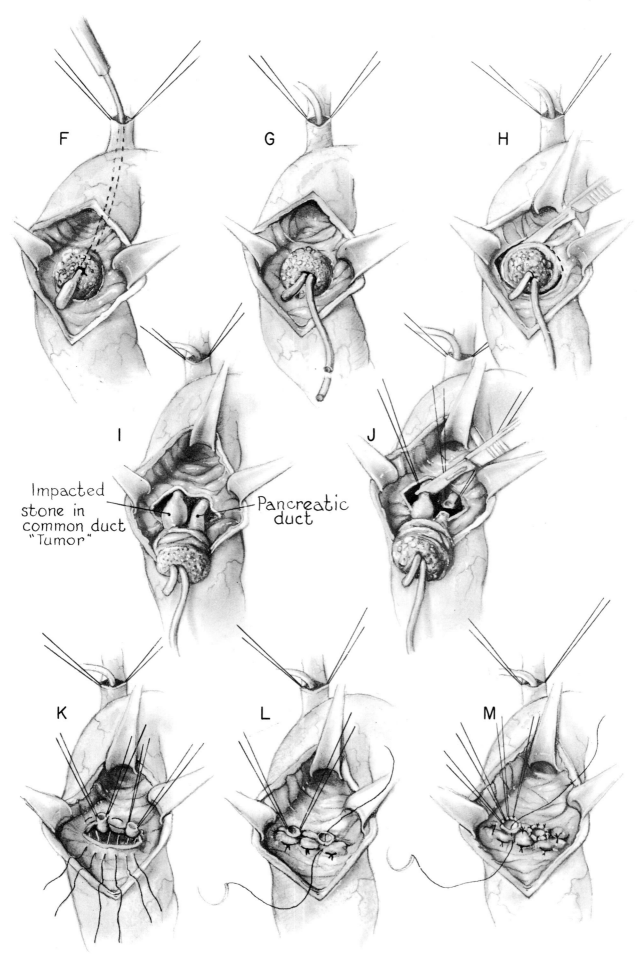

F

G

H

I

Impacted
stone in
common duct
"Tumor"

Pancreatic
duct

J

K

L

M

N. A catheter (14 F) is inserted in the common duct through its terminal reconstructed orifice into the duodenum. A second catheter (14 F) is inserted transduodenally through the new orifice of the pancreatic duct into its lumen.

O. The longitudinal incision in the duodenum is closed transversely using interrupted sutures of silk (000). These sutures commencing at either end are inserted alternately from the "inside out" to the "outside in" so that, when tied, the knots are on the inside of the lumen and the serosal layers are inverted.

P, Q. A second reinforcing layer of seroserosal mattress sutures of silk (000) are inserted (P) and tied (Q) about the protruding pancreatic duct catheter.

R, S. By traction on the terminal mattress sutures anteriorly, the bowel wall is rotated on its longitudinal axis, and a layer of seroserosal mattress sutures of silk (000) is inserted (R) and tied (S) to reinforce the line of closure posteriorly.

T. The completed closure of the duodenum and the protruding pancreatic duct catheter are shown.

U. The operative field immediately prior to the closure of the abdominal incision is shown. The catheters (14 F) in the common and pancreatic ducts respectively and the Penrose drain in the foramen of Winslow have their exit through the line of closure of the incision rather than separate stab wound drainage sites.

DISCUSSION–DR. WALTER L. MERSHEIMER. Patients with tumors of the ampulla of Vater often present clinical and laboratory evidence of obstructive jaundice and occasionally melena.

If of sufficient length, the right paramedian muscle-retracting incision illustrated, affords excellent exposure, particularly in the patient with a narrow costal margin. I prefer a right subcostal incision located so that it can be extended to the left across the midline if necessary for better exposure. Patients are more comfortable postoperatively with the transverse incision, and they have a lower incidence of wound complications, particularly disruption and evisceration.

Careful exploration of the peritoneal cavity should localize the lesion to the extrahepatic biliary system. Note should be made of any evidence of additional pathologic findings either allied or unrelated. In most instances of tumors of the papilla of Vater the gallbladder and common duct will be dilated. This may not be true if there is concomitant cholecystitis and cholelithiasis, as the diseased gallbladder may be incapable of dilating.

Dr. Madden has illustrated two very important points of technic that assure adequate exposure of the common duct. (1) Incision of the phrenocolic ligament permits the hepatic flexure of the colon to be displaced down and to the left. (2) Mobilization of the duodenum and head of the pancreas by the "Kocher maneuver" exposes the retroduodenal portion of the common duct. A linear incision in the common duct between guy sutures should be of ample length. In the presence of a dilated common duct, absence of stones and inability to pass catheters or dilators through the ampulla into the duodenum demand a duodenotomy either to demonstrate or negate the presence of a lesion. An impacted stone, stricture of the duct, stenosis of the ampulla, or tumor of the papilla of Vater may be difficult to palpate. Once the duodenum is opened, elevation of the papilla by means of a dilator or probe inserted through the opening in the common duct will aid in its identification.

When the diagnosis of a tumor of the papilla of Vater is established, a decision must be made to proceed with one of the following operations: (1) pancreaticoduodenectomy, (2) local excision of the tumor and decompression of the biliary tract as the first of a two-stage operation, or (3) local excision only.

If an immediate and conclusive diagnosis of a malignant tumor is established by frozen section, preference should be given to pancreaticoduodenectomy, provided that the patient's general condition is satisfactory and there is no distal spread of the tumor. If the tumor is proved benign, local excision is the definitive procedure. When at operation it is doubtful whether the tumor is benign or malignant and the frozen sections are equivocal, local excision is advised. However, if the subsequent histopathologic studies prove that the tumor is malignant, pancreaticoduodenectomy may be performed as a secondary operation, should it be deemed justifiable. Malignant adenomas of the papilla of Vater respond well to local excision, as do the benign lesions.

Following completion of the operation (local excision), a long T-tube is inserted in the common duct and its lower end extends through the choledochoduodenostomy into the duodenum. The use of a separate catheter in the pancreatic duct, emerging through the wall of the duodenum, as illustrated by Dr. Madden, has not been practiced. However, it is believed a valuable step in the procedure.

The technic of elliptical excision of the tumor of the papilla and the exposure of the terminal portion of the common bile duct and pancreatic duct are beautifully illustrated and concisely described. Similarly, the details of reanastomosis of the ducts to the duodenum are clearly depicted, and, accordingly, further comment is believed unnecessary.

Plate 241

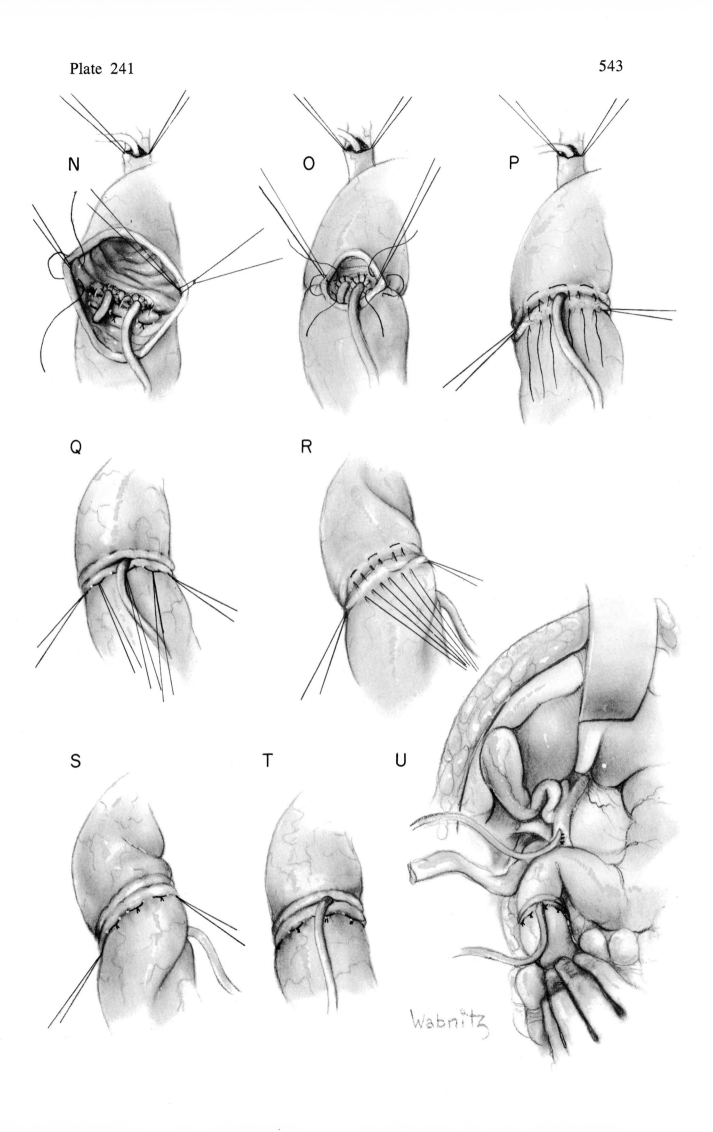

PANCREATICODUODENECTOMY

A. The upper right paramedian muscle-splitting incision is outlined.

A₁. The wound layers are separated, and the incision in the anterior parietal peritoneum is depicted.

B. The peritoneal cavity is entered, and the large distended gallbladder, which was easily palpable on abdominal examination, is seen. To obtain maximum exposure, the falciform ligament is serially clamped and severed as indicated.

B₁. Inset showing a trocar being inserted into the lumen of the enlarged gallbladder for suction decompression. In obstruction caused by a carcinoma of the head of the pancreas, the material aspirated is usually greenish-black in color and molasses-like in consistency. Preliminary decompression of the distended gallbladder is considered a techni-

cal expediency in the performance of a pancreaticoduodenectomy.

C. Traction is maintained on the pursestring suture (00 silk) that occludes the opening previously made into the lumen of the gallbladder, and the areolar tissue attachments to the transverse colon are severed by scissor dissection.

C₁. The decompressed and mobilized gallbladder is covered with a moist gauze pad and retracted to show the freeing of the hepatic flexure of the colon by severance (broken line) of the right phrenocolic ligament.

C₂. The mobilized segment of colon is reflected downward and medialward, exposing a portion of the duodenal "loop" and the encirclement of the dilated common bile duct with a rubber tissue tape.

Plate 242

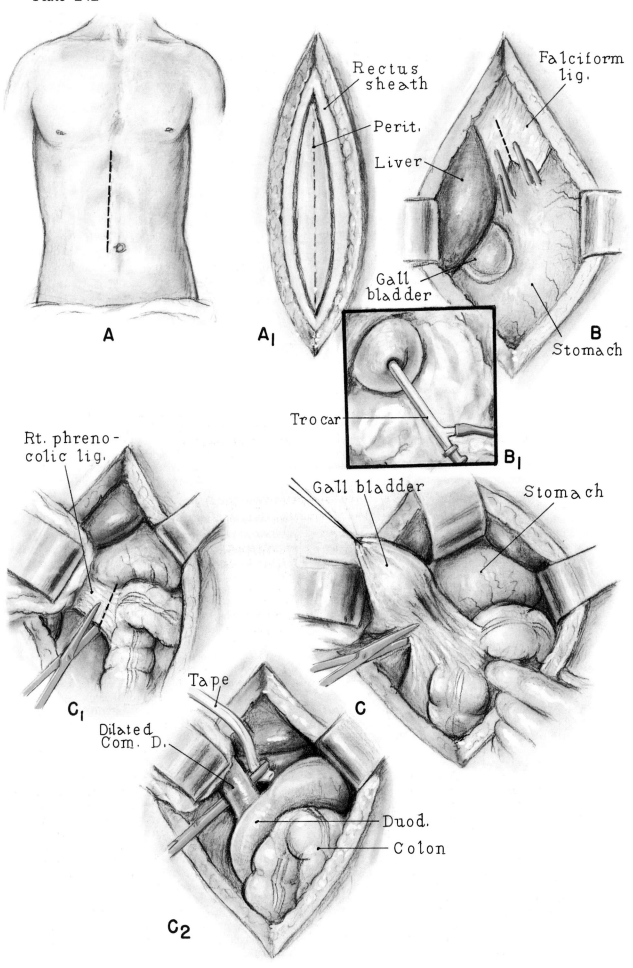

A

A₁

Rectus sheath

Perit.

Liver

Gall bladder

Falciform lig.

B

Stomach

Trocar

B₁

Rt. phreno- colic lig.

C₁

Gall bladder

Stomach

C

Tape

Dilated Com. D.

C₂

Duod.

Colon

D. The duodenal "loop" is now visible, and the avascular areolar tissue attachments between the head of the pancreas and the transverse mesocolon are severed by scissor dissection.

D₁. The anterior surface of the head of the pancreas is exposed, and the pancreatic tributaries of the superior mesenteric vein are seen. The uppermost tributary, doubly ligated in continuity (000 silk), is being transected with scissors.

D₂. Upon retraction of the ends of the transected tributary, the formation of a common venous trunk with a deeper-lying tributary is visible. The pancreatic tributaries are each in turn doubly ligated in continuity (000 silk) and severed with scissors as in-

dicated. These tributaries as shown are constant anatomic structures that are not in general accurately depicted in the standard texts and atlases of anatomy.

To minimize blood loss, exposure, ligation, and severance of the tributary veins, as indicated, are believed mandatory.

D₃. The operative field on completion of the ligation and transection of the pancreatic tributaries is shown.

D₄. The mobilized superior mesenteric vein is retracted medialward and elevated to show the course of the duodenum beneath it. The whole of the duodenal "loop" in relation to the surrounding structures is now visible.

DISCUSSION—DR. ALEXANDER BRUNSCHWIG. When this operation was first described in 1937, it was called "pancreatoduodenectomy," not "pancreaticoduodenectomy" (*Surg., Gynec. & Obst.,* 65:681-685, 1937). Over the years the latter designation has crept into the literature but would seem inappropriate because one does not say "gastricoenterostomy" or "cholecysticogastrostomy" or "enterenticoenterostomy."

Emphasis on careful dissection of the vessels, especially the smaller thin-walled veins about the head of the pancreas, is a point well made, because the serious hemorrhage that might be encountered if this were not done might greatly complicate the procedure and delay the progress of the operation for some time.

I usually do not resect as much stomach as depicted here but transect about 3 to 4 in. proximal to the pylorus. I do not recall any instance of stoma ulcer in the jejunum following this procedure.

In transecting the common duct, it is well to first expose the cystic duct in order to be sure that at the time the common duct is divided, this is carried out below the entrance of the cystic duct.

Ordinarily I do not greatly expose the superior mesenteric artery, just the vein. In transecting the neck of the pancreas, I attempt to mobilize it to the maximal degree first by careful attempts to insert the right index finger above it and the right thumb beneath it and try to have them meet under it so that it (the neck) may be "picked up" from the anterior aspect of the superior mesentery vein. No attempt is made to *force* the digits together. A Kocher grooved dissector is bent slightly and passed carefully beneath the neck. The latter is divided, and the head and neck are very gently retracted to the right. In this step great care is taken to avoid tearing thin-walled veins coursing from the deep surfaces of the neck and head into the superior mesenteric veins. As soon as dis-

covered they are clamped and ligated *with silk.*

I concur with the method depicted of mobilizing the jejunum and bringing it up to the common duct for anastomosis. In addition, I like to have a normal gallbladder in order to anastomose it, side-to-side with the jejunum below the choledochojejunal anastomosis. In this way facilities for bile drainage into the gut are appreciably enhanced.

In regard to implantation of the body of the pancreas into the jejunal loop, I have never performed this for the following reasons: (1) It is an extra step, consumes time and creates a potential added source of fistula. (2) It has been demonstrated that the human being can get along quite well without external pancreatic secretion (if stools are loose, pancreatin is given by mouth). This point of view is based upon the observation of six personal cases surviving 19, 18, 17, 9, 7, and 5 years, to say nothing of 1- to 3-year survivors who died of recurrences.

Upon transecting the neck of the pancreas, I identify the main pancreatic duct, apply a small clamp, ligate it with silk, insert interlocking mattress sutures of silk to firmly compress the surrounding pancreatic parenchyma, and suture a layer of mesentery over the neck. The area is drained.

A pancreatic fistula often does develop, but in the absence of infection there is no digestion. The fistula soon heals and its presence does not prolong hospitalization. The patients are discharged with instructions for self-care (dressing changes as needed). (3) Even if the pancreatojejunal anastomosis is done, there is every reason to assume cicatrization will often occur, and the pancreatic juice becomes occluded anyway.

Since the level of transection of the stomach is lower than shown in the diagrams, I do not have the problem of narrowing the outlet and so carry out a straight gastrojejunostomy using two rows of interrupted silk.

Plate 243

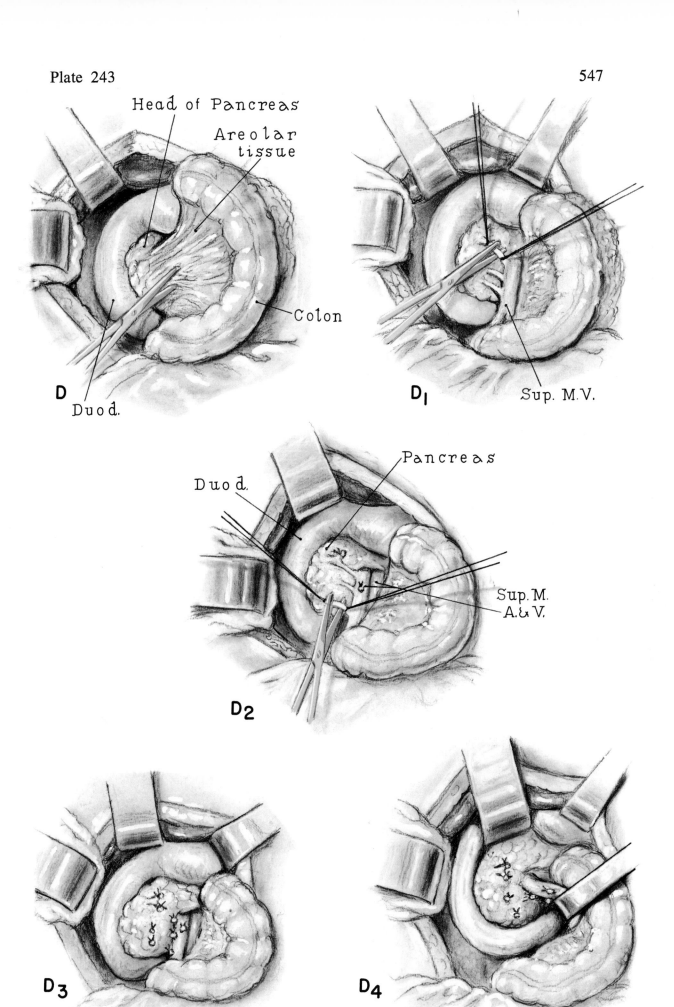

Head of Pancreas

Areolar tissue

Colon

D

Duod.

D₁

Sup. M.V.

Duod.

Pancreas

D₂

Sup. M.
A. & V.

D₃

D₄

E. The duodenal "loop" and the head of the pancreas are mobilized and elevated to facilitate the cutting of the areolar tissue attachments between the transverse or third portion of the duodenum and the mesentery of the colon adjacent. As the dissection proceeds medialward, caution must be observed to avoid opening into the general peritoneal cavity.

E_1. The duodenum is completely mobilized, and its relation to the mesenteric vascular stalk and adjacent structures is seen.

F. The duodenum and head of the pancreas are retracted toward the midline to show the related structures posteriorly. The retroduodenal and retropancreatic portions of the common bile duct and the enlarged common duct lymph node may be clearly seen, as well as the inferior vena cava and the

spermatic (or ovarian) vein, which drains eccentrically into the vena cava at the level of the midportion of the second part of the duodenum.

G. The transverse colon is manually retracted upward, and as traction is maintained, the ligament of Treitz is severed (broken line) to mobilize the duodenojejunal junction.

G_1. The left hand is placed beneath the gastrocolic ligament, and its relatively avascular attachments to the transverse colon are cut with scissors. The gastroepiploic arch cephalad may be seen. Although not performed in this patient, the usual procedure is to elevate the apron of greater omentum and enter the lesser sac by severance of its avascular attachments to the transverse colon. The segment of omentum thus mobilized is included in the resected specimen.

DISCUSSION—DR. CHARLES G. CHILD, III. My comments upon Doctor Madden's technic of pancreaticoduodenectomy will firmly support the view that few are the operations that cannot be done well in more than one way. In brief, I perform this operation differently.

Although vertical incisions (A) are useful for some operations, they are not, in my opinion, appropriate to pancreaticoduodenectomy. An oblique incision extending from the mid-left costal margin to deep in the right flank provides more adequate access to the body and tail of the pancreas as well as greater technical freedom in the right upper quadrant.

In commencing mobilization of the pancreas and duodenum, I prefer to depress the transverse colon and to work through the gastrocolic ligament rather than laterally by mobilizing the hepatic flexure as illustrated (C_1 through F). The reason for this difference in surgical philosophy and technic resides in the conviction that operability should be determined at the earliest possible moment of the procedure. For this reason, the hepatoduodenal and right third of the gastrohepatic ligaments are skeletonized shortly after entering the abdomen. By this maneuver, freedom of the common duct, hepatic artery, and cephalad portal vein from tumor invasion is determined.

Next, the base of the transverse mesocolon is explored to prove that neither of these structures nor the superior mesenteric vessels are invaded by tumor.

Having completed these two basic maneuvers, the following questions concerning operability are answered: (1) Is the portal vein free of invading tumor? (2) Is the base of the mesocolon uninvaded? (3) Are the regional lymph nodes free of tumor?

With these challenges to operability resolved, the duodenum is mobilized (much as in F), and, if found unattached by cancer to aorta and vena cava, the operation may proceed with reasonable assurance that the tumor at hand is resectable.

One critical question still remains unanswered, however: Is there invasion of the superior mesenteric artery? To obtain an answer to this question, the stomach and pancreas are transected and the resectability of the tumor is determined—namely, whether or not the superior mesenteric artery is free of invading cancer. This requires, of course, that the pancreas be divided farther to the left than is shown in L. There is an additional reason for dividing the pancreas at the junction of body and tail rather than at junction of body and head: the smaller stump of pancreas provided can be invaginated into the open end of jejunum far easier than can the bulkier junction of body and head.

If the superior mesenteric artery and adjacent aorta are invaded by cancer, the operation can be abandoned gracefully at this point with gastrogastrostomy, pyloroplasty, and distal pancreatectomy and splenectomy. If the superior mesenteric artery is free of tumor, pancreaticoduodenectomy is completed much as outlined (H-K and M-N). As the distal segment of the stomach, the duodenum, and the head and body of the pancreas fall toward the patient's right side, the portal vein is freed from the uncinate process of pancreas, and the inferior pancreaticoduodenal artery is severed.

Enteric continuity is not broken by transecting the duodenum as shown in O but by severance of the jejunum some centimeters distal to the ligament of Treitz. The entire duodenum and upper jejunum are then delivered from left to right from behind the superior mesenteric vessels. At this point, the stomach, duodenum, upper jejunum, head, uncinate process, and body of the pancreas constitute the specimen, anchored only by the common duct. This is dissected free, together with adjacent nodes and fat to a point just below the junction of the right and left hepatic ducts. The gallbladder, cystic duct, and a 2 cm. segment of common hepatic duct are then removed en bloc with the specimen. These structures should not be

Plate 244   549

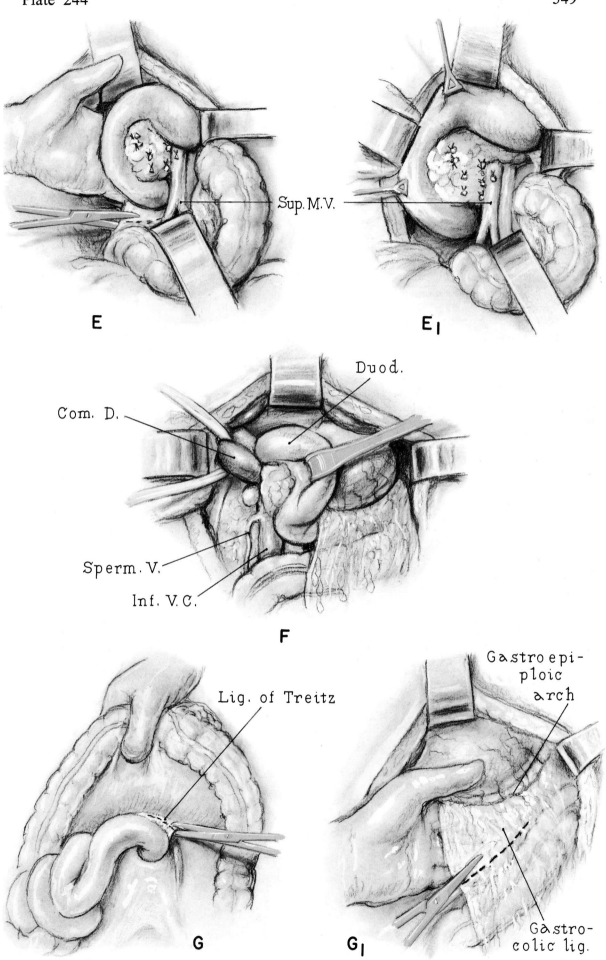

E

E₁

Sup. M.V.

Duod.

Com. D.

Sperm. V.

Inf. V.C.

F

Lig. of Treitz

G

Gastro epi-
ploic
arch

Gastro-
colic lig.

G₁

H. The right gastric artery, a branch of the hepatic propria artery, having been doubly ligated in continuity, is being cut with scissors between the ligatures. The large lymph node that characteristically overlies the hepatic artery is visible.

H₁, H₂. A ligature of silk (00) is being withdrawn beneath the gastroduodenal artery (H₁), which is ligated in continuity and then transected (H₂). The arch which is formed by the gastroduodenal artery with its parent trunk, the hepatic artery, is an excellent anatomic landmark for the location of the portal vein. This vein, just after its formation by the union of the superior mesenteric and splenic veins, passes cephalad beneath this arch in an obliquity of

approximately 45° (H₁; see also Frontispiece).

I. The gastrocolic ligament and its contained gastroepiploic arch are serially clamped and severed (broken line) subjacent to the site of transection of the stomach.

J. The descending branch of the left gastric artery and its accompanying veins along the lesser curvature of the stomach are mobilized by blunt dissection and elevated on the left index finger.

J₁, J₂, J₃. The left gastric vessels are doubly clamped, severed and ligated (J₁, J₂), and the "bare" aserosal segment of the lesser gastric curvature is reperitonized with interrupted sutures of 000 silk (J₂, J₃).

DISCUSSION—DR. CHILD (cont.)

left behind for the lymphatics about them are often invaded by tumor. Furthermore, the removal of these structures is generally accomplished with ease.

Re-establishment of enteric continuity (Q, R, U) is, in my opinion, less than ideal. There is no need to retain jejunum in a position behind the superior mesenteric vessels. Furthermore, the common duct may not be dilated to a point where it is equivalent in size to the open end of the jejunum. For these reasons, the jejunum is passed through the already established rent in the transverse mesocolon and end-to-end pancreaticojejunostomy is performed by invaginating the stump of the pancreas into the open end of jejunum. Since the pancreas has been severed near its tail, it is small enough to invaginate easily into the open end of the jejunum using two layers of silk and cotton sutures. I do not imply that an end to side pancreaticojejunostomy (R, R₁, R₂, R₃, R₄) is not possible, but only that end-to-end pancreaticojejunostomy is uncomplicated and efficient. Choledochojejunostomy is next performed in the end-

to-side position and an antecolic gastrojejunostomy completes the operation.

In summary, I would outline the important disagreements with the illustrated technic of Doctor Madden for the performance of a one-stage radical pancreaticoduodenectomy: (1) determination of resectability early in the operation so that it can be abandoned gracefully if one or more of the following structures are invaded by tumor: base of mesocolon, portal vein, aorta, vena cava, or superior mesenteric artery; (2) inclusion in the resected specimen, the gallbladder, cystic duct, common duct and the common hepatic duct up to its bifurcation; (3) re-establishment of enteric continuity first by retrocolic end-to-end pancreaticojejunostomy, then by end-to-side choledochojejunostomy with the jejunal loop anterior to the superior mesenteric vessels, and, finally, by an antecolic, long loop gastrojejunostomy; and (4) hemigastrectomy and vagotomy should always be considered and added to the operation if reasonable.

DISCUSSION—DR. CLARENCE DENNIS. Several basic physiologic considerations must be borne in mind in the performance of this procedure. In the experience of Dennis and Varco (*Surgery*, 20:72, 1946), more than half of these patients are achlorhydric. An occasional patient has high gastric acid and may get into trouble with marginal ulcer after resection. It is therefore important that a gastric analysis be done before operation, in order to establish the amount of stomach that must be resected in order to avoid this complication.

In contrast to the technic outlined, I prefer not to dissect the first portion of the duodenum or the pyloric area away from the head and neck of the pancreas, lest seeding of tumor be rendered more likely.

In view of the frequency with which recurrent tumor is seen to involve the common bile duct and of the frequency with which careful serial sections

of the common bile duct show rather far-reaching direct extension of tumors of the ampulla and head of the pancreas, together with the frequency with which the cystic duct lumen does not join the common duct lumen for a considerable distance below the apparent external junction, the gallbladder and all of the common duct are routinely removed, and the jejunal anastomosis is made to the common hepatic duct.

The patterns of technic for anastomosis of the pancreatic duct to the intestine are varied. That technic devised by Varco (*Surgery*, 18:569, 1945) was employed in a series of patients by Dennis and Varco and is the only reported technique that has had no incidence of fistula formation. This consists in placement of a catheter for several centimeters into the dilated pancreatic duct, securing it in position by a 000 catgut pursestring suture at the cut end of the pancreas, placement of

Plate 245

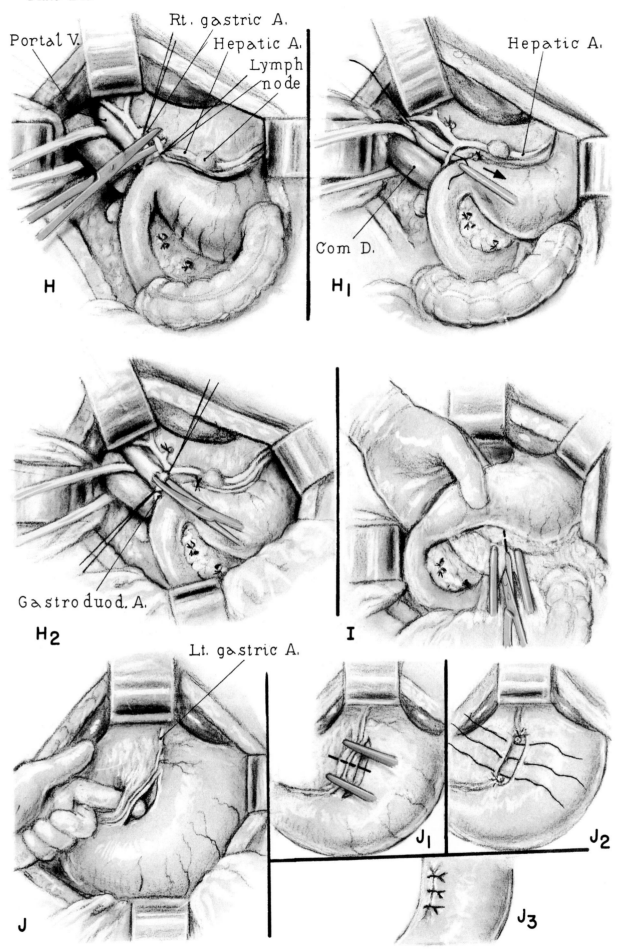

Portal V.

Rt. gastric A.

Hepatic A.

Lymph node

H

Hepatic A.

Com D.

H₁

Gastro duod. A.

H₂

I

Lt. gastric A.

J

J₁

J₂

J₃

K. The serosal layer of the stomach at the level of its transection is incised, and the underlying vessels in the submucosal layer are undersewn proximally for hemostasis with ligatures of 000 silk. An opening into the gastric lumen anteriorly on the greater curvature side is visible. The stomach is cross-clamped (Payr) distally to prevent both retrograde bleeding and the escape of any contained gastric material. In operations upon the gastrointestinal tract, occlusive clamps are not applied to any tissues that are to be anastomosed.

K₁, K₂. The opening previously made into the lumen of the stomach is extended by scissor dissection (K_1), and upon its completion, the posterior wall of the stomach is transected (K_2).

K₃, K₄. The cut margins of the open proximal end of the stomach are temporarily approximated with clamps of the Babcock type (K_3, K_4), and the cross-clamped distal transected end of the stomach is covered with a large moist pad and retracted laterally (K_4). This exposes a large surface area of the pancreas and its relation to the surrounding structures. The relation between the origin of the portal vein and the arch (now transected) formed by the hepatic artery and its gastroduodenal branch is again visible (K_4).

DISCUSSION—DR. DENNIS (cont.)

the catheter through a stab wound into the intestine, and mattress suture approximation of the pancreatic capsule to the wall of the jejunum encircling this stab wound. The length of the intra-intestinal catheter may be 10 cm. but not longer, as there has been one occasion of knotting of the catheter after passage, with intestinal obstruction secondary thereto.

The pattern of gastrojejunostomy is apparently important. Dennis first proposed (*Surgery*, 12:201, 1942) the utilization of a 40 cm. segment of jejunum between the biliary anastomosis and the lower-lying gastrojejunostomy in order to prevent reflux of gastric content into the biliary tree. In the series later reported by Dennis and Varco (*Surgery*, 39:92, 1956), only two instances of transient cholangitis were observed; in each of these it did not appear until more than five years after pancreaticoduodenectomy. The technic without this loop, recommended first by H. E. Pearse (*Surg., Gynec. & Obst.*, 75:333, 1942), omitted this 40 cm. segment and was characterized by a high later incidence of cholangitis. Subsequent experimental studies by Pearse, Radakovich, and Cogbill (*Ann. Surg.*, 129:57, 1949) indicated that

this length of segment is essential to avoidance of regurgitation.

In this procedure, the closed anastomosis is routinely employed for gastrojejunostomy, inasmuch as it lessens the risk of postoperative hemorrhage and permits a smaller inverted cuff of tissue at the suture line.

The extent of pancreatic loss superimposed upon the damage resulting from pancreatic obstruction has been sufficient to cause some of these patients to behave like diabetics for several days after operation. It is therefore well worthwhile to utilize a careful pattern of diabetic supervision in the early postoperative period.

Although carcinoma of the ampulla and carcinoma of the head of the pancreas are not infrequently considered to be lesions not susceptible to surgical cure, particularly with the extent of the operative procedure employed and the attendant operative mortality, Dennis and Varco nevertheless indicated that a surgical mortality risk no higher than 10 per cent should be possible, and reported five-year survival of 5 patients out of 14 subjected to such radical procedures.

DISCUSSION—DR. MAURICE MERCADIER. The method we have adopted for pancreaticoduodenectomy differs appreciably from John Madden's in its technic and even more so in some of the technical details. Our procedure, which is more systematic, comprises five stages taken up in precise chronologic order, so that, if necessary, we can always withdraw without causing any damage. The five stages of the intervention are:

1. Exposure and exploration of the abdominal structures.
2. Mobilization.
3. Section of the viscera and blood vessels.
4. Freeing of the head of the pancreas and of the retromesenteric and retroportal segments of the pancreas.
5. Reconstruction.

Rather than describe each one of the steps of the operation, we should like to stress a few points. First, we attach considerable importance to adequate exposure and thorough exploration of the gland. In order to do this, we begin by opening the lesser omentum so as to have access to the celiac region and the suprapancreatic groups of lymph nodes; the greater omentum is then divided or detached over its full width, which enables one to deflect the stomach upward and bring into view the whole of the supramesocolic portion of the pancreas.

A leftward extension of the tumor and fixation of the posterior surface of the pancreas are contraindications to proceeding any further. We attach the same importance to the invasion of the root of the upper mesenteric pedicle by lymph nodes—

Plate 246

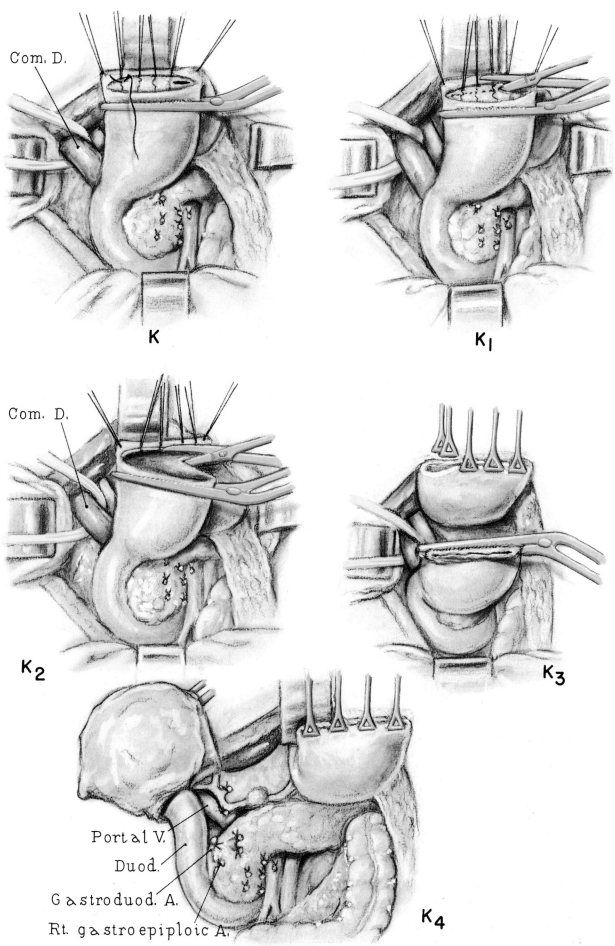

Com. D.

K

K₁

Com. D.

K₂

K₃

Portal V.

Duod.

Gastroduod. A.

Rt. gastroepiploic A.

K₄

L. A rubber tissue tape has been withdrawn beneath the neck of the pancreas, which is being transected with a scalpel. The severed ends of the pancreatic duct, eccentric in position, are visible.

L_1. The transected ends of the pancreas are compressed with Babcock clamps and retracted to show the junction of the superior mesenteric and splenic veins to form the portal vein. In this patient, the inferior mesenteric vein was a tributary of the superior mesenteric vein. Equally common, it may be a tributary of the splenic vein or empty into the angle of junction of the superior mesenteric and splenic veins.

M. The proximal transected end of the neck of the pancreas is retracted laterally and the superior mesenteric vein medially to show the dissection of the uncinate process. The resection of this portion of the pancreas is the most tedious and time-consuming part of the operation. In most of the surgical texts, only one artery, the inferior pancreaticoduodenal branch of the superior mesenteric artery, is commonly illustrated. However, as shown in the subsequent illustrations, a multiplicity of arterial branches, five in number, required ligation and severance before the uncinate process was mobilized completely. The first arterial branch to be exposed is doubly ligated in continuity (00 silk) and transected with scissors.

M_1, M_2. Three arterial branches to the uncinate process have been ligated and cut, and a fourth branch, both large and tortuous, is doubly ligated in continuity (00 silk) and transected (broken line).

M_3. The remaining arterial branch, the fifth and largest, enters the apex of the uncinate process and is mobilized by both clamp and digital dissection before being ligated and cut.

N. The apex of the uncinate process is elevated on the left index finger and with digital traction maintained its last arterial branch from the superior mesenteric artery is severed between ligatures of silk (00). The multiplicity of arterial branches to the uncinate process precludes their exact identification. However, the first one ligated was believed to be the inferior pancreaticoduodenal.

N_1. The uncinate process is completely mobilized, and the mesentery of the jejunum, which has been partially withdrawn beneath the mesenteric vascular stalk, is clamped and severed as depicted.

DISCUSSION—DR. MERCADIER (cont.)

which are impossible to remove properly—and to the existence of segmentary portal hypertension in the territory of the splenic vein (splenomegaly) or of the mesenteric veins (venous distention in the region of the mesentery), since such pathologic findings are signs of a compression or invasion of the portal trunk or its afferent tributaries.

The second step in the operation is that of the mobilization of the pancreaticoduodenal block and of the tumor. First, the precephalic vessels (i.e., below and on the right: the right lower pancreaticoduodenal vessels; above and on the left: the right gastro-epiploic vessels) are isolated and clamped. Then the right portion of the transverse mesocolon is pushed toward the root of the mesenteric pedicle, so as to liberate completely the anterior aspect of the duodenum. Freeing of the posterior aspect of the pancreaticoduodenal block is then carried out to the left, as far as the left border of the aorta, so that practically the whole pancreas can be brought up to the level of the surgical opening.

The third step of the procedure described by Madden comprises the section of the viscera in the following order: section of the right gastric artery (H, H_1) section of the gastroduodenal artery (H_2); section of the epiploic arch (I); section of the vascular arch of the lesser curvature of the stomach (J); section of the neck of the pancreas (L) and finally, freeing of the lesser pancreas (M) and section of the jejunum (O).

We prefer to follow a different order and begin by freeing the portal vein from the neck of the pancreas; this is the most perilous stage of the operation. First the superior mesenteric vein is exposed at the base of the mesenteric pedicle; from then on we proceed carefully from the bottom upward, using a small sponge for dissection. If the adhesions are not too dense, the dissection is carried out progressively up to the neck of the pancreas, where a transverse incision is made in the peritoneum. An oiled tape is passed between the pancreas and the portal trunk, and the pancreatic parenchyma is incised, the incision being carried from the top downward, over the support provided by the oiled tape. The adhesions are sometimes important enough to constitute an insuperable obstacle; in this eventuality, we would rather give up than risk injuring a vein, which may be difficult to repair or having to resect a segment of the axial veins. The prognosis in such cases is extremely poor.

Once the pancreas has been incised, the next steps are section of the stomach at the junction of its lower and middle thirds; section of the vessels at the base of the hepatic pedicle, i.e., the right

Plate 247   555

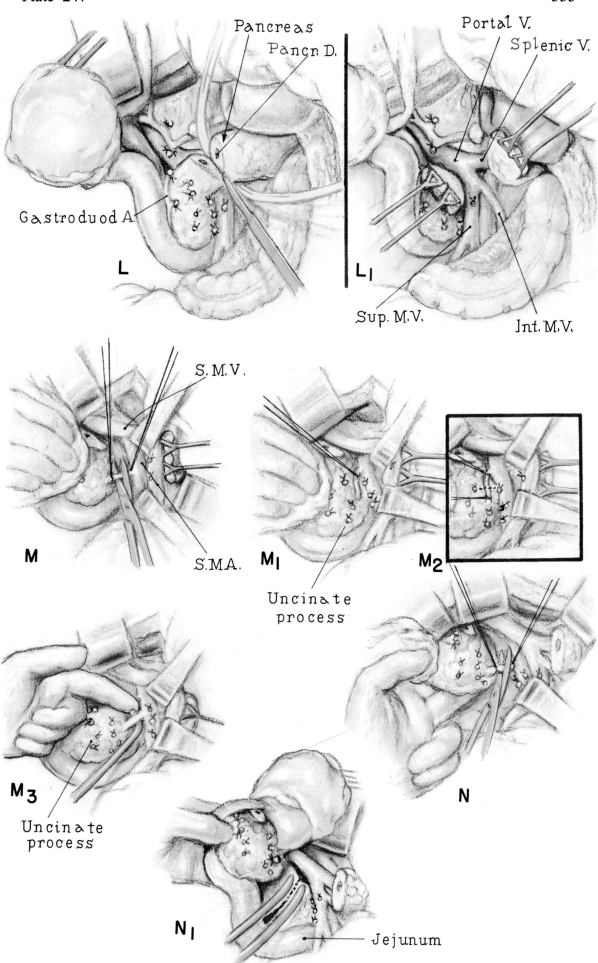

Pancreas

Pancn D.

Portal V.

Splenic V.

Gastroduod A.

L

L₁

Sup. M.V.

Inf. M.V.

S. M.V.

M

S.M.A.

M₁

Uncinate process

M₂

M₃

Uncinate process

N

N₁

Jejunum

O. The jejunum, after severance of its mesentery, is doubly cross-clamped and transected (broken line). The distal clamp is not locked. The jaws of the clamp are approximated with only the force that is required to hold the jejunum while it is being transected.

O₁. Guy sutures of arterial silk (00000) are inserted in the medial and lateral walls of the lower portion of the common duct, which is elevated on the left index finger as it is cut across (broken line) with scissors just proximal to the superior border of the duodenum. The common bile duct is not clamped, and the bile, as it flows into the operative field, is removed by suction as depicted.

O₂. The transection of the common duct, the final step in the pancreaticoduodenectomy, permits the removal of the operative specimen (P₂). The operative field on removal of the specimen is shown. The proximal cut end of the common duct is temporarily occluded with a series of Babcock clamps and retracted upward. A probe is seen inserted into the lumen of the pancreatic duct. The distal transected and open end of the jejunum and its relation to the mesenteric vascular stalk may also be seen.

P, P₁. The operative field just before the performance of the first and most proximal anastomosis, the end-to-end choledochojejunostomy, is shown. In P₁, the superior mesenteric vein is retracted to expose a portion of the superior mesenteric artery, which is beneath and medial to the vein.

P₂. This is a view of the surgical specimen on completion of the pancreaticoduodenectomy.

Q. The jejunum is partially mobilized beneath the mesenteric vascular stalk and its transected end is held in anatomic forceps which are used to aid its approximation to the common duct when the sutures, which form the posterior layer of the anastomosis, are tied.

Q₁. The posterior layer of the anastomosis is completed, and the "angle" sutures of the first anterior layer are inserted but not tied.

Q₂. The first anterior layer of sutures is completed and the last of the mattress sutures, which form the second anterior layer, is being inserted.

Q₃. The mattress sutures are tied to complete the end-to-end choledochojejunostomy. Because of the extent of dilatation of the common duct, there was no discrepancy in the lumen size of the respective viscera.

DISCUSSION—DR. MERCADIER (cont.)

gastric vessels, the right upper gastroduodenal and pancreaticoduodenal vessels, section of the common duct, freeing of the duodenojejunal angle, and section of the first jejunal loop, followed by passage of the small bowel behind the mesenteric pedicle.

The fourth step of the operation—a particularly arduous one—consists in liberating the veins from the head of the pancreas, the retromesenteric and retroportal portions of the pancreas (which in 12 to 25 per cent of the cases are found to extend as far as the superior mesenteric artery). The danger lies in the proximity of the venous axis collaterals. These veins are not easily identified, except for the inferior pancreaticoduodenal arch, with its upper extremity opening into the portal trunk and its lower extremity in the mesenteric vein. A satisfactory exposure of the veins is obtained by deflecting the pancreaticoduodenal block to the right;

the veins are thereby adequately stretched and can be ligated from top to bottom and from bottom to top with little risk of injury.

The reconstitution of the abdominal structures is the last stage of the operation. We resort to the technic described by Child and modified by Waugh—our personal contribution to the procedure being that the suture is made in one layer with nonabsorbable material (silk 000) for the anastomosis. The mounting is effected by diverting the second jejunal loop which is made to pass anteriorly to the superior mesenteric pedicle and passed through an avascular opening in the supramesocolic portion of the transverse mesocolon. When we started applying this technic, we used to drive the jejunal loop behind the superior mesenteric pedicle, but we had some unfavorable results, such as obstruction or occlusion syndromes, and so gave up this method.

Plate 248

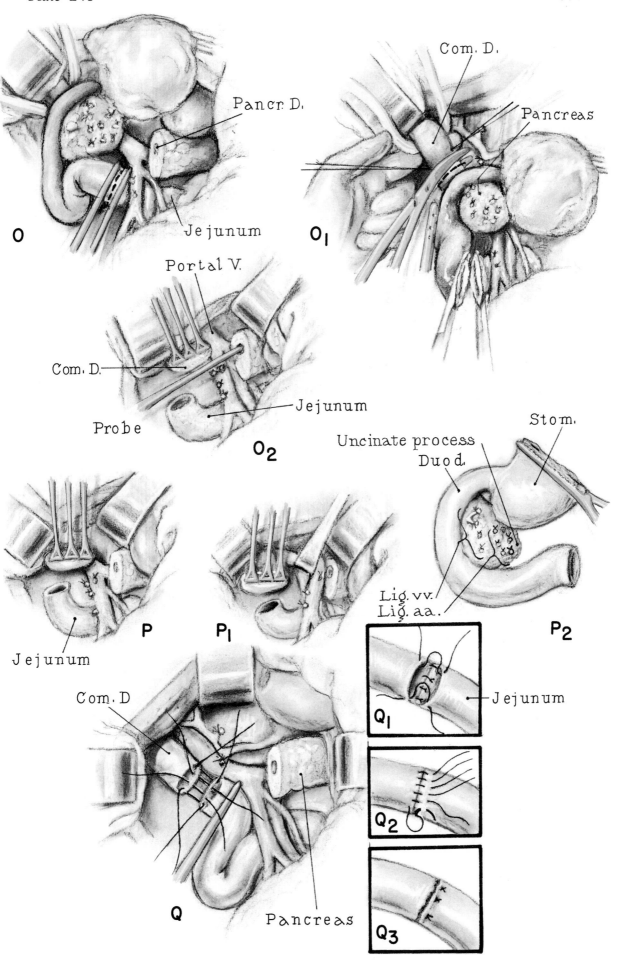

O

Pancr. D.

Jejunum

O₁

Com. D.

Pancreas

Portal V.

Com. D.

Jejunum

Probe

O₂

Uncinate process

Duod.

Stom.

P

P₁

P₂

Jejunum

Lig. vv.

Lig. aa.

Com. D

Q₁

Jejunum

Q₂

Q

Pancreas

Q₃

R. A short loop of jejunum is interposed between the first anastomosis, the end-to-end choledochojejunostomy, and the second anastomosis, the end-to-side pancreaticojejunostomy. An opening previously made into the lumen of the jejunum for anastomosis to the pancreatic duct is shown.

R₁. This close-up view shows the completion of the insertion of the interrupted sutures of 00000 silk that form the posterior layer of the anastomosis.

R₂. The sutures posteriorly are tied, and the insertion of the first anterior layer of sutures (00000 silk) is completed.

R₃, R₄. The mattress sutures of silk (0000) that form the second anterior layer are first all inserted (R₃) and then tied to complete the end-to-side pancreaticojejunostomy (R₄). The advisability of performing a pancreaticojejunostomy is often questioned because of the belief that the anastomosis rarely remains patent. However, it is believed that a careful mucosa-to-mucosa apposition, using fine sutures of silk (00000), will maintain patency of the anastomosis in most patients.

S. Preparatory to its anastomosis with the jejunum, the gastric stoma is decreased in size by the insertion of a series of inversion sutures (000 silk) along the lesser gastric curvature. These sutures are inserted from the inside-out to the outside-in, so that, when tied, the knots are on the inside of the lumen. Three such sutures usually suffice. The inverted fold of the lesser curvature is visible within the stomach.

S₁. A two-layer inversion (optional) is obtained by the insertion of a series of interrupted seroserosal mattress sutures of 000 silk.

S₂. The inversion of the lesser gastric curvature and the insertion of the first posterior layer (000 silk) of sutures are completed.

The sutures (000 silk) which form the second posterior layer are all inserted but not tied.

S₃. The anastomosis posteriorly is completed and the sutures forming the first anterior layer are inserted. The first anterior suture on the lesser curvature side of the gastrojejunostomy, the so-called W stitch, is a seroserosal approximation suture that seals this angle of the anastomosis. This suture proceeds from the outside-in to the inside-out on the jejunal side, and on the stomach side from the outside-in (posterior gastric wall) to inside-out (anterior gastric wall).

T. An alternate method for the insertion of the first anterior layer of sutures makes use of a series of interrupted inverting sutures. Each suture (000 silk) is inserted alternately from either angle of the anastomosis toward the center, where the last two sutures terminate. Inward traction on the suture previously inserted as the succeeding suture is tied, facilitates the inversion of the tissue layers.

T₁. A row of interrupted seroserosal (Lembert) sutures of silk (000) is being inserted to complete the second anterior layer of the anastomosis.

U. The operative field upon completion of the three anastomoses is shown. Each anastomosis is separated by a short loop of jejunum, the end-to-side gastrojejunostomy (isoperistaltic) being the lowest of the three. This arrangement is believed to minimize the regurgitation of gastrointestinal contents into the stomas of the two anastomoses proximally. The jejunum distally maintains a position posterior to the mesenteric vascular stalk. Before closure of the wound, a new ligament of Treitz is formed by anchorage of the jejunum to the base of the transverse mesocolon, using interrupted sutures of 000 silk. The wound, which is closed in layers, using interrupted sutures of silk (00), is not drained.

Plate 249

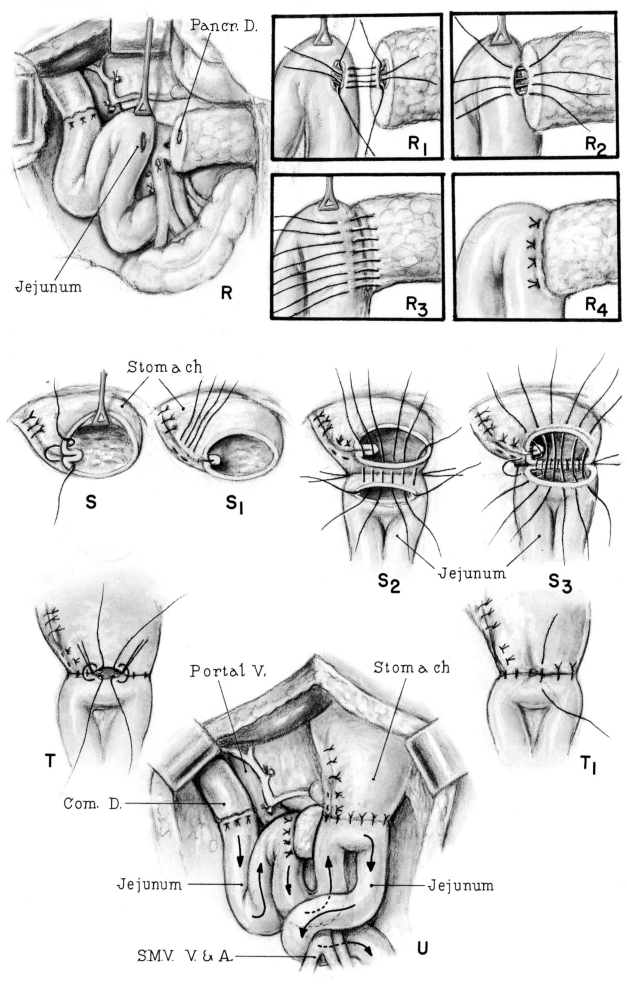

Pancr. D.

Jejunum

R

R₁

R₂

R₃

R₄

Stomach

S

S₁

S₂

S₃

Jejunum

Portal V.

Stomach

Com. D.

Jejunum

Jejunum

T

T₁

S.M.V. V. & A.

U

BILATERAL ADRENALECTOMY—ANTERIOR APPROACH

A. The upper right paramedian incision is outlined and crosshatched to facilitate later closure.

B. The incision is deepened through the rectus sheath, and the rectus muscle is retracted laterally to expose the opening made into the peritoneal cavity.

C, D. The peritoneal cavity is entered, and the mobilized hepatic flexure of the colon is retracted downward and medially to expose the duodenal "loop." The posterior parietal peritoneum is incised (C, broken line), and the mobilized duodenum and head of the pancreas are retracted toward the midline (D) to show the underlying retroperitoneal structures.

E. The right kidney is mobilized and manually retracted downward as the posterior parietal peritoneum is severed (broken line) with scissors toward the base of the retracted liver. This is necessary to obtain proper exposure of the adrenal gland.

Plate 250   561

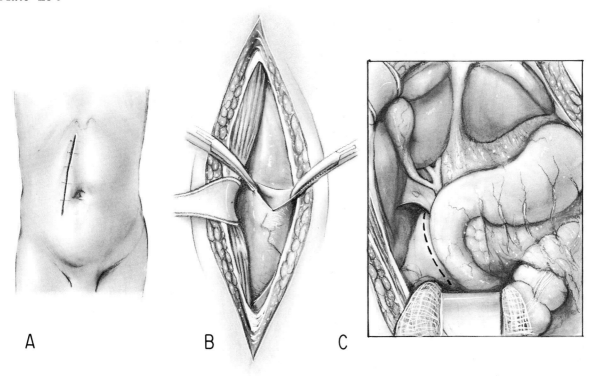

A   B   C

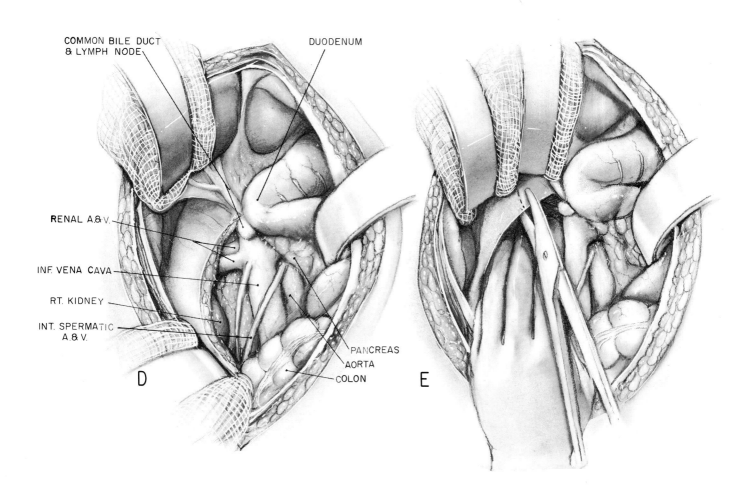

COMMON BILE DUCT
& LYMPH NODE   DUODENUM

RENAL A.& V.

INF. VENA CAVA

RT. KIDNEY

INT. SPERMATIC
A.& V.

PANCREAS
AORTA
COLON

D   E

F. The mobilization of the kidney and the downward rotation and retraction of its superior pole are essential technical maneuvers to obtain proper exposure of the adrenal gland. However, to achieve clarity relative to the operative field, this maneuver is not depicted. The isolated right adrenal vein, a tributary of the inferior vena cava, is doubly ligated (000 silk) in continuity and is being transected with scissors. Its entrance into the vena cava is more posterior than illustrated.

G, H, I. A second and smaller adrenal vein was similarly doubly ligated in continuity (G, H), severed (H), and the right adrenal gland removed (I).

Plate 251

563

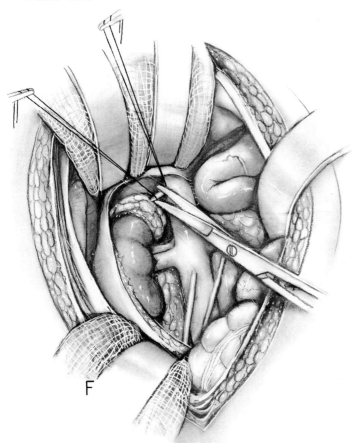

F

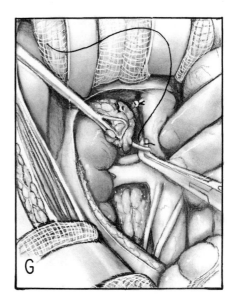

G

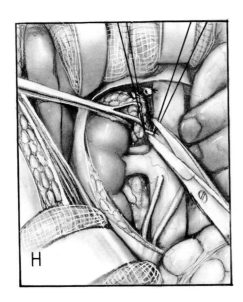

H

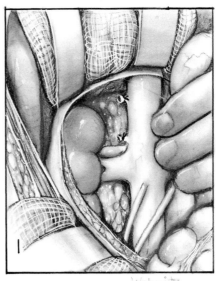

I

Wabnitz

J. To expose the left adrenal gland, the lesser sac is entered by serially clamping and severing the gastrocolic ligament cephalad to the gastroepiploic arch. The mobilized greater curvature and posterior wall of the stomach are retracted upward and the transverse colon downward to demonstrate the gastropancreatic fold of peritoneum and its contained left gastric vessels. These vessels are isolated, triply clamped, and severed (broken line) between the two uppermost clamps.

K. The two lowermost clamps are replaced by a ligature (00 silk) and suture ligature (000 silk), respectively.

L. An opening is made in the posterior parietal peritoneum and subsequently extended (broken line) by scissor dissection. The celiac axis and its branches in relation to the surrounding structures are readily visible. An anatomic fact that has not been emphasized sufficiently is the close approximation of the left adrenal gland to the celiac axis, particularly its left gastric and splenic branches.

M. The left adrenal gland is mobilized and held upward in a Babcock clamp modified on the Potts principle.* The use of this clamp minimizes trauma and is particularly suitable for fragile tissues. In mobilizing the gland relatively few vessels, and mostly veins, require severance. Hemostasis is readily and most easily obtained with the use of silver clips (Cushing brain clips). The relation of the adrenal gland to the celiac axis and the left kidney is visible. The left adrenal vein, a tributary of the left renal vein, is uniformly large and prominent and longer than the right adrenal vein. It is doubly ligated (000 silk) in continuity and transected (broken line) between the ligatures to complete the removal of the gland.

---

* Manufactured by Edward Weck & Co., Long Island City, N.Y.

Plate 252   565

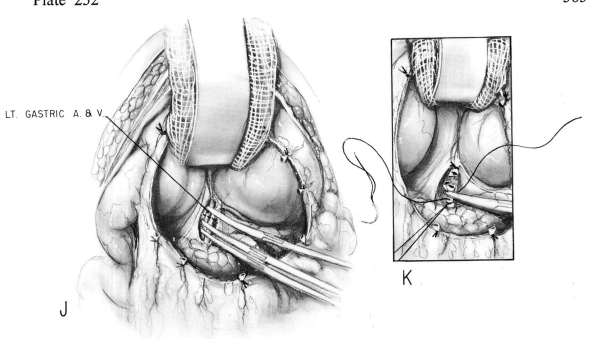

LT. GASTRIC A. & V.

J

K

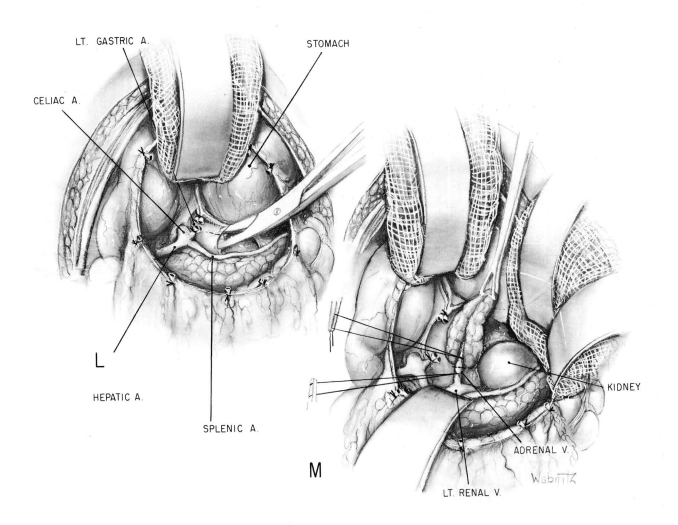

LT. GASTRIC A.

CELIAC A.

STOMACH

HEPATIC A.

L

SPLENIC A.

KIDNEY

ADRENAL V.

M

LT. RENAL V.

Wabritz

BILATERAL ADRENALECTOMY—POSTERIOR APPROACH

A. General endotracheal anesthesia, using nitrous oxide, oxygen, and ether, is employed, and the patient, when anesthetized, is turned and placed in the prone, "jack-knife" position. The outline of the incision on the left side may be seen.

B. The incisions used are those advocated by the late Hugh Young of Baltimore for the one-stage bilateral exposure of the adrenal glands. Each incision is located approximately 5 cm. lateral to the midline of the vertebral column and extends downward and outward in a curvilinear direction from the level of the tenth rib to the level of the superior border of the iliac crest.

C. The incision on the left side is shown deepened through the subcutaneous fatty tissue layer, and the wound margins are retracted to expose the latissimus dorsi muscle and its origin from the posterior lamella of the lumbodorsal fascia. A small segment of the fibers of this muscle and its fascia of origin have been incised cephalad, and the incision is continued caudad in a curvilinear direction, as indicated by the broken line. A portion of the underlying sacrospinalis muscle is visible through the opening made in the fascia.

D. The cut margins of the lumbodorsal fascia (posterior lamella) are clamped and retracted to show a broad expanse of the sacrospinalis muscle and fascia. This muscle is frequently mistaken for the latissimus dorsi; in fact, in the illustrations of the original article by Young (1936) it is incorrectly labeled as such. If one remembers that the latissimus dorsi muscle is flat and relatively thin, that it arises from and is superficial to the lumbodorsal fascia, and that its fibers are directed upward and lateral in a fanwise direction, there should be no mistaken identity with the sacrospinalis muscle. The sacrospinalis muscle, located beneath the lumbodorsal fascia, is thick and round in contour, and its fibers course in a cephalad-caudad direction. It has a broad fascial attachment, and the muscle fibers are perforated by multiple small blood vessels and the posterior lumbar nerves. The ligated ends of the severed vessels are shown, and one of the posterior lumbar nerves is being transected with scissors.

Plate 253

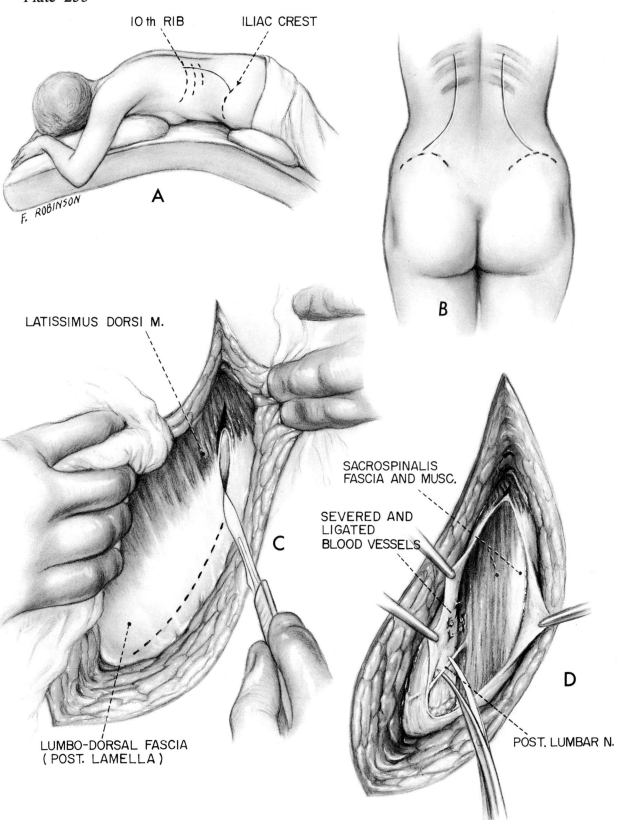

10th RIB   ILIAC CREST

F. ROBINSON

A

B

LATISSIMUS DORSI M.

C

LUMBO-DORSAL FASCIA
(POST. LAMELLA)

SACROSPINALIS
FASCIA AND MUSC.

SEVERED AND
LIGATED
BLOOD VESSELS

D

POST. LUMBAR N.

E. The sacrospinalis muscle is retracted toward the midline, and its pedicle attachment to the lower border of the twelfth rib is being severed with scissors. The relation of the posterior and middle layers (lamellae) of the lumbodorsal fascia that encase the sacrospinalis muscle is shown.

F. The middle lamella of the lumbodorsal fascia is being incised, and, through the opening, a portion of the quadratus lumborum muscle and the transversalis fascia (anterior lamella of the lumbodorsal fascia) are visible. The line of the incision in the periosteum of the twelfth rib preparatory to its resection is indicated in broken outline. A portion of the posterior serratus inferior muscle, which is partially covered by the latissimus dorsi muscle and its fascial origin, may also be seen.

G. The index finger is inserted beneath the incised middle layer of the lumbodorsal fascia to displace the pleura upward from the posterior aspect of the twelfth rib. The subsequent severance of the posterior subcostal ligament is indicated by the broken line.

H. The thinned-out fibers of attachment of the diaphragm posteriorly are being transected with scissors. The relation of these fibers to the subjacent intercostal vessels and nerve (subcostal or twelfth) is visible. The location of the quadratus lumborum muscle between the middle and anterior lamellae of the lumbodorsal fascia is also depicted.

DISCUSSION—DR. JAMES D. HARDY. Most surgeons use either the anterior or the posterior approach in performing bilateral subtotal adrenalectomy, but the lateral loin or "kidney" exposure is still occasionally employed. The posterior approach, so well presented in the illustrations, has the advantage that relatively little dissection is required to expose the adrenals, since they lie far posteriorly, adjacent to the aorta on the left and the vena cava and spinal column on the right. In this way the thick panniculus of fat in the abdominal wall is avoided, and a relatively shallow posterior wound is substituted for a usually deep abdominal wound.

Even so, the posterior approach has never gained widespread acceptance among general surgeons, and I have rarely used it. Perhaps this is because doubt so often exists preoperatively regarding the type of lesion that will be encountered. Cushing's syndrome is produced by either a tumor or hyperplasia, and a catechol amine-producing tumor may lie not only in either adrenal but also on either side of the spine along the sympathetic chains. The anterior or transverse abdominal incision permits initial exploration through a small wound, which is then extended to either the right or the left if a tumor is palpated in one or the other adrenal gland. Furthermore, if an unanticipated tumor is discovered, the abdominal incision can be extended into the thorax if necessary, to excise the neoplasm completely without rupturing its capsule because of limited exposure. The anterior approach permits inspection of the uterus and biopsy of the ovaries, if desired, and it allows the anesthesiologist to ventilate the patient in the supine rather than in the prone position imposed by the posterior approach. In addition, I usually transplant a portion of each totally excised adrenal gland to the corresponding thigh when the operation is performed for Cushing's disease, as it usually is, and for this procedure the patient must lie in the supine position. Adrenal venous blood samples are available with either the anterior or the posterior approach.

Yet the anterior approach also has disadvantages. As noted, the obesity of Cushing's disease requires the division of much fat in the abdominal wall, and similar fat deposits must be divided or retracted within the abdomen. The right adrenal gland must be exposed where it lies flush against the vena cava beneath the liver, and a tear in the vena cava, in the depths of the wound, can require considerable surgical poise for precise closure with fine sutures while avoiding excessive blood loss. This point that the right adrenal vein must be carefully handled and vena caval injury expertly managed has been properly emphasized by Dr. Madden. It is perhaps the most serious operative hazard of adrenalectomy, because of the limited accessibility of the vena cava at this level. On the left the anterior incision requires mobilization of the tail of the pancreas, with the result that postoperative pancreatitis occasionally results. Since this may not develop until the patient has been discharged from the hospital, on a low maintenance dose of replacement steroid, the abrupt and unmet increase in steroid requirement imposed by the pancreatitis can prove disastrous.

As for anesthesia, I prefer halothane or some other nonexplosive agent, for the cautery scalpel is very useful in dividing fatty and areolar tissues surrounding the adrenal glands.

Lastly, regardless of the operative approach employed, consistently successful bilateral adrenalectomy requires a total surgical effort in which competent surgical technic is combined with experience in postoperative care.

Plate 254

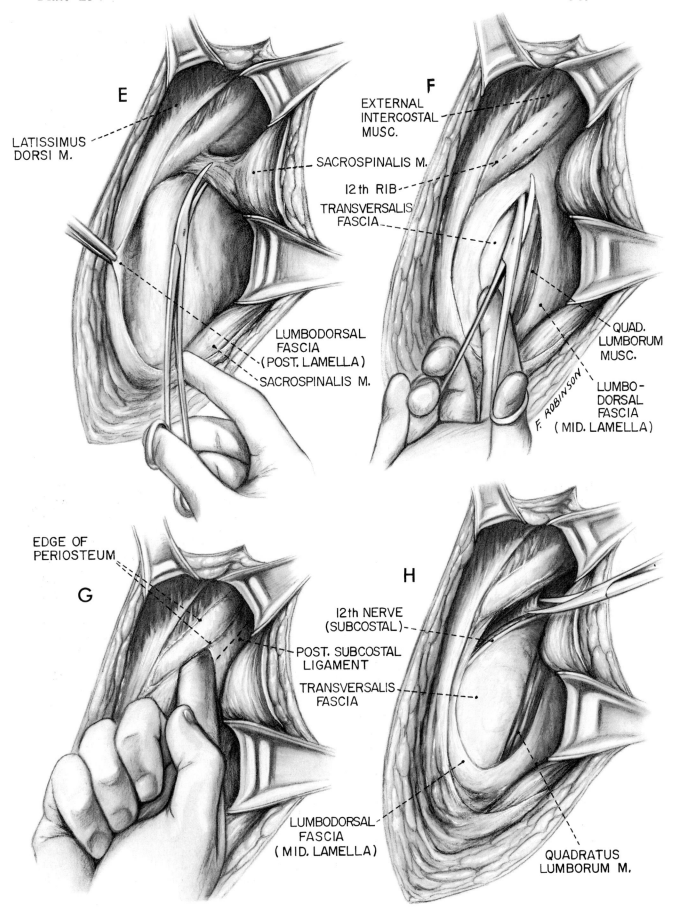

E

LATISSIMUS
DORSI M.

LUMBODORSAL
FASCIA
(POST. LAMELLA)

SACROSPINALIS M.

F

EXTERNAL
INTERCOSTAL
MUSC.

SACROSPINALIS M.

12th RIB

TRANSVERSALIS
FASCIA

QUAD.
LUMBORUM
MUSC.

LUMBO-
DORSAL
FASCIA
(MID. LAMELLA)

F. ROBINSON

G

EDGE OF
PERIOSTEUM

LUMBODORSAL
FASCIA
(MID. LAMELLA)

H

12th NERVE
(SUBCOSTAL)

POST. SUBCOSTAL
LIGAMENT

TRANSVERSALIS
FASCIA

QUADRATUS
LUMBORUM M.

I, J. The twelfth rib is resected (I), and the opening in the anterior lamella of the lumbo-dorsal fascia (transversalis fascia) is being enlarged cephalad to the subcostal vessels and nerve (twelfth) by scissor dissection (J). The relation of the pleural reflection and the severed attenuated fibers of the diaphragm to this fascial layer is evident. A thin layer of retroperitoneal (para-nephric) fat is visible beneath the fascia.

J$_1$. The posterior layer of the renal fascia (Gerota's) is being severed with scissors, and the underlying perinephric fat is seen partly herniated through the opening.

K. The left kidney is manually depressed, and downward traction is placed on the cut margin of the diaphragm, to show its relation to the overlying lung encased within its pleural covering.

DISCUSSION—DR. MARK A. HAYES. Adrenalectomy for diseases of the adrenocortex requires a bilateral simultaneous exposure as illustrated. The experience reported from the Yale Clinic (1) indicated that in about half of the patients with surgically correctible diseases of the adrenocortex, there was either preoperative unlocalizable unilateral disease or unsuspected contralateral disease. Since the time of that report, cited further experience in adults and children has continued to support these facts. Additional benefits accrue to the patients from an extraperitoneal posterior or posterolateral approach: prompt return of gastrointestinal function, absence of prolonged ileus, intake of a normal diet earlier, early time of ambulation and shortened length of hospital stay.

Though not shown completely in Dr. Madden's presentation, positioning of the patient is very important. It is essential that the normal anterior lumbar curve of the spine be flattened, and the knees should be flexed to reduce venous pooling in the lower extremities during the operative procedure. The incision employed in the Yale Clinic is designed to be lateral to the large sacrospinalis mass of muscle, since medial retraction of that muscle mass is prohibited by the transverse processes of the lumbar vertebrae. After an incision is made through the latissimus dorsi muscle, it is extended through the junction of the anterior and posterior layers of the lumbodorsal fascia, thus

avoiding the vessels perforating the paravertebral muscles. Subjacent to these structures is the lateral edge of the quadratus lumborum muscle and the transversalis fascia (often incorrectly called the anterior layer of the lumbodorsal fascia).

In G the posterior subcostal ligament (often referred to as the posterior lumbocostal ligament) is an important landmark. It marks the posterior inferior reflection of the pleura. Careful division of this ligament, reflection of the pleura, and removal of the twelfth rib may be all that is necessary for adrenal surgery in thin patients or children, without opening the pleura. In patients with typical Cushing's syndrome, however, there is no objection to removing all of the twelfth rib and a segment of the eleventh rib, with incision of the diaphragm and pleura to facilitate the removal of large glands or tumors.

It is wise to follow the advice of Munro in dividing nerves with a cutaneous distribution, attempting to avoid annoying paresthesias and causalgic states. This is done by applying three fine crushing hemostats close together. The center clamp is removed and the division of the nerve is made sharply through the crushed area. The transected ends are ligated with fine silk as the remaining clamps are removed.

The use of neurosurgical clips with long clip-applying forceps is an absolutely essential part of the armamentarium. The connective tissue inti-

Plate 255

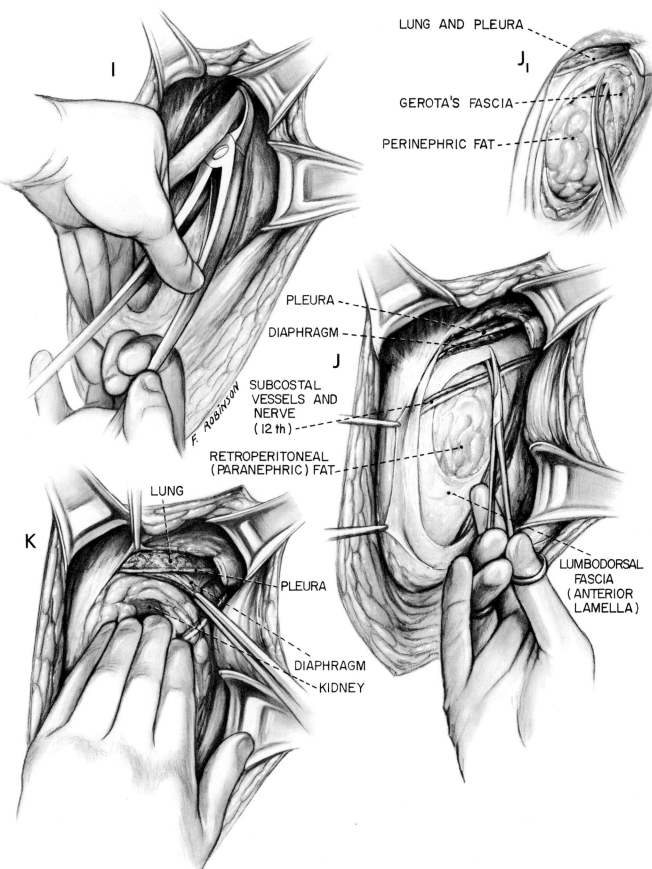

I

J₁

LUNG AND PLEURA

GEROTA'S FASCIA

PERINEPHRIC FAT

PLEURA

DIAPHRAGM

J

SUBCOSTAL
VESSELS AND
NERVE
(12 th)

RETROPERITONEAL
(PARANEPHRIC) FAT

LUMBODORSAL
FASCIA
(ANTERIOR
LAMELLA)

F. ROBINSON

K

LUNG

PLEURA

DIAPHRAGM

KIDNEY

L. Manual depression of the kidney is maintained as the fatty tissue about the partially exposed adrenal gland is dissected with scissors. From the posterior approach, the adrenal gland is more superficially located than is generally realized and can be readily identified from the surrounding fatty tissue by its characteristic golden-brown color.

M. The superior pole of the kidney has been mobilized and rotated downward and backward, a maneuver that facilitates the exposure of the adrenal gland. The displaced superior pole of the kidney, covered by a moist gauze sponge, is manually retracted, and one of the multiple tributary veins is being occluded by both clamp and clip (Cushing). The friability of the gland and the ease with which these small delicate veins may be avulsed make the use of the metallic clips for hemostasis a desirable technical aid in the performance of an adrenalectomy. The arterial branches to the adrenal gland are rarely recognized as such during its dissection.

N. The mobilization of the adrenal gland is continued, and the larger tributary veins are doubly clamped, severed with scissors, and subsequently occluded with ligatures of silk (000).

Discussion—Dr. Hayes (cont.)

mately associated with the pseudocapsule of the gland carries a multitude of fine vessels that, in pathologic glands can cause annoying bleeding. The use of special cautery scissors,* insulated except at the tip, can facilitate the dissection and mobilization of the gland immeasurably.

It is obligatory that absolutely no forceps or clamp, even those of the atraumatic Babcock variety, be applied to the gland. Diseased glands are exceptionally friable, and any break in its structure can cause difficulties of many varieties: bleeding, very difficult to control, may obscure the field for the remainder of the procedure; spilling and auto-implantation of a few cells, particularly the histologically bizarre cell types of children's tumors, provide the possibility of recurrent disease comparable to splenosis after a ruptured spleen and in recurrent malignancy. It is customary to manipulate the gland by using the adventitia or the perisuprarenal fascia (2) as a convenient handle, using flat Wangensteen forceps.

It is not always possible to obtain the beautifully illustrated visualization of the adrenal veins for ligation and suture. The careful placement of the neurosurgical clips can be advantageously used in this location also.

In the event of the undesirable occurrence of a tear in either the renal vein or the inferior vena cava and an accompanying inability to suture the rent as described by the authors, another useful procedure is available. Because of the low pressure venous system, an open-end suction tip can be applied to the rent. With careful traction the rent can be functionally closed. Another suction tip can be used to clear the field for accurate visualization and the application of a closely placed row of silver clips at right angles to the tear.

The pleural cavities, both having been opened in most adult cases, are closed over suction catheters, which are withdrawn as the incision in the diaphragm is closed in one layer. In this clinic no drainage of the operative site or the pleural cavities is ever employed. A portable postoperative roentgenogram of the chest is obtained in the recovery room.

References

1. Hayes, M. A., and Goldenberg, I. S. Operative treatment of adrenal cortical hyperfunctioning diseases, Ann. Surg., Supplement, 154:33, 1961.
2. Hayes, M. A. Abdominopelvic fasciae, Am. J. Anat., 87:119, 1950.

---

* Available from Edward Weck & Co., Long Island City, N.Y.

Plate 256

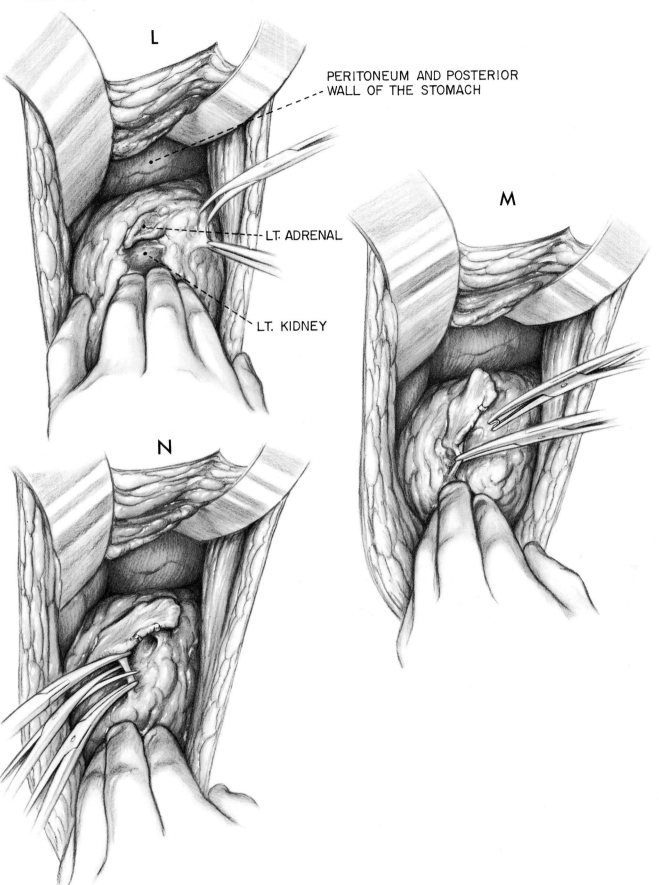

L

PERITONEUM AND POSTERIOR
WALL OF THE STOMACH

M

LT. ADRENAL

LT. KIDNEY

N

O. The left adrenal gland, completely mobilized from its surrounding structures, is held up in forceps, and a lymph node is being removed from the base of the adrenal vein as a biopsy specimen.

P. Upward traction with clamps (Babcock) is maintained as the left adrenal vein, uniformly large, is being encircled with a ligature of silk (00) at its entrance into the left renal vein.

Q. The adrenal vein, clamped proximally and ligated (00 silk) distally is being occluded

between with a transfixion suture ligature of 000 silk.

R, S. The adrenal vein is severed between the clamp and ligatures (R), and the specimen is removed (S).

T, U. On completion of the operation on the left side, a moist gauze pad is placed in the "bed" of the adrenal gland (T). After repositing the kidney, it is covered with a moist gauze pad and the retractors are withdrawn (U). The operator now goes to the opposite side for the removal of the right adrenal gland.

In the performance of bilateral adrenalectomy the selection of the operative approach, whether anterior (transabdominal or transperitoneal) or posterior (extraperitoneal), is dependent upon the experience and preference of the surgeon. The purported advantages of the transabdominal approach are (1) that both adrenal glands are readily examined, (2) that bilateral oophorectomy, when indicated, may be performed as a complimentary procedure, and (3) that ectopic adrenal tissue may be present and its removal is easily accomplished.

Despite the stated advantages of the anterior approach, and after an equal experience in the use of both the anterior and posterior approaches, the posterior or extraperitoneal exposure is preferred. It is believed much less shocking and is particularly suited to the obese patient. Furthermore, the glands are more readily exposed, and, should bleeding occur, hemostasis is believed more easily obtained. Also, the duration of operation is not unduly, if at all, prolonged.

In the use of the posterior approach it should be emphasized that once the renal fascia (Gerota's) is severed, the adrenal gland is located more superficially in the surrounding areolar tissue than is usually expected. The gland is identified by its distinctive yellowish-brown color, which differentiates it from the surrounding fatty tissue in which it is embedded.

In the preoperative preparation of the patient for bilateral adrenalectomy, and in the postoperative management, the method advised by Huggins, with but minor modifications, is prescribed. The morning of the day preceding operation, 50 mg. of cortisone acetate is given

Plate 257   575

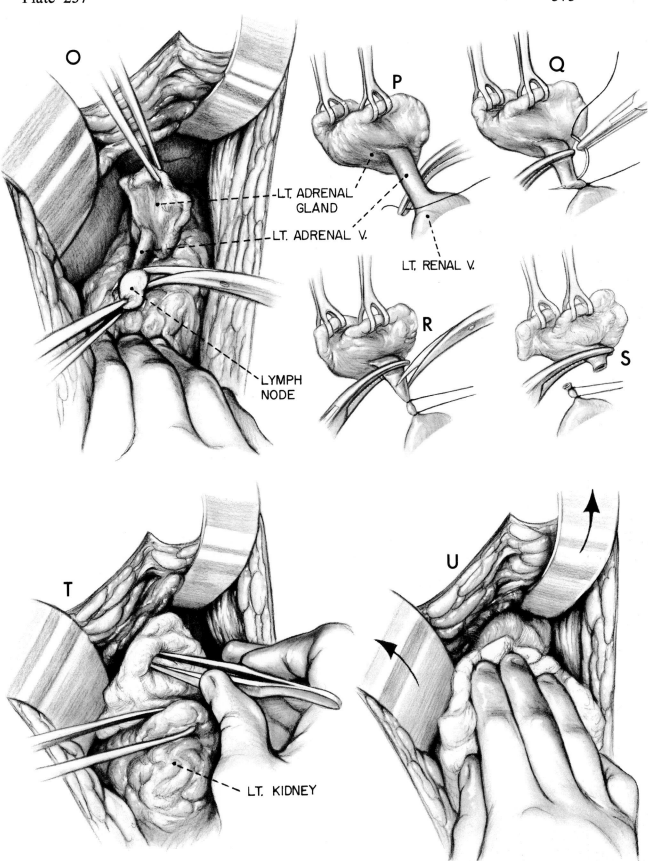

O

LT. ADRENAL GLAND

LT. ADRENAL V.

P

Q

LT. RENAL V.

R

S

T

LT. KIDNEY

U

V. The exposure of the operative field for the removal of the right adrenal gland is obtained as previously illustrated for the left adrenal gland. The mobilized gland is held upward in clamps (Babcock), and the uniformly short and wide right adrenal vein, emptying into the inferior vena cava, is visible. The relation of these structures to the right kidney, peritoneum, and liver may also be seen.

W, X, Y. The adrenal vein is encircled with a ligature of 000 silk (W) and ligated in continuity (X). A transfixion suture ligature is inserted proximal to the ligature (X), and the vein is transected between this ligature and a clamp (Y). The shortness of the right adrenal vein precludes the application of a clamp prior to the insertion of the transfixion suture ligature (X). It also predisposes to an avulsion tear and serious hemorrhage from the inferior vena cava. If this should occur, experience has demonstrated that it is best controlled by compression with small gauze pads held in dressing forceps ("stick sponges"). The vena cava is occluded by compression both cephalad

and caudad to the site of tear, and the wound is toiletted by repeated irrigations with warm saline solution and suction siphonage of the fluid. The tear in the inferior vena cava is next located and closed with interrupted sutures of 00000 arterial silk. When the closure is completed, the "stick sponges" are slowly removed as the closure is observed for adequacy of hemostasis. If bleeding recurs, it may be controlled by simply compressing the bleeding site with a dry gauze sponge. Rarely, the insertion of additional sutures may be necessary. It cannot be overemphasized that the application of clamps blindly into an operative field flooded with blood usually results in more extensive damage to the vena cava, thereby endangering the life of the patient. Since venous blood loss at this juxtacentral level is poorly tolerated, hemostasis should be obtained quickly and effectively. The method just described has proved most satisfactory.

Z. The incisions on completion of the wound closures are shown.

intramuscularly, and every four hours subsequently 25 mg. (I.M.) is administered until 6:00 A.M. on the day of operation. In addition, 1 g. of potassium chloride (orally) every eight hours is also prescribed.

On the morning (6:00 A.M.) of the day of operation, 200 mg. of cortisone acetate is administered intramuscularly (100 mg. in each buttock) and in the operation room an infusion of Solu-Cortef, 100 mg. in 1000 cc. of 10 per cent glucose in water is begun. This is administered as a slow drip (30 drops per minute) during the operation.

Postoperatively, cortisone acetate (100 mg.) is administered every six hours throughout the day of operation and decreased to 50 mg. every six hours for the first day, and 50 mg. every eight hours for the second and third days after operation. From the third through the fifth postoperative days, the dosage is further decreased to 25 mg. every six hours. For the next four days 12.5 mg. every six hours is prescribed. Subsequent to the ninth postoperative day, the patient is given an oral maintenance dose of 25 mg. of cortisone acetate twice daily and 1 g. of potassium chloride, also twice daily. These drugs are continued as permanent medications. In some patients cortisone acetate causes severe nausea and anorexia, which are promptly relieved when Decadron (0.75 mg.) is substituted. One-half tablet or one tablet twice daily is prescribed, dependent upon the maintenance requirements of the patient.

The primary indications for total ablation of adrenal function are (1) Cushing's disease and (2) metastases, especially osseous, secondary to a primary cancer of the breast. Unilateral adrenalectomy is performed for tumors, benign or malignant, of the adrenal cortex or medulla.

Plate 258 577

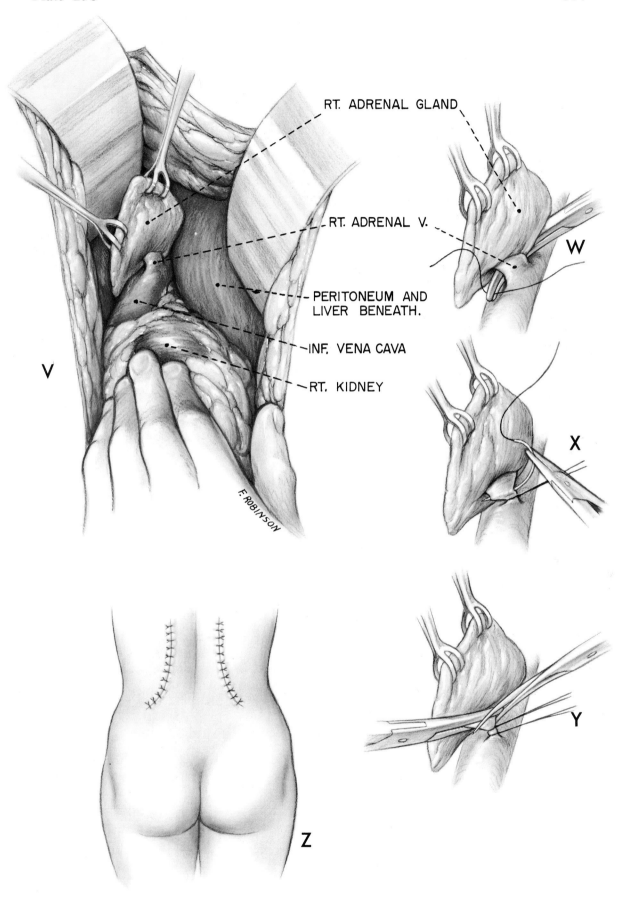

RT. ADRENAL GLAND

RT. ADRENAL V.

PERITONEUM AND
LIVER BENEATH.

INF. VENA CAVA

RT. KIDNEY

V

W

X

Y

Z

F. ROBINSON

TOTAL HYSTERECTOMY

A. The left paramedian incision is outlined and crosshatched to facilitate later closure.

A₁. Severed vessels in the rectus muscle layer are occluded with suture ligatures of silk (000). This technic is preferred to the use of clamps and ligatures because it is less traumatic and utilizes the hemostatic qualities inherent in muscle tissue.

B. The deep epigastric vessels are doubly clamped, severed, and ligated with ligatures of fine silk (000). The adjacent structures are depicted.

C. The anterior parietal peritoneum, tented with forceps, is being incised with a scalpel.

D, E. The cut margins of the peritoneum are grasped in forceps, and a protective moist gauze pad is inserted into the peritoneal cavity. The opening in the peritoneum is then extended caudad (D) with scissors and cephalad (E) with a scalpel. This particular sequence facilitates entrance into the peritoneal cavity with minimal change in the position of the operator standing on the left side of the operation table.

Plate 259   579

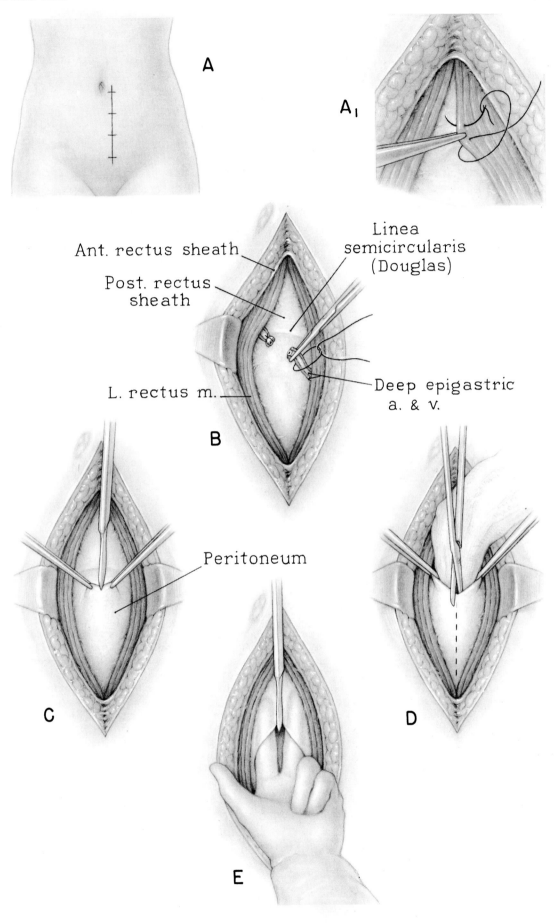

A

A₁

Ant. rectus sheath

Post. rectus sheath

Linea semicircularis (Douglas)

L. rectus m.

Deep epigastric a. & v.

B

Peritoneum

C

D

E

F, F₁. The patient is placed in the Trendelenburg position, and the small intestine, elevated on the palm of the left hand, is enclosed in moist gauze pads and displaced upward into the peritoneal cavity.

G, G₁. Clamps (Kocher) are applied to the cornua of the uterus, and upward traction is maintained to tense the round ligaments. The round ligament on the right is ligated and severed, and the one on the left is being encircled with a ligature of 000 silk (G).

A clamp is applied proximally, and the round ligament is severed with scissors between the clamp and the ligature (G₁).

H, H₁. The openings on each side between the leaves of the broad ligament are enlarged toward the bladder by scissor dissection (H) preliminary to the elevation of the bladder reflection of peritoneum by digital dissection (H₁). The fingers are ideally suited for this maneuver, which is an important initial step in the operation.

DISCUSSION—DR. JOHN S. WELCH. Total abdominal hysterectomy is a fundamental operative procedure. It is performed by surgeons with varied training in pelvic surgery and for a variety of lesions. A soundly conceived operation with built-in safety factors is a prime requisite.

The incision illustrated in A represents an unusual incision for pelvic operations. I prefer a lower midline incision, which can be extended to the left or the right of the umbilicus. With a midline incision no portion of the rectus abdominis needs to be denervated and no major vessels are encountered. The ability to perform transverse incisions, including the Pfannenstiel incision, is an essential part of the technical training of the surgeon who does pelvic surgery.

Since exposure in the pelvis often is limited, it is well to apply as few instruments as possible to the structures to be removed as well as those to be preserved. G and G₁ demonstrate an unnecessary step and an unnecessary application of forceps. A sound grasp on the uterus may be obtained with straight forceps applied bilaterally to incorporate the round ligament, the fallopian tube, and the utero-ovarian ligament. Forceps applied laterally from these basic instruments offer control of the severed pedicles, which may then be ligated without resort to the suture ligature. After division of the round ligaments, traction cephalad on the uterine clamps will facilitate the dissection of the anterior cul-de-sac peritoneum under direct vision by elevating it with Mayo-Russian forceps and undermining it slightly with long-handled scissors. I prefer to delay the division of the vesical peritoneum until all structures attached to the uterine fundus have been separated; hence, there is no restraining influence on the movement of the uterine fundus by the shortness of the ovarian pedicle (H, H₁, I, I₁).

As noted in I and I₁, the bladder must be re-

Plate 260   581

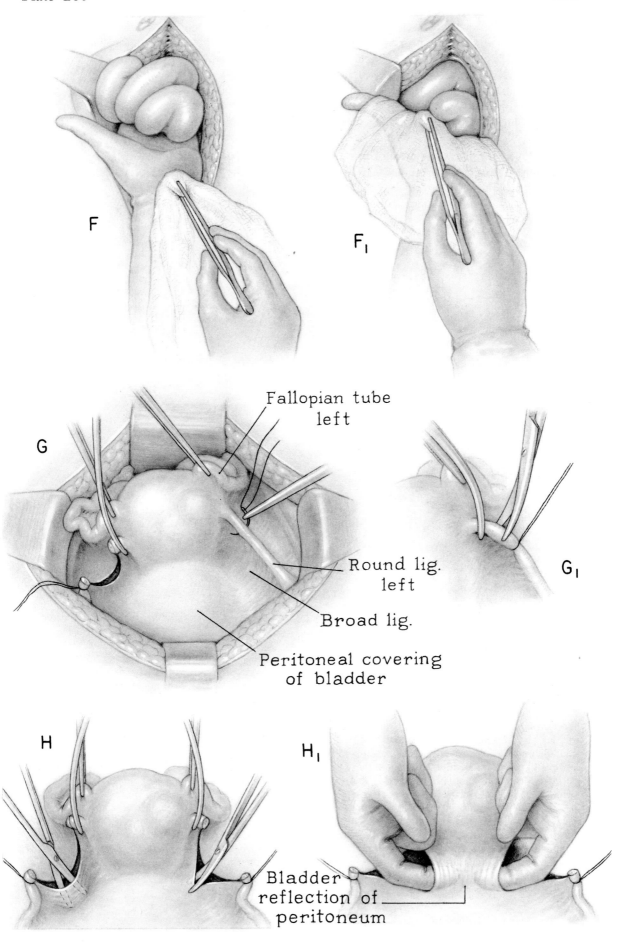

F

F₁

G

Fallopian tube
left

Round lig.
left

G₁

Broad lig.

Peritoneal covering
of bladder

H

H₁

Bladder
reflection of
peritoneum

I, I₁. The mobilized bladder reflection layer of peritoneum is severed (broken line) with scissors (I), and the bladder is bluntly dissected with a gauze pledget on a clamp from the anterior surface of the cervix (I₁). The tip of the Foley catheter within the bladder lumen is visible in broken outline.

J. For clarity of the surrounding structures, the sigmoid colon is eliminated from the operative field. The ureter on each side crosses over the bifurcation of the common

iliac artery and is located medial to and parallels the infundibulopelvic ligament. The infundibulopelvic ligament is first mobilized by blunt digital dissection and then triply clamped.

J₁-J₇. The infundibulopelvic ligament is severed between the two distal clamps (J₁) and the proximal end is occluded with a ligature (J₂, J₃) and suture ligature (J₃-J₇) of 00 and 000 silk, respectively.

DISCUSSION—DR. WELCH (cont.)

flected downward if one is to accomplish safely a total abdominal hysterectomy. The vesical wall need not be pressed downward much farther than the terminal portion of the cervix, and substantial venous bleeding may thus be avoided.

J, J₁, and J₇ demonstrate a vital portion of any complete pelvic procedure. Although the ureter is nearly always in anatomic position at the pelvic brim, it may be drawn medially lower in the pelvis by chronic inflammatory disease, endometriosis, or malignant lesions. The second most common position of ureteral damage occurs near the infundibulopelvic ligament if the surgeon picks up a large bundle without first identifying the position of the ureter. My preference is to isolate the in-

fundibulopelvic or ovarian pedicle after identifying the ureter and to simply clamp it doubly, dividing the pedicle between clamps for simple ligation. The ovarian pedicle, like any clamped pedicle, must have sufficient cuff distal to the applied clamp to prevent its slipping from the forceps during ligation. The double clamping technic shown is an additional safeguard of definite use for the young surgeon, but I prefer a simple double ligature. One note of caution at this point concerns the brittleness of the vessels in the ovarian pedicle: excessive tension or twisting may result in their breakage, with subsequent development of a retroperitoneal collection of blood.

Similar comments apply to my own method

Plate 261

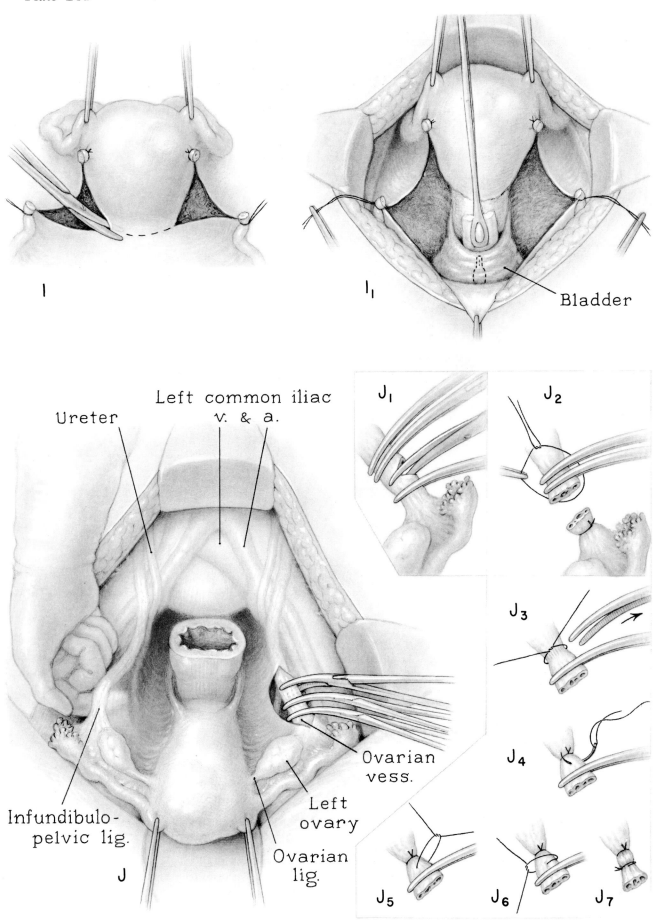

I

I₁

Bladder

Ureter

Left common iliac
v. & a.

J₁

J₂

J₃

J₄

Infundibulo-
pelvic lig.

J

Ovarian
vess.

Left
ovary

Ovarian
lig.

J₅

J₆

J₇

K, K₁. When the tube and ovary are to be preserved, an opening is made in the broad ligament below the tube and ovarian ligament by a combination of blunt (digital) and sharp (scalpel) dissection (K). The tube and ovarian ligament are triply clamped and severed (K₁) and subsequently ligated in the same manner as previously described for the infundibulopelvic ligament (J₁-J₇).

L. The severance and ligation of the infundibulopelvic ligaments are completed, and the relation of the severed ends on the right side to the surrounding structures is visible. The right ureter is seen to pass over the bifurcation of the right common iliac artery and then course downward beneath the uterine artery to terminate ultimately in the bladder.

DISCUSSION—DR. WELCH (cont.)

when the ovary and the tube are to be preserved. It is highly important for the surgeon to grasp an adequately developed pedicle, as demonstrated in K and K₁, so that ligatures may be applied accurately.

The passage of the ureter beneath the uterine artery is demonstrated in L. Traction on the straight forceps previously applied to the sides of the uterine fundus will raise the uterus and attached structures out of the pelvis and demonstrate the broad ligament for what it is—a double layer of peritoneum with some enclosed areolar tissue. This peritoneum can be cut sharply, as shown in M, or it can be merely wiped down with a sponge to demonstrate the region of the uterine artery.

The so-called cardinal ligament with its associated and enclosed uterine artery is better managed, in my opinion, by a technic akin to the "blind" method demonstrated in O₁ and O₂. An Ochsner forceps is used to clamp all structures remaining in the cardinal ligament, including the uterine artery and its branches. It is vital in the application of this clamp that the uterus be drawn

contralaterally so that structures are placed on tension. The points of the forceps applied are caused to slide off the cervix to incorporate all structures immediately alongside. The ligament may then be severed, together with the uterine artery and its branches; the uterus is released, and a small window is opened in the endopelvic fascia that immediately surrounds the cervix. Although the ureter is not routinely demonstrated at this time, it is easily palpable 1.5 to 2 cm. lateral to the single clamp so placed. Double and triple clamping seems unnecessary, since there is relatively little back bleeding from the nearly detached uterus and adequate precautions are made to leave a cuff distal to the applied Ochsner forceps. After similarly detaching the cardinal ligament on the opposite side, the two windows of the endopelvic fascia may be connected anteriorly, severing, as a smooth layer, the so-called pubocervical fascia. It is important that this fascia be preserved and utilized in reconstruction of the vaginal vault.

Most gynecologists do not ligate the uterosacral ligaments. I prefer to clamp them, since they occasionally contain briskly bleeding vessels. They

Plate 262   585

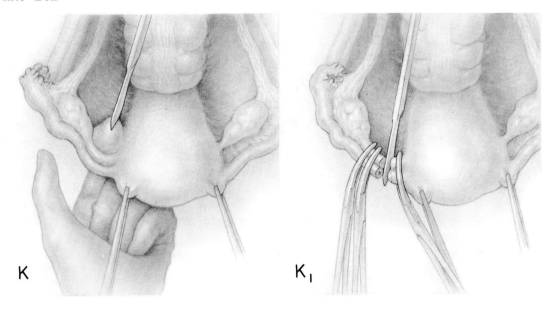

K   K₁

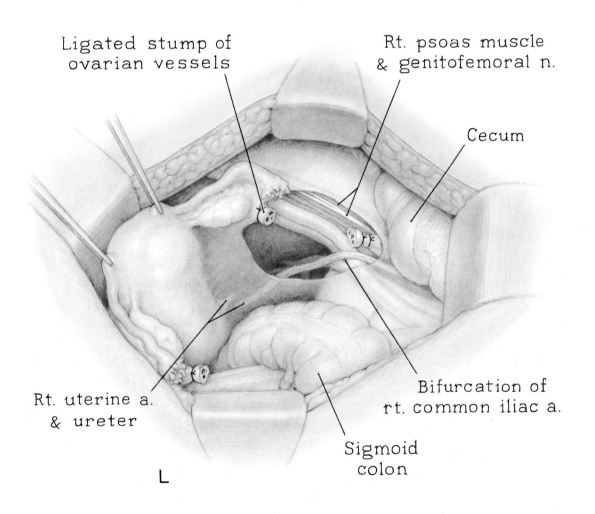

Ligated stump of
ovarian vessels

Rt. psoas muscle
& genitofemoral n.

Cecum

Rt. uterine a.
& ureter

Bifurcation of
rt. common iliac a.

Sigmoid
colon

L

M. The relation of the ureter and the uterine artery on the right side is depicted. On the left side the fibroareolar tissue layer is being dissected with scissors to expose the uterine artery as seen on the right side.

N. The uterus is displaced anteriorly, and the scissor dissection posteriorly toward the related uterosacral ligament is shown.

O, O₁, O₂. The uterine arteries on either side are clearly visible, as are their ascending and descending branches (O). The dissection, isolation, and clamping of each uterine artery under direct vision is preferred to the "blind" triple clamp method illustrated (O_1, O_2). This method, though faster, does not comply with the basic tenets of vascular surgery as related to the ligation of blood vessels. Accordingly, slipping of the hemostatic ligatures is more apt to occur.

O₃-O₈. These sequential illustrations depict two technics for the severance and ligation of the isolated uterine artery. The uterine artery may be ligated (00 silk) in continuity and its ascending branches doubly clamped and severed (O_3, O_4), or the uterine artery alone may be triply clamped, severed, and ligated (O_5-O_8).

DISCUSSION—DR. WELCH (cont.)

are severed, as demonstrated, at the same time that the posterior peritoneum is incised, clearly demonstrating the closely apposed rectum and demonstrating the posterior layer of the endopelvic fascia, the so-called rectovaginal fascia, which likewise must be preserved and utilized in the reconstruction of the vaginal vault.

Some sort of traction is needed on the vaginal vault after detachment of the uterine cervix. Henrotin vulsella in the four quadrants do this nicely in my practice.

Reconstruction of the vaginal vault assumes the highest priority in the prevention of its subsequent prolapse. It is a basic tenet that the round ligaments offer little if any permanent support to the vaginal vault; indeed, many gynecologic surgeons do not utilize them except for their function in reperitonization. For this reason I disagree with the depicted attachment of the round ligaments into the vagina (S, S₁-S₄) for two reasons: they will offer no permanent support, and the raw ligated end will be troublesome in the postoperative period, leading to the formation of granulation tissue and also offering an opening from the vagina into the clean retroperitoneal tissues. I close the vaginal vault in a double layer, the first row of sutures approximating the severed edges of the vagina and the second layer approximating, over the top of the vault, the anterior and posterior endopelvic fascial layers previously isolated. The uterosacral thickenings together with the cardinal ligament stumps may then be anchored to the corners of the vaginal vault, much as one attempts to do with a vaginal hysterectomy. To facilitate reperitonization thereafter, the round ligaments may be anchored to the closed vaginal vault, not for support but because they draw the attached peritoneum medially. Reperitonization may then be accomplished by interrupted sutures or a continuous suture, as demonstrated in T and U.

It should be stressed that thorough abdominal exploration will have been accomplished prior to the pelvic procedure. Usually I remove the appendix as an incidental procedure.

Plate 263   587

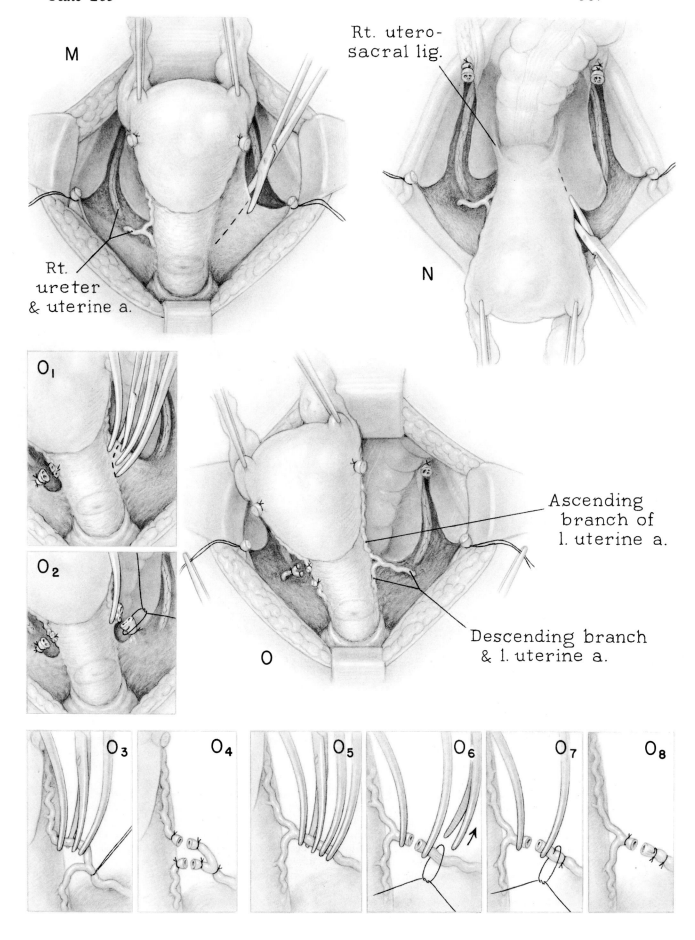

M

Rt. utero-
sacral lig.

N

Rt.
ureter
& uterine a.

O₁

O₂

O

Ascending
branch of
l. uterine a.

Descending branch
& l. uterine a.

O₃   O₄   O₅   O₆   O₇   O₈

P. The uterus is again displaced anteriorly, and each uterosacral ligament is ligated (00 silk) in continuity and severed proximal to the ligature. The peritoneum overlying the vaginal vault posteriorly is then incised (broken line).

Q. The mobilized uterus is displaced to the right, and the mobilized left vaginal artery and its relation to the severed stump of the left uterine artery are shown (Q). The vaginal artery may be isolated, doubly clamped, and severed (Q₁), or the "blind"

method may be used (Q₂), in which a portion of the cardinal ligaments is included with the artery.

R, R₁, R₂. Traction sutures of silk (000) are inserted on either side of the vaginal vault, and the vaginal lumen is entered by a stab incision with a scalpel (R). The opening is enlarged anteriorly by scissor dissection (R₁), and with the cervix grasped in a tenaculum forceps, the vaginal wall posteriorly is severed with scissors (R₂).

DISCUSSION—DR. JAMES PRATT MARR. Many gynecologists are convinced that a Pfannenstiel incision, with a transverse fascial incision, is a logical approach to the pelvic organs. This incision is anatomic, physiologic, and cosmetic and, when used with the O'Sullivan-O'Connor retractors, gives adequate exposure. Another nicety is available in utilizing Bissel pads, composed of 8-in. rubber envelopes enclosing a damp laparotomy pad to pack intestinal coils upward.

I am in complete accord with the illustrated steps of this operation through O₈. Each step is deliberate, exact, and essential to a proper approach to the uterine vessels. However, for a number of years, I have abandoned the steps illustrated from P through to S₄, believing that the cervix may be released from the vaginal vault by dissection within a pericervical fascial cuff, thereby avoiding any injury to the uterus, bladder, or bowel.

Before ligating the uterine vessels, is is essential that one should palpate the length of the cervix. This structure varies in length with individuals and multiparity. It is at this level of the ligated uterine vessels that the transverse cervical ligaments (cardinal or Mackenrodt's) envelop the cervix. They may be recognized by a dense, glistening layer of fibroareolar connective tissue, which completely surrounds the lower segment of the uterus, the cervix, and the vault of the vagina. The posterior surface of the cervix is covered with a layer of parietal peritoneum, into which the uterosacral ligaments are inserted.

A transverse incision on the anterior surface of the cervix, at the level of the ligated uterine vessels, may reveal a line of cleavage between the cervix and its fascial covering. When defined, the edges of this cuff of tissue are picked up in Allis forceps, and with the aid of blunt scissors, the cuff is further dissected down to the vaginal vault.

Plate 264

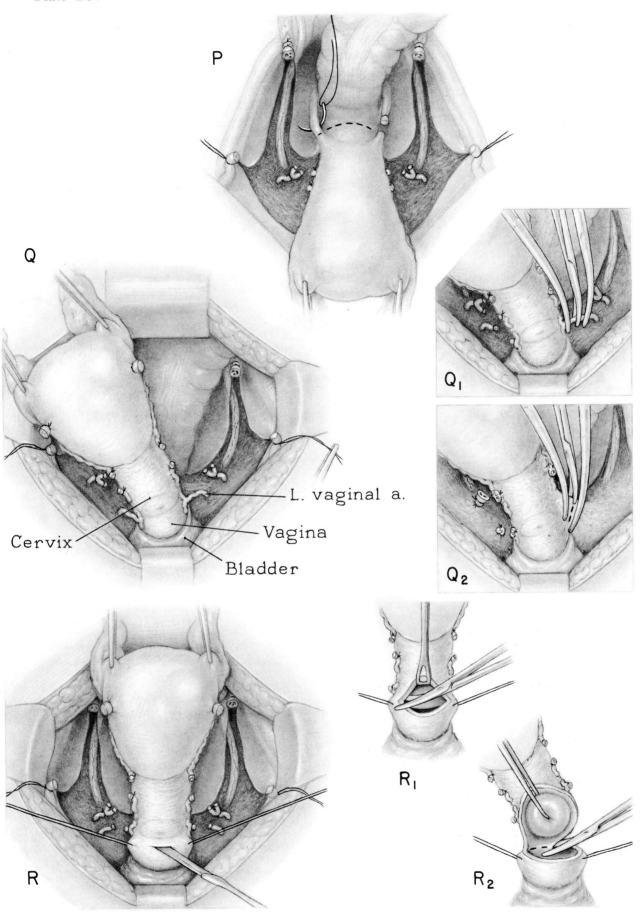

P

Q

Q₁

Q₂

Cervix

L. vaginal a.

Vagina

Bladder

R

R₁

R₂

S. The insertion of the angle suture on the left side, which incorporates the severed distal end of the round ligament, is completed. The angle suture on the right side is being inserted.

S₁, S₂, S₃, S₄. These illustrations show in detail the insertion of the angle suture on the right side. The suture is essentially a figure of 8, which is inserted from the center behind to the angle in front, then from the angle in front through the angle behind, and then through the stump of the round ligament (S₁) to the center in front (S₂). When the suture is tied, the stump of the round ligament is incorporated in the angle closure (S₃). Upon completion of the angle closures, the cut margins of the anterior and posterior walls of the vagina are approximated with a continuous interlocking suture of 0 chromic catgut or 00 silk (S₄).

T. The cut margins of the posterior parietal peritoneum are approximated with a continuous suture of 00 chromic catgut. The suture commences on the right side just cephalad to the ligated stump of the infundibulopelvic ligament and terminates just to the left of the midline anteriorly. In the approximation anteriorly, three sutures are taken in the bladder reflection of the peritoneum for each suture in the peritoneum posteriorly to compensate for its redundancy. A second peritoneal closure suture (00 chromic catgut) is started on the left side just proximal to the ligated stump of the left infundibulopelvic ligament and is continued downward to meet its opposite fellow in juxtaposition to the midline anteriorly, where the sutures are tied to each other.

U. The operative field on completion of the insertion of the reperitonizing sutures is shown. The relation of the ureters to the peritoneal closure and the supporting effect of the round ligaments incorporated in the closure of the vaginal vault are also visible.

DISCUSSION—DR. MARR (cont.)

The same procedure at the same level is performed posteriorly, where the separation is easier because of an abundance of fibroareolar tissue. Kocher clamps are now applied to each cardinal ligament within the cuff and to the inside of the uterine vessel stumps. The cardinal ligaments are severed between the clamps with a scalpel and doubly ligated, as they contain the descending branches of the uterine arteries.

The cervix, now liberated from its fascial attachment, may be raised. With the thumb and index finger, the cervix is squeezed away from the vagina, much like squeezing a pea from a pod, thus permitting a given amount of the vaginal vault to be excised by scissor dissection.

Following the removal of the uterus, each lateral angle suture is inserted from the inside-out on the vagina, runs through the stump of the Cardinal ligament, is reinserted into the vagina from the outside-in, and is tied. The incorporation of the Cardinal ligaments in the angle sutures gives support and elasticity to the vagina.

The vaginal mucosa is approximated with a continuous suture of 00 chromic catgut, followed by the approximation of the fascial cuff as a second layer and by a similar suture. The proximal ends of the round, utero-ovarian or infundibulopelvic ligaments *are never fixed to the vaginal vault* to either facilitate peritonization or as a support for the vagina. Furthermore, we believe that the blood supply to the ovaries is improved by permitting them to be retracted to the lateral pelvic walls. When the ovaries are drawn down toward the midline, they tend to prolapse into the cul-de-sac, causing both discomfort and dyspareunia.

The contraindications for the type of abdominal hysterectomy I have described is in carcinoma of the cervix with involvement of the fascial cuff and/or the base of the bladder. In such circumstances, Dr. Madden's illustrated technic is superior.

Plate 265   591

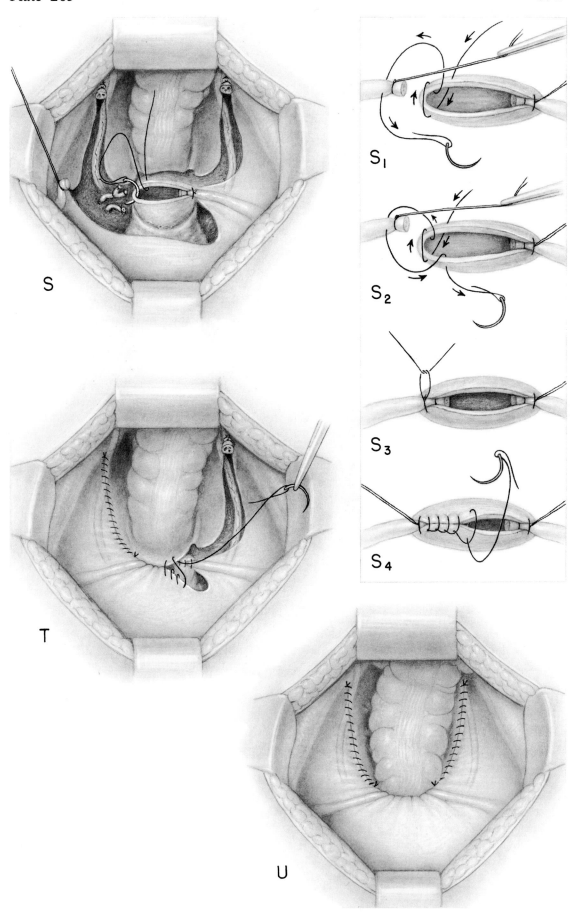

S

S₁

S₂

S₃

S₄

T

U

AORTOCAVAL NODE DISSECTION FOR CANCER
OF THE UTERINE CERVIX

The patient, a 39-year-old married white woman, was admitted to the hospital with the complaint of intermittent vaginal bleeding of 11 months duration. Pelvic examination revealed an extensive cancer of the cervix, with extension into each fornix with foreshortening of the vaginal vault. At operation, huge masses of matted nodes were observed, which obscured the pelvic vessels and extended cephalad to cover the abdominal aorta and inferior vena cava. The size of the nodes and the associated phlegmonous edema made it impossible to elicit by palpation the pulsations in the common iliac arteries.

Following the aortocaval-iliac node dissection as depicted, a total hysterectomy and bilateral salpingo-oophorectomy, with wide excision of the parametria and partial vaginectomy, was performed. The postoperative convalescence was satisfactory, and the patient was completely well for a period of seven months. At this time the patient complained of severe headache, nausea and vomiting, and was readmitted to the hospital. Pelvic examination showed no evidence of recurrence. The condition of the patient rapidly worsened and was associated with a progressive oliguria, elevation of the blood urea, and coma, which terminated in the death of the patient. Necropsy showed bilateral ureteral obstruction secondary to recurrent metastatic disease.

This is the third patient with cancer of the cervix in whom I have observed metastases to the aortocaval nodes. The other two were previously mentioned in the discussion of radical right hemicolectomy (page 400). Accordingly, it is apparent that pelvic lymphadenectomy concomitant with radical extirpation of the uterus for carcinoma of the cervix is incomplete as it fails to include the whole of the lymphatic drain. To be complete, the nodal dissection must of anatomic necessity include the aortocaval nodes immediately cephalad to the renal veins, just as it does for cancer of the testicle, colon, and stomach.

The technics for aortocaval node dissection in the radical operations for gastric and colonic cancer are depicted elsewhere in this volume.

A. The patient is in the supine position, and the left rectus paramedian muscle-splitting (inner third) incision is outlined and cross-hatched to facilitate later closure.

B. The peritoneal exposure is enlarged for clarity in depicting the anatomic and pathologic structures. The proximal jejunal segment is manually elevated, and the relation of the duodenojejunal junction to the inferior mesenteric vein is visible. The broken line that extends obliquely downward from the duodenojejunal junction to encircle the attached cecum indicates the line of incision to mobilize the root of the small bowel mesentery and the cecoascending colon. An opening is made in the posterior parietal peritoneum to show more clearly the right ureter and the cephalad stump of the infundibulopelvic ligament in relation to the mass of metastatically invaded lymph nodes overlying the right common iliac artery and its bifurcation. These nodes covered completely the aorta and inferior vena cava and their branches and tributaries respectively within the pelvis.

C. The right side of the colon is mobilized and retracted toward the midline to show the retrocolic portion of the duodenum and the head of the pancreas in relation to the surrounding retroperitoneal structures and the aortocaval nodal mass.

Plate 266   593

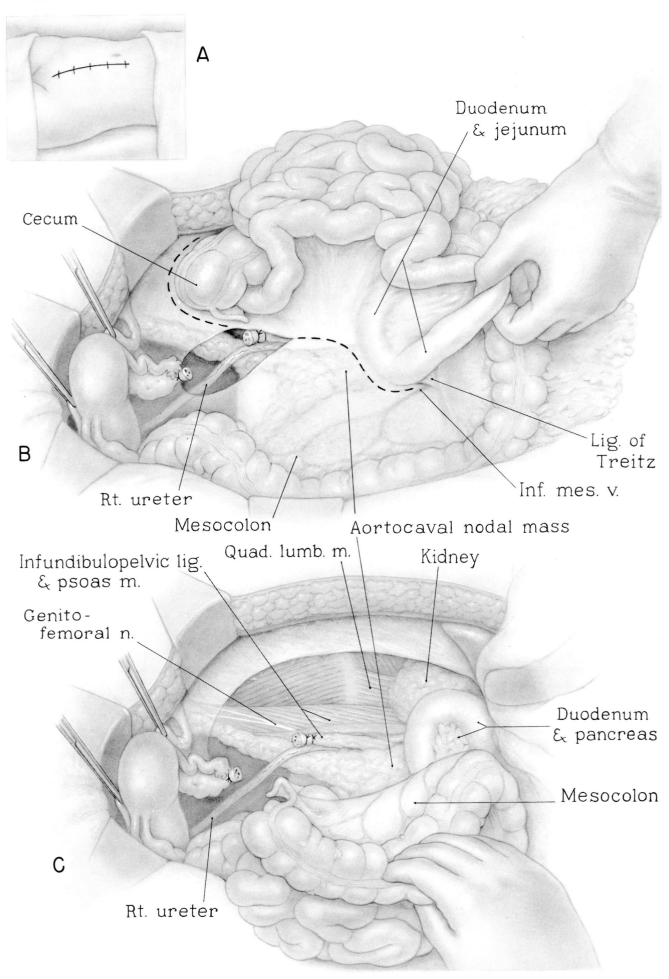

A

Duodenum
& jejunum

Cecum

Lig. of
Treitz

B

Inf. mes. v.

Rt. ureter

Mesocolon   Aortocaval nodal mass

Quad. lumb. m.   Kidney

Infundibulopelvic lig.
& psoas m.

Genito-
femoral n.

Duodenum
& pancreas

Mesocolon

C

Rt. ureter

D. The sigmoid colon is mobilized, and an opening is made in the base of its mesocolon to show the ureter as it crosses the nodal mass, which obscures the left common iliac artery and its bifurcation. The third or horizontal portion of the duodenum is elevated by a retractor to show its relation to the cephalad extension of the aortocaval nodal mass.

E. The duodenum is retracted upward to show the beginning of the dissection with scissors of the metastatic nodal mass from the inferior vena cava and aorta.

Plate 267   595

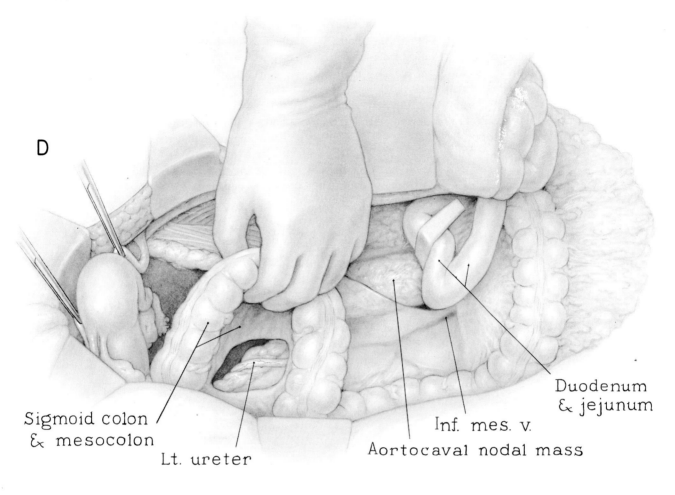

D

Sigmoid colon
& mesocolon

Lt. ureter

Inf. mes. v.

Aortocaval nodal mass

Duodenum
& jejunum

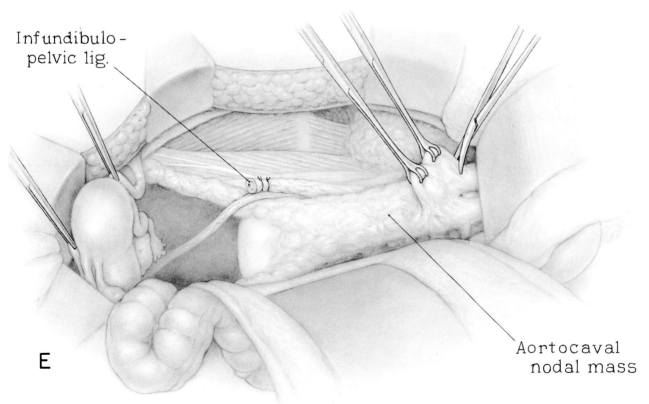

Infundibulo-
pelvic lig.

Aortocaval
nodal mass

E

F. The aortocaval node dissection is continued, and the attachment of the nodal
mass to the aorta and its inferior mesenteric
arterial branch is being freed by scissor dissection. In this patient the renal arteries
were paired bilaterally and the left renal
vein was posterior to the aorta rather than
in its usual anterior location.

G. The aorta and its bifurcation are cleared,
and the dissection of the nodal mass is continued along the left common iliac artery
and its bifurcation.

H. This illustration depicts the near completion of the aortocaval node dissection as
the remaining attachments of the metastatic
nodes along the right external iliac artery
are being severed by scissor dissection. The
relation of the completed aortocaval node
dissection to the surrounding structures is
clearly depicted.

Plate 268   597

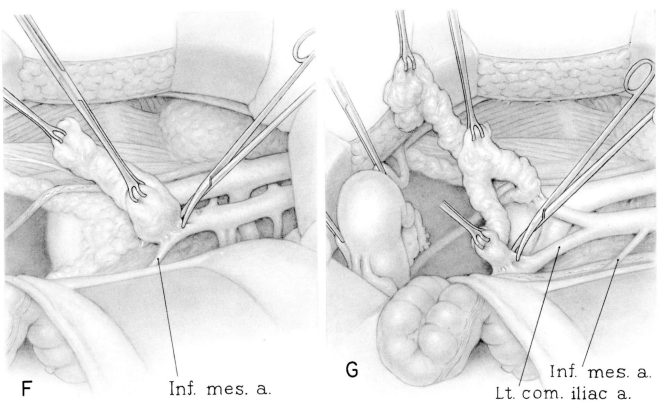

F   Inf. mes. a.

G   Inf. mes. a.
                                      Lt. com. iliac a.

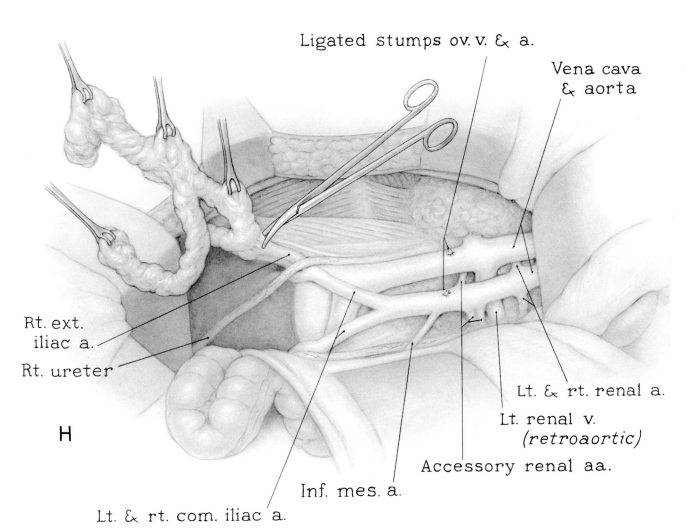

Ligated stumps ov. v. & a.

Vena cava
& aorta

Rt. ext.
iliac a.

Rt. ureter

Lt. & rt. renal a.

Lt. renal v.
(retroaortic)

Accessory renal aa.

H

Inf. mes. a.

Lt. & rt. com. iliac a.

SALPINGO-OOPHORECTOMY

A. The patient is in the supine position, and the protuberance of the abdomen caused by a large right ovarian cyst is apparent. The left paramedian incision is outlined and crosshatched to facilitate later closure.

B. The peritoneal cavity is entered, and the right infundibulopelvic ligament, devoid of its peritoneal covering, is triply clamped and severed between the two lowermost clamps. The oval-shaped bodies within the ligament are dilated lymphatic vessels. The right ureter, located medial to the infundibulopelvic ligament, characteristically courses over the right common iliac artery at its bifurcation; this constant finding serves as an identifying anatomic landmark for the isolation of the ureter. The ovarian cyst, partially compressed by a retractor, and its relation to the surrounding structures is visible.

B₁. The lower transected end of the infundi-

bulopelvic ligament is ligated (00 silk), and its proximal end is tied with a ligature and suture ligature of 00 and 000 silk, respectively.

C. To facilitate dissection of the cyst, it is first decompressed. A trocar and cannula are inserted, and the trocar is withdrawn. Suction decompression is then obtained through the cannula by the removal of approximately 1200 cc. of a clear fluid.

D. The opening in the cyst after removal of the cannula is occluded with a clamp. Through this clamp, upward traction on the wall of the collapsed cyst is maintained as scissor dissection is being performed within the "leaves" of the broad ligament to isolate the uterine end of the Fallopian tube and the ovarian ligament. The relation of this dissection to the round ligament anteriorly is visible.

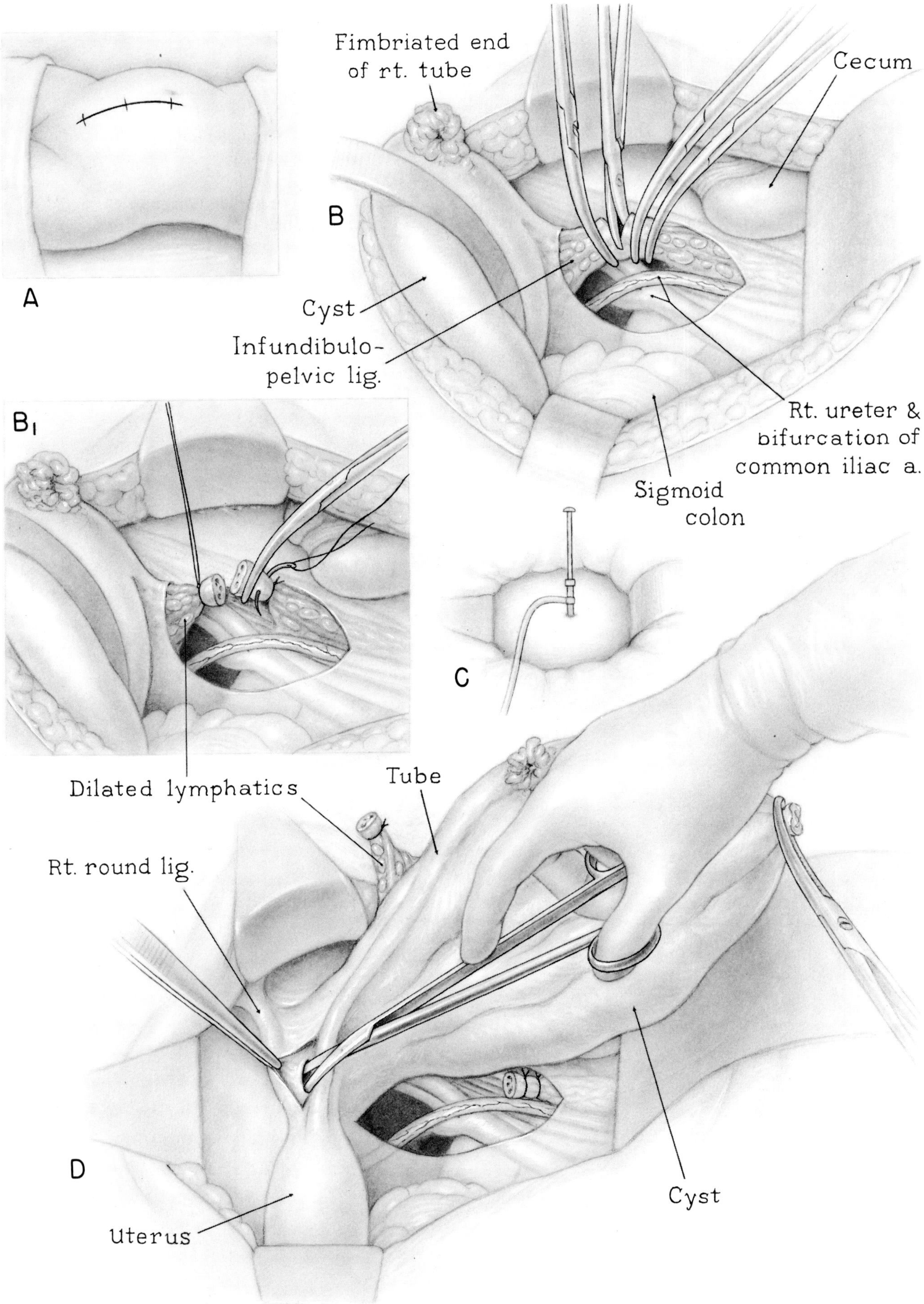

Plate 269

A

Fimbriated end
of rt. tube

Cecum

B

Cyst

Infundibulo-
pelvic lig.

Rt. ureter &
bifurcation of
common iliac a.

Sigmoid
colon

B₁

C

Dilated lymphatics

Tube

Rt. round lig.

Cyst

D

Uterus

E. The cyst is elevated out of the peritoneal cavity, and by blunt dissection a clamp (Mixter) is inserted through the posterior "leaf" of the broad ligament beneath the uterine end of the Fallopian tube and the ovarian ligament. The broken line indicates the line of severance of the remaining peritoneal attachment of the ovary.

E₁, E₂. The tube and ovarian ligament in juxtaposition to the cornu of the uterus are triply clamped and severed between the two distal clamps and the specimen is removed (E_1). The two clamps remaining are replaced with a ligature (proximal) and suture ligature (distal) of 00 and 000 silk, respectively (E_2). The relation of the psoas muscle and the genitofemoral nerve to the operative field is depicted.

F. The salpingo-oophorectomy is completed, and reperitonization of the operative area is begun, using a continuous suture of 00 chromic catgut.

G. The reperitonization is completed, and its relation to the surrounding anatomic structures may be seen.

H. The wound closure is in layers, the skin margins being approximated with a series of straight needles, which are all first inserted, withdrawn individually, and the sutures (000 silk) tied.

Plate 270

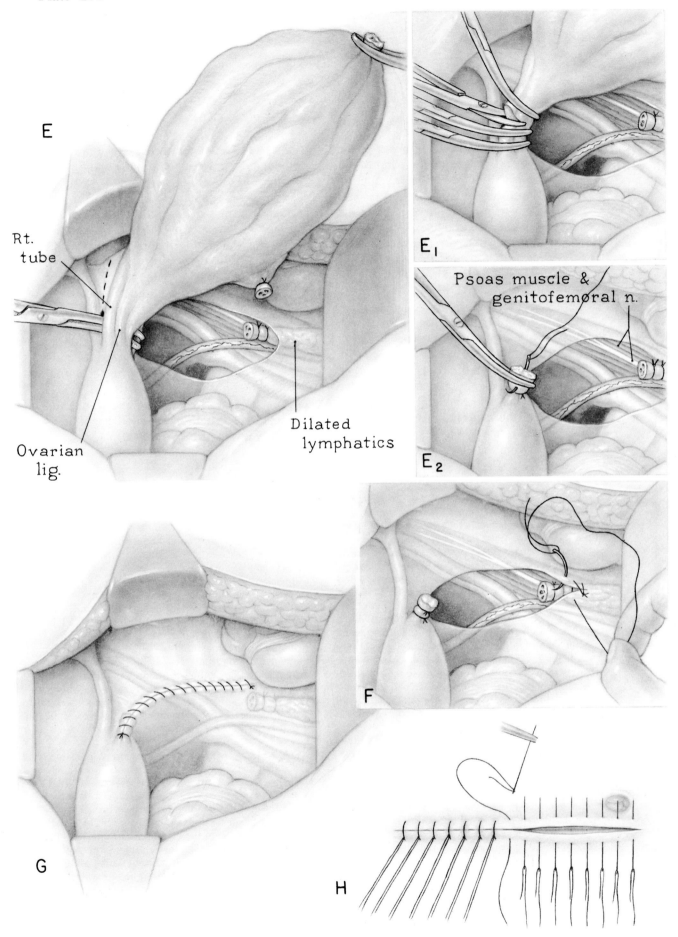

E

Rt.
tube

Ovarian
lig.

Dilated
lymphatics

E₁

Psoas muscle &
genitofemoral n.

E₂

F

G

H

TENDON GRAFT

A. The elliptical incision for removal of the previous operative scar on the palm of the hand is shown in dotted outline. Similarly, the incision in the wrist to obtain the palmaris longus tendon as a free graft and the lateral hinge flap incision to expose the digital portion of the flexor tendon are also shown in dotted outline. Prior to making the incisions depicted and following preparation of the operative field, the upper extremity is elevated for approximately three minutes before the inflation of the previously applied tourniquet. A tourniquet is routinely employed in operations upon tendons, with maintenance of the tourniquet pressure at a level of 250 mm. of mercury.

B. The elevation of the palmar flap is completed, and the digital flap is being raised by scalpel dissection. The scar tissue mass, incorporated in the distal palmar aspect of the flexor digitorum profundus tendon to the middle finger, and the surrounding anatomic structures are visible.

C. Traction is applied to a cotton tape, which encircles the bridge of tissue in the distal aspect of the palm overlying the flexor tendons of the middle finger, to expose the transection of the flexor profundus tendon in the palm proximal to the scar tissue mass. If scar tissue is present in the proximal cut end of the tendon, it is transected farther cephalad until normal tendon tissue is obtained. A sterile tongue depressor is placed beneath the tendon at its site of transection to prevent accidental injury to the subjacent structures.

D. The proximal segment of the transected tendon is secured on either side by the insertion of guy sutures of 0000 silk.

DISCUSSION—DR. J. WILLIAM LITTLER. The successful outcome of a tendon graft used to restore continuity of the disrupted flexor tendon mechanism of the thumb or fingers depends greatly upon the proper selection of cases, strict attention to surgical technic, and postoperative management. In general, when both flexor tendons of the finger have been divided in the region of the distal palm or proximal phalanx, a primary repair often fails because the tendon juncture becomes incorporated in the surrounding damaged fixed structures and the necessary tendon amplitude for finger flexion is lost. In order to overcome this, it is necessary to resort to a free tendon graft whereby the tendon junctures can be placed advantageously in the soft tissue of the proximal palm and at the terminal phalanx, thereby leaving an intact tendon running through the zone of injury.

Prior to the placing of the tendon graft, the interphalangeal joints of the finger should be mobile, good coverage should be present, and sensation should be intact on at least one side of the finger. Quite often the sensory nerves are divided together with the flexor tendons. In general, when both nerves have been divided, a primary nerve suture is indicated followed by a secondary free tendon graft at a time when sensation has returned to the finger. If, however, only one digital nerve is divided together with the flexor tendons, only the skin at the base of the finger need be sutured, and in the future, when the tissues have softened, a secondary tendon graft can be placed and the one digital nerve sutured.

It is essential, as pointed out by Dr. Madden, to carry out the secondary tendon grafting in a bloodless field provided through a brachial tourniquet inflated to approximately 250 mm. of mercury and maintained for a period of no longer than one-and-one-half hours. Prior to tourniquet inflation, the arm is drained by elevation or through the use of a rubber Martin bandage.

Incisions are of prime importance in the hand, and in general they should be made in the fingers midlateral to the interphalangeal joints and, in the palm, should parallel the flexion creases. However, as illustrated, the curved palmar incision can be carried proximally along the inner border of the hypothenar eminence without transgressing the flexion creases at a right angle. The palmaris longus tendon can be removed either through two small transverse incisions made at the wrist and in the midforearm or through a longitudinal incision, as illustrated. However, the longitudinal incision, especially in women, is disfiguring.

Exposure of the palmar structures is gained through a division of the vertical septa of the palmar fascia to the ulnar side of the flexor tendon in question. Care must be taken not to damage the neurovascular bundles which lie with the lumbricals between the flexor tendons. The fibrous tendon sheath which extends from the distal palmar crease to the distal interphalangeal crease should be totally resected except for pertinent pulleys which are to be left at the base of the proximal phalanx and in the midportion of the middle phalanx, to prevent bowstringing. A bridge of pulley approximately 0.5 cm. in width is desirable. Exposure of the fibrous tendon sheath in the finger can be made through the midlateral incision, as illustrated, carrying the neurovascular bundle with the volar flap, or by dissecting the

Plate 271

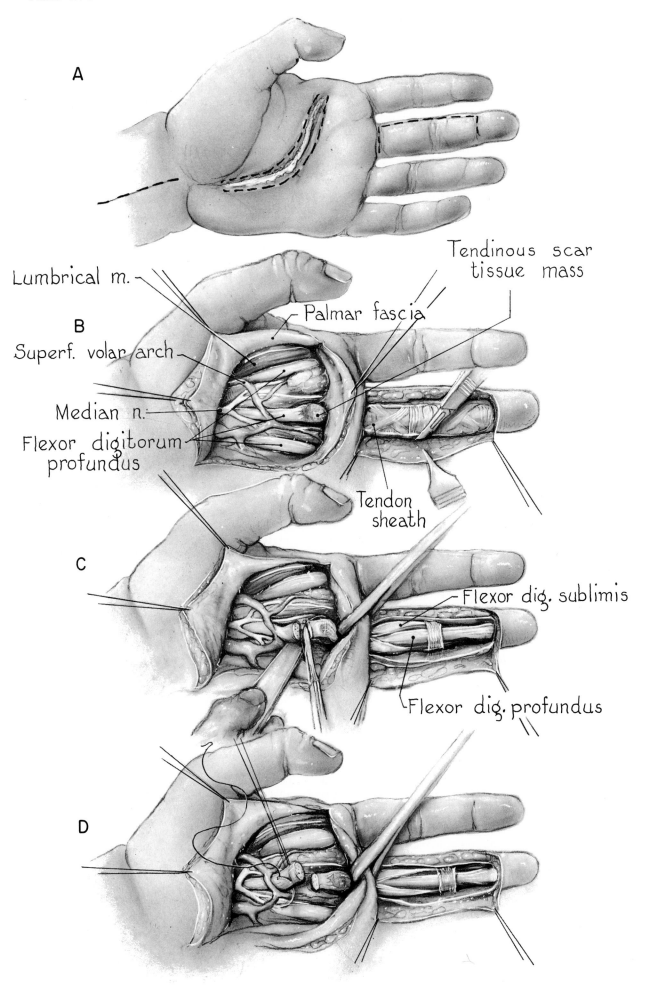

A

Lumbrical m.

B

Superf. volar arch

Median n.

Flexor digitorum profundus

Palmar fascia

Tendinous scar tissue mass

Tendon sheath

C

Flexor dig. sublimis

Flexor dig. profundus

D

E, F. By blunt dissection, a clamp is inserted beneath the proximal portion of the digital segment of the flexor digitorum profundus tendon (E), and, by upward traction through the clamp, the tendinous scar tissue mass and the distal transected end of the palmar portion of the flexor digitorum profundus tendon are delivered from beneath the overlying bridge of tissue (F). Clamp traction is maintained on the transected end of the tendon just proximal to the scar tissue mass as it is severed distally over an underlying sterile tongue depressor (F).

G. A moist gauze pad is placed in the open wound in the palm of the hand, and the incision on the volar aspect of the wrist and overlying the palmaris longus tendon is being made with a scalpel.

H, I. The wound margins are retracted to show a segment of the palmaris longus tendon elevated on a clamp preparatory to its mobilization (H). The distal transected end of the palmaris longus tendon, secured by guy sutures of silk (0000), is retracted upward as the tendon, encased in its shiny and filmy mesotenon, is mobilized proximally by scalpel dissection (I).

DISCUSSION—DR. LITTLER (cont.)

digital flap off the bundle. The lateral skin ligaments which arise in the region of the interphalangeal joint and attach to the skin are known as Cleland's ligament and must be divided to permit easy entry into the finger. The tendon remnants are removed leaving a short stump of the profundus distally and a 1 cm. stump of the sublimis in the region of the proximal interphalangeal joint, to prevent a recurvatum deformity.

The palmaris longus tendon is favored as a graft; a toe extensor or a small sublimis tendon, liberated in the palm and withdrawn at the wrist, may also be used. The graft should be sutured proximally to the profundus tendon at the level of the lumbrical muscle, specifically at its distal border. This will place the proximal profundus graft juncture deep in the palm in soft tissue. The graft is then threaded through the proximal and middle phalangeal pulleys and secured to the stump of the profundus tendon at the terminal phalanx by an end-to-end suture, as illustrated, or secured with a Bunnell pull-out wire into a cortical recess gouged from the ventral cortex of the terminal phalanx between the split profundus tendon stump. The pull-out wire is passed through the finger nail where it is secured with a button. The proper tension to be placed on the graft is readily determined by placing the finger in question in the functional position with the wrist neutral and adjusting the tension on the graft so that it has just a little more tone than an adjacent normal finger. The tendon junctures can be made as indicated with 0000 silk or with stainless steel wire. It is the consensus that 00000 braided wire used at the proximal juncture is less reactive than silk. If a pull-out wire is to be used, No. 34 or 35 monofilament stainless steel wire is preferred.

In children end-to-end junctures are made both proximally and distally, and no pull-out wire is used. The skin in the very young can be closed with 000000 catgut, making it unnecessary to remove sutures at the end of a three-and-one-half to four-week period of immobilization. At the end of this period, active exercises on the part of the child can be permitted. Little postoperative care is necessary in the very young. In adults, the skin is closed with either silk, nylon, or wire sutures. The hand should be immobilized with the wrist and fingers semiflexed using a dorsal plaster mold. In young children the plaster should be carried above the flexed elbow to insure its remaining in place. In the older individual the sutures should be removed on or about the 12th day; however, there is no urgency to remove either wire or nylon sutures in the hand and they can remain in place during the entire three-and-one-half to four-week period of immobilization, at which time active and passive exercises are started.

It is important for the patient with a free tendon graft to learn the value of immobilizing the proximal phalanx with the opposite hand and directing his effort toward interphalangeal flexion. If the metacarpophalangeal joint is not supported in extension, the adherent tendon graft will flex only this joint and power will not be transmitted distally. A good result following a tendon graft is generally manifest by the end of the third month. The results depend to a large degree upon the original condition of the finger, the surgical technic, and the effort expended on the part of the patient.

Plate 272

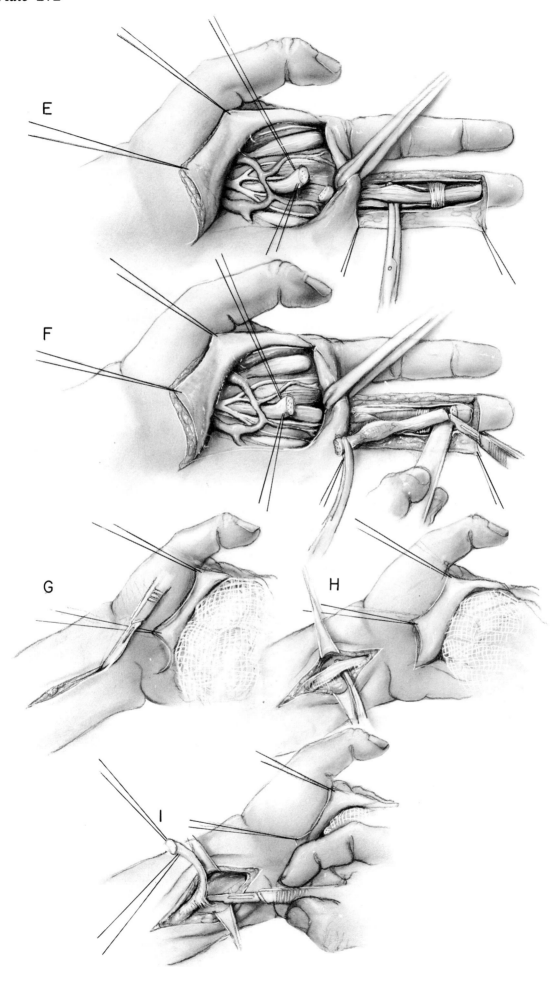

E

F

G

H

I

J, J¹. The transfixion mattress sutures (Bunnell) are inserted in the proximal ends of both the flexor digitorum profundus tendon and the tendon graft. Two of the strands of the opposing sutures are being tied (J) to approximate the ends of the tendons. The inset (J¹) shows more clearly the completion of the insertion of the Bunnell type of suture employed.

K, L. The transfixion mattress sutures are tied to approximate the proximal end of the tendon graft to the proximal end of the host tendon. The line of approximation is reinforced by interrupted sutures which are first inserted (K) and then tied (L).

M. By use of the long strands of the mattress sutures (a, b), axial rotation of the tendon ends is obtained to allow the insertion of a series of interrupted sutures of silk (0000) posteriorly.

N. The completion of the anastomosis of the tendon graft to the host tendon proximally is shown.

O. In like manner, an anastomosis of the tendon graft with the host tendon distally is performed to complete the insertion of the graft. The incised margins of the tendon sheath are being approximated with sutures of silk (0000).

P. The closure of the three skin incisions with interrupted sutures of silk (0000) is shown. Following the application of a fluff gauze dressing and a firm but not too tight compressive bandage, a plaster splint is applied to the extensor aspects of the forearm, wrist, and hand respectively, with the fingers in a flexed position and the forearm midway between pronation and supination. Immobilization in this manner is maintained for a period of four weeks.

Plate 273

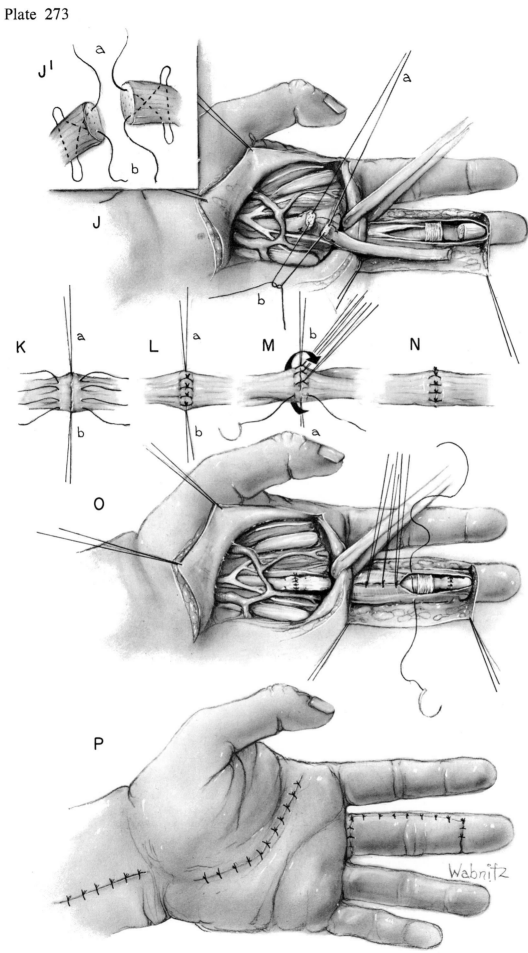

STENOSING TENOSYNOVITIS AT THE RADIOSTYLOID PROCESS (DE QUERVAIN'S DISEASE)

A. The longitudinal incision (4-5 cm.) along the dorsal aspect of the radial border of the right wrist is indicated by the broken line. If preferred, a transverse skin incision may prove equally satisfactory.

B. The incision is deepened through the subcutaneous fatty tissue layer, and the wound margins are retracted to expose the superficial fascia, the superficial (dorsal cutaneous) branch of the radial nerve, and its accompanying vein. Injury to the nerve should be avoided. The site of incision in the fascia is shown (broken line).

C. The superficial fascia layer is incised, and the underlying tendon sheath in relation to the muscle fibers proximally and the dorsal carpal ligament (extensor retinaculum) distally is visible.

D. The tendon sheath, which was thickened, hyperemic, and edematous, is opened, and the contained abductor pollicis longus and extensor pollicis brevis are exposed. Because of the markedly thickened tendon sheath distally, it was thought that simple incision alone might not release completely the constriction effect on the tendons. Accordingly, an excision (broken line) of a segment of the indurated portion of the sheath was deemed advisable.

E. The appearance of the operative field after the excision of a portion of the thickened tendon sheath is shown.

F, G. The closure of the fascia layer (F) and skin (G) with interrupted sutures of 000 silk completes the operation.

DISCUSSION—DR. KAZUO YANAGISAWA. This condition, first described by de Quervain in 1895, is characterized by pain on active flexion and abduction movements of the thumb. The pain is usually at the radial aspect of the thenar eminence and the distal portion of the radial aspect of the forearm. In addition to pain, there is difficulty in holding objects in the hand.

On examination the following symptoms are noted: (1) tenderness to pressure distally over the tendon sheath of the extensor pollicis brevis and abductor pollicis longus, which is frequently thickened and bulbous, (2) pain on attempting to extend and abduct the thumb against resistance, and (3) forced abduction of the thumb across the palm with concomitant forced flexion, causing pain at the annulus (Finkelstein's sign).

The manifest symptoms are due to a tenosynovitis (tendovaginitis), which exerts a constrictive and binding effect upon the encased tendons (abductor pollicis longus and extensor pollicis brevis).

The treatment of tendovaginitis may be either conservative or surgical. In the conservative treatment, immobilization of the involved hand and wrist in a plaster cast for three to four weeks is prescribed and may result in the complete relief of symptoms. An alternate method would be the local infiltration of procaine (1 per cent) into the tendon sheath beneath the annulus. If desired, hydrocortone (1 cc.) may be combined with the procaine.

In those patients in whom symptoms persist after an adequate trial of conservative measures, operation is advised. Both the annulus and the underlying tendon sheath are incised. This effects the immediate release of pressure, but a recurrence of symptoms is likely if the tendon sheath reattaches its cut edges. To obtain the best result, therefore, excision of the thickened portion of the sheath is recommended.

On opening the tendon sheath, fluid, gelatinous mucoid material or simply scar tissue may be encountered. Occasionally, one may see a bulbous swelling of the annulus, which causes a palpable click on flexion of the thumb. This is relieved by excision of the annulus. Also, an aberrant tendon slip of the abductor pollicis longus attached to the distal end of the radius may be present. This should be looked for and, if present, excised, as it serves no useful purpose and may cause persistence of pain.

In A the longitudinal incision (broken line) 3-4 cm. in length along the lateral aspect of the radial border of the right wrist is shown. A transverse incision may prove equally satisfactory; if used, care should be taken to avoid the radial vessels and the dorsal cutaneous branch of the radial nerve. Palpation of the tendons of the abductor pollicis longus and the extensor pollicis brevis at the lateral border of the distal end of the radius is the anatomic landmark for the incision.

The technic illustrated should prove entirely satisfactory. Excision of the thickened tendon sheath as indicated in E is particularly advised. Postoperatively, active mobilization of the thumb is begun on the first postoperative day, and grasping exercises are practiced by the fifth postoperative day. The skin sutures are removed ten days after operation, and normal activities are permitted thereafter.

Plate 274   609

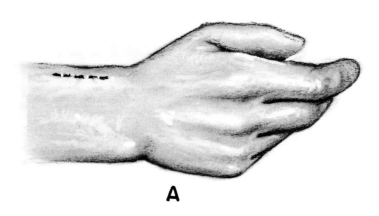

A

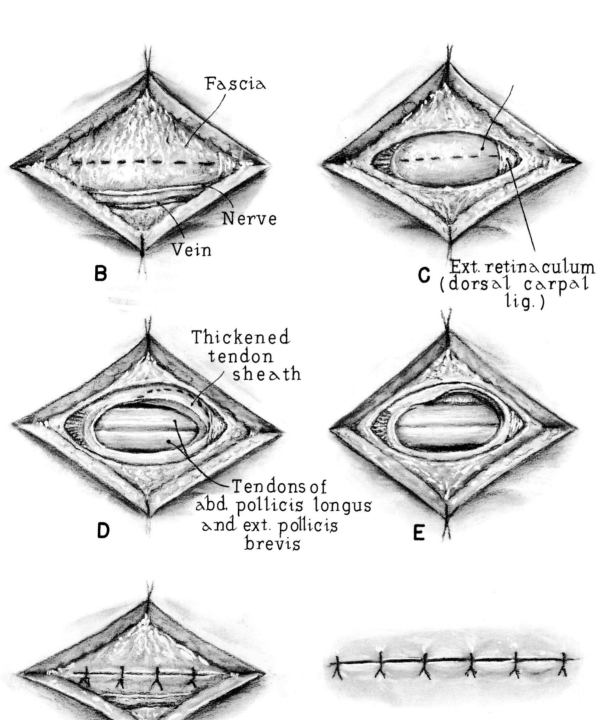

Fascia

Nerve

Vein

B

Ext. retinaculum
(dorsal carpal
lig.)

C

Thickened
tendon
sheath

Tendons of
abd. pollicis longus
and ext. pollicis
brevis

D

E

F

G

SUPRACONDYLAR AMPUTATION—FEMUR, RIGHT

A. The incision to form the anterior flap is made and crosshatched to facilitate later closure. The vertical portions of the incision begin and terminate approximately 5 cm. cephalad to either femoral condyle. The convex border of the lowermost portion courses just distal to the superior border of the patella.

B. The incision is deepened through the subcutaneous tissue layer, and the underlying fascia is incised at the level of retraction of the upper flap.

C. The mobilization of the anterior flap of skin, fat, and fascia is completed, and the formation of the posterior flap is begun by incising transversely the skin and subcutaneous tissue overlying the medial aspect and distal portion of the thigh. This incision is continued posteriorly and is joined by a similar incision from the lateral aspect of the thigh.

D, E. The adductor canal is entered by digital dissection (D), and the mobilized neurovascular bundle is elevated on the fingers (E) preparatory to the application of clamps.

Plate 275   611

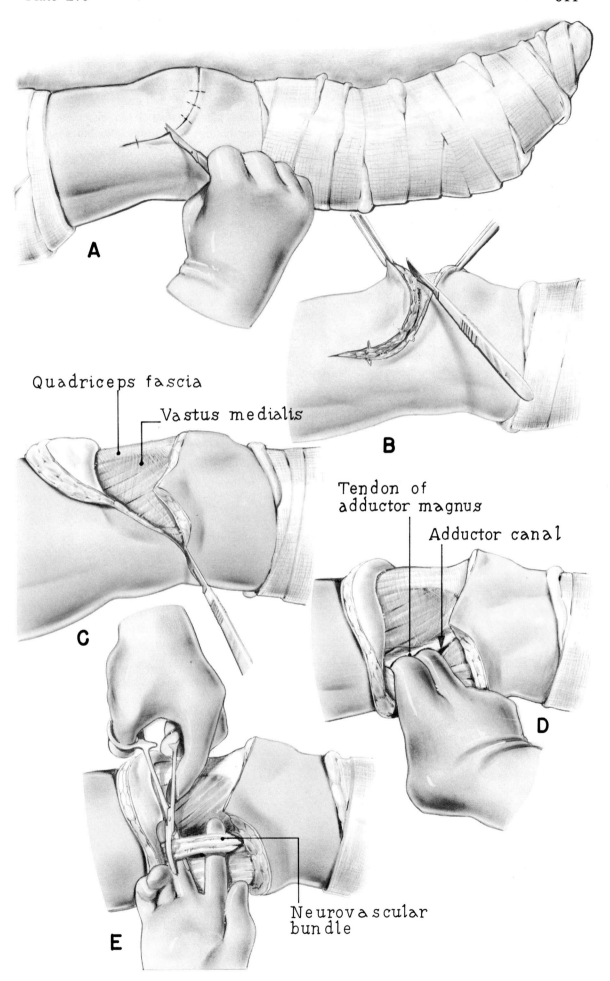

Quadriceps fascia

Vastus medialis

Tendon of
adductor magnus

Adductor canal

Neurovascular
bundle

A

B

C

D

E

F. The neurovascular bundle is triply clamped and severed between the two distal clamps.

F₁, F₂. The two clamps proximally are replaced by a ligature (F_1) and suture ligature (F_2), respectively, of 00 silk.

G, H. The vastus medialis muscle is transected (G, broken line), and then the tendon of the quadriceps femoris muscle is incised (H). The suprapatellar bursa underlies and is intimately adherent to the tendon. Accordingly, it is routinely entered (H) when the tendon is transected.

I, J. The cephalad portion of the incised bursa is grasped in a clamp, and as traction is maintained, it is mobilized first by scissor (I) and then by scalpel (J) dissection from its tendinous and muscle attachments.

J'. On completion of the mobilization of the suprapatellar bursa, the vastus lateralis is transected (broken line) at the same level of transection as the vastus medialis.

Plate 276

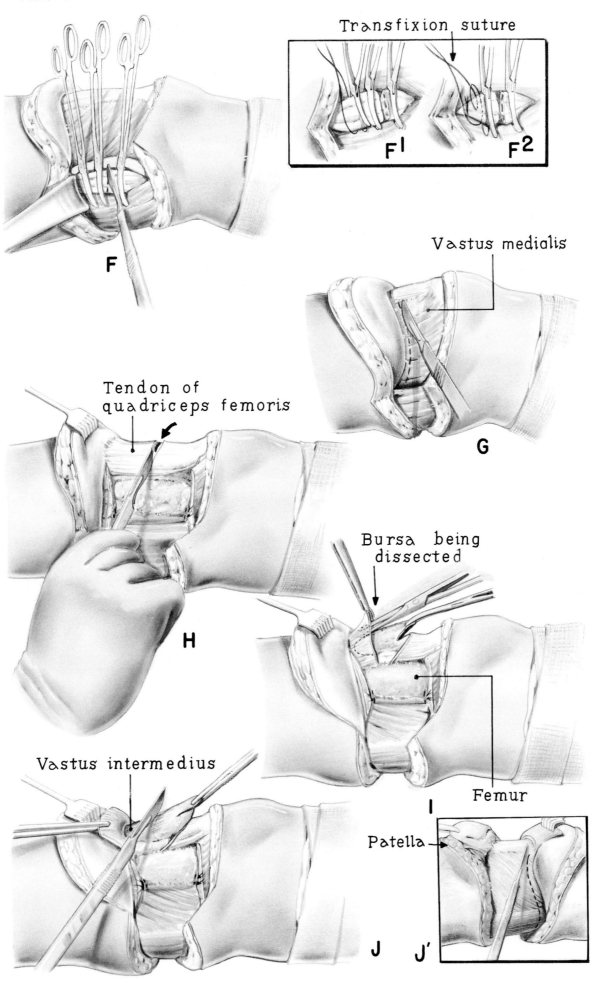

Transfixion suture

F1

F2

F

Vastus medialis

G

Tendon of
quadriceps femoris

H

Bursa being
dissected

Femur

I

Vastus intermedius

Patella

J

J'

K. This is again the medial aspect of the thigh. The previously mobilized sciatic nerve is being clamped distally.

L. The sciatic nerve is doubly clamped, and rhexis of the neural bundles is accomplished by repeated forceful rotation of the clamps in opposite directions. This is done in the belief that it may possibly lessen the incidence of phantom limb pain. After the nerve is transected (broken line), caudal traction is maintained on the proximal clamp, and the ligature that encircles the nerve is tied. The nerve is then severed just distal to the ligature and allowed to retract cephalad deep to the plane of muscle transection. The sciatic nerve is always ligated for hemostasis because of the relatively large blood vessel that accompanies it.

M. The transected surfaces of the thigh cephalad and caudad are covered with moist gauze pads, and the periosteum at the site of transection of the femur is visible. This site corresponds to the level of retraction of the severed muscle bundles.

N, O. The periosteum distally is separated from the femur (M), which is then transected with a hand saw flush with the proximal cut rim of periosteum (O). This transection is facilitated by keeping the area continually moistened with sterile saline.

Plate 277

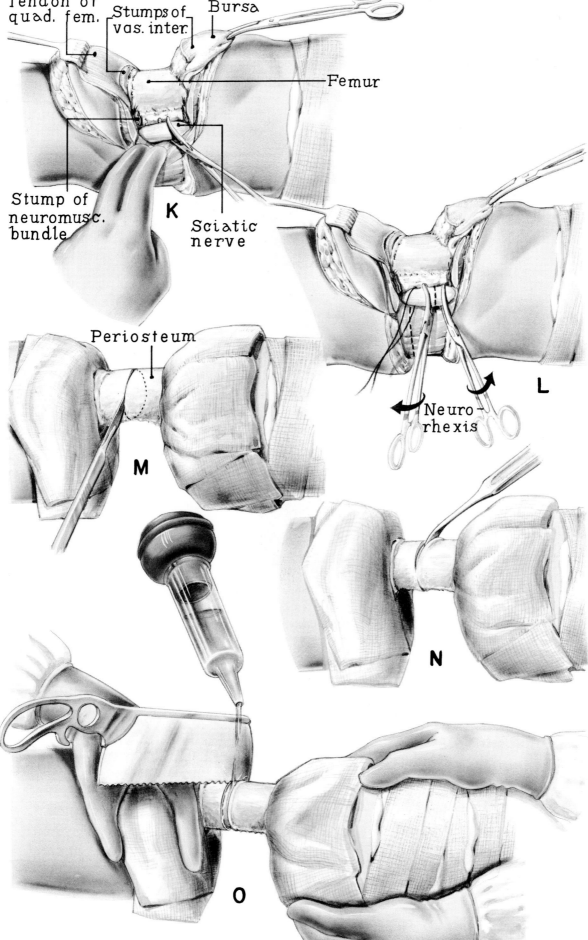

Tendon of quad. fem.

Stumps of vas. inter.

Bursa

Femur

Stump of neuromusc. bundle

Sciatic nerve

K

Periosteum

M

Neuro-rhexis

L

N

O

P, Q. The amputation completed, the medullary cavity is shown being curetted (P), subsequent to which the rough spicules of bone are removed by a rasp (Q). Curettage of the medullary cavity is not practiced as a routine. It was done in this patient because of persistent bleeding.

R. The medullary cavity is being wiped with dry sterile gauze held in a clamp preparatory to closure of the stump. The relation of the surrounding structures to the cut end of the femur is depicted.

S, T. The palms of the second assistant are placed on the anterior and posterior surfaces of the thigh stump (H) and compressed toward each other as concomitant downward traction is effected (S). The subcutaneous fascia layer (S) and the skin (T) are approximated with interrupted sutures of 000 silk. A rubber tissue drain has its exit just lateral to the center of the line of closure of the skin.

U, V. The closure of the stump is completed (U), and a large "fluff" compression dressing is secured by the application of a roller gauze bandage (V).

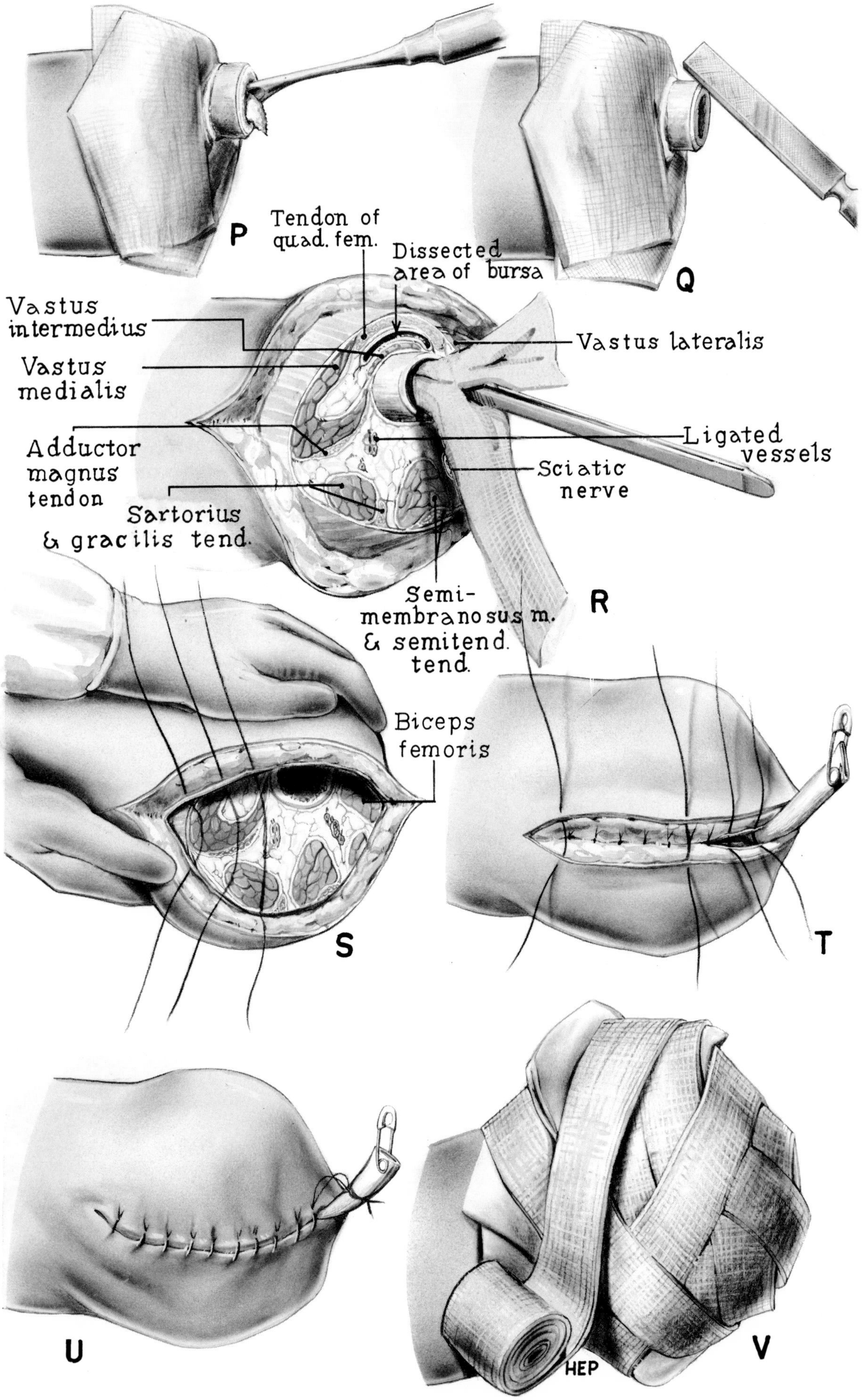

Plate 278

P

Q

Tendon of
quad. fem.

Dissected
area of bursa

Vastus
intermedius

Vastus lateralis

Vastus
medialis

Ligated
vessels

Adductor
magnus
tendon

Sciatic
nerve

Sartorius
& gracilis tend.

R

Semi-
membranosus m.
& semitend.
tend.

Biceps
femoris

S

T

U

HEP

V

TRANSTHORACIC, SUPRADIAPHRAGMATIC RESECTION OF THE VAGUS NERVES

A. The patient is placed in the direct right lateral prone position, and a relatively short incision in the eighth interspace, extending from the anterior to the posterior axillary lines, is outlined.

B, C. The incision is deepened through the underlying muscle layers and the left pleural cavity is entered (D).

D. The adjacent rib margins are retracted and the entrance into the posterior mediastinal space through an incision in the reflection of the pleura forming the inferior pulmonary ligament is shown.

d'. An inset to demonstrate an alternate method of incising the inferior pulmonary ligament between suture ligatures of silk (000).

E. The cut margins of the posterior mediastinal pleura are reflected by guy sutures of silk (0000), and by blunt scissor dissection, an opening is made in the avascular fatty areolar tissue overlying the esophagus.

F. The esophagus is displaced posteriorly, and the left or anterior vagus nerve is mobilized on a nerve hook. This nerve, smaller than the right, is always in close approximation to the anterior surface of the esophagus.

Plate 279

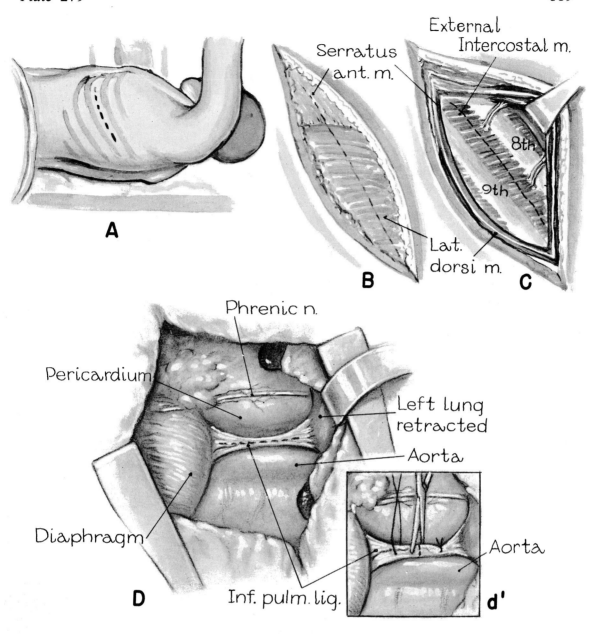

A

Serratus
ant. m.

External
Intercostal m.

8th

9th

Lat.
dorsi m.

B

C

Phrenic n.

Pericardium

Left lung
retracted

Aorta

Diaphragm

Aorta

D

Inf. pulm. lig.

d'

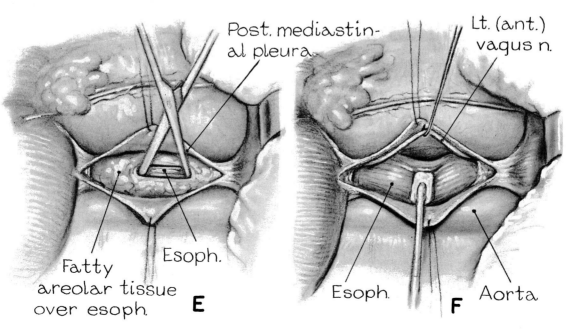

Post. mediastin-
al pleura

Lt. (ant.)
vagus n.

Fatty
areolar tissue
over esoph.

Esoph.

E

Esoph.

F

Aorta

G, H. A segment of the left (anterior) vagus nerve is removed between demarcating silver clips. A communicating branch of the vagus nerve is visible.

I, J, K. The esophagus is displaced anteriorly to visualize the right (posterior) vagus nerve which lies in the fatty areolar tissue plane posterior and medial to the esophagus. Similarly, as previously demonstrated, a segment of this nerve is resected.

L. The communicating branch is mobilized on a nerve hook preliminary to its severance. Subsequently careful digital exploration of the complete circumference of the esophagus is performed to detect and sever all of the additional nerve fibers which may be present. The importance of this maneuver cannot be overemphasized since the success of the operation is dependent upon the completeness of the vagal denervation of the stomach.

M, N, O. The layer closure of the incision is illustrated. Just prior to the completion of the closure the water-seal drainage catheter is removed. Two periosteal flaps are raised at the lower border of the ninth rib to permit the insertion of the pericostal sutures (No. 2 silk) without impingement upon the subjacent intercostal nerve. It is believed that the use of this technic may lessen the incidence of post-thoracotomy pain. If preferred, heavy sutures of chromic catgut may be used for the pericostal sutures.

Plate 280

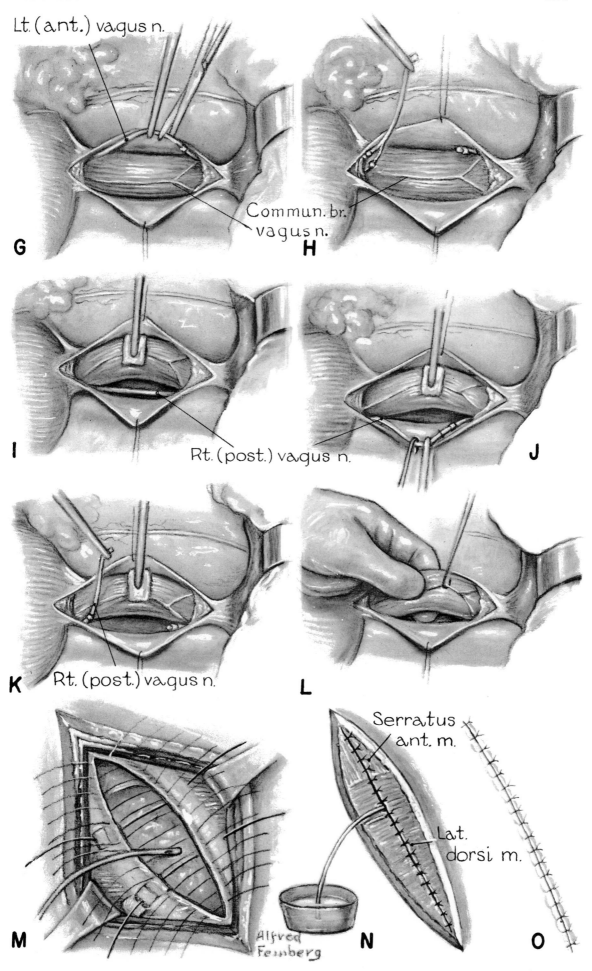

Lt. (ant.) vagus n.

Commun. br. vagus n.

G

H

Rt. (post.) vagus n.

I

J

Rt. (post.) vagus n.

K

L

Serratus ant. m.

Lat. dorsi m.

M

Alfred Feinberg

N

O

REFERENCES

Pre- and Postoperative Care

Abbott, W. E. Nutrition, body fluids, shock, and burns, Surg., Gynec. & Obst., 116:141, 1963.

Alican, F., Dalton, M. L., Jr., and Hardy, J. D. Experimental endotoxin shock: circulatory changes with emphasis upon cardiac function, Am. J. Surg., 103:702, 1962.

Altemeier, W. A., and Cole, W. R. Nature and treatment of septic shock, Arch. Surg., 77:498, 1958.

Arturson, G. Pathophysiological aspects of the burn syndrome with special reference to liver injury and alterations of capillary permeability, Acta. chir. scandinav. (supp.) 274:1, 1961.

Barnett, W. O., and Hardy, J. D. Shock in peritonitis—Mechanism and management, S. Clin. North America, 42:1101, 1962.

Becker, J. M., and Artz, C. P. The treatment of burns in children, A.M.A. Arch. Surg. 73:207, 1956.

Boba, A. Acute hemorrhage, Ann. Surg., 152:51, 1960.

Brown, J. B., and Fryer, M. P. Postmortem homografts to reduce mortality in extensive burns, J.A.M.A., 156:1163, 1954.

Churchill, E. D. Etiology and mechanisms of shock; wound shock, Symposium on Shock, Washington, D.C., Army Med. Ser. Grad. Schl., 1951, p. 1–1.

Clowes, G. H. A., Jr., Sabga, C. A., Konitaxis, A., Tomin, R., Hughes, M., and Simeone, F. A. Effects of acidosis on cardiovascular function in surgical patients, Ann. Surg., 154:524, 1961.

Cole, W. H., and Laws, J. F. Symposium on recent advances in surgery; Electrolytes in surgery, S. Clin. North America, 32:3, 1952.

Cope, O., and Moore, F. D. The redistribution of body water and the fluid therapy of the burned patient, Ann. Surg., 126:1010, 1947.

Davies, D. D. Noradrenaline in shock due to visceral perforation, Brit. M. J., 1:261, 1957.

Elman, R., Lemmer, R. A., Weichselbaum, T. E., Owen, J. G., and Yore, R. W. Minimum postoperative maintenance requirements for parenteral water, sodium, potassium, chloride and glucose, Ann. Surg., 130:703, 1949.

Evans, E. I. Potassium deficiency in surgical patients; its recognition and management, Ann. Surg., 131:945, 1950.

Gollub, S., Ulin, A. W., Winchell, H. S., Ehrlich, E., and Weiss, W. Hemorrhagic diathesis associated with massive transfusion, Surgery, 45:204, 1959.

Grant, R. T. Mechanisms of shock, Symposium on Shock, Washington, D.C., Army Med. Ser. Grad. Schl., 1951.

Hardaway, R. M., and Drake, D. C. Prevention of "irreversible" hemorrhagic shock with fibrinolysin, Ann. Surg., 157:39, 1963.

Holman, S. P., Shaya, E. S., Hoffmeister, F. S., and Edgerton, M. T., Jr. Studies on burns: the exposure method vs. occlusive dressings in local treatment of experimental burns, Ann. Surg., 143:49, 1956.

Jorgensen, H. E., and Schlegel, J. U. Studies in metabolism of Trauma. III. Postoperative sodium retention, Surg., Gynec. & Obst., 108:339, 1959.

Lauson, H. D., Bradley, S. E., and Cournand, A. Renal circulation in shock, J. Clin. Invest., 23:381, 1944.

Lehr, H. B., Rhoads, J. E., Rosenthal, O., and Blakemore, W. S. The use of intravenous fat emulsions in surgical patients, J.A.M.A., 181:745, 1962.

MacLean, L. D. Pathogenesis and treatment of bacteremic shock, Surg., Gynec. & Obst., 115:307, 1962.

McNair, R. D., Quigley, W., and O'Donnell, D. Protein nutrition in surgical patients. II. A comparison of the nitrogen-sparing action of glucose, invert sugar and fructose, Ann. Surg., 143:448, 1956.

Mollison, P. L. The investigation of hemolytic transfusion reactions, Brit. M. J., 1:529, 1943.

Moore, F. D., Peacock, W., Blakely, E., and Cope, O. The anemia of thermal burns, Ann. Surg., 124:811, 1946.

——— Langohr, J. L., Ingebretsen, M., and Cope, O. The role of exudate losses in the protein and electrolyte imbalance of burned patients, Ann. Surg., 132:1, 1950.

——— Metabolic care of the surgical patient. Philadelphia, W. B. Saunders, 1959.

Rabelo, A., Litwin, M. S., Brady, M. P., and Moore, F. D. A comparison of the effects of the several osmotic diuretic agents after acute hemorrhage in the dog, Surg., Gynec. & Obst., 115:657, 1962.

Shires, T., and Jackson, D. E. Postoperative salt tolerance, Arch. Surg., 84:703, 1962.

Shoemaker, W. C., and Fitch, L. B. Hepatic lesion of hemorrhagic shock, Arch. Surg., 85:492, 1962.

Stead, E. A. Physiology and methods of measurement of shock; circulation dynamics in shock. Symposium on Shock, Washington, D.C., Army Med. Ser. Grad. Schl., 1951, p. VII–1.

Zimmermann, B., and Wangensteen, O. H. Observations on water intoxication in surgical patients, Surgery, 31:654, 1952.

ABDOMINAL INCISIONS

Battle, W. H. Modified incision for removal of the vermiform appendix, Brit. M. J., 2:1360, 1895.

Carrel, A. Process of wound healing, Proc. Inst. Med. Chicago, 8:62, 1930.

Cherney, L. S. Modified transverse incision for low abdominal operations, Surg., Gynec. & Obst., 72:92, 1941.

Farr, R. E. Abdominal incisions, Lancet, 32:561, 1912.

Gurd, F. B. Abdominal Incisions in Operative Surgery, edited by Bancroft, F. W., New York, D. Appleton-Century Co., 1941, pp. 417–463.

Haight, C., and Ransom, H. K. Observations on the prevention of atelectasis and bronchopneumonia, Ann. Surg., 114:243, 1941.

Holman, E. An incisional approach for cholecystectomy and choledochotomy designed to reduce injuries to the common duct, Surg., Gynec. & Obst., 97:344, 1953.

Kammerer, F. Modified incision for quiescent appendicitis, Ann. Surg., 26:225, 1897.

Kehr, H. Ueber den Bauchdeckenschnitt, die Bauchnaht und die Tamponade bei Gallenstein-operationen, Arch. f. klin. Chir., 97:74, 1912.

Marwedel, G. Die Aufklappung des Ripperbogens für Erleichterung Operativer Eingriffe in Hypochondrium und im Zwerchfellkuppetraum, Zentralbl. f. Chir., 35:938, 1903.

Masson, J. C. Exposure in gallbladder surgery, Ann. Surg., 69:422, 1919.

Maylard, A. E. Direction of abdominal incisions, Brit. M. J., 2:895, 1907.

McBurney, C. The incision made in the abdominal wall in cases of appendicitis with a description of a new method of operating, Ann. Surg., 20:38, 1894.

Pfannensteil, J. Ueber die Vortheile des Supra-symphysären Fascienquershnitts für die gynäkologischen Koliotomien, zugleich ein Beitrag zu der Indikations-stellung der Operationswege, Samml. klin. Votr., No. 268 (gynäk. No. 97): 1735, 1900.

Reid, M. R., Zinninger, M. M., and Merrell, P. Closure of the abdomen with through-and-through silver wire sutures in cases of acute abdominal emergencies, Ann., Surg., 98:890, 1933.

Rockey, A. E. Transverse incision in abdominal operations, M. Rec., 68:779, 1905.

Sokolov, S. Postoperative rupture of abdominal wounds with protrusion or prolapse of the viscera, Vestnik. Chir., No. 65, 66:219, 1931. Abst.: Internat. Abstr. Surg., 55:157, 1932.

Southam, A. H. A comparative study of abdominal incisions, Brit. M. J., 1:513, 1924.

Stevenson, J. M., and Reid, M. R. The Fundamental Principles of Surgical Technic in Operative Surgery, edited by Bancroft, F. W., New York, D. Appleton-Century Co., 1941, pp. 241–304.

Thompson, W. D., Ravdin, I. S., and Frank, I. L. Effect of hypoproteinemia on wound disruption, Arch. Surg., 36:500, 1938.

Wangensteen, O. H. Cancer of the Esophagus and the Stomach, New York, 1951, American Cancer Society.

Weir, R. F. An improved operation for acute appendicitis or for quiescent cases with complications, M. News, 76:241, 1900.

Whipple, A. O., and Elliot, R., Jr. The repair of abdominal incisions, Ann. Surg., 108:741, 1938.

HERNIORRHAPHY

Andrews, Edmund. A method of herniotomy utilizing only white fascia, Ann. Surg., 80:225, 1924.

———— Imbrication method for inguinal hernia, S. Clin. North America, 14:919, 1934.

Andrews, Edward W. Imbrication or lap joint method. A plastic operation for hernia, Chicago M. Rec., 9:67, 1895.

———— Technique of the Andrews operation for hernia, Surg., Gynec. & Obst., 11:89, 1906.

Anson, B. J., and McVay, C. B. Inguinal hernia: anatomy of region, Surg., Gynec. & Obst., 66:186, 1938.

———— Morgan, E. H., and McVay, C. B. The anatomy of the hernia regions: I. inguinal hernia, Surg., Gynec. & Obst., 89:417, 1949.

Bartlett, W., Jr. Observations on concept of inguinal hernia repair, Surg., Gynec. & Obst., 83:55, 1946.

Bassini, E. Ueber die Behandlung des Leistenbruches, Arch. f. klin. Chir., 40:429, 1890.

———— Neue Operationsmethode zur Radicalbehandlung der Schenkelhernie, Arch. f. klin. Chir., 47:1, 1894.

Bloodgood, J. C. The transplantation of the rectus muscle or sheath for the cure of inguinal hernia when the conjoined tendon is obliterated, Ann. Surg., 70:81, 1919.

Burton, C. C. Rationale and factors for consideration in Cooper's ligament hernioplasty, Internat. Abstr. Surg., 85:1, 1947.

Carlson, R. I. The historical development of the surgical treatment of inguinal hernia, Surgery, 39:1031, 1956.

Casten, D., and Bodenheimer, M. Strangulated hernia reduced en masse, Surgery, 9:561, 1941.

Cheatle, G. L. An operation for the radical cure of inguinal and femoral hernia, Brit. M. J., 2:68, 1920.

———— An operation for inguinal hernia, Brit. M. J., 2:1025, 1921.

Clark, J. H., and Hashimoto, E. I. Utilization of Henle's ligament, iliopubic tract, aponeurosis transversus abdominis and Cooper's ligament in inguinal herniorrhaphy: a report of 162 consecutive cases, Surg., Gynec. & Obst., 82:480, 1946.

Connell, F. G. Radical operation for the cure of oblique inguinal hernia, Surg., Gynec. & Obst., 7:481, 1908.

———— The repair of the internal ring in oblique inguinal hernia, J.A.M.A., 52:1087, 1909.

Herniorrhaphy (cont.)

—— Repair of internal ring in oblique hernia, Surg., Gynec. & Obst., 46:113, 1928.

Downes, W. A. Management of direct inguinal hernia, Arch. Surg., 11:455, 1924.

Edwards, H. Inguinal hernia, Brit. J. Surg., 31: 172, 1943.

Fallis, L. S. Inguinal hernia: a report of 1600 operations, Ann. Surg., 104:403, 1936.

—— Recurrent inguinal hernia; analysis of 200 operations, Ann. Surg., 106:363, 1937.

—— Direct inguinal hernia, Ann. Surg., 107: 572, 1938.

Farris, J. M., Ettinger, J., and Weinberg, S. A. The hernia problem with reference to a modification of the McVay technique, Surgery, 24:293, 1948.

Ferguson, A. H. Oblique inguinal hernia, J.A.M.A., 33:6, 1899.

Gallie, W. E., and Le Mesurier, A. B. The use of living sutures in operative surgery, Canad. M. A. J., 11:504, 1921.

Halsted, W. S. The radical cure of hernia, Bull. Johns Hopkins Hosp., 1:12, 1889.

—— The cure of the more difficult as well as the simpler inguinal ruptures, Bull. Johns Hopkins Hosp., 14:208, 1903.

Harkins, H. N., and Schug, R. H. Hernial repair using Cooper's ligament; follow-up studies on three hundred and sixty-seven operations, Arch. Surg., 55:689, 1947.

—— The repair of groin hernias: progress in the past decade, S. Clin. North America, 29: 1457, 1949.

Henry, A. K. Operation for femoral hernia by a midline extraperitoneal approach, with preliminary note on use of this route for reducible inguinal hernia, Lancet, 1:531, 1936.

Hesselbach, F. C. De Ortu Herniarum, Wurzburg, 1816.

Hoguet, J. P. Direct inguinal hernia, Ann. Surg., 72:671, 1920.

Keith, A. On the origin and nature of hernia, Brit. J. Surg., 11:455, 1924.

Koontz, A. R. Hernia, New York, Appleton-Century-Crofts, 1963.

La Roque, E. P. The permanent cure of inguinal and femoral hernia, Surg., Gynec. & Obst., 29:507, 1919.

Lytle, W. J. The internal inguinal ring, Brit. J. Surg., 32:441, 1945.

—— Inguinal hernia, Ann. Roy. Coll. Surgeons, England, 9:245, 1951.

MacGregor, W. W. Demonstration of true internal inguinal sphincter and its etiologic role in hernia, Surg., Gynec. & Obst., 49:510, 1929.

Marcy, H. O. Radical cure of hernia by antiseptic use of carbolized catgut ligature, Tr. A.M.A. Philadelphia, 29:295-305, 1878.

—— The cure of hernia by antiseptic use of animal ligature. Transactions of the Seventh Session of the International Medical Congress, London, August 2nd to 9th, 1881, Vol. II, pp. 446–448.

—— The cure of hernia, J.A.M.A., 8:589-592, 1887.

—— The Anatomy and Surgical Treatment of Hernia. New York, D. Appleton, 1892.

McGregor, A. L. Third inguinal ring, Surg., Gynec. & Obst., 49:273, 1929.

McVay, C. B., and Anson, B. J. A fundamental error in current methods of inguinal herniorrhaphy, Surg., Gynec. & Obst., 74:746, 1942.

Mikklesen, W. P., and Berne, C. F. Femoral hernioplasty: suprapubic extraperitoneal (Cheatle-Henry) approach, Surgery, 35:743, 1954.

Nyhus, L. M., Condon, R. E., and Harkins, H. N. Clinical experiences with preperitoneal hernial repair for all types of hernia of the groin; with particular reference to the importance of transversalis fascia analogues, Am. J. Surg., 100: 234, 1960.

Ogilvie, W. H. Hernia, Baltimore, Williams & Wilkins, 1959.

Patrick, W. Recurrent hernia, Brit. J. Surg., 31: 231, 1944.

Pearse, H. E., Jr. Strangulated hernia reduced en masse, Surg., Gynec. & Obst., 53:822, 1931.

Pitzman, M. A fundamentally new technic for inguinal herniotomy, Ann. Surg., 74:610, 1921.

Potts, W. J., Riker, W. L., and Lewis, S. E. The treatment of inguinal hernia in infants and children, Ann. Surg., 132:566, 1950.

Ryan, E. A. Recurrent hernias, Surg., Gynec. & Obst., 96:343, 1953.

Seelig, M. G., and Chouke, K. S. A fundamental factor in recurrence of inguinal hernia, Arch. Surg., 7:553, 1923.

Stetten, De W. Modified technic for the radical cure of inguinal hernia in the male, Ann. Surg., 71:744, 1920.

Summers, J. E. Classical herniorrhaphies of Bassini, Halsted and Ferguson, Am. J. Surg., 73:87, 1947.

Usher, F. C. A new technique for repairing large abdominal wall defects, Arch. Surg., 82:870, 1961.

—— Hernia repair with marlex mesh: an analysis of 541 cases, Arch. Surg., 84:325, 1962.

Watson, L. F. Hernia, St. Louis, The C. V. Mosby Co., 1938.

Zimmerman, L. M. Inguinal hernia; surgical treatment of direct inguinal hernia, Surg., Gynec. & Obst., 66:193, 1938.

—— Symposium on recent advances in surgery of inguinal hernia, S. Clin. North America, 32:135, 1952.

Sliding Hernia

Bevan, A. D. Sliding hernias of the ascending colon and caecum, the descending colon and sigmoid, and of the bladder, Ann. Surg., 92: 754, 1930.

Graham, R. R. The operative repair of sliding hernia of the sigmoid, Ann. Surg., 102:784, 1935.

Sliding Hernia (cont.)

La Roque, G. P. The intra-abdominal method of removing inguinal and femoral hernia, Arch. Surg., 24 [No. 2]: 189–203, Feb., 1932.

Moschcowitz, A. V. The rational treatment of sliding hernias, Ann. Surg., 81:330–334, 1925.

Williams, C. Repair of sliding inguinal hernia through the abdominal (La Roque) approach, Ann. Surg., 126:612, 1947.

Femoral Herniorrhaphy

Annandale, T. Case in which a reducible oblique and direct inguinal and femoral hernia existed on the same side, and were successfully treated by operation, Edinburgh M. J., 21:1087, 1875–1876.

Anson, B. J., Reimann, A. F., and Swigart, La Vern L. The anatomy of hernial regions, II. Femoral hernia, Surg., Gynec. & Obst., 89:753, 1949.

Buckley, J. P. The etiology of the femoral hernial sac, Brit. J. Surg., 12:60, 1924.

Cooper, A. P. The Anatomy and Surgical Treatment of Abdominal Hernia. In Two Parts, 2nd ed. by C. A. Key, London, Longman, Rees, Orme, Brown & Green, 1827.

De Gimbernat, A. Nuevo Método de Operar en la Hernia Crural, Madrid, 1793.

Dennis, C., and Varco, R. L. Femoral hernia with gangrenous bowel, Surgery, 22:312, 1947.

Henry, A. K. Operation for femoral hernia by a midline extraperitoneal approach, Lancet, 1:531, 1936.

Hull, H. C., and Ganey, J. B. The Henry approach to femoral hernia, Ann. Surg., 137:57, 1953.

La Roque, G. P. The permanent cure of inguinal and femoral hernia, Surg., Gynec. & Obst., 29:507, 1919.

Lotheissen, G. Zur Radikaloperation de Schenkelhernien, Centralbl. f. Chir., 25:548, 1898.

Lytle, W. J. Femoral hernia, Ann. R. Coll. Surg. Engl., 21:244, 1957.

——— Operative treatment of herniae, Proc. Roy. Soc. Med., 54:967, 1961.

McClure, R. D., and Fallis, L. S. Femoral hernia: report of ninety operations, Ann. Surg., 109:987, 1939.

McVay, C. B., and Anson, B. J. Inguinal and femoral hernioplasty, Surg., Gynec. & Obst., 88:473, 1949.

Moschcowitz, A. Femoral hernia; a new operation for the radical cure, New York State J. Med., 7:396, 1907.

Musgrove, J. E., and McCready, F. J. The Henry approach to femoral hernia, Surgery, 26:608, 1949.

Shelly, H. J. Femoral hernias: a study of two hundred and thirty-eight hernias and two hundred and twenty-six repairs, Arch. Surg., 41:1229, 1940.

Umbilical Hernia

Barrington-Ward, L. I. The Abdominal Surgery of Children, London, Oxford University Press, 1937.

Cattell, R. B. Repair of incisional hernia, S. Clin. North America, 29:787 (June), 1949.

Gross, R. E. A new method for surgical treatment of large omphaloceles, Surgery, 24:277, 1948.

Iason, A. H. Congenital eventration at umbilicus, Surgery, 16:950, 1944.

Koontz, A. R. Preliminary report on the use of tantalum mesh in the repair of ventral hernias, Ann. Surg., 127:1079, 1948.

Lam, C. R., Szilagyi, D. E., and Puppendahl, M. Tantalum gauze in the repair of large postoperative ventral hernias, Arch. Surg., 57:234, 1948.

Mahorner, H. Umbilical and midline ventral herniae, Ann. Surg., 111:979, 1940.

Mayo, W. J. An operation for the radical cure of umbilical hernia, Ann. Surg., 34:276, 1901.

——— Further experience with the vertical overlapping operation for the radical cure of umbilical hernia, J.A.M.A., 41:225, 1903.

Michelson, E., and Raffel, W. Repair of large umbilical hernia, Surgery, 10:999, 1941.

Nuttall, H. C. Rectus transplantation for midline incisional herniae, Brit. J. Surg., 25:344, 1937.

Power, R. W. Preservation of umbilicus in radical cure of umbilical hernias in children, Brit. M. J., 2:353, 1934.

Russo, A. G., and Mazzini, E. J. B. Preoperative pneumoperitoneum in surgical therapy of large hernias and eventrations with report of cases, Bol. y. trab., Soc. argent. de cirujanos, 5:1071, 1944.

Stone, Harvey B. Umbilical hernia; a method of operative treatment, Arch. Surg., 10:404, 1926.

Watson, L. F. Hernia, 2nd ed., St. Louis, C. V. Mosby Co., 1938.

Combined Operation for Congenital Inguinal Hernia and Undescended Testicle

Browne, D. Some anatomical points in operation for undescended testicles, Lancet, 1:460, 1933.

Carroll, W. A. Malignancy in cryptorchidism, J. Urol., 61:396, 1949.

——— The treatment of the undescended or maldescended testis associated with inguinal hernia, Ann. Surg., 48:321, 1908.

——— Operative treatment of undescended and maldescended testis with especial reference to end results, Surg., Gynec. & Obst., 28:452, 1919.

Deming, C. L. The evaluation of hormonal therapy in cryptorchidism, J. Urol., 68:354, 1952.

Duckett, J. W. Treatment of congenital inguinal hernia, Ann. Surg., 135:879, 1952.

Eccles, W. McA. The anatomy, physiology and

COMBINED OPERATION FOR CONGENITAL
INGUINAL HERNIA AND UNDESCENDED
TESTICLE (cont.)

pathology of the imperfectly descended testis, Lancet, 1:569, 1902.

———— Value of imperfectly descended testis, Brit. M. J., II:1314, 1902.

Hansen, T. S. Fertility on operatively treated and untreated cryptorchidism, Proc. Roy. Soc. Med., 42:645, 1945.

Hart, D. B. The nature and cause of the physiological descent of the testis: descent in man, J. Anat. & Physiol., 44 (3rd series): 4 (first part), 1909–1910.

Hunter, R. H. The etiology of congenital inguinal and abnormally placed testis, Brit. J. Surg., 14:125, 1926.

Keetley, C. B. Medical Society of London: (1) Two cases of retained testis presenting points of special interest; (2) Exhibited two cases of retained testis illustrating new mode of operating, Lancet, 1:1008, 1894.

———— Temporary fixation of testis to thigh. A series of 25 cases operated on for undescended testis, Lancet, 2A:279–281, 1905.

Koop, C. E. Symposium on Pediatrics: Undescended testicles: differential diagnosis and management, M. Clin. North America, 36:779, 1952.

Lewis, L. G. Cryptorchism, J. Ural., 60:345, 1948.

MacCollum, D. W. Clinical study of spermatogenesis of undescended testicles, Arch. Surg., 31:290, 1935.

Mayer, H. W. Undescended testicle, with special reference to Torek's method of orchiopexy, Surg., Gynec. & Obst., 44:53, 1927.

Moschcowitz, A. V. The anatomy and treatment of undescended testis with especial reference to the Bevan operation, Ann. Surg., 52:821, 1910.

Rea, C. E. Treatment of undescended testicle, Tr. West. Surg. Assn., Chicago, 56:95, 1949.

Torek, F. The technique of orchiopexy, New York M. J., 90:948, 1909.

Womack, G. B., and Koch, F. C. Studies on extraction of testicular hormone from tissues and on its quantitative distribution therein, Endocrinology, 16:267, 1932.

HYDROCELECTOMY

Andrew, E. W. The "Bottle Operation". Method for the radical cure of hydrocele, Ann. Surg., 46:915, 1907.

Longuet, L. De la transposition extra sereuse du testicule, ses applications à l'hydrocele et au varicocele, Le Progress Medical, Sept. 21, 1901, p. 177.

Rolnick, H. C. Hydrocele, spermatocele, varicocele, S. Clin. North America, 15:757, 1935.

Young, H. H. Radical cure of hydrocele by excision of serous layer of sac, Surg., Gynec. & Obst., 70:807–812, 1940.

EXCISION OF PILONIDAL CYST

Cattell, R. B. Technic of operation for pilonidal sinus, S. Clin. North America, 14:1289, 1934.

Dunphy, J. E., and Matson, D. D. The treatment of pilonidal sinus, Surg., Gynec. & Obst., 75:737, 1942.

Fox, S. L. The origin of pilonidal sinus, Surg., Gynec. & Obst., 60:137, 1935.

Gage, M. Pilonidal sinus, Arch. Surg., 31:175, 1935.

———— Pilonidal sinus, Ann. Surg., 109:291, 1939.

Holman, E. Pilonidal sinus—treatment by primary closure, Surg., Gynec. & Obst., 83:94, 1946.

Kleiman, A. Pilonidal cyst: a comparison of treatments, Surgery, 28:851, 1950.

Lahey, F. H. A further suggestion for the operative treatment of pilonidal sinuses, Surg. Gynec. & Obst., 54:521, 1932.

MacFee, W. F. Pilonidal cysts and sinuses; method of wound closure, Ann. Surg., 116:687, 1942.

Rogers, H., and Hall, M. G. Pilonidal sinus, Arch. Surg., 31:742, 1935.

Shute, F. C., Jr., Smith, T. E., Levine, M., and Burch, J. C. Pilonidal cysts and sinuses, Ann. Surg., 118:706, 1943.

Stone, H. B. The origin of pilonidal sinus, Ann. Surg., 94:317, 1931.

EXCISION OF MAMMARY DUCT PAPILLOMA

Adair, F. E. Sanguineous discharge from nipple and its significance in relation to cancer of the breast, Ann. Surg., 91:197, 1930.

Babcock, W. W. The removal of benign tumors of the breast without visible scars, Surgery, 5:226, 1939.

Campbell, O. J. The bleeding nipple, Surgery, 19:40, 1946.

Copeland, M. M., and Higgins, T. G. Significance of discharge from the nipple in nonpuerperal mammary condition, Ann. Surg., 151:638, 1960.

Handley, W. S. Hunterian lecture on papilloma and its menace, Lancet, 1:1383, 1930.

Howard, M. A., and Rosenblatt, M. S. Management of intraductal papilloma; its relationship to cancer of breast, Am. J. Surg., 92:142, 1956.

McLaughlin, C. W., Jr., and Coe, J. D. A study of nipple discharge in the nonlactating breast, Ann. Surg., 157:810, 1963.

RADICAL MASTECTOMY

Ackerman, L. An evaluation of the treatment of cancer of the breast at the University of Edinburgh (Scotland), under the Direction of Dr. Robert McWhirter, Cancer, 8:883, 1955.

Andreassen, M., and Dahl-Iversen, E. Recherches sur les métastases microscopiques des ganglions

RADICAL MASTECTOMY (cont.)

lymphatiques sus-claviculaires dans le cancer du sein, J. internat. chir., 9:27, 1949.

Auchincloss, H. Significance of location and number of axillary metastases in carcinoma of the breast: a justification for a conservative operation, Ann. Surg., 158:37–46, 1963.

Baclesse, F. A method of pre-operative roentgen therapy by high doses, followed by radical operation for carcinoma of the breast (showing survivals up to 10 years) (Skinner Lecture), J. Fac. Radiologists, 6:233, 1955.

Bateman, J. C., and Carolton, H. N. Role of chemotherapy in the treatment of breast cancer, Surgery, 47:895, 1960.

Berger, S. M., and Gershon-Cohen, J. The roentgenographic diagnosis of carcinoma of the breast, J. Internat. Coll. Surgeons, 36:750, 1961.

Britton, R. C., and Nelson, P. A. Causes and treatment of postmastectomy lymphedema of the arm: report of 114 cases, J.A.M.A., 180:95, 1962.

Brooks, B., and Daniel, R. A., Jr. The present status of the "radical operation" for carcinoma of the breast, Ann. Surg., 111:68, 1940.

Butcher, H. R., Jr. Effectiveness of radical mastectomy for mammary cancer: an analysis of mortalities by the method of probits, Ann. Surg., 154:383, 1961.

Byrd, B. F., Jr., and Connerly, D. B., Jr. The role of simple mastectomy in treatment of carcinoma of the breast, Ann., Surg., 141:477, 1955.

Cade, S. Adrenalectomy for breast cancer (Hunterian Lecture, abridged), Brit. M.J., 1:1, 1955.

Cheatle, G. L., and Cutler, M. Tumours of the Breast, Philadelphia, J. B. Lippincott Co., 1931.

Dahl-Iversen, E. Recherches sur les métastases parasternaux dans le cancer du sein, J. internat. chir., 11:492, 1951.

Deaver, J. B., and McFarland, J. The Breast: Its Anomalies, Its Diseases, and Their Treatment, pp. 567–636, Philadelphia, P. Blakiston's Son and Co., 1917.

Egan, R. L. Mammography, an aid to diagnosis of breast carcinoma, J.A.M.A., 182:839, 1962.

——— Mammography, Amr. J. Surg., 106:421, 1963.

Galante, M., Rukes, J. M., Forsham, P. H., Wood, D. A., and Bell, H. G. Bilateral adrenalectomy for advanced carcinoma of the breast with preliminary observations on the effect of the liver on the metabolism of adrenal cortical steroids, Ann. Surg., 140:502, 1954.

Gershon-Cohen, J., Berger, S. M., and Hermel, M. B. Roentgenography and management of breast cancer, Am. J. Roentgenol., 89:51, 1963.

Greenough, R. B., and Simmons, C. C. End results in cancer cases: cancer of breast, Boston Med. and Surg. J., 185:253, 1921.

Haagensen, C. D. A technique for radical mastectomy, Surgery, 19:100, 1946.

——— Diseases of the Breast, Philadelphia, W. B. Saunders Co., 1956.

——— and Stout, A. P. Carcinoma of the breast, results of treatment, Ann. Surg., 116:801, 1942.

——— and Stout, A. P. Carcinoma of the breast, criteria of operability, Ann. Surg., 118:859 and 1032 (Nov. and Dec.), 1943.

——— and Stout, A. P. Carcinoma of the breast, J.A.M.A., 138:195 and 279 (Sept. 18 and 25), 1948.

——— (with twelve additional contributors). Treatment of early mammary carcinoma: A cooperative international study, Ann. Surg., 157:157–179, 1963.

Halsted, W. S. The results of operation for the cure of cancer of the breast, Ann. Surg., 20:497, 1894.

——— The swelling of the arm after operation for cancer of the breast (elephantiasis chirurgica), its cause and prevention, Bull. Johns Hopkins Hosp., 32:309, 1921.

Handley, R. S., and Thackray, A. C. The internal mammary lymph chain in carcinoma of the breast: study of 50 cases, Lancet, 2:276, 1949.

——— Patey, D. H., and Hand, B. H. Excision of internal mammary chain in Radical Mastectomy. Results in 57 cases. Lancet, 1:457, 1956.

——— Observations and reflections on breast cancer, J. Roy. Coll. Surg., Edinburgh, 6:1, 1960.

Handley, W. S. Cancer of the Breast and Its Operative Treatment, London, John Murray, 1922.

Hendrick, J. W. Results of treatment of carcinoma of the breast—five to 18 years, Ann. Surg., 146:728, 1957.

Holman, C. C. Cancer of breast; principles of surgical treatment, Lancet, 1:174, 1954.

Horsley, J. S. III, and Horsley, G. W. Twenty years' experience with prophylactic bilateral oophorectomy in the treatment of carcinoma of the breast, Ann. Surg., 155:935, 1962.

Jackson, J. N. A new technique for breast amputation, J.A.M.A., 46:627–633, 1906.

Jennings, J. E. Dissection of the axilla in radical operations for cancer of the breast, Ann. Surg., 83:770, 1926.

Kaae, J., and Johansen, H. Breast cancer, a comparison of the results of simple mastectomy with postoperative roentgen irradiation by the McWhirter method with those of extended radical mastectomy, Acta. Radio Suppl., 181:155, 1959.

Kennedy, B. J., and Nathanson, I. T. Effects of intensive sex steroid hormone therapy in advanced breast cancer; report to Council on Pharmacy and Chemistry from Committee on Research, J.A.M.A., 152:1135, 1953.

Klinger, H. M., and Buffington, R. Breast carcinoma, Arch. Surg., 84:439, 1962.

Kocher, T. Chirurgische Operationslehre, 4th ed., pp. 239–245, Jena, Gustav Fischer, 1902.

Kraft, R. O. An approach to the problems of mammary cancer, S. Clin. North America, 41:1219, 1961.

Leis, H. P., Jr. The hormonal therapy of ad-

RADICAL MASTECTOMY (cont.)

vanced carcinoma of the breast, J. Internat. Coll. Surgeons, 36:225, 1961.

Lenz, M. Tissue dosage in roentgen therapy of mammary cancer, Acta radiol., 28:583, 1947.

Lewis, F. S. Extended or super-radical mastectomy for cancer of the breast, Minnesota Med., 36:763, 1953.

Lewison, E. F. The surgical treatment of breast cancer, Surgery, 34:904, 1953.

MacDonald, I. Resection of the axillary vein in radical mastectomy: its relation to the mechanism of lymphedema, Cancer, 1:618, 1948.

——— Mammary carcinoma: review of 2636 cases, Surg., Gynec. & Obst., 74:75, 1942.

MacFee, W. F. A submaxillary incision for radical mastectomy, Ann. Surg., 137:850, 1953.

Margottini, M., and Bucalossi, P. Le metastasi linfoghiandolari mammarie interne nel cancro della mammella, Oncologia, 23:70, 1949.

Marshall, J. F. Lymphangiosarcoma of the arm following radical mastectomy, Ann. Surg., 142:871, 1955.

McWhirter, R. Cancer of the breast, Am. J. Roentgenol., 62:335, 1949.

——— The treatment of cancer of the breast, Proc. Roy. Soc. Med. 41:122, 1948.

——— Simple mastectomy and radiotherapy in the treatment of breast cancer, Brit. J. Radiol., 28:128, 1955.

Meyer, A. C., Dockerty, M. B., and Harrington, S. W. Inflammatory carcinoma of the breast, Surg., Gynec. and Obst., 87:417, 1948.

Meyer, W. An improved method of the radical operation for carcinoma of the breast, Med. Rec., 46:746, 1894.

——— Ten years experience with my method of radical operation, J.A.M.A., 45:297, 1905.

——— Cancer of the breast, Surg., Gynec. and Obst., 24:553, 1917.

Monroe, C. W. Lymphatic spread of carcinoma of the breast, Arch. Surg., 57:479, 1948.

Murphey, D. R., Jr. The use of atmospheric pressure in obliterating axillary dead space following radical mastectomy, South. Surgeon, 13:372, 1947.

Nathanson, I. T., Adair, F. E., Allen, W. M., and Engle, E. T. Estrogens and androgens in mammary cancer, J.A.M.A., 135:987, 1947.

Noer, R. J. Thio-tepa with radical mastectomy in the treatment of breast cancer, Amer. J. Surg., 106:405, 1963.

Orr, T. G. Incision for complete breast amputation, Ann. Surg., 106:454, 1937.

Peters, M. V. Carcinoma of the breast associated with pregnancy, Radiology, 78:58, 1962.

Phaler, G. E., and Keefer, G. P. The object, the value, and the technique of preoperative and postoperative X-ray treatment in carcinoma of the breast, Surg., Gynec. and Obst., 85:35, 1942.

Ratkowski, E., and Hochman, A. Survival of patients with "Recurrent" or inoperable carcinoma of the breast with special consideration

of the effect of hormonal treatment, Cancer, 14:300, 1961.

Rodman, J. S. Skin removal in radical breast amputation, Ann. Surg. 118:694, 1943.

Rodman, W. L. Cancer of the breast, J.A.M.A., 53:1648, 1909.

Sanger, G. An aspect of internal mammary metastases from carcinoma of the breast, Ann. Surg., 157:180, 1963.

Senstrom, K. W., and Baggenstoss, O. J. Results of surgery and radiation for carcinoma of the breast with axillary metastases, Acta radiol., 28:623, 1947.

Smith, B. B. The use of full thickness grafts and suction following radical mastectomy, Am. J. Surg., 102:532, 1961.

Smith, R. R. A two-flap incision for cancer of the breast, Surg., Gynec. and Obst., 43:95, 1926.

Sorensen, B. Recherches sur la localisation des ganglions lymphatique parasternaux, J. internat. chir., 11:50, 1951.

Sternby, N. H., Gynning, I., and Hogeman, K. E. Postmastectomy angiosarcoma, Acta. Chir. Scandinav., 121:420, 1961.

Stewart, F. T. Amputation of the breast by a transverse incision, Ann. Surg., 62:250, 1915.

Stewart, F. W., and Treves, N. Lymphangiosarcoma in post-mastectomy lymphedema; a report of 6 cases in elephantiasis chirurgica, Cancer, 1:64: 1948.

Stibbe, E. P. Internal mammary lymphatic glands, J. Anat., 52:257 (April), 1918.

Taylor, G. W., and Daland, E. M. The Greenough technique of radical mastectomy, Surg., Gynec. and Obst., 65:807, 1937.

——— and Wallace, R. H. Carcinoma of the breast; 50 years experience at the Massachusetts General Hospital, Ann. Surg., 132:833, 1950.

Urban, J. A. Radical excision of the chest wall for mammary cancer, Cancer, 4:1263, 1951.

——— Radical mastectomy in continuity with en bloc resection of internal mammary lymph node chain: new procedure for primary operable cancer of breast, Cancer, 5:992, 1952.

——— Current trends in breast cancer treatment, N. Y. J. Med., 61:3120, 1961.

——— Extended radical mastectomy for breast cancer, Amer. J. Surg., 106:399, 1963.

Veal, J. R. The pathologic basis for swelling of the arm following radical amputation of the breast, Surg., Gynec. and Obst., 67:752, 1938.

Vermund, H., and Kline, J. C. Current trends in radiotherapy of breast cancer, Amer. J. Surg., 106:430, 1963.

Wangensteen, O. H. In discussion of H. Glenn Bell, "cancer of the breast," Ann. Surg., 130:310, 1949.

Warren, J. C. The operative treatment of cancer of the breast, Ann. Surg., 40:805, 1904.

Watson, G. W., and Turner, R. L. Surgery plus chemotherapy in the treatment of breast cancer, Brit. M. J., 1:1315, 1959.

White, T. T. Prognosis of breast cancer for pregnant and nursing women. Analysis of 1413 cases, Surg., Gynec. and Obst., 100:661, 1955.

RADICAL MASTECTOMY (cont.)

——— and White, W. C. Breast cancer and pregnancy, Ann. Surg., 144:384, 1956.

White, W. C. The problem of local recurrence after radical mastectomy for carcinoma, Surgery, 19:149, 1946.

——— Comparison of radical and less extensive surgery in cancer of the breast, Amer. Surg., 22:942, 1956.

TRACHEOSTOMY

Abbey, P. Laryngostomy in acute laryngeal obstruction, Lancet, 1:573, 1963.

Carter, B. N., and Giuseffi, J. The use of tracheotomy in the treatment of crushing injuries of the chest, Surg., Gynec. & Obst., 96:55, 1953.

Cawthorne, T. Tracheotomy, Surg., Gynec. & Obst., 68:782, 1939.

Colvin, E. M., and Morrison, W. M. The value of tracheotomy in acutely ill surgical patients, Surg., Gynec. & Obst., 96:338, 1953.

Conley, J. J. Diagnosis and treatment of encrustations in trachea, J.A.M.A., 154:829, 1954.

Davis, H. S., Kretchmer, H. E., and Bryce-Smith, R. Advantages and complications of tracheotomy, J.A.M.A., 153:1156, 1953.

Dickman, M. D., and Baronofsky, I. D. Tracheotomy—one solution for pulmonary problems in the critically ill patient, Journal Lancet, 71:43, 1951.

Jackson, C., and Jackson, C. L. Tracheotomy, Am. J. Surg., 46:519, 1939.

Kofman, S., Lepper, M. H., Jackson, G. G., and Dowling, H. F. Effect of proteolytic enzymes on physical and chemical characteristics of tracheobronchial secretion of patients with poliomyelitis, Am. J. M. Sc., 228:426, 1954.

Lahey, F. H., and Hoover, W. B. Tracheotomy after thyroidectomy, Ann. Surg., 133:65, 1951.

Lepper, M. H., Kofman, S., Blatt, N., Dowling, H. F., and Jackson, G. G. Effect of eight antibiotics used singly and in combination on tracheal flora following tracheotomy in poliomyelitis, Antibiotics & Chemother., 4:829, 1954.

Lichtenstein, M. E. Acute injuries to the neck involving the food and air passages, Surg., Gynec. & Obst., 85:734, 1947.

Negus, V. E. Some disorders of the larynx. Hunterian Lecture, Lancet, 2:581 (Sept. 19), 1925.

Nelson, T. G. Tracheotomy: a clinical and experimental study: part I, The American Surgeon, Vol. 23, No. 7, July, 1957; part II, The American Surgeon, Vol. 23, No. 8, August, 1957; part III, The American Surgeon, Vol. 23, No. 9, September, 1957.

Plum, F., and Dunning, M. F. Technics for minimizing trauma to the tracheobronchial tree after tracheotomy, New England J. Med., 254:193, 1956.

Steigman, A. J., and Scott, C. H. Trypsin in poliomyelitis patients with tracheotomy, J.A.M.A., 150:1403, 1952.

Thomson, St. Clair. Tranquil tracheotomy by injecting cocaine within the windpipe, Brit. M. J., 2:460 (Oct. 11), 1919.

——— and Negus, V. E. Diseases of the Nose and Throat, New York, D. Appleton-Century Co., 1937, pp. 868–885.

Ulin, A. W., Olsen, A. K., and Martin, W. L. Factors determining mortality in patients with acute head injury, J.A.M.A., 157:496, 1955.

Waitaker H. T., and Lee, S. S. Indications for tracheotomy, Ann. Surg., 145:974, 1957.

Waldapfel, R. The opening of the anterior tracheal wall in tracheotomy, Surg., Gynec. & Obst., 71:191, 1940.

Watts, J. McK. Tracheostomy in modern practice, Brit. J. Surg., 50:954, 1963.

Wilhelm, D. L. Regeneration of tracheal epithelium, J. Path. & Bact., 65:543, 1953.

Williams, M. H. Multiple rib fractures: an indication for tracheotomy, Surgery, 30:664, 1951.

SCALENOTOMY

Adson, A. W., and Coffey, J. R. Cervical rib; a method of anterior approach for the relief of symptoms by division of the scalenus anticus, Ann. Surg., 85:839, 1927.

——— Surgical treatment for symptoms produced by cervical ribs and the scalenus anticus muscle, Surg., Gynec. & Obst., 85:687, 1947.

Craig, W., and Knepper, P. A. Cervical rib and the scalenus anticus syndrome, Ann. Surg., 105:556, 1937.

Donald, J. M., and Morton, B. F. The scalenus anticus syndrome with and without cervical rib, Ann. Surg., 111:709, 1940.

McGowan, J. M. Cervical rib: the role of the clavicle in occlusion of the subclavian artery, Ann. Surg., 124:71, 1946.

Naffziger, H. C. The scalenus syndrome, Surg., Gynec. & Obst., 64:119, 1937.

——— and Grant, W. T. Neuritis of the brachial plexus mechanical in origin, the scalenus syndrome, Surg., Gynec. & Obst., 67:722, 1938.

Ochsner, A., Gage, M., and DeBakey, M. Scalenus anticus (Naffziger) syndrome, Am. J. Surg., 28:669, 1935.

Patterson, R. H. Cervical ribs and the scalenus muscle syndrome, Ann. Surg., 111:531, 1940.

Spurling, R. G., and Bradford, F. K. Scalenus neurocirculatory compression, Ann. Surg., 107:708, 1938.

Telford, E. D., and Stofford, J. S. B. The vascular complications of cervical rib, Brit. J. Surg., 18:557, 1930–1931.

——— Cervical rib and hyperhidrosis, Brit. M. J., 2:96, 1942.

White, J. C., Poppel, M. H., and Adams, R. Congenital malformation of the first thoracic rib, Surg., Gynec. & Obst., 81:643, 1945.

EXCISION OF THYROGLOSSAL DUCT CYST

Clute, H. M., and Cattell, R. B. Thyroglossal cysts and sinuses, Ann. Surg., 92:57, 1930.

EXCISION OF THYROGLOSSAL DUCT CYST (cont.)

Fallon, J. A method for resection of the thyroglossal duct, Surg., Gynec. & Obst., 93:107, 1951.

Gross, R. E., and Connerley, M. C. Thyroglossal cysts and sinuses, New England J. Med., 223:616, 1940.

Hill, D. P. Papillary carcinoma arising in a thyroglossal tract, Canad. M.A.J., 85:791, 1961.

Lahey, F. H., and Nelson, H. F. Branchial cysts and sinuses, Ann. Surg., 113:508, 1941.

Marshall, S. F., and Becker, W. F. Thyroglossal cysts and sinuses, Ann. Surg., 129:642, 1949.

——— Thyroglossal cysts and sinuses, S. Clin. North America, 33:633, 1953.

Nachlas, H. E. Thyroglossal duct cysts, Ann. Otol., Rhin., & Laryng., 59:381, 1950.

Pemberton, J. de J., and Stalker, L. K. Cysts, sinuses and fistulae of the thyroglossal duct, Ann. Surg., 111:950, 1940.

Sistrunk, W. E. The surgical treatment of cysts of the thyroglossal tract, Ann. Surg., 71:121, 1920.

Ward, G. E., Hendrick, J. W., and Chambers, R. G. Thyroglossal tract abnormalities—cysts and fistulas; report of 105 cases from Johns Hopkins Hospital observed during years 1926 to 1946, Surg., Gynec. & Obst., 89:727, 1949.

THYROIDECTOMY

Adams, H. D. Transthoracic thyroidectomy, J. Thoracic Surg., 19:741, 1950.

Astwood, E. B. Thiouracil treatment in hyperthyroidism, J. Clin. Endocrinol., 4:229, 1944.

Bartels, E. C. Hyperthyroidism—An evaluation of treatment with antithyroid drugs followed by subtotal thyroidectomy, Ann. Int. Med., 37:1123, 1952.

——— Bell, G. O., and Geokas, M. C. Evaluation of the thyroid nodule, S. Clin. North America, 42:655, 1962.

Beahrs, O. H., Pemberton, J. de J., and Blake, B. M. Nodular goiter and malignant lesions of the thyroid gland, J. Clin. Endocrinol., 11:1157, 1951.

Black, B. M. Surgical treatment of carcinoma of the thyroid gland, J. Clin. Endocrinol., 9:1422, 1949.

——— Surgical treatment of thyroidal carcinoma, S. Clin. North America, 43:1107, 1963.

Block, M. A., Horn, R. C., and Brush, B. E. The place of total thyroidectomy in surgery for thyroid carcinoma, Arch. Surg., 81:236, 1960.

Blumgart, H. L., Levine, S. A., and Berlin, D. D. Congestive heart failure and angina pectoris. The therapeutic effect of thyroidectomy on patients without clinical or pathologic evidence of thyroid toxicity, Arch. Int. Med., 51:866, 1933.

Bowden, R. E. M. The surgical anatomy of the recurrent laryngeal nerve, Brit. J. Surg., 43:153, 1955.

——— The surgery of the recurrent laryngeal nerve, Proc. Roy. Soc. M. Lond., 48:437, 1955.

Bressler, S., and Thompson, S. A. Posterior mediastinal goiter, Am. J. Surg., 85:237, 1953.

Cattell, R. B. Indications for neck dissection in carcinoma of the thyroid, J. Clin. Endocrinol., 10:1099, 1950.

——— Indications for neck dissection in carcinoma of the thyroid, J. Clin. Endocrinol., 10:1099, 1950.

——— Neck dissection for carcinoma of the thyroid, S. Clin. North America, 897–907, June, 1953.

Chesky, V. E., Dresse, W. C., and Hellwig, C. A. Invasive adenoma of the thyroid, Surg., Gynec. & Obst., 98:581, 1954.

Clark, D. E., and Rule, J. H. Radioactive iodine or surgery in the treatment of hyperthyroidism, J.A.M.A., 159:995, 1955.

Clark, R. L., Jr., White, E. C., and Russell, W. O. Total thyroidectomy for cancer of the thyroid: significance of intra-glandular dissemination, Ann. Surg., 149:858, 1959.

Cole, W. H., Majarakis, J. D., Slaughter, D. P. Incidence of carcinoma of the thyroid in nodular goiter, J. Clin. Endocrinol., 9:1007–1011, 1949.

Cope, O., Dobyns, B. M., Hamlin, E., and Hopkirk, J. What thyroid nodules are to be feared? J. Clin. Endocrinol., 9:1012, 1949.

Crile, G. Problems in the surgery of the thyroid gland, Surg., Gynec. & Obst., 67:363, 1938.

Crile, G., Jr., and Dempsey, W. S. Indications for removal of non-toxic nodular goiters, J.A.M.A., 139:1247, 1949.

——— Cancer of the thyroid, J. Clin. Endocrinol., 10:1152, 1950.

——— Suhrer, J. G., Jr., and Hazard, J. B. Results of conservative operations for malignant tumors of thyroid, J. Clin. Endocrinol., 15:1422, 1955.

——— The danger of surgical dissemination of papillary carcinoma of the thyroid, Surg., Gynec. & Obst., 102:161, 1956.

Cutler, E. C., and Zollinger, R. The surgical procedure for total thyroidectomy, Surg., Gynec. & Obst., 67:69, 1938.

Dorsey, J. M., and McKinnon, A. Surgical management of intrathoracic goiter through the sternum-splitting approach, Arch. Surg., 65:570, 1952.

Ehrenhaft, J. L., and Buckwalter, J. A. Mediastinal tumors of thyroid origin, Arch. Surg., 71:347, 1955.

Ellenberg, A. H., Goldman, L., Gordan, G. S., and Lindsay, S. Thyroid carcinoma in patients with hyperparathyroidism, Surgery, 51:708, 1962.

Ellis, F. H., Good, C. A., and Seybold, W. S. Intrathoracic goiter and roentgen diagnosis, Radiology, 53:227, 1949.

Frazell, E. L., and Foote, F. W., Jr. Natural history of thyroid cancer; review of 301 cases. J. Clin. Endocrinol., 9:1063, 1949.

——— and Foote, F. W., Jr. Papillary thyroid cancer: pathologic findings in cases with and without clinical evidence of cervical node involvement, Cancer, 8:1164, 1955.

THYROIDECTOMY (cont.)

Graham, A. Riedel's Struma in contrast to struma lymphomatosa, West. J. Surg., 39:681, 1931.
——— Malignant adenoma of the thyroid. Local recurrences in the veins of the neck, Surg., Gynec. & Obst., 66:577, 1938.

Hashimoto, H. Zur Kenntniss der lymphomatösen Veränderung der Schilddrüse (Struma Lymphomatosa), Arch. f. clin. Chir., 97:219, 1912.

Hinton, J. W., and Lord, J. W., Jr. Is surgery indicated in all cases of nodular goiter toxic and non-toxic? J.A.M.A., 129:695, 1945.

Horn, R. C., Welty, R. F., Brooks, F. P., Rhoads, J. E., and Prendergrass, E. P. Carcinoma of the thyroid, Ann. Surg., 126:140, 1947.
——— Pathologic physiology of carcinoma of thyroid, S. Clin. North America, 35:1669, 1955.

Johnston, J. H., Jr., and Twente, G. E. Surgical approach to intrathoracic (Mediastinal) goiter, Ann. Surg., 143:572, 1956.

Joll, C. A. Pathology, diagnosis and treatment of Hashimoto's disease (Struma Lymphomatosa), Brit. J. Surg., 27:351, 1939.

Kalliomaki, J. L., Turunen, M., and Viikaii, S. J. Ligation of inferior thyroid arteries in thyroidectomy and the post-operative parathyroid function, Acta chir. scandinav. 122:57, 1961.

King, W. L. M., and Pemberton, J. deJ. So-called lateral aberrant thyroid tumors, Surg., Gynec. & Obst., 74:991, 1942.

Lahey, F. H., Bartels, E. C., Warren, S., and Meissner, W. A. Thiouracil—its use in the preoperative treatment of severe hyperthyroidism, Surg., Gynec. & Obst., 81:425, 1945.
——— and Bartels, E. C. The use of thiouracil, thiobarbital and prophylthiouracil in patients with hyperthyroidism, Ann. Surg., 125:572, 1947.
——— Technic of subtotal thyroidectomy, S. Clin. North America, 29:641 (June), 1949.
——— and Hare, H. F. Malignancy in adenomas of the thyroid, J.A.M.A., 145:689, 1951.

MacDonald, I., and Kotin, P. Surgical management of papillary carcinoma of the thyroid gland—the case for total thyroidectomy, Ann. Surg., 137:156, 1953.

MacFee, W. F. The surgical treatment of carcinoma of the thyroid gland, S. Clin. North America, 33:361 (April), 1953.

Marine, D. Iodine in diseases of thyroid gland, Medicine, 6:121, 1927.
——— The use and abuse of iodine in the treatment and prevention of goitre, Ann. Clin. Med., 5:942, 1927.

Marshall, S. F., Meissner, W. A., and Smith, D. C. Chronic Thyroiditis, New England J. Med., 238:758, 1948.
——— and Meissner, W. A. Struma lymphomatosa (Hashimoto's disease), Ann. Surg., 141:737, 1955.

Martin, H. Surgery of thyroid tumors, Cancer, 7:1063, 1954.

Maurer, E. R. The surgical treatment of retro-tracheal intrathoracic goiter, Arch. Surg., 71:357, 1955.

McClintock, J. C., and Wright, A. W. Riedel's struma and struma lymphomatosa (Hashimoto); comparative study, Ann. Surg., 106:11, 1937.

McCort, J. J. Intrathoracic goiter. Its incidence, symptomatology and roentgen diagnosis, Radiology, 53:337, 1949.

McSwain, B., and Moore, S. W. Struma lymphomatosa (Hashimoto's disease), Surg., Gynec. & Obst., 76:562, 1943.
——— and Diveley, W. Malignant tumors of the thyroid gland, Surgery, 23:525, 1948.

Moran, R. E., and Castro, A. F. The superior laryngeal nerve in thyroid surgery, Ann. Surg., 134:1018–1021, 1951.

Morris, K. N. Posterior mediastinal goiter: Report of 11 cases, Australian & New Zealand. J. Surg., 24:241, 1955.

Pemberton, J. de J. Surgery of substernal and intrathoracic goiters, Arch. Surg., 2:1, 1921.
——— Malignant lesions of the thyroid gland. A review of 774 cases, Surg., Gynec. & Obst., 69:417, 1939.

Penick, R. M., Jr. Use of thyroid extract without thiouracil in the preparation of the thyrotoxic patient, Ann. Surg., 125:582, 1947.

Plummer, H. S., and Boothby, W. M. Value of iodine in exophthalmic goiter, J. Iowa M. Soc., 14:66, 1924.
——— and Boothby, W. M. Value of iodine in exophthalmic goiter, Illinois M. J., 46:401, 1924.
——— and Boothby, W. M. The Administration of thyroid preparations, J.A.M.A., 83:1333–1335, 1924.

Portmann, U. V. Malignant tumors of the thyroid gland, Surg., Gynec. & Obst., 70:185, 1940.

Reeve, T. S., Rundle, F. F., Hales, I. B., Epps, R. G., Thomas, I. D., Indyk, J. S., Myhill, J., and Oddie, T. H. The investigation and management of intrathoracic goiter, Surg., Gynec. & Obst., 115:223, 1962.

Riedel, B. M. C. L. Die Chronische, zur Bildung eisenharter Tumoren führende Entzündung der Schilddrüse, Verhandl. d. deutsch. Gesellsch. f. Chir., 25:101, 1896.

Rustad, W. H., Lindsay, S., and Dailey, M. E. Comparison of the incidence of complications following total and subtotal thyroidectomy for thyroid carcinoma, Surg., Gynec. & Obst., 116:109, 1963.

Sloan, L. W. Of the origin, characteristics and behavior of thyroid cancer, J. Clin. Endocrinol., 14:1309, 1954.

Sokal, J. E. Surgical statistics on malignant goiter, Surg., Gynec. & Obst., 99:108, 1954.

Statland, H., Wasserman, M. M., and Vickery, A. L. Struma lymphomatosa (Hashimoto's struma): review of 51 cases with discussion of endocrinologic aspects, A.M.A. Arch. Int. Med., 88:659, 1951.

Sweet, R. H. Intrathoracic goiter located in the posterior mediastinum, Surg., Gynec. & Obst., 89:57, 1949.

Thyroidectomy (cont.)

Wade, J. S. H. Vulnerability of the recurrent laryngeal nerves at thyroidectomy, Brit. J. Surg., 43: 164, 1955.

Ward, R. Cancer of the thyroid in children, Am. J. Surg., 90:338, 1955.

Warren, S. Significance of invasion of blood vessels in adenomas of the thyroid gland, Arch. Path., 11:255, 1931.

——— and Meissner, W. A. Tumors of the thyroid gland, Washington, D.C., Armed Forces Institute of Pathology, 1953.

Williams, A. C., Davis, J. M., and Kiely, A. A. Thyroid cancer in 1330 cases of surgical goiter, Am. J. Surg., 104:672, 1962.

Winship, T., and Chase, W. W. Thyroid carcinoma in children, Surg., Gynec. & Obst., 101:217, 1955.

Zimmerman, L. M., Wagner, D. H., Perlmutter, H. R., and Amromin, G. D. Benign and malignant epithelial tumors of the thyroid gland, Arch. Surg., 60:1183, 1950.

Radical Neck Dissection

Barber, K. W., Jr., and Beahrs, O. H. Bilateral radical dissection of the neck: surgical treatment for carcinoma of the mouth and larynx, Arch. Surg., 83:388, 1961.

Barclay, T. H. C., Peltier, L. F., and Kremen, A. J. Neck dissections in the treatment of cancers of the head and neck, Ann. Surg., 134:828, 1951.

Beahrs, O. H. Radical dissection of structures of the neck: How radical should it be? Preliminary report, J.A.M.A., 157:794, 1955.

Gossel, J. D., and Hollinshead, W. H. Technic and surgical anatomy for radical neck dissection, Am. J. Surg., 90:490, 1955.

——— Devine, K. D., and Henson, S. W., Jr. Treatment of carcinoma of the tongue: End results in 168 cases, A.M.A. Arch. Surg., 79: 399, 1959.

——— and Barber, K. W., Jr. The value of radical dissection of structures of the neck in the management of carcinoma of the lip, mouth, and larynx, A.M.A. Arch. Surg., 85:49, 1962.

Black, J. I., Shaw, H. J., and Ellis, M. Discussion on block dissection of the neck, Proc. R. Soc. M., Lond., 52:415, 1959.

Block, M. A., Miller, J. M., and Brush, B. E. Place of radical neck surgery in thyroid carcinoma, Arch. Surg., 78:706 (discussion), 712, 1959.

——— and Miller, J. M. Modified neck dissection for thyroid carcinoma, Am. J. Surg., 101: 349, 1961.

Brown, J. B., and McDowell, F. Neck dissections for metastatic carcinoma, Surg., Gynec. & Obst., 79:115, 1944.

Cade, S., and Lee, E. S. Cancer of the tongue: study based on 653 patients, Brit. J. Surg., 44: 433, 1957.

Carveth, S. W., Devine, K. D., and ReMine,

W. H. Laryngectomy with radical neck dissection in extensive cancer of larynx, Am. J. Surg., 104:705, 1962.

Conley, J. J., and Pack, G. T. Surgical procedure for lessening the hazard of carotid bulb excision, Surgery, 31:845, 1952.

——— Swallowing dysfunctions associated with radical surgery of the head and neck, Arch. Surg., 80:602, 1960.

——— The use of regional flaps in head and neck surgery, Trans. Amer. Laryng. Assn., 81:95, 1960.

Corso, P. F., and Gerold, F. P. Use of autogenous dermis for protection of the carotid artery and pharyngeal suture lines in radical head and neck surgery, Surg. Forum, 12:483, 1961.

Crile, G. W. Excision of cancer of the head and neck, with reference to the plan of dissection based on one hundred and thirty-two operations, J.A.M.A., 47:1780 (discussion), 1785, 1906.

——— Technique of operations upon the head and neck, Ann. Surg., 44:464, 1906.

Cunning, D. S. Diagnosis and treatment of laryngeal tumors, J.A.M.A., 142:73, 1950.

Duffy, J. J. Treatment of cervical nodes in intraoral cancer. Surg., Gynec. & Obst., 71:664, 1940.

Fischel, E. Unilateral block resection of the lymph nodes of the neck for carcinoma, Am. J. Surg., 30:27, 1935.

Frazell, E. L., Harrold, C. C., and Rasmussen, L. Bilateral chylothorax: An unusual complication of radical neck dissection, Ann. Surg., 134:135, 1951.

Gaisford, J. C., Hanna, D. C., Atwell, R. B., and Terry, J. L. Evaluation of radical neck dissections and jaw resections, Plast. Reconstr. Surg., 25:39, 1960.

Gius, J. A., and Grier, D. H. Venous adaptation following bilateral radical neck dissection with excision of the jugular veins, Surgery, 28:305 (discussion), 319, 1950.

Harrington, S. W., Clagett, O. T., and Dockerty, M. B. Tumors of carotid body: clinical and pathologic considerations of twenty tumors affecting nineteen patients (one bilateral), Ann. Surg., 114:820, 1941.

Jackson, C., and Jackson, C. L. Cancer of the Larynx, Philadelphia, W. B. Saunders, 1939.

Kennedy, R. H. Epithelioma of lower lip: a suggested routine for treatment with description of operative excision of submental and submaxillary lymph nodes, Ann. Surg., 106:577–583, 1937.

King, G. D. The case against antibiotic prophylaxis in major head and neck surgery, Laryngoscope 72:647, 1961.

Lahey, F. H., and Warren, K. W. Long term appraisal of carotid body tumors with remarks on their removal, Surg., Gynec. & Obst., 92:481, 1951.

Lewis, G. K. Skin Flaps in reconstruction of head and neck following excision of malignant lesions, Trans. Amer. Acad. Ophthal. and Otolaryng., 64:660, 1960.

RADICAL NECK DISSECTION (cont.)

MacFee, W. F. Transverse incisions for neck dissection, Ann. Surg., 151:279, 1960.

Martin, H. The treatment of cervical metastatic cancer, Ann. Surg., 114:972 (discussion), 983, 1941.

———— and Morfit, H. M. Cervical metastasis as first sign of cancer, Surg., Gynec. & Obst., 78: 133, 1944.

———— Del Valle, B., Ehrlich, H., and Cahan, W. G. Neck dissection, Cancer, 4:441, 1951.

———— Radical neck dissection, Clin. Symposia (CIBA), 13:103, 1961.

McClure, R. D., and Lam, C. R. Should neck nodes be dissected in patients with carcinoma of the lip? Ann. Surg., 125:658, 1947.

Moore, O., and Smith, R. A. A case of one-stage bilateral neck dissection with recovery, Cancer, 4:1337, 1951.

———— and Baker, H. W. Carotid artery ligation in surgery of head and neck, Cancer, 8: 912, 1955.

Morfit, H. M. Simultaneous bilateral radical neck dissection: Total ablation of both internal and external jugular venous systems at one sitting, Surgery, 31:216, 1952.

Nahum, A. M., Mullally, W., and Marmor, L. A syndrome resulting from radical neck dissection, Arch. Otolaryng., 74:424, 1961.

Noble, A. B. Some aspects of anaesthesia for head and neck surgery, Canad. Anaesth. Soc. J., 7: 269, 1960.

Ogura, J. H. Supraglottic subtotal laryngectomy and radical neck dissection for carcinoma of the epiglottis, Laryngoscope, 68:983, 1958.

———— Watsons, R. K., and Jurema, A. A. Partial pharyngectomy and neck dissection for posterior hypopharyngeal cancer. Immediate reconstruction with preservation of voice, Laryngoscope, 70:1523, 1960.

O'Keefe, J. J. Evaluation on laryngectomy with radical neck dissection, Trans. Amer. Laryng., Rhinol., & Otol. Soc., 1959:671.

Peltier, L. F., Thomas, L. B., Barclay, T. H. C., and Kremen, A. J. Incidence of distant metastases among patients dying with head and neck cancer, Surgery, 30:857, 1951.

Perzik, S. L. Simultaneous bilateral radical neck dissection with recovery, Surgery, 31:297, 1952.

Pressman, J. J. Extended retrohyoid radical neck dissection for cancer of the oral cavity and neck, Surg., Gynec. & Obst., 100:329, 1955.

Putney, F. J. Elective versus delayed neck dissection in cancer of the larynx, Surg., Gynec. & Obst., 112:736, 1961.

Reed, G. F., Mueller, W., and Snow, J. B., Jr. Radical neck dissection. A clinico-pathological study of 200 cases. Trans. Amer. Laryng., Rhinol., & Otol. Soc., 1959:628.

Royster, H. P. Radical neck dissection, S. Clin. North America, 37:1535, 1957.

Schwartz, A. W., Hollinshead, W. H., and Devine, K. D. Laryngectomy: anatomy and technique, S. Clin. North America, 43:1063, 1963.

Semken, G. H. Surgery of the neck, in Nelson's Loose-Leaf Surgery, Vol. II, 1941, pp. 843–897.

Sisson, G. A. Problems and complications in head and neck surgery, Laryngoscope, 70:1142, 1960.

Slaughter, D. P. Neck dissections: Indications and technics, S. Clin. North America, 26:102, 1946.

———— and Trevino, E. T. Elective neck dissection for intraoral cancer, Arch. Surg., 80:905, 1960.

Southwick, H. W., and Slaughter, D. P. Neck dissection: Complications and safeguards, S. Clin. North America, 35:31, 1955.

Staley, C., and Scanlon, E. F. Bilateral radical neck dissection, Am. J. Surg., 98:851, 1959.

———— A muscle cover for the carotid artery after radical neck dissection, Am. J. Surg., 102: 815, 1961.

Sugarbaker, E. D. The surgical problem of cancer lymph nodes, Surgery, 18:608, 1945.

Till, H. J., and Cameron, J. M. A method of reconstruction of the neck after esophagectomy and laryngectomy, Surg., Gynec. & Obst., 114: 121, 1962.

Ward, G. E., Edgerton, M. T., Chambers, R. G., and McKee, D. M. Cancer of the oral cavity and pharynx and results of treatment by means of the composite operation (in continuity with radical neck dissection), Ann. Surg., 150:202, 1959.

LARYNGECTOMY

Babcock, W. W. Laryngectomy for carcinoma of the larynx, S. Clin. North America, 11:1207, 1931.

Clerf, L. H. Laryngectomy, Surg., Gynec. & Obst., 86:197, 1948.

———— Putney, F. J., and O'Keefe, J. J. Carcinoma of the larynx, Tr. Am. Laryng. Rhinol., & Otol. Soc., p. 482, 1948.

Crile, G. W. Laryngectomy for cancer, Tr. Am. S. A., 33:259, 1933.

Harris, W., Silverstone, S. M., and Kramer, R. Therapy for cancer of the larynx and laryngopharynx. Twenty years' experience, Am. J. Roentgenol., 71:813, 1954.

Jackson, C. L., and Norris, C. M. Surgical treatment of cancer of the larynx, Tr. Am. Laryngol. Rhinol., & Otol. Soc., p. 45, 1945.

MacKenty, J. E. Operation of total laryngectomy for the care of intrinsic cancer of the larynx, Ann. Otol. Rhin., & Laryng., 31:110, 1922.

Martin, H. The incidence of total and partial laryngectomy, 1947 and 1952, Cancer 8:1122, 1955.

McGavran, M. H., Bauer, W. C., and Ogura, J. H. The incidence of cervical lymph node metastases from epidermoid carcinoma of the larynx and their relationship to certain characteristics of the primary tumor: A study based on the clinical and pathological findings for 96 patients treated by en bloc laryngectomy and radical neck dissection, Cancer, 14:55, 1961.

LARYNGECTOMY (cont.)

New, G. B. Surgical treatment of cancer of the larynx, Surg., Gynec. & Obst., 68:462, 1939.
———— Figi, F. A., Haven, F. Z., and Erich, J. B. Carcinoma of the larynx, Surg., Gynec. & Obst., 85:623, 1947.
Thomson, St. C., and Colledge, L. Cancer of Larynx, New York, Macmillan, 1930.

RESECTION OF
PHARYNGOESOPHAGEAL DIVERTICULUM

Adams, H. D. Diverticula of the thoracic esophagus, J. Thoracic Surg., 17:639–645, 1948.
Barrett, N. R. Diverticula of the thoracic esophagus, Lancet, 1:1009, 1933.
Bell, C. Surgical Observations, London, Longman, Rees, Orme, Brown & Green, 1816, pp. 64–70.
Bergmann, E. Ueber den Oesophagusdivertikel und seine Behandlung, Arch. klin. Chir., 43: 1–30, 1892.
Bevan, A. D. Pulsion diverticulum of esophagus— cure by the Sippy-Bevan operation, Surg. Clin. Chicago, 1:449–457, 1917.
Crile, G. W., and Dinsmore, R. Diverticula of esophagus, S. Clin. North America, 4:863, 1924.
Crile, G., Jr., and Robnett, A. H. Treatment of pharyngoesophageal diverticulum by inversion of the sac, Cleveland Clin. Quart., 18:42, 1951.
Gants, R. T., and Cohen, A. A thyroidectomy type (transverse) incision for excision of pharyngoesophageal diverticula, Surg., Gynec. & Obst., 104:373, 1957.
Goldmann, E. E. Die zweizeitige Operation von Pulsiondivertikeln der Speiseroehre, Beitr. klin. Chir., 61:741–749, 1909.
Harrington, S. W. Pulsion diverticulum of the hypopharynx at pharyngoesophageal junction: surgical treatment in 140 cases, Surgery, 18:66, 1945.
Hill, W. Pharyngeal pouch treated by diverticulopexy, Proc. R. Soc. M. Lond. (Sect. Laryng.), 11:60, 1917–1918.
Kausel, H. W., and Lindskog, G. E. Epiphrenic diverticulum of the esophagus. A review of its surgical treatment and report of a case, Dis. of Chest, 21:334, 1952.
King, B. T. New concepts of the etiology and treatment of diverticula of the esophagus, Surg., Gynec. & Obst., 85:93, 1947.
Kocher, T. Das Oesophagus divertikel und dessen Behandlung, Cor.-Bl. f. schweiz. Aerzte, 22: 233–244, 1892.
Lahey, F. H. Technique of the two stage operation for pulsion oesophageal diverticulum, Surg., Gynec. & Obst., 43:359–365, 1926.
———— Esophageal diverticula, Arch. Surg., 41: 1118–1140, 1940.
———— Pharyngo-esophageal diverticulum; its management and complications, Ann. Surg., 124:617–636, 1946.
———— and Warren, K. W. Esophageal diverticula, Surg., Gynec. & Obst., 98:1–28, 1954.

Ludlow, A. Obstructed deglutition, from a preternatural dilatation of, and bag formed in, the pharynx, Med. Obs. Soc. Physicians, London, 3:85–101, 1762–1767.
McNealy, R. W., and McCallister, J. W. The surgical management of esophageal diverticula, S. Clin. North America, 31:71, 1951.
Negus, V. E. Pharyngeal diverticula. Observations on their evolution and treatment, Brit. J. Surg., 38:129–146, 1950.
Nicoladoni, K. Behandlung der Oesophagusdivertikel, Wien. med. Wschr., 27:606–607, 1877.
Niehans, cited by Zesas, G. Beitrag zur chirurgischen Behandlung des Speisenroehren-Divertikels, Deutsche Ztschr. f. Chir., 82:577, 1906.
Shallow, T. A., and Clerf, L. H. One stage pharyngeal diverticulectomy, Surg., Gynec. & Obst., 86:317, 1948.
Sweet, R. H. Pulsion diverticulum of the pharyngoesophageal junction: technic of the one-stage operation. A preliminary report, Ann. Surg., 125:41, 1947.
———— Thoracic Surgery, 2nd ed., Philadelphia, W. B. Saunders, 1954.
von Bergmann, E. Uber das Oesophagusdivertikel und seine Behandlung, Arch. f. klin. Chir., 43:1, 1892.
Warren, K. W. Am. J. Surg., 93:205–217, 1957.
Zenker, F. A., and Zeimssen, H. Krankheiten des Oesophagus, in Handbuch der speciellen Pathologie und Therapie, Leipzig, F. C. Vogel, Vol. 7 (supp.), pp. 50–87.

ESOPHAGUS

Benson, C. D., Mustard, W. T., Ravitch, M. A., Snyder, W. H., Jr., and Welch, K. J. The esophagus. Congential esophageal atresia and tracheosophageal fistula, Pediatric Surgery, Year Book Medical Publishers, Inc., 1962, Section 2, p. 266.
Carter, B. N., Stevenson, J., and Abbott, O. A. Transpleural esophagogastrostomy for carcinoma of the esophagus and for carcinoma of the cardiac portion of the stomach; report of two cases, Surgery, 8:587, 1940.
Dodge, O. G. The surgical pathology of gastrooesophageal carcinoma, Brit. J. Surg., 49:121, 1961.
Eggers, C. Treatment of carcinoma of the esophagus, Surg., Gynec. & Obst., 63:54, 1936.
Faure, J. L. Cancer de la portion thoracique de l'oesophage. Extirpation du neoplasme par la voie mediastinale posterieure directe combinée à une incision cervicale, Rev. de chir., 27:401, 1903.
Meyer, W. Cancer of the esophagus from the standpoint of intrathoracic surgery; report of four resections, Surg., Gynec. & Obst., 15:639, 1912.
Ochsner, A., and DeBakey, M. Surgical aspect of carcinoma of the esophagus: Review of the literature and report of four cases, J. Thoracic Surg., 10:401, 1941.

ESOPHAGUS (cont.)

Santy, P., Ballivert, M., and Berard, M. Thoracic esophagectomy for cancer; report of two successful cases, J. Thoracic Surg., 12:397, 1943.

Tuffier, M. Sur la résection de l'oesophage thoracique, Presse med., 11:364, 1903.

Turner, G. G. Excision of the thoracic oesophagus for carcinoma, with construction of the extra-thoracic gullet, Lancet, 2:1315, 1933.

ESOPHAGOCARDIOMYOTOMY

Adams, C. W. M., Brain, R. H. F., Ellis, F. G., Kauntze, R., and Trounce, J. R. Achalasia of the cardia, Guy's Hospital Rep., 110:191, 1961.

Alvarez, W. C. A simple explanation for cardiospasm and Hirschsprung's disease, Gastroenterology, 13:442, 1949.

Barrett, N. R., and Franklin, R. H. Concerning the unfavourable late results of certain operations performed in treatment of cardiospasm, Brit. J. Surg., 37:194, 1949.

Browse, N. L., and Carter, S. J. The late results of Heller's operation in the treatment of achalasia, Brit. J. Surg., 49:59, 1961-62.

Effler, D. B., and Rogers, J. W. Megaesophagus, Arch. Surg., 71:551, 1955.

Frobese, A. S., Stein, G. N., and Hawthorne, H. R. Hiatal hernia as a complication of the Heller operation, Surgery, 49:599, 1961.

Gröndahl, N. B. Cardioplastik ved Cardiospasmus, Nord. med. Ark., 49:236, 1916.

Heller, E. Extramukose Cardioplastik beim chronischen Cardiospasmus mit Dilatation des Oesophagus, Mitt. a. d. Grenzgeb. d. Med. u. Chir., 27:141-149, 1913.

Hertz, A. F. Case of achalasia of the cardia (so-called cardiospasm), Proc. Roy. Soc. Med., 8:22 (Dec.), 1914.

———— Achalasia of the cardia, Quart. J. Med. (Oxford), 8:300, 1915.

Heyrovsky, H. Casuistir und Therapie der idiopathischen Dilatation der Speiseröhre; Oesophagogastroanastomose, Arch. f. klin. Chir., 100:703, 1913.

Laimer, E. Beitrag zur Anatomie des Oesophagus, Wien, Med. Jahrbucher, Jahrg., 333-338, 1883.

Lerche, W. The Esophagus and Pharynx in Action, Springfield, Charles C Thomas, 1950.

Maingot, R. Abdominal Operations, New York, Appleton-Century-Crofts, Inc., 1948, pp. 343-347.

———— Surgical treatment of cardiospasm, Postgrad. Med., 5:351, 1949.

Ochsner, A., and De Bakey, M. Surgical considerations of achalasia, Arch. Surg., 41:1146, 1940.

Olsen, A. M., Ellis, F. H., and Creamer, B. Cardiospasm (achalasia of the cardia), Am. J. Surg., 93:299, 1957.

Petrovsky, B. V. Cardiospasm and its surgical correction, Ann. Surg., 155:60, 1962.

Puppel, I. D. The role of esophageal motility in the surgical treatment of mega-esophagus, J. Thoracic Surg., 19:371, 1950.

Rake, G. W. On the pathology of achalasia of the cardia, Guy's Hosp. Rep., 77:141, 1927.

Sweet, R. H. A consideration of certain benign lesions of the esophagus, Surgery, 40:447, 1956.

Vinson, P. P. Diagnosis and treatment of cardiospasm, Postgrad. Med., 3:13-18, 1948.

Von Mikulicz, J., Jr. Zur Pathologie und Therapie des Cardiospasms, Deutsche med. Wchnschr., 30:17, 1904.

Wangensteen, O. H. A physiologic operation for mega-esophagus (dystonia, cardiospasm, achalasia), Ann. Surg., 134:301, 1951.

———— Technique of achieving an adequate extramucosal myotomy in mega-esophagus (achalasia, cardiospasm, dystonia), Surg., Gynec. & Obst., 105:339, 1957.

Wendel, W. Zur Chirurgie des Oesophagus, Arch. f. klin. Chir., 93:311, 1910.

Wolf, S., and Almy, T. Experimental observations on cardiospasm in man, Gastroenterology, 13:401, 1949.

Wooler, G. H. Cardiospasm, Thorax, 3:53, 1948.

ESOPHAGEAL HIATUS HERNIA

Adler, R. H. Hiatal hernia and esophagitis, Surg., Gynec. & Obst., 116:1, 1963.

Allison, P. R. Reflux esophagitis, sliding hiatal hernia, and the anatomy of repair, Surg., Gynec. & Obst., 92:419, 1951.

———— Observations on conservative approach to nonmalignant lesions at the cardia, J. Thoracic Surg., 32:150, 1956.

Barrett, N. R. Benign structure in the lower esophagus, J. Thoracic & Cardiovasc. Surg., 43:703, 1962.

Bowden, L., and Miller, C. J. Massive hematemesis from hiatus hernia, Arch. Surg., 63:143, 1951.

Brick, I. B. Incidence of hiatus hernia and associated lesions diagnosed by roentgen rays, Arch. Surg., 58:419, 1949.

Carey, J. M., and Hollinshead, W. H. An anatomic study of the esophageal hiatus, Surg., Gynec. & Obst., 100:196, 1955.

Dunhill, T. Diaphragmatic hernia, Brit. J. Surg., 22:475, 1935.

Effler, D. B., and Ballinger, C. S. Complications and surgical treatment of hiatus hernia and short esophagus, J. Thoracic Surg., 22:235, 1951.

———— and Groves, L. K. Short esophagus, Arch. Surg., 75:639, 1957.

Harrington, S. W. Diaphragmatic hernia in children, Ann. Surg., 115:705, 1942.

———— Surgical treatment of the more common types of diaphragmatic hernia; esophageal hiatus, traumatic, pleuroperitoneal hiatus, congenital absence and foramen of Morgagni. Report of 404 cases, Ann. Surg., 122:546, 1945.

———— Various types of diaphragmatic hernia treated surgically; report of 430 cases, Surg., Gynec. & Obst., 86:735, 1948.

———— Esophageal hiatal diaphragmatic hernia, Surg., Gynec. & Obst., 100:277, 1955.

ESOPHAGEAL HIATUS HERNIA (cont.)

Humphreys, G. H., II, Ferrer, J. M., Jr., and Wiedel, P. D. Esophageal hiatus hernia of the diaphragm. An analysis of surgical results, J. Thoracic Surg., 34:749, 1957.

Johnsrud, R. L. The repair of the phrenoesophageal ligament in surgical treatment of hiatal hernia, Surg., Gynec. & Obst., 103:708, 1956.

Kirklin, B. R. Roentgenologic diagnosis of diaphragmatic hernia, Postgrad. Med., 4:501, 1948.

Lam, C. R., and Kenny, L. G. The problem of the hiatus hernia of the diaphragm, J. Thoracic Surg., 27:1, 1954.

Lawler, R. H., West, J. W., and Lawler, E. G. Treatment of diaphragmatic hernia in the newborn, Am. J. Dis. Child., 84:79, 1952.

Madden, J. L. Anatomic and technical considerations in the treatment of esophageal hiatal hernia, Surg., Gynec. & Obst., 102:187, 1956.

Merendino, K. A., Varco, R. L., and Wangensteen, O. H. Displacement of the esophagus into a new diaphragmatic orifice in the repair of paraesophageal and esophageal hiatus hernia, Ann. Surg., 129:185, 1949.

Miller, C. Carcinoma of thoracic esophagus and cardia: Review of 405 cases, Brit. J. Surg., 69:507, 1962.

Morton, J. J. Herniation through the diaphragm, Surg., Gynec. & Obst., 68:257, 1939.

Neville, W. E., and Clowes, G. H. A., Jr. Surgical treatment of reflux esophagitis, Arch. Surg., 83:534, 1961.

Olsen, A. M., and Harrington, S. W. Esophageal hiatal hernia of the short esophagus type: Etiologic and therapeutic considerations, J. Thoracic Surg., 17:189, 1948.

Plachta, A. Benign tumors of esophagus: Review of literature and report of 99 cases, Am. J. Gastroenterol, 38:639, 1962.

Pories, W. J., Gerle, R. D., Sherman, C. D., and Hinshaw, J. R. The danger of esophageal replacement with antiperistaltic loops of small bowel, Am. Surg., 1956:68, 1962.

Rives, J. D., and Baker, D. O. Anatomy of the attachments of the diaphragm. Their relation in the problems of the surgery of diaphragmatic hernia, Ann. Surg., 115:745, 1942.

Sweet, R. H. The repair of hiatus hernia of the diaphragm by the supradiaphragmatic approach. Technic and results, New England J. Med., 238:649, 1948.

——— Esophageal hiatus hernia of the diaphragm: The anatomical characteristics, technic of repair and results of treatment in 111 consecutive cases, Ann. Surg., 135:1, 1952.

——— Experience with 500 cases of hiatus hernia: a statistical survey, J. Thoracic & Cardiovas. Surg., 44:145, 1962.

Truesdale, P. E. Diaphragmatic hernia. Its varieties and surgical treatment of the hiatus type, Am. J. Surg., 32:204, 1936.

Wangensteen, O. H., and Leven, N. L. Gastric resection for esophagitis and stricture of acid-peptic origin, Surg., Gynec. & Obst., 88:560, 1949.

Young, D. Esophageal-hiatus hernia, Rev. Gastroenterol., 9:345, 1942.

STOMACH AND DUODENUM

Abbott, W. E., Krieger, H., and Levey, S. Technical surgical factors which enhance or minimize postgastrectomy abnormalities, Ann. Surg., 148:567, 1958.

Amendola, F. H. The management of massive gastroduodenal hemorrhage, Ann. Surg., 129:47, 1949.

Barber, K. W., Jr., Waugh, J. H., and Priestley, J. T. Operation in one stage for gastrojejunocolic fistula, S. Clin. North America, 42:1443, 1962.

Cammock, E. E., Hallett, W. Y., Nyhus, L. M., and Harkins, H. N. Diagnosis and therapy in gastrointestinal hemorrhage, Arch. Surg., 86:608, 1963.

Chinn, A. B., Littell, A. S., Badger, G. F., and Beams, A. J. Acute hemorrhage from peptic ulcer: follow-up study of 310 patients, New England J. Med., 255:973, 1956.

Cole, W. H. Surgical treatment of bleeding peptic ulcers, S. Clin. North America, 31:271, 1951.

Colp, R., and Druckerman, L. J. Rational approach to surgery of high gastric ulcer, S. Clin. North America, 27:231, 1947.

Cooper, W. A. End results in the treatment of peptic ulcer by posterior gastroenterostomy, Surgery, 23:425, 1948.

Dragstedt, L. R. A concept of the etiology of gastric and duodenal ulcer, Gastroenterology, 30:208, 1956.

Drapanas, T., McDonald, J. C., and Stewart, J. D. Serotonin release following instillation of hypertonic glucose into proximal intestine, Ann. Surg., 156:528, 1962.

Edkin, J. S. The chemical mechanism of gastric secretion, J. Physiol., 34:133, 1906.

——— and Tweedy, M. The natural channels of absorption evoking the chemical mechanism of gastric secretion, J. Physiol., 38:263, 1909.

Finsterer, H. Surgical treatment of acute profuse gastric hemorrhages, Surg., Gynec. and Obst., 69:291, 1939.

Garlock, J. H., and Lyons, A. S. The surgical therapy of duodenal ulcer, Surgery, 25:352, 1949.

Gilbertsen, V. A., and Hollenberg, M. The results of surgery for cancer of the stomach, Surg., Gynec. & Obst., 115:543, 1962.

Gilchrist, R. K. Surgical treatment of high-lying gastric ulcer, J.A.M.A., 162:1039, 1956.

Gilmore, J. Prognosis and treatment in acute perforated peptic ulcer: review of 206 cases, Lancet, 2:870, 1953.

Glenn, F. Present status of the surgical treatment of peptic ulcer, J.A.M.A., 145:11, 1951.

Gordon-Taylor, G. The problem of the bleeding peptic ulcer, Brit. J. Surg., 25:403, 1937.

Stomach and Duodenum (cont.)

Gray, H. K., Shands, W. C., and Thuringer, C. Problem of massive gastrointestinal hemorrhage from undetermined source, S. Clin. North America, 34:495, 1954.

Gray, S. J., Benson, J. A., Jr., Reifenstein, R. W., and Spiro, H. M. Chronic stress and peptic ulcer: I. Effect of corticotropin (ACTH) and cortisone on gastric secretion, J.A.M.A., 147:1529, 1951.

———— Ramsey, C. L., and Reifenstein, R. W. Clinical use of the urinary uropepsin determination in medicine and surgery, New England J. M., 251:835, 1954.

Guiss, L. W. Collective review: end results from gastric cancer; 2891 cases, Surg., Gynec. & Obst., 93:313, 1951.

Hampton, A. O. A safe method for roentgen demonstration of bleeding duodenal ulcers, Am. J. Roentgenol., 38:565, 1937.

Harvey, H. D., Titherington, J. B., Stout, A. P., and St. John, F. R. Gastric carcinoma: experience from 1916 to 1949 and present concepts, Cancer, 4:717, 1951.

Hay, L. J., Varco, R. L., Code, C. F., and Wangensteen, O. H. The experimental production of gastric and duodenal ulcers in laboratory animals by the intramuscular injection of histamine in bees wax, Surg., Gynec. & Obst., 75:170, 1942.

Irvine, W. T. The liver's role in histamine absorption from the alimentary tract, Gut, 1:83, 1960.

Johnson, H. D., and Orr, I. M. Surgical policy for peptic ulcer, Lancet, 1:253, 1953.

Johnson, L. P., Sloop, R. D., Jesseph, J. E., and Harkins, H. N. Serotonin antagonists in experimental and clinical "dumping," Ann. Surg., 156:537, 1962.

Kay, A. W. Effect of large doses of histamine on gastric secretion HCl; augmented histamine test, Brit. M. J., 2:77, 1953.

Kirtley, J. A., Jr., Riddell, H., and Smith, E. I. Upper gastrointestinal hemorrhage of obscure origin, Ann. Surg., 145:789, 1957.

Klug, T. J., Zollinger, R. M., and Ellensohn, J. Long term evaluation of two conservative surgical procedures for duodenal ulcer, Am. J. Surg., 105:370, 1963.

Kozoll, D. D., and Meyer, K. A. Massively bleeding gastroduodenal ulcers: general factors influencing incidence and mortality, Arch. Surg., 86:445, 1963.

Lewison, E. F. Bleeding peptic ulcer, Surg., Gynec. & Obst., 90:1, 1950.

Mann, F. C., and Williamson, C. S. The experimental production of peptic ulcer, Ann. Surg., 77:409, 1923.

Mayo, H. W. The physiological basis of operations for duodenal, gastric and gastrojejunal ulcer, Surgery, 26:251, 1949.

McCleery, R. S., Kesterson, J. E., and Proffitt, J. H. The technic and results of a dependent greater curvature gastroenterostomy, Ann.

Surg., 134:844, 1951.

McNeer, G., Sunderland, D. A., McInnes, G., Vandenberg, H. J., and Lawrence, W. A more thorough operation for gastric cancer. Anatomical basis and description of technique, Cancer, 4:957, 1951.

Meulengracht, E. Fifteen years experience with free feeding of patients with bleeding peptic ulcer, Arch. Int. Med., 80:697, 1947.

Moore, J. R., and Morton, H. J. Gastric carcinoma, Ann. Surg., 141:185, 1955.

Nicoloff, D. M., Griffen, W. O., Jr., Salmon, P. A., Peter, E. T., and Wangensteen, O. H. Local gastric hypothermia in the management of massive gastro-intestine hemorrhage, Surg., Gynec. & Obst., 114:495, 1962.

Ochsner, A., and Blalock, J. Carcinoma of the stomach. Necessity for re-evaluation of therapeutic philosophy, J.A.M.A., 151:1377, 1953.

Olsson, O., Westerborn, A., and Endresen, R. Results of treatment of gastric cancer: 15 years experience with 201 resections, Acta chir. Scandinav., 111:1, 1956.

Orr, I. M. Selective surgery for peptic ulcer: a review, Gut, 3:97, 1962.

Pack, G. T., and McNeer, G. End results in the treatment of cancer of the stomach, Surgery, 24:769, 1948.

Pavlov, I. P. The Work of the Digestive Glands, London, Charles Griffin and Co., Ltd., 1902.

Pridgen, J. E. Leiomyosarcoma of the stomach, Ann. Surg., 153:971, 1961.

Ransom, H. K. Cancer of the stomach, Surg., Gynec. & Obst., 96:275, 1953.

ReMine, W. H., Walters, W., Priestley, J. T., Waugh, J. M., Judd, E. S., Ferris, D. O., Hallenbeck, G. A., and Adson, M. A. Report of surgery of the stomach and duodenum for 1958 and 1959, Proc. Mayo Clin., 36:529, 1961.

———— Dockerty, M. B., and Priestley, J. T. Some factors which influence prognosis in surgical treatment of gastric carcinoma, Ann. Surg., 138:311, 1953.

———— Priestley, J. T., and Berkson, J. Cancer of the stomach, Philadelphia and London, W. B. Saunders Co., 1964.

Ryan, E. P., and Beal, J. M. The development of carcinoma of the stomach in patients with duodenal ulcer, Surgery, 42:271, 1957.

Schechter, D. C., and Swan, H. Levin and his tube, Surgery, 51:415, 1962.

Stone, H. B. The limitations of radical surgery in the treatment of cancer, Surg., Gynec. & Obst., 97:129, 1953.

Sunderland, D. A., McNeer, G., Ortega, L. G., and Pearce, L. S. The lymphatic spread of gastric cancer, Cancer, 6:987, 1953.

Tanner, N. C. The surgical treatment of peptic ulcer, Brit. J. Surg., 51:5, 1964.

Thompson, J. C., and Peskin, G. W. The gastric antrum in the operative treatment of duodenal ulcer, Int. Abstr. Surg., 112:205, 1961.

Thompson, J. C., Tramontana, J. A., Lerner, H. J., and Stallings, J. O. Physiologic scope of the

STOMACH AND DUODENUM (cont.)

antral inhibitory hormone, Ann. Surg., 156:550, 1962.

Visalli, J. A., and Grimes, O. F. Embryologic and anatomic approach to treatment of gastric cancer, Surg., Gynec. & Obst., 103:401, 1956.

Walters, W. Developments in peptic ulcer surgery at the Mayo Clinic, Arch. Surg., 82:260, 1961.

Wangensteen, O. H., Peter, E. T., Bernstein, E. F., Walder, A. I., Sosin, H., and Madsen, A. J. Can physiological gastrectomy be achieved by gastric freezing? Ann. Surg., 156:579, 1962.

———— Varco, R. L., Hay, L., Walpole, S., and Trach, B. Gastric acidity before and after operative procedures with special reference to role of pylorus and antrum; preliminary report of clinical and experimental study, Ann. Surg., 112:626, 1940.

Welch, C. E., and Allen, A. W. Carcinoma of stomach, New England J. Med., 238:583, 1948.

Woodward, E. R., Bigelow, R. R. and Dragstedt, L. R. Effect of resection of antrum of stomach on gastric secretion in Pavlov pouch dogs, Am. J. Physiol., 162:99, 1954.

Zinninger, M. N., and Collins, W. T. Extension of carcinoma of the stomach into the duodenum and esophagus, Ann. Surg., 130:557, 1949.

Zollinger, R. M., and Ellison, E. H. Nutrition after gastric operations, J.A.M.A., 154:811, 1954.

PARTIAL GASTRECTOMY

Brunschwig, A., and Simandl, E. The first successful pylorectomy for cancer. Case history, Surg., Gynec. & Obst., 92:375–379, 1951.

Capper, W. M., and Welbourn, R. B. Billroth I gastric resection, Lancet, 2:193, 1954.

Clagett, O. T., and Waugh, J. M. Indications for and advantages of Schoemaker-Billroth I gastric resection, Arch. Surg., 56:758, 1948.

Colp, R., Klingenstein, P., Druckerman, L. J., and Weinstein, V. A. A comparative study of subtotal gastrectomy with and without vagotomy, Ann. Surg., 128:470, 1948.

———— Surgical management of the duodenal ulcer, Surg., Gynec. and Obst., 91:306, 1950.

Devine, H. B. Basic principles and supreme difficulties in gastric surgery, Surg., Gynec. & Obst., 40:1, 1925.

———— Gastric exclusion, Surg., Gynec. & Obst., 47:239, 1928.

Dunphy, J. E., and Hoerr, S. O. The indication for emergency operation in severe hemorrhage from gastric or duodenal ulcer, Surgery, 24:231, 1948.

Eastman, W. H., and Cole, W. H. Precautions and results in gastrectomy, Arch. Surg., 59:768, 1949.

Everson, T. C. Experimental comparison of protein and fat assimilation after Billroth II, Billroth I, and segmental types of subtotal gastrec-

tomy, Surgery 36:525, 1954.

———— Hutchings, V. Z., Eisen, J., and Witanowski, M. F. Comparative evaluation of dumping syndrome after parial gastrectomy and after vagotomy with gastroenterostomy, Ann. Surg., 145:182, 1957.

———— Hutchings, V. Z., Eisen, J., and Witanowski, M. F. Partial gastrectomy versus vagotomy with gastroenterostomy in treatment of duodenal ulcer, Arch. Surg., 74:547, 1957.

Farmer, D. A., Howe, C. W., Porell, W. J., and Smithwick, R. H. The effect of various surgical procedures upon the acidity of the gastric contents of ulcer patients, Ann. Surg., 134:319, 1951.

Finney, J. M. T. A new method of gastroduodenostomy. End-to-side, South. Surg. Transactions, 36:576, 1923.

Goligher, J. C., Moir, P. B., and Wrigley, J. H. The Billroth I and Polya operations for duodenal ulcer: a comparison, Lancet, 1:230, 1956.

Harkins, H. N., Schmitz, E. J., Nyhus, L. M., Kanar, E. A., Zech, R. K., and Griffith, C. A. The Billroth I gastric resection: experimental studies and clinical observations on 291 cases, Ann. Surg., 140:405, 1954.

Harvey, H. D. The nutritional status of patients after partial gastrectomy with gastrojejunostomy for duodenal ulcer, Surg., Gynec. & Obst., 105:559, 1957.

———— Safety in performing partial gastrectomy, for peptic ulcer, Ann. Surg., 153:256, 1961.

———— Twenty-four years of experience with elective gastric resection for duodenal ulcer, Surg., Gynec. & Obst., 112:203–210, 1961.

Herrington, J. L., Edwards, W. H., and Edwards, L. W. Re-evaluation of the surgical treatment of duodenal ulcer, Surgery, 49:540, 1961.

———— Consideration of the factors responsible for obstruction following a Billroth I anastomosis, Arch. Surg., 157:83, 1963.

Hickinbotham, P. The Billroth I gastrectomy, Brit. J. Surg., 44:206, 1956.

Hinton, J. W. The evaluation of end results in physiologic versus pathologic operative procedures: for chronic duodenal ulcer during the past two decades, Ann. Surg., 132:641, 1950.

Hodgson, P. E., and Hunter, D. C. Protection of a duodenal stump closure, S. Clin. North America, 41:1323, 1961.

Horsley, G. W., and Barnes, W. C. Twenty-five years' experience with Billroth I gastric resection, Ann. Surg., 145:758, 1957.

Jordan, G. L., Jr., de Bakey, M. E., and Cooley, D. A. Role of resective therapy in management of acute gastroduodenal perforation, Am. J. Surg., 105:396, 1963.

Kelling, G. Ueber die operative behandling des chronischen ulcus ventriculi, Arch. klin. chir., 109:775, 1918.

Lahey, F. H. The removal of the ulcer in subtotal gastrectomy for duodenal ulcer, S. Clin. North America, 32:6, 1952.

Localio, S. A. Adequate gastric resection with

PARTIAL GASTRECTOMY (cont.)

gastroduodenostomy, Surg., Gynec. & Obst., 101:269, 1955.

Marshall, S. F. Partial gastric resection for peptic ulcer, S. Clin. North America, 29:767, 1949.

Mathieson, A. J. H. Billroth I recurrent ulcer, Brit. J. Surg., 50:251, 1963.

Maynard, A. De L., and Prigot, A. Gastroduodenal perforation: a report of 120 cases over a five and one-half year period with consideration of the role of primary gastrectomy, Ann. Surg. 153:261, 1961.

Mayo, H. W., Jr., Owens, J. K., and Weinberg, M. A critical evaluation of radical subtotal gastric resection as a definite procedure for antral gastric carcinoma, Ann. Surg., 141:830, 1955.

McKittrick, L. S., Moore, F. D., and Warren, R. Complications and mortality in subtotal gastrectomy for duodenal ulcer, Ann. Surg., 120:531, 1944.

McNeer, G., Vandenberg, H. J., Donn, F. Y., and Bowden, L. A critical evaluation of subtotal gastrectomy for the cure of cancer of the stomach, Ann. Surg., 134:2, 1951.

Moore, H. G., Jr., and Harkins, H. N. The Billroth I Gastric Resection: With Particular Reference to the Surgery of Peptic Ulcer, Boston, Little, Brown and Co., 1954.

Morris, G. C., Jr., Greenfield, L. J., Jordan, G. L., Jr., Peddie, G. H., Gordon, J. R., and DeBakey, M. E. Physiologic considerations in the dumping syndrome, Ann. Surg., 150:90, 1959.

Morton, C. B., II, Alrich, E. M., and Hill, L. D., III. Internal hernia after gastrectomy, Ann. Surg., 141:759, 1955.

Newton, St. E. III, and Judd, E. S. Long term follow-up proves Billroth I gastric resection inadequate for permanent control of duodenal ulcer, Surg., Gynec. & Obst., 116:170, 1963.

Ordahl, N. B., Ross, F. P., and Baker, D. V., Jr. The failure of partial gastrectomy with gastroduodenostomy in the treatment of duodenal ulcer, Surgery, 38:158, 1955.

Pack, G. T., and Livingston, E. M. General technique of operations for gastric carcinoma, Am. J. Surg., 45:167–218, 1939.

Palumbo, L. T., and Sharpe, W. S. Partial gastrectomy for chronic duodenal ulcer with hemorrhage: results in 450 cases, Surgery, 49:585, 1961.

Patel, J. C. Les desinsertions accidentelles de la papille au cours des gastroduodenectomies, J. chir., 84:441, 1962.

Polak, M., Pontes, J. F. The cause of post-gastrectomy steatorrhea, Gastroenterol, 30:489, 1956.

Priestley, J. T., and Gibson, R. H. Gastrojejunal ulcer: clinical features and late results, Arch. Surg., 56:625, 1948.

Pulvertaft, C. N. Results of partial gastrectomy for peptic ulcer, Lancet, 1:225, 1952.

Ransom, H. K. Treatment of jejunal ulcer, Arch. Surg., 58:684, 1949.

Stafford, E. S., and Finney, G. G. Results of sur-

gical treatment of peptic ulcer, Ann. Surg., 155:687, 1962.

Stammers, F. A. A clinical approach to an analysis and treatment of post-gastrectomy syndromes, Brit. J. Surg., 42:28, 1961.

Stevens, A. R., Pirzio-Biroll, G., Harkins, H. N., Nyhus, L. M., and Finch, C. A. Iron metabolism in patients after partial gastrectomy, Ann. Surg., 149:534, 1959.

Stewart, J. D., Rudman, I., Citret, C., and Hale, H. J. The definite treatment of bleeding peptic ulcer, Ann. Surg., 132:681, 1950.

——— Cosgriff, J. H., and Gray, J. G. Experience with treatment of acutely massively bleeding peptic ulcer by blood replacement and gastric resection, Surg., Gynec. & Obst., 103:409, 1956.

Thal, A. P., Perry, J. F., Jr., and Wangensteen, O. H. Physiologic effects of various types of gastrectomy on gastric acid production with special reference to function of denervated gastric antrum, Surgery, 41:576, 1957.

von Haberer, H. Terminolaterale Gastroduodenostomie bei der Resektions Methode nach Billroth I, Zentrabl. f. Chir., 40:1321, 1922.

Wallensten, S., and Gothman, L. An evaluation of the Billroth I operation for peptic ulcer, Surgery, 33:1, 1953.

——— Results of surgical treatment of peptic ulcer by partial gastrectomy according to Billroth I and II methods: a clinical study based on 1256 operated cases, Acta chir. scandinav. (Suppl.), 191:1, 1954.

Walters, W., and Lynn, T. E. Results of 237 Billroth I gastric resections for peptic ulcer: a 6- to-15 year follow up, Ann. Surg., 144:464, 1956.

Wangensteen, O. H. The problem of surgical arrest of massive hemorrhage in duodenal ulcer, Surgery, 8:275, 1940.

Welch, C. E., and Rodkey, G. V. Partial gastrectomy for duodenal ulcer, Ann. Surg., 105:338, 1963.

Zollinger, R. M., and Ellison, E. H. Nutrition after gastric operations, J.A.M.A., 154:811, 1954.

RESECTION OF VAGUS NERVES ALONE
AND COMBINED

Bachrach, W. H. Laboratory criteria for completeness of vagotomy, Am. J. Digest Dis., 7:1071, 1962.

Beattie, A. D. Vagotomy and partial pylorectomy, Lancet, 1:525, 1950.

Burge, H. The hepatic vagal plexus, Lancet, 2: 899, 1961.

——— and Clark, P. A. Post-vagotomy diarrhoea: its cause and prevention, Brit. M. J., 1:1142, 1959.

——— and Vane, J. B. Method of testing for complete nerve section during vagotomy, Brit. M. J., 1:615, 1958.

RESECTION OF VAGUS NERVES ALONE
AND COMBINED (cont.)

——— Vagotomy in the treatment of peptic ulceration, Postgrad. Med. J., 36:2, 1960.

——— Vagal nerve section in chronic duodenal ulceration, Ann. Roy. Coll. Surgeons England, 26:231, 1960.

Coffey, R. J., and Lazaro, E. J. Vagotomy, hemigastrectomy and gastroduodenostomy (Finney–Von Haberer) in the treatment of duodenal ulcer, Ann. Surg., 141:862, 1955.

Crile, G., Jr., Jones, T. E., and Davis, J. B. Surgical treatment of duodenal ulcer—comparison of results with and without vagotomy, Ann. Surg., 130:31, 1949.

Dorton, H. E. Vagotomy and pyloroplasty for duodenal ulcer: evaluation of 15 years' experience, J. Kentucky M.A., 61:39, 1963.

Dorton, H. E. Vagotomy pyloroplasty and suture —a safe and effective remedy for the duodenal ulcer that bleeds, Ann. Surg., 153:378, 1961.

Dragstedt, L. R., and Owens, F. M., Jr. Supra diaphragmatic section of the vagus nerves in the treatment of duodenal ulcer, Proc. Soc. Exper. Biol. & Med., 53:152, 1943.

——— Clarke, J. R., Harper, P. V., Jr., Woodward, E. R., and Tovee, E. B. Supra diaphragmatic section of the vagus nerves to the stomach in gastrojejunal ulcer, J. Thoracic Surg., 16:26, 1947.

——— Harper, P. V., Jr., Tovee, E. B., and Woodward, E. R. Section of the vagus nerves to the stomach in the treatment of peptic ulcer. Complications and end results after four years, Ann. Surg., 126:687, 1947.

——— Oberhelman, H. A., Jr., and Smith, C. A. Experimental hyperfunction of the gastric antrum with ulcer formation, Ann. Surg., 134:332, 1951.

——— and Woodward, E. R. Appraisal of vagotomy for peptic ulcer after seven years, J.A.M.A., 145:11, 1951.

——— Oberhelman, H. A., Jr., and Woodward, E. R. Physiology of gastric secretion and its relation to the ulcer problem, J.A.M.A., 147:17, 1951.

——— Oberhelman, H. A., Jr., Evans, S. O., and Rigler, S. P. Antrum hyperfunction and gastric ulcer, Ann. Surg., 140:396, 1954.

——— Ragins, R., Dragstedt, L. R., II, and Evans, S. O., Jr. Stress and duodenal ulcer, Ann. Surg., 144:450, 1956.

Edwards, L. W., Herrington, J. L., Jr., Stephenson, S. E., Jr., Carlson, R. I., Phillips, R. J., Jr., Cote, W. R., Jr., and Scott, H. W., Jr. Duodenal ulcer: treatment by vagotomy and removal of gastric antrum, Ann. Surg., 145:738, 1957.

——— Edwards, W. H., Sawyers, J. L., Gobbel, W. G., Jr., Herrington, J. L., Jr., and Scott, H. W., Jr. The surgical treatment of duodenal ulcer by vagotomy and antral resection, Am. J. Surg., 105:352, 1963.

Farmer, D. A., Howe, C. W., Porell, W. S., and

Smithwick, R. H. The effect of various surgical procedures upon the acidity of the gastric contents of ulcer patients, Ann. Surg., 134:319, 1951.

Farris, J. M., and Smith, G. K. Role of pyloroplasty in the surgical treatment of gastric ulcer, Ann. Surg., 154 (Supp.):293, 1961.

——— and Smith, G. K. Treatment of gastric ulcer (in situ) by vagotomy and pyloroplasty: a clinical study, Ann. Surg., 1958:461, 1963.

——— and Smith, G. K. Vagotomy and pyloroplasty for bleeding duodenal ulcer, Am. J. Surg., 105:388, 1963.

Feggetter, G. Y., and Pringle, R. Long-term results of bilateral vagotomy and gastrojejunostomy for chronic duodenal ulcer, Surg., Gynec. & Obst., 116:175, 1963.

Franksson, C. Proceedings of Meeting of Svensk kiruryisk förening, Stockholm, October 24, 1947.

——— Selective abdominal vagotomy, Acta, Chir. Scandinav., 96:409, 1948.

Gillespie, I. E., and Kay, A. W. Effect of medical and surgical vagotomy on the augmented histamine test in man, Brit. M. J., 1:1557, 1961.

Griffith, C. A. Selective gastric vagotomy. Part I. Eliminating the occurrence of incomplete gastric vagotomy by refined technics of total abdominal and selective gastric vagotomy, West. J. Surg., 61:316, 1953.

——— and Harkins, H. N. Partial gastric vagotomy: an experimental study. Gastroenterology, 32:96, 1957.

——— Gastric vagotomy vs. total abdominal vagotomy, Arch. Surg., 81:781, 1960.

——— Selective gastric vagotomy. Part II. Eliminating undesirable sequelae of total abdominal vagotomy by selective gastric vagotomy, West. J. Surg., 70:175, 1962.

——— Stavney, L. S., Kato, T., and Harkins, H. N. Selective vagotomy combined with hemigastrectomy and Billroth I anastomosis, Am. J. Surg., 105:362, 1963.

Grimson, K. S., Taylor, H. M., Trent, J. C., Wilson, D. A., and Hill, H. C. The effect of transthoracic vagotomy upon the functions of the stomach and upon the early clinical course of patients with peptic ulcer, South. M. J., 39:460, 1946.

——— Rowe, C. R., Jr., and Taylor, H. M. Results of vagotomy during seven years, Ann. Surg. 135:5, 1952.

Hamilton, J. E., Harbrecht, P. J., Robbins, R. E., and Kinnaird, D. W. A comparative study of vagotomy and emptying procedure versus subtotal gastrectomy used alternately in the treatment of duodenal ulcer, Ann. Surg., 153:934, 1961.

Harkins, H. N., Stevenson, J. K., Jesseph, J. E., and Nyhus, L. M. The "combined" operation for peptic ulcer, Arch. Surg., 80:743, 1960.

——— Zech, R. K., Nyhus, L. M., Moore, H. G., Sauvage, L. R., and Griffith, C. A. The relative effects of different gastric drainage proce-

RESECTION OF VAGUS NERVES ALONE
AND COMBINED (cont.)

dures on the hormonal phase of gastric secretion, Surg. Forum, 5:281, 1954.

———— and Jones, T. W. The mechanism of inhibition of gastric acid secretion by the duodenum, Gastroenterology, 37:81, 1959.

———— Jesseph, J. E., Stevenson, J. K., and Nyhus, L. The "combined" operation for peptic ulcer, Arch. Surg., 80:743, 1960.

———— Stavney, L. S., Griffith, C. A., Savage, L. E., Kato, T., and Nyhus, L. M. Selective gastric vagotomy, Ann. Surg., 158:448, 1963.

Hartzell, J. B. The effect of section of the vagus nerves on gastric acidity, Am. J. Physiol., 91–92:161, 1929.

Hoerr, S. O., Brown, C. H., Ramsey, E. W., and Crile, G., Jr. Results of treatment of duodenal ulcer with vagus resection and gastroenterostomy, J.A.M.A., 149:16, 1952.

Hollander, F. The insulin test for the presence of intact nerve fibers after vagal operations for peptic ulcer, Gastroenterology, 7:607, 1946.

Howe, C. W., and Porell, W. J. Effect of fifty per cent gastrectomy alone and combined with vagotomy, Arch. Surg., 65:714, 1952.

Jackson, R. G. Anatomic study of the vagus nerves, with a technique of transabdominal selective gastric vagus resection, Arch. Surg., 57:333, 1948.

Jordan, G. L. The afferent loop syndrome, Surgery, 38:1027, 1955.

———— Quast, D., and Johnston, R. Hemigastrectomy and vagotomy for the treatment of duodenal ulcer, Am. J. Gastroenterol., 35:546, 1961.

Klein, E. Left vagus section and partial gastrectomy for duodenal ulcer with hyperacidity, Ann. Surg., 90:65, 1929.

Kraft, R. O., Fry, W. J., and Ransom, H. K. Selective gastric vagotomy, Arch. Surg., 85:687, 1962.

———— and Fry, W. J. Operative technic of selective gastric vagotomy, Am. J. Surg., 105:423, 1963.

Lake, N. C. Aftermath of gastrectomy, Brit. M. J., 1:285, 1948.

Latarjet, A. Note préliminaire sur l'innervation et l'énervation de l'estomac, Lyon méd., 130:166–167, 1921.

———— Résection des nerfs de l'estomac. Technique opératoire. Résultats Cliniques, Bull. Acad. de méd., Paris, 87:681, 1922.

MacKelvie, A. A. Vagal resection in treatment of duodenal ulcer, Brit. M. J., 1:321, 1957.

Moore, F. D., Chapman, W. P., Schulz, M. D., and Jones, C. M. Transdiaphragmatic resection of the vagus nerves for peptic ulcer, New England J. Med., 234:241, 1946.

———— Vagus resection for ulcer: an interim evaluation, I. Operative technique and hospital management, Arch. Surg., 55:164, 1947.

———— Vagus resection for ulcer: an interim evaluation, II. Clinical results, Ann. Surg., 126:664, 1947.

———— Follow-up of vagotomy in duodenal ulcer, Gastroenterology, 11:442, 1948.

Nyhus, L. M., Kanar, E. A., Moore, H. G., Jr., Sauvage, L. R., Schmitz, E. J., Storer, E. H., and Harkins, H. N. Gastrojejunostomy and Finney pyloroplasty: their effects upon Heidenhain pouch secretion in vagotomized and nonvagotomized dogs, Surg. Forum, 4:346, 1953.

Schiassi, B. The role of the pyloro-duodenal nerve supply in the surgery of duodenal ulcer, Ann. Surg., 81:939, 1925.

Smith, G. K., and Farris, J. M. Some observations upon selective gastric vagotomy, Arch. Surg., 86:716, 1963.

Walters, W., Neibling, H. A., Bradley, W. F., Small, J. T., and Wilson, J. W. A study of the results, both favorable and unfavorable, of section of the vagus nerves in the treatment of peptic ulcer, Ann. Surg., 126:679, 1947.

———— and Mobley, J. E. Five-to-ten-year follow up of 162 cases of duodenal ulcer treated by vagotomy with and without associated gastric operations, Ann. Surg., 145:753, 1957.

Weinberg, J. A. Treatment of the massively bleeding duodenal ulcer by ligation, pyloroplasty and vagotomy, Am. J. Surg., 102:158, 1961.

———— Vagotomy and pyloroplasty in the treatment of duodenal ulcer, Am. J. Surg., 105:347, 1963.

TOTAL GASTRECTOMY, SPLENECTOMY,
AND PARTIAL PANCREATECTOMY

Allen, A. W. Cancer of the stomach, Editorial, Surg., Gynec. & Obst., 92:757, 1951.

Amann, W., and Brunschwig, A. Importance of gastric mucosal patch in continuity with alimentary canal following total gastrectomy. Experimental study, Ann. Surg., 144:428, 1956.

Beal, J. M., Briggs, J. D., and Longmire, W. P., Jr. The use of jejunal segment to replace the stomach following total gastrectomy, Am. J. Surg., 88:194, 1954.

Berry, R. E. L., and Rottschafer, W. Lymphatic spread of cancer of stomach observed in operative specimens removed by radical surgery including total pancreatectomy, Surg., Gynec. & Obst., 104:269, 1957.

Boerema, I. The technique of our method of transabdominal total gastrectomy in cases of gastric cancer, Arch. Chir. Neerlandicum, 6:95, 1954.

———— The resectability of gastric carcinoma, Ann. Surg., 142:228, 1955.

Brigham, C. B. Case of removal of entire stomach for carcinoma, Boston M. & S. J., 138:415, 1898.

TOTAL GASTRECTOMY, SPLENECTOMY,
AND PARTIAL PANCREATECTOMY (cont.)

Brunschwig, A. Five-year survivors following pan-
creato-spleno-total gastrectomy for "advanced"
cancer of the stomach, Ann. Surg., 141:62,
1955.

Castleman, B. Extension of gastric carcinoma into
the duodenum, Ann. Surg., 103:348, 1936.

Coller, F. A., Kay, E. B., and MacIntyre, R. S.
Regional lymphatic metastases of carcinoma of
the stomach, Arch. Surg., 43:748, 1941.

Eker, R. Carcinoma of the stomach. Investigation
of the lymphatic spread from gastric carcinoma
after total and partial gastrectomy, Acta chir.
Scandinav., 101:112, 1951.

Everson, T. C. Nutrition following total gastrectomy; with particular reference to fat and protein assimilation, Surg., Gynec. & Obst., 95:209,
1952.

Farris, J. M., Ransom, H. K., and Coller, F. A.
Total gastrectomy. Effects upon nutrition and
hematopoiesis, Surgery, 13:823, 1943.

Finney, J. M. T., and Rienhoff, W. F., Jr. Gastrectomy, Arch. Surg., 18:140, 1929.

Garlock, J. H. Technical problems in the surgical
treatment of carcinoma of the esophagus and
upper stomach, J. Thoracic Surg., 16:215, 1947.

Giberson, R. G., Dockerty, M. B., and Gray, H.
K. Leiomyosarcoma of the stomach; a clinico-
pathologic study of 40 cases, Surg., Gynec. &
Obst., 98:186, 1954.

Graham, R. R. A technique for total gastrectomy,
Surgery, 8:257, 1940.

Harvey, H. D., Titherington, J. B., Stout, A. P.,
and St. John, F. B. Gastric carcinoma experience from 1916 to 1949 and present concepts,
Cancer, 4:717, 1951.

Harvie, J. B. Report of a case of recovery after
gastrectomy for carcinoma, Ann. Surg., 31:344,
1900.

Hoerner, M. T. Total gastrectomy, Am. J. Surg.,
86:646, 1953.

Hunnicutt, A. J. Replacing stomach after total
gastrectomy with right ileocolon, Arch. Surg.,
65:1, 1952.

Hunt, C. J. Construction of food-pouch-form segment of jejunum as substitute for stomach in
total gastrectomy, Arch. Surg., 64:601, 1952.

Judd, E. S., Jr., and Hoon, J. R. An investigation
of the merits of end to end esophagoduodenostomy, Arch. Surg., 61:102, 1950.

Lahey, F. H. Complete removal of the stomach
for malignancy with a report of five surgically
successful cases, Surg., Gynec. & Obst., 67:212,
1938.

——— and Marshall, S. F. Indications for, and
experiences with, total gastrectomy, Ann. Surg.,
119:303, 1944.

Lee, C. M., Jr. Transposition of a colon segment
as a gastric reservoir after total gastrectomy,
Surg., Gynec. & Obst., 92:456, 1951.

Longmire, W. P., Jr. Total gastrectomy for carci-

noma of the stomach, Surg., Gynec. & Obst.,
84:21, 1947.

——— and Beal, J. Construction of a substitute
gastric reservoir following total gastrectomy,
Ann. Surg., 135:637, 1952.

MacDonald, G. C. Total removal of stomach for
carcinoma of the pylorus: recovery, J.A.M.A.,
31:538, 1898.

MacDonald, R., Inglefinger, F. J., and Belding,
H. W. Late effects of total gastrectomy in man,
New England J. Med., 237:887, 1947.

——— Inglefinger, F. J., and Kotin, P. Predeter-
minism in gastric carcinoma as the limiting
factor of curability, Surg., Gynec. & Obst., 98:
148, 1954.

Marshall, S. F., and Uram, H. Total gastrectomy
for gastric cancer: effects upon mortality, morbidity, and curability, Surg., Gynec. & Obst., 99:
657, 1954.

McCorkle, H. J., and Harper, H. A. The problem
of nutrition following complete gastrectomy,
Ann. Surg., 140:467, 1954.

Nakayama, K. Evaluation of the various operative
methods for total gastrectomy, Surgery, 40:488,
1956.

Neibling, H. A., and Walters, W. Total gastrectomy with esophagoduodenal anastomosis, Proc.
Staff Meet., Mayo Clin., 21:449–453, 1946.

Pack, G. T., and McNeer, G. Total gastrectomy
for cancer: a collective review of the literature
and an original report of twenty cases, Surg.,
Gynec. & Obst., 77:265, 1943.

——— McNeer, G., and Booher, R. J. Principles
governing total gastrectomy: a report of 41
cases, Arch. Surg., 53:457, 1947.

Priestley, J. T., and Kumpuris, F. Total gastrectomy with esophagoduodenal anastomosis, Arch.
Surg., 56:145, 1948.

Ransom, H. K. Total gastrectomy, Arch. Surg.,
55:13, 1947.

ReMine, W. H., and Priestley, J. T. Late results
of total gastrectomy, Surg., Gynec. & Obst., 94:
519, 1952.

Richardson, M. H. A successful gastrectomy for
cancer of the stomach, Boston M. & S. J., 139:
381, 1898.

Roeder, C. A. Total gastrectomy, Ann. Surg., 98:
221, 1933.

Schlatter, C. Oesophago-enterostomy after extirpation of the stomach, Lancet, I:141, 1898.

Scott, H. W., Jr., and Longmire, W. P., Jr. Total
gastrectomy: report of 63 cases, Surgery, 26:
488, 1949.

State, D., Barclay, T. H. C., and Kelly, W. D.
Total gastrectomy with utilization of a segment
of transverse colon to replace the excised stomach, Ann. Surg., 134:1035, 1951.

Sweet, R. H. Total gastrectomy by the transthoracic approach, Ann. Surg., 118:816, 1943.

——— Total gastrectomy by the transthoracic approach; a subsequent report, Ann. Surg., 138:
297, 1953.

Wangensteen, O. H. Technical suggestions in the

TOTAL GASTRECTOMY, SPLENECTOMY, AND PARTIAL PANCREATECTOMY (cont.)

performance of total gastrectomy, Surgery, 25: 766, 1949.

Waugh, J. M., and Fahland, G. T. R. Total gastrectomy, S. Clin. North America, 25:903, 1945.

ULCEROGENIC TUMORS OF PANCREAS (ZOLLINGER-ELLISON SYNDROME)

Davis, C. E., Jr., Smith, P., Jr., and Davalos, X. S. Ulcerogenic tumor of the pancreas, Ann. Surg., 155:669, 1962.

Ellison, E. H. Ulcerogenic tumor of pancreas, Surgery, 40:147, 1956.

Gregory, R. A., Tracy, H. J., French, J. M., and Sircus, W. Extraction of a gastrin-like substance from a pancreatic tumor in the case of Zollinger-Ellison Syndrome, Lancet, 1:1045, 1960.

Oberhelman, H. A., Jr., Nelson, T. S., Johnson, A. N., Jr., and Dragstedt, L. R. II. Ulcergenic tumors of the duodenum. 153:214, 1961.

Potter, J. F., and Sabesin, S. M. Intractable peptic ulceration associated with islet cell carcinoma of the pancreas (Zollinger-Ellison Syndrome) and with endocrine adenomatosis, Ann. Surg., 154: 885, 1961.

Wermer, P. Genetic aspects of adenomatosis of endocrine glands, Am. J. Med., 16:363, 1954.

Zollinger, R. M., and Ellison, E. H. Primary peptic ulceration of the jejunum associated with islet cell tumors of the pancreas, Ann. Surg., 142: 709, 1955.

——— Technic of vagotomy, hemigastrectomy and Billroth I anastomosis, Am. J. Surg., 105: 413, 1963.

——— and Craig, T. V. Ulcergenic tumors of the pancreas, Am. J. Surg., 99:424, 1960.

——— Elliott, D. W., Endahl, G. L., Grant, G. N., Goswitz, J. T. and Taft, D. A. Origin of the ulcerogenic hormone in endocrine induced ulcer, Ann. Surg., 156:570, 1962.

PYLOROMYOTOMY (FREDET-WEBER-RAMSTEDT OPERATION)

Abt, I. A., and Strauss, A. A. Clinical study of 221 operative cases of hypertrophic congenital pyloric stenosis, M. Clin. North America, 9: 1305–1315, 1926.

Akin, J. T., Jr., and Forbes, E. B. Congenital hypertrophic pyloric stenosis, Surgery, 21:512, 1947.

Benson, C. D., and Lloyd, J. R. Infantile pyloric stenosis. A review of 1,120 cases, Am. J. Surg., 107:429, 1964.

Davis, H. H. Right rectus gridiron incision in congenital hypertrophic pyloric stenosis, Surg., Gynec. & Obst., 78:213, 1944.

Donovan, E. J. Congenital hypertrophic pyloric stenosis in infancy, Ann. Surg., 95:174–182, 1932.

——— Congenital hypertrophic pyloric stenosis, Am. J. Surg., 39:377–381, 1938.

——— Congenital hypertrophic pyloric stenosis, Surg., Gynec. & Obst., 83:261, 1946.

Downes, W. A. The operative treatment of pyloric obstruction in infants, Surg., Gynec. & Obst., 22:251–271, 1916.

Dufour, H., and Frédet, P. La sténose hypertrophique du pylore chez le nourisson et son traitement chirurgical, Rev. de chir., Paris, 37:208–253, 1908.

Findlay, L. Radiology in the diagnosis of hypertrophic pyloric stenosis, Arch. Dis. Childhood, 13:145–151, 1938.

Fleming, H. T. Pyloric obstruction following Ramstedt's operation, Brit. M. J., 2:995, 1939.

Hayes, M. A., and Goldenberg, I. S. The problems of infantile pyloric stenosis, Surg., Gynec. & Obst., 104:105, 1957.

Horgan, E. The use of a transverse abdominal incision in, and comments on, the surgical treatment of infantile pyloric stenosis, Surgery, 18: 399, 1945.

Jacoby, N. M. Pyloric stenosis. Selective medical and surgical treatment, Lancet, 2:748, 1944.

Judd, E. S., and Thompson, H. L. Hypertrophic stenosis of the pylorus in adults, S. Clin. North America, 13:801, 1933.

Keeley, J. L. Transverse incision for pyloromyotomy, Surg., Gynec. & Obst., 89:748, 1949.

Ladd, W. E., Ware, P. F., and Pickett, L. K. Congenital hypertrophic pyloric stenosis, J.A.M.A., 131:647, 1946.

Lanman, T. H., and Mahoney, P. J. Congenital hypertrophic stenosis of the pylorus; a study of four hundred and twenty-five cases treated by pyloromyotomy, Surg., Gynec. & Obst., 56:205–209, 1933.

Lynn, H. B. The mechanism of pyloric stenosis and its relationship to preoperative preparation, Arch. Surg., 81:453, 1960.

Mack, H. C. A history of hypertrophic pyloric stenosis and its treatment, Bull. Hist. Med., 12: 465, 595, 666, 1942.

McClure, C. C. Hypertrophy of the pyloric muscle in adults, Surg., Gynec. & Obst., 52:945–952, 1931.

McNamee, E. P. Pyloric stenosis with hypertrophy of the pyloric muscle in the adult, Am. J. Roentgenol., 29:24–29, 1933.

Miller, D. R., and Friesen, S. R. Hypertrophic pyloric stenosis: clinical analysis of 87 cases with special reference to etiologic factors, Am. Surgeon, 22:108, 1956.

Mouriquand, G., and Weill, L. Remarques concernant le diagnostic et le traitement de trente-trois sténoses pyloriques du nourrisson, Bull. Acad. de méd., Paris, 118:803–806, 1937.

——— and Weill, L. À propos du diagnostic de la sténose pylorique du nourrisson. Valeur de l'examen radioscopique, Lyon méd., 161:543, 547, 1938.

PYLOROMYOTOMY
(FREDET-WEBER-RAMSTEDT OPERATION) (cont.)

Pollack, W. F., and Norïis, W. J. Dr. Conrad Ramstedt and pyloromyotomy, Surgery, 42: 966, 1957.

Ramstedt, C. Zur Operation der angeborenen Pylorusstenose, Med. Klin., 8:1702–1705, 1912.

———— Zur Behandlung des Pylorospasmus der Säuglinge, Deutsche med. Wchnschr., 56:348, 350, 1930.

———— Ist die Pyloromyotomie beim kindlichen Pylorospasmus die Methode der Wahl? Chirurg., 3:449–451, 1931.

———— Die operative Behandlung der hypertrophischen Pylorusstenose der Säuglinge, Ergebn. d. Chir. u. Orthop., 27:54–105, 1934.

Rheinlander, H. F., and Swenson, O. The diagnosis and management of congenital hypertrophic pyloric stenosis, J. Pediat., 41:314–319, 1952.

Robertson, D. E. Congenital pyloric stenosis, Ann. Surg., 112:687–699, 1940.

Scudder, C. L. Stenosis of the pylorus in infancy, Ann. Surg., 59:239–257, 1914.

Szilagyi, D. E., and McGraw, A. B. The problems of infantile pyloric stenosis with particular reference to surgical treatment, Surgery, 13:764, 1943.

Thomson, J. Observations on congenital hypertrophy of the pylorus, Edinburgh M. J., 25:1–20, 1921.

Twining, E. W. Chronic hypertrophic stenosis of the pylorus in adults, Brit. J. Radiol., 6:644–655, 1933.

Varden, A. E. Hypertrophic pyloric stenosis in twins, J. Pediat., 3:493–497, 1933.

Weber, W. Ueber eine technische Neuerung bei der Operation der Pylorusstenose des Säuglings, Klin. Wchnschr., 47:763–765, 1910.

Wolfson, W. L. A modified Ramstedt operation, Ann. Surg., 101:965–968, 1935.

Wyatt, O. S. Hypertrophic pyloric stenosis: a review of 100 cases, Journal Lancet, 59:233, 1939.

PERFORATED DUODENAL ULCER

Auchincloss, H., Jr. Immediate subtotal gastrectomy for acute perforated peptic ulcer, Ann. Surg., 135:134, 1952.

Barber, R. F., and Madden, J. L. Acute gastroduodenal perforation, Am. J. Surg., 59:484, 1943.

Baritell, A. L. Perforated gastroduodenal ulcer, Surgery, 21:29, 1947.

Bedford-Turner, E. W. Conservative treatment of duodenal ulcer, Brit. M. J., 1:457, 1945.

Blackford, J. M. Panel discussion on ulcer, J.A.M.A., 120:825, 1942.

Bowers, W. F., Geer, T. M., and Hughes, C. W. Perforated duodenal ulcer; Results of individualized care, Arch. Surg., 82:293, 1961.

Byrd, B. F., and Carlson, R. I. Simple closure of peptic ulcer, Ann. Surg., 143:708, 1956.

Cellan-Jones, C. J. A rapid method of treatment in perforated duodenal ulcer, Brit. M. J., 1: 1076, 1929.

Cooley, D. A., Jordan, G. L., Brockman, H. L., and DeBakey, M. E. Gastrectomy in acute gastroduodenal perforation: analysis of 112 cases, Ann. Surg., 141:840, 1955.

Cope, V. Z. Discussion on the treatment of perforated peptic ulcer, Proc. Roy. Soc. Med., 31: 465, 1938.

Davison, M., Aries, L. J., and Pilot, I. A bacteriological study of the peritoneal fluid in perforated peptic ulcers, Surg., Gynec. & Obst., 68:1017, 1939.

DeBakey, M. E. Acute perforated gastroduodenal ulceration, Surgery, 8:852 and 1028, 1940.

Forty, F. One hundred cases of perforated peptic ulcer, with analysis of immediate and remote results of simple closure, Brit. M. J., 1:790, 1946.

Graham, R. R. Treatment of perforated duodenal ulcers, Surg., Gynec. & Obst., 64:235, 1937.

———— and Tovee, E. B. The treatment of perforated duodenal ulcers, Surgery, 17:704, 1945.

———— Treatment of acute perforation of duodenal ulcer, Am. J. Surg., 72:802, 1946.

Harvey, H. D. Acute massive hemorrhage and acute perforation in peptic ulcer, S. Clin. North America, 35:369, 1955.

Hastings, H., and Machida, R. Perforated peptic ulcer, results after simple surgical closure, Am. J. Surg., 102:136, 1961.

Jones, F. A., and Doll, R. Treatment and prognosis of acute perforated peptic ulcer, Brit. M. J., 1:122, 1953.

Keetley, C. B. The surgery of nonmalignant gastric ulcer and perforation, Lancet, 1:885, 1902.

Lowdon, A. G. R. The treatment of acute perforated peptic ulcer by primary partial gastrectomy, Lancet, 1:1270, 1952.

Mage, S., and Payson, B. A consideration of the present status of simple suture in the treatment of acute perforated gastroduodenal ulceration, Surg., Gynec. & Obst., 94:581, 1952.

Magladry, G. W., Jr., Herrod, C. E., and Mathewson, C., Jr. Perforations of gastroduodenal ulcers, analysis of two hundred two cases, Arch. Surg., 66:810, 1953.

Martinis, A. J., Olson, H. H., and Harkins, H. N. Treatment of perforated peptic ulcer: report of 437 surgical cases, West. J. Surg., 65:72, 1957.

Matheson, A. T. Perforated peptic ulcer: immediate and long term sequelae, Brit. J. Surg., 43: 641, 1956.

McCaughan, J. J., Jr., and Bowers, R. F. Simple closure for perforated peptic ulcer, Surgery, 42:476, 1957.

Mikulicz, J. Die chirurgische Behandlung des chronischen Mageneschwuers, Zentrabl. f. Chir., 24:69, 1897.

Miller, E. M., Mersheimer, W. L., and Silverstein, M. E. Management of acute gastroduode-

PERFORATED DUODENAL ULCER (cont.)

nal perforations, Am. J. Surg., 86:688, 1953.

Moore, H. G., Jr., Harkins, H. N., and Merendino, K. A. The treatment of perforated peptic ulcer by primary gastric resection, Surg., Gynec. & Obst., 98:105, 1954.

Noordijk, J. A. Perforated peptic ulcer, the results of treatment in The Netherlands (1934–1950). An analysis of 2,551 cases, Acta chir. Neerlandicum, 5:262, 1953.

Rea, C. E. Conservative versus operative treatment of perforated peptic ulcer, Surgery, 32:654, 1952.

Reid, R. Perforated peptic ulcer treated without operation, Lancet, 2:734, 1946.

Saegesser, F. The treatment of perforations of gastric, duodenal and jejunal ulcers, Surg., Gynec. & Obst., 102:157, 1956.

Seeley, S. F. Nonoperative treatment of perforated duodenal ulcer, Postgrad. Med., 10:359, 1951.

———— and Campbell, D. Nonoperative treatment of perforated peptic ulcer: a further report, Surg., Gynec. & Obst., 102:435, 1956.

Stabins, S. J. The aftermath of perforated duodenal ulcer, Surgery, 34:614, 1953.

Strauss, A. Primary gastric resection for perforated gastroduodenal ulcers, Ann. Surg., 120:60, 1944.

Taylor, H. Peptic ulcer perforation treated without operation, Lancet, 2:441, 1946.

———— Aspiration treatment of perforated ulcers, Lancet, 1:7, 1951.

———— and Warren, R. P. Perforated acute and chronic peptic ulcer: conservative treatment, Lancet, 1:397, 1956.

Turner, F. P. Acute perforations of stomach, duodenum and jejunum, Surg., Gynec. & Obst., 92:281, 1951.

von Haberer, H. Zur therapie akuter Geschwurs-perforationen des Magens und Duodenums in die freie Bauchhole, Wien. klin. Wchnschr., 32:413, 1919.

Wangensteen, O. H. Non-operative treatment of localized perforations of the duodenum, Minnesota Med., 18:477, 1935.

Zinninger, M. M. Should operation be discarded in treating perforated peptic ulcer? Surg., Gynec. & Obst., 91:244, 1950.

DUODENAL STENOSIS, ATRESIA, AND
DIAPHRAGMATIC OCCLUSION

Able, L. E. Duodenal obstruction in infants, Texas State J. Med., 48:11, 748–754, (Nov.) 1952.

Bachmann, K. D. Über die angeborene Duodenalstenose und ihre Umwandlung zur funktionellen Atresie, Ztschr. f. Kinkerh., Bd. 73:287–293, 1953.

Benson, C. D., and Coury, J. J. Congenital intrinsic obstruction of the stomach and duodenum in the newborn, Arch. Surg., 62:856–866 (June) 1951.

Bill, A. H., Jr., and Pope, W. M. Congenital duodenal diaphragm, Surgery, 35:482–486, 1954.

Billard, C. M. Traité des Maladies des Enfants, 3rd ed., 375–377, Paris, 1837.

Bland-Sutton, J. Imperforate ileum, Am. J. M. Sc., 98:457–462, 1889.

Bodian, M., White, L. L. R., Carter, C. O., and Louw, J. H. Congenital duodenal obstruction and mongolism, Brit. M. J., 1:4749, (Jan.) 1952.

Bolling, R. W. Complete congenital obstruction of the duodenum. Duodeno-jejunostomy at nine days, Ann. Surg., 83:543–544, 1926.

Boyd, R. Description of a malformation of the duodenum, Lancet, 1:648, 1845.

Braun, H. Angeborene Duodenalstenose bei einem Kind und bei einem 49 jahrigen Mann, Virchow's Arch. f. path. Anat., 302:618–626, 1938.

Brody, H. Ruptured diverticulum of the stomach in a newborn infant, associated with a congenital membrane occluding the duodenum, Arch. Path., 29:125–128, 1940.

Buchanan, G. Malformation of duodenum in a child, Tr. Path. Soc. London, 12:121–129, 1861.

Calder, J., Jr. Two examples of children born with preternatural conformations of the guts, Med. Essays & Observations, Edinburgh, 1:203–206, 1733.

Cannon, P. R., and Halpert, B. Congenital stenosis of the third portion of the duodenum with acute occlusion and rupture of the stomach, Arch. Path., 8:611–621, 1929.

Champneys, F. H., and Powers, D'A. Occlusion of the duodenum by complete membranous septum, Brit. M. J., 1:718, 1897.

De Sanctis, A. G., and Craig, J. D. Congenital duodenal stenosis and atresia, Am. J. Dis. Child., 37:818–831, (April) 1929.

Duckett, J. W. Intestinal obstruction in the newborn, Ann. Surg., 116:321–333, 1942.

Ernst, N. P. A case of congenital atresia of the duodenum treated successfully by operation, Brit. M. J., 1:644–645, (May 6) 1916.

Evans, H. M. On the development of the aortae, cardinal and umbilical veins, and the other blood vessels of vertebrate embryos from capillaries, Anat. Rec., 3[No. 9]:498–518, 1909.

Fanconi, G. Fünf Fälle von angeborenem Darmverschluss, Virchow's Arch. f. path. Anat., Bd. 229, 1921.

Farber, S. C. Congenital atresia of the alimentary tract: diagnosis by microscopic examination of the meconium, J.A.M.A., 150:1753, 1933.

Fockens, P. Ein operativ geheilter Fall von kongenitaler Dünndarmatresie, Zentralbl, f. Chir., 38:532–535, (April 15) 1911.

Forshall, I. Duodenal obstruction in the newborn with a description of four cases, Brit. J. Surg., 35:58–69, (July) 1947.

Forssner, H. Die angeborenen Darm- und Oesophagusatresien, Anat. Hefte, 34:1–160, 1907.

Fox, P. F. Duodenal obstruction in infants and

DUODENAL STENOSIS, ATRESIA, AND
DIAPHRAGMATIC OCCLUSION (cont.)

children, Arch. Surg., 67:475–489, 1953.

Galton, J. Congenital occlusion of the duodenum, Guy's Hosp. Rep., 50:221, 1893.

Garvin, J. A. Congenital occlusion of the duodenum by a complete diaphragm, Am. J. Dis. Child., 35:109–112, (Jan.) 1928.

Glaser, S. Congenital occlusion of the duodenum, Brit. M. J., 2:712–713, (Oct.) 1948.

Glover, D. M., and Hamman, C. A. Congenital obstruction in the newborn due to congenital anomalies, Ohio State M. J., 36:833–840, 1940.

——— and Barry, F. M. Intestinal obstruction in the newborn, Ann. Surg., 130:480–511, 1949.

Gomez, F., and Lozoya, J. Duodenal occlusion due to atresia with diaphragm in duodenojejunal angle, Bol. Méd. del Hosp. Inf. Mexico, 2:143–151, 1945.

Gordon, L. A case of congenital stenosis of the duodenum, Brit. J. Surg., 18:331–333, (Oct.) 1930.

Hamperl, H. Zur Kenntnis der angeborenen Duodenalstenose und ihrer operativen Behandlungsmöglichkeiten, Wien. klin. Wchnschr., 65:737–738, (Sept.) 1953.

Hicken, N. F., Snow, S., Couray, Q. B., and Jackson, E. G. Complete duodenal obstruction in the newborn, Am. J. Surg., 71:461–469, 1946.

Kautz, F. G., Lisa, J. R., and Kraft, E. Congenital duodenal obstruction, Radiology, 46:334–342, (April) 1946.

Keith, A. Constrictions and occlusions of the alimentary tract of congenital or obscure origin, Brit. M. J., 1:301–304, 1910.

Kreuter, E. Zur Aetiologie der congenitalen Atresien des Darms und Oesophagus, Arch. f. klin. Chir., 88:303–309, 1909.

Krieg, E. G. Duodenal diaphragm, Ann. Surg., 106:33–41, (July) 1937.

Ladd, W. E. Congenital obstruction of the duodenum in children, New England J. Med., 206:277–283, 1932.

——— Congenital duodenal obstruction, Surgery, 1:878–885, (June) 1937.

——— Personal communication.

Lampson, O. F. Duodenal septum, West. J. Surg., 54:384–389, 1946.

Lanman, T. H. Personal communication.

Madden, J. L., and McCann, W. J. Congenital diaphragmatic occlusion of the duodenum with a report of three cases, Surg., Gynec. & Obst., 103:1, 1956.

Maris, E. P., McGuiness, A. C., Lee, H. F., Rhoades, J. E., and Lee, W. E. Pre- and postoperative use of metal tipped gastroduodenal tube as aid in surgical treatment of duodenal obstruction in newborn, Ann. Surg., 117:348–354, 1943.

Menzes, H. Cited by Lampson.

Moore, N. Multiple diverticula of the small intestine with congenital stricture of the duodenum, Tr. Path. Soc. London, 35:202–204, 1884.

Morton, J. J. Atresia of duodenum and right internal hernia, Am. J. Dis. Child., 25:371–378, 1923.

——— Surgical care of patients in the extremes of life, Am. J. Surg., 30:92–108, 1935.

——— and Jones, T. B. Obstructions about the mesentery in infants, Ann. Surg., 104:864–891, (Nov.) 1936.

Nagel, C. E. Duodenal diaphragm as a cause of intestinal obstruction, J. Internat. Coll. Surgeon, 2:315, 327, 1939.

Nagel, G. W. Unusual conditions in the duodenum and their significance, Arch. Surg., 11:529–549, 1925.

Nakata, I. Zwei Fälle von angeborenem Darmstenose, Mitt. d. med. Gesellsch. zu Tokio, 52:622, 1938.

Nelson, W. I. Congenital diaphragm of the duodenum, Minnesota Med., 30:745–752, (July) 1947.

Peterson, E. W. In discussion of paper by Bolling, Ann. Surg., 83:543, 1926.

Preisich, K. Angeborener doppeltr Klappenverschluss des Duodenum, Jahrb. f. Kinder Heilk. 57:346–349, 1903.

Richter, H. M. Surgery of the Gastrointestinal Tract in Children. Abt's Pediatrics, Philadelphia, W. B. Saunders & Co., 1924, Vol. 3, p. 512.

Roe, W. F., and Shaw, E. H. A case of congenital atresia of the duodenum, Lancet, 2:947, 1911.

St. John, L., and Tamoney, H. Partial intestinal obstruction caused by an intraduodenal septum, Am. J. Dis. Child., 84:4, 439–441, (Oct.) 1952.

Santulli, T. V., and Blanc, W. A. Congenital atresia of the intestine: Pathogenesis and treatment, Ann. Surg., 154:939, 1961.

Saunders, J. B. de C. M., and Lindner, H. H. Congenital anomalies of the duodenum, Ann. Surg., 112:321–338, (Sept.) 1940.

Schaefer, M. Cited by Billard.

Schmid, F. Seltene angeborene Dünndarmverschlüsse, Kinderärztliche Praxis, 18:481–485, 1950.

Schridde, H. Über die Epithelproliferationen in der embrionalen menschlichen Speiseröhre, Virchow's Arch. f. path. Anat., 191:179–192, 1908.

Schroeder, C. H. Congenital obstruction of the duodenum; report of a case, J.A.M.A., 28:1039–1041, (April) 1922.

Schuier, F. L. Duodenalstenose bei neugeborenen, Kinderärztliche Praxis, 21:8, 354–358, (Aug.) 1953.

Schwegler, R. A., Jr., and Boyden, E. A. The development of the pars intestinalis of the common bile duct in the fetus with special reference to the origin of the ampulla of Vater and the sphincter of Oddi, Anat. Rec., 67:459, 1937.

Seidlin, S. M. Congenital Duodenal Septum with Obstruction. Bull. Johns Hopkins Hosp., 37:328–339, (Nov.) 1925.

Shaw, H. L. K., and Baldauf, L. K. Congenital stenosis of the duodenum; report of case, Arch. Pediat. 24:813–818, 1907.

DUODENAL STENOSIS, ATRESIA, AND
DIAPHRAGMATIC OCCLUSION (cont.)

Sheldon, W. P. H. Congenital atresia of the alimentary tract, Arch. Dis. Childhood, 1:279–284, (Oct.) 1926.

Silcock, A. Q. Epithelioma of the ascending colon; enterocolitis; congenital duodenal septum with internal diverticulum, Trans. Path. Soc. London, 36:207, 1885.

Smellie, J. M. Three cases of congenital duodenal occlusion, Brit. J. Child. Dis., 21:192–195, (July) 1924.

Spriggs, N. I. Congenital intestinal occlusion; an account of twenty-four unpublished cases with remarks based thereon and upon the literature of the subject, Guy's Hosp. Rep., 66:143–218, 1912.

Stetten, De W. Duodenojejunostomy for congenital intrinsic total atresia at the duodenojejunal junction; successful result in three-day old, one month premature infant weighing four pounds two ounces, Ann. Surg., 3:583–596, 1940.

Sumner, W. C., and Morris, K. A. Duodenal atresia in the newborn, Am. J. Surg., 68:120–123, (April) 1945.

Sweet, G. B., and Robertson, C. Case of congenital atresia of jejunum with recovery, Arch. Dis. Childhood, 2:186–188, (June) 1927.

Tandler, J. Zur Entwicklungsgeschichte des menschlichen Duodenums in fruhen Embryonalstadiem, Morphol. Jahrb., 29:187–216, 1902.

Terry, W. I., and Kilgore, A. R. Congenital stenosis of the duodenum in an adult, J.A.M.A., 66:1774–1776, (June 3) 1916.

Thorndike, A., Jr. Duodenal atresia and stenosis in infancy; important diagnosis: case reports, Boston M. & S. J., 196:763–768, 1927.

Turner, E. K. A case of congenital intrinsic obstruction of the duodenum, with associated malrotation of the gut, successfully treated by operation, M. J. Australia, 1:369–371, (March) 1950.

Walz: Cited by W. Weber, Med. Klin., 6:1294 and 1334, 1910.

Webb, C. H., and Wangensteen, O. H. Congenital intestinal atresia, Am. J. Dis. Child., 41:262–284, (Feb.) 1931.

Weber, G. Zur Diagnose und Klinik der angeborenen Duodenalstenose, Monatschr. f. Kinderh., 45:208–224, 1929.

Weber, W. Zur Kasuistik der angeborenen Atresie des Duodenum, Med. Klin., 6:1294 and 1334, 1910.

White, C. S., and Collins, J. L. Congenital duodenal obstruction, Arch. Surg., 43:858–865, 1941.

Wilkie, D. P. D. Duodenal diverticula and Duplicature of the duodenal wall, Edinburgh M. J., 11:219–229, 1913.

Wyss, M. O. Ueber kongenitale duodenal Atresien, Bruns Beitrage z. Klin. Chir., 26:631–666, 1900.

Young, E. R., and Mueller, J. J. Atresia of the duodenum, J. Iowa M. Soc., 28:240–243, (June) 1938.

MALROTATION OF THE COLON
AND VOLVULUS OF THE MIDGUT

Bardeen, C. R. The critical period in the development of the intestines, Am. J. Anat., 16:427, 1914.

Brenner, E. C. Total volvulus, Am. J. Surg., 16:34, 1932.

Brown, R. B., and Ross, D. Congenital abnormalities of intestinal rotation and mesenteric attachment—a cause of intestinal obstruction in the adult, Ann. Surg., 134:88, 1951.

Bush, J. A., Lenox, C. C., and Myers, H. C. Volvulus neonatorum, South. Surgeon, 13:204, 1947.

Del Junco, T., and Franco, R. Midgut volvulus with rectal hemorrhage in the newborn, Ann. Surg., 147:112, 1958.

Dott, N. M. Abnormalities of intestinal rotation: Their embryology and surgical aspects, with report of five cases, Brit. J. Surg., 11:251, 1923.

Duckett, J. W. Intestinal obstruction in the newborn, Ann. Surg., 16:321, 1942.

Elman, R. Ladd's operation for the cure of incomplete rotation and volvulus of the small intestine producing duodenal obstruction in infancy, Ann. Surg., 112:234, 1940.

Frazer, J. E., and Robbins, R. H. On the factors concerned in causing rotation of the intestine in man, J. Anat. & Physiol., 50:75, 1915.

Gardner, C. E., Jr., and Hart, D. Anomalies of intestinal rotation as a cause of intestinal obstruction: Report of two personal observations; Review of one hundred and three reported cases, Arch. Surg., 29:942, 1934.

——— The surgical significance of anomalies of intestinal rotation, Ann. Surg., 131:879, 1950.

Glover, D., and Barry, F. M. Intestinal obstruction in the newborn, Ann. Surg., 130:480, 1949.

Gripenburg, Lars. On the anomalies of intestinal rotation, Acta chir. Scandinav., 104:261, 1952.

Hamann, C. A. Faulty rotation of the intestine, Ann. Surg., 76:491, 1922.

Jones, T. B., and Morton, J. J. Congenital malformations of the intestine in children, Am. J. Surg., 39:382, 1938.

Ladd, W. E. Congenital obstruction of the small intestine, J.A.M.A., 101:1453, 1933.

——— Congenital duodenal obstruction, Surgery, 1:878, 1937.

——— and Gross, R. E. Abdominal Surgery of Infancy and Childhood, Philadelphia, W. B. Saunders Co., 1941.

Mall, F. P. Development of the human intestine and its position in the adult, Bull. Johns Hopkins Hosp., 9:197, 1898.

McIntosh, R., and Donovan, E. J. Disturbances of rotation of the intestinal tract; Clinical picture based on observation in twenty cases, Am. J. Dis. Child., 57:116, 1939.

Miller, E. M. Bowel obstruction in the newborn, S. Clin. North America, 27:73, 1947.

Mole, R. H. Congenital non-rotation of the intestine, Brit. J. Surg., 17:670, 1930.

Morton, J. J., and Jones, T. B. Obstructions about

MALROTATION OF THE COLON AND VOLVULUS OF THE MIDGUT (cont.)

the mesentery in infants, Ann. Surg., 104:864, 1936.

Nelson, W. The embryology of the midgut and its relation to midgut anomalies, Am. Surg., 18:579, 1952.

Raymond, H. E., and Dragstedt, L. R. Anomalies of intestinal rotation: A review of the literature with report of two cases, Surg., Gynec. & Obst., 53:316, 1931.

Rixford, E. Failure of primary rotation of the intestine (left sided colon) in relation to intestinal obstruction, Ann. Surg., 72:114, 1920.

Snyder, W. H., Jr., and Chaffin, L. Malrotation of the intestine, S. Clin. North America, 36:1479, 1956.

——— and Chaffin, L. Embryology and pathology of the intestinal tract: Presentation of 40 cases of malrotation, Ann. Surg., 140:368, 1954.

Stewart, J. S. Congenital extrinsic duodenal obstruction in the newborn, South. Surgeon, 14:15, 1948.

Summers, J. E. The dilated duodenum, Ann. Surg., 88:576, 1928.

Swenson, O., and Ladd, W. E. Surgical emergencies of alimentary tract of newborn, New England J. Med., 233:660, 1945.

Thompson, H. C., Jr. Intestinal obstruction in newborn due to volvulus, Arch. Pediat., 57:234, 1940.

Wakefield, E. G., and Mayo, C. W. Intestinal obstruction produced by mesenteric bands in association with failure of intestinal rotation, Arch. Surg., 33:47, 1936.

Wang, Chiu-an, and Welch, C. E. Anomalies of intestinal rotation in adolescents and adults, Surgery, 54:839, 1963.

Waugh, G. E. Congenital malformation of the mesentery: A clinical entity, Brit. J. Surg., 15:438, 1928.

Wikle, H. T. Congenital obstruction of small intestine, Am. J. Surg., 51:429, 1941.

Wright, R. D. B. Volvulus in 48-hour old baby, operation, recovery, Brit. M. J., 2:773, 1947.

EXCISION OF DUODENAL DIVERTICULA

Ackerman, W. Diverticula and variations of duodenum, Ann. Surg., 117:403, 1943.

Basch, S. Diverticulum of the duodenum with a report of a case diagnosed during life and successfully operated on, Am. J. M. Sc., 153:833, 1917.

Blegen, H. M., Swanberg, A. V., and Cox, W. B. Entrance of common bile duct into duodenal diverticulum: report of a case corrected by surgery, J.A.M.A., 148:195, 1952.

Boland, F. K., Jr. Acute perforated duodenal diverticulum: case report, Surgery, 6:65, 1939.

Case, J. T. Roentgen observations on the duodenum with special reference to lesions beyond the first portion, Am. J. Roentgenol., 3:314, 1916.

Cattell, R. B., and Mudge, T. J. The surgical significance of duodenal diverticula, New England J. Med., 246:317, 1952.

Chitamber, I. A. Duodenal diverticula, Surgery, 33:768, 1953.

Dunstan, E. M., Lowance, M. I., and Jones, E. C. The clinical importance of duodenal diverticula, South. M. J., 42:460, 1949.

Edwards, H. C. Diverticula of duodenum, Surg., Gynec. & Obst., 60:946, 1935.

Elstner, L., and Waugh, J. M. Duodenal and jejunal diverticula, Surgery, 41:674, 1957.

Ferguson, L. K., and Cameron, C. S., Jr. Diverticula of the stomach and duodenum: treatment by invagination and suture, Surg., Gynec. & Obst., 84:292, 1947.

Finney, J. M. T., Jr. Duodenal diverticula: their significance and treatment, South. Surgeon, 11:543, 1942.

Forssell, G., and Key, E. Ein Divertikel an der Pars descendens duodeni mittels Röntgenuntersuchung diagnostiziert und operativ entfernt, Fortschr. a. d. Geb. d. Röntgenstrahlen, 24:48, 1916–1917.

Greenler, J., and Curtis, C. Duodenal diverticula, Arch. Surg., 60:1011, 1950.

MacLean, N. J. Diverticulum of the duodenum: with report of a case in which the diverticulum was imbedded in the head of the pancreas, and a method for its removal, Surg., Gynec. & Obst., 37:6, 1923.

Mahorner, H., and Kisner, W. H. Diverticula of the duodenum and jejunum, Surg., Gynec. & Obst., 85:607, 1947.

——— Diverticula of the duodenum: a report of eight surgical cases, Ann. Surg., 133:697, 1951.

Mino, R. A., and Livingstone, R. G. A technic of exposure for diverticula of the third and fourth parts of the duodenum, Ann. Surg., 129:235, 1949.

Morrison, T. H., and Feldman, M. A case of carcinoma in a duodenal diverticulum: with a consideration of duodenal diverticulosis, Ann. Clin. Med., 4:403, 1925.

Morton, J. J. Surgical treatment of primary duodenal diverticula, Surgery, 8:265, 1940.

Ogilvie, R. F. Duodenal diverticula and their complications with particular reference to acute pancreatic necrosis, Brit. J. Surg., 28:362, 1941.

Pappalardo, C., and Sherwin, C. S. Duodenal diverticulitis with perforation: Report of three cases, Ann. Surg., 154:107, 1961.

Patterson, R. H., and Bromberg, B. Surgical significance of duodenal diverticula, Ann. Surg., 134:834, 1951.

Pearse, H. E. Surgical management of duodenal diverticula, Surgery, 15:705, 1944.

Waugh, J. M., and Johnston, E. V. Primary diverticula of the duodenum, Ann. Surg., 141:193, 1955.

Weintraub, S., and Tuggle, A. Duodenal diverticula, Radiology, 36:297, 1941.

Whitmore, W. H. Duodenal diverticula with ulceration, Am. J. Roentgenol., 59:343, 1948.

Excision of Duodenal Diverticula (cont.)

Zeifer, H. D., and Goersch, H. Duodenal diverticulitis with perforation, Arch. Surg., 82:746, 1961.

Zinninger, M. M. Diverticula of the duodenum: Indications for and technique of surgical treatment, Arch. Surg., 66:846, 1953.

Segmental Resection of the Small Intestine

Barnes, J. P. A safe, simple and efficient method of intestinal anastomosis, Surg., Gynec. & Obst., 80:656, 1945.

Botsford, T. S. Benign and malignant tumors of the small intestine, New England J. Med., 236:683, 1947.

Connell, F. G. Intestinal sutures, some old, some not so old, and a new one, Philadelphia Monthly M. J., 1:37, 1899.

———— Through-and-through intestinal suture, with report of additional cases, Am. Med., 5:135, 1903.

Cushing, H. W. The "right angle" continuous intestinal suture, Tr. Am. S. A., 17:297, 1899.

Foreman, R. C. Carcinoid tumors; a report of 38 cases, Ann. Surg., 136:838, 1952.

Halsted, W. S. Circular suture of the intestine—an experimental study, Am. J. M. Sc., 94:436, 1887.

Haymond, H. E. Massive resection of the small intestine, Surg., Gynec. & Obst., 61:693, 1935.

Kerr, H. H. The development of intestinal surgery, J.A.M.A., 51:641 (Aug. 25), 1923.

Lembert, A. Memoire sur l'enterorrphie—Rep. gen. d'anat. et de physiol., 2:104, 1826.

Madelung, O. W. Enterorrhaphy; its history, technique and present status, J.A.M.A., 21:215, 1893.

Maunsell, H. W. A new method of intestinal suture, Am. J. M. Sc., 130:245, 1892.

Morton, J. J. Factors determining the selection of operation in obstruction of the small intestine, Surgery, 1:848, 1937.

Murphy, J. B. Cholecysto-intestinal, gastro-intestinal, entero-intestinal anastomosis and approximation without sutures (original research), Chicago Med. Rec., 3:803, 1892.

Owings, J. C., and Stone, H. B. Technique of anastomosis using the stone clamp, Surg., Gynec. & Obst., 68:95, 1939.

Parker, E. M., and Kerr, H. H. Intestinal anastomosis without open incisions by means of basting stitches, Bull. Johns Hopkins Hosp., 19:132, 1908.

Rankin, F. W., and Mayo, C., II. Carcinoma of the small bowel, Surg., Gynec. & Obst., 50:939, 1930.

Rochlin, D. B., and Longmire, W. P., Jr. Primary tumors of the small intestine, Surgery, 50:586, 1961.

Sako, K., and Blackman, G. E. The use of a reversed jejunal segment after massive resection of the small bowels: an experimental study, Am. J. Surg., 103:202, 1962.

Scarff, J. E. Aseptic end-to-end suture of intestine, Ann. Surg., 83:490, 1926.

Summers, J. E. The treatment of annular gangrene of the small bowel by invagination versus resection, Surg., Gynec. & Obst., 44:374, 1927.

Ileo-Entectropy

Neumann, C. G., Braunwald, N. W., and Hinton, J. W. The absorption of ascitic fluid by a pedicled flap of intestinal mucosa exposed within the peritoneal cavity, Plast. & Reconstruct. Surg., 17:189, 1956.

———— Adie, G. C., and Hinton, J. W. The absorption of ascitic fluid by means of ileo-entectropy in patients with advanced cirrhosis, Ann. Surg., 146:700, 1957.

———— and Richman, H. Studies on the mechanisms of the control of ascites by means of ileo-entectropy, Plast. & Reconstruct. Surg., 20:379, 1957.

Intussusception

Benson, C. D., Lloyd, J. R., and Fischer, H. Intussusception on infants and children: Analysis of 300 cases, Arch. Surg., 86:745, 1963.

Bolling, R. W. Acute intussusception in infants, Ann. Surg., 78:349, 1923.

Brown, H. P., Intussusception in children, Ann. Surg., 81:637, 1925.

Clubbe, C. P. B. The Diagnosis and Treatment of Intussusception, 2nd ed., London, Oxford University Press, 1921.

Dennis, C. Resection and primary anastomosis in the treatment of gangrenous or non-reducible intussusception in children, Ann. Surg., 126:788, 1947.

Dennison, W. M. Acute intussusception in infancy and childhood, Glasgow M. J., 29:71, 1948.

Dowd, C. N. Resection of one-third of the colon for irreducible intussusception in an infant five days old, Ann. Surg., 57:713, 1913.

Goldenberg, I. S. Intussusception, Surgery, 36:732, 1954.

Gross, R. E., and Ware, P. F. Intussusception in childhood: experiences from 610 cases, New England J. Med., 239:645, 1948.

———— The Surgery of Infancy and Childhood, Philadelphia and London, W. B. Saunders Co., 1953.

Harkins, H. N. Intussusception due to invaginated Meckel's diverticulum, Ann. Surg., 98:1070, 1933.

Hays, D. M., Geller, F. C., Norris, W. J., and Snyder, W. H. A review of the management of intussusception in a pediatric center (1938–1958), Arch. Surg., 70:788, 1960.

Hipsley, P. L. Intussusception and its treatment by hydrostatic pressure. M. J. Australia, 2:201, 1926.

———— The treatment of intussusception, Surgery, 1:825, 1937.

INTUSSUSCEPTION (cont.)

Hogg, B. M., and Donovan, E. J. Acute intussusception, Ann. Surg., 124:262, 1946.

Hutchinson, J. A successful case of abdominal section for intussusception, Tr. Roy. Med.-Chir. Soc. Glasgow, 57:31, 1874.

Kahle, H. R., and Thompson, C. T. Diagnostic and therapeutic considerations of intussusception, Surg., Gynec. & Obst., 97:693, 1953.

Kirsner, J. B., and Miller, J. F. Roentgen diagnosis of intussusception, Radiology, 31:658, 1938.

Ladd, W. E., and Gross, R. E. Intussusception in infancy and childhood, Arch. Surg., 29:365, 1934.

Lawrence, G. H., and Ulfelder, H. Intussusception: a review of experience at The Masssachusetts General Hospital, 1937–1951, New England J. Med., 247:499, 1952.

Monrad, S. Acute invagination of the intestine in small children, Acta paediat., 6:31, 1926.

Montgomery, A. H. The treatment of irreducible intussusception in children, Surg., Gynec. & Obst., 51:415, 1930.

Nordentoft, J. M., and Hansen, H. Treatment of intussusception in children, Surgery, 38:311, 1955.

Peck, D. A., Lynn, H. B., and DuShane, J. W. Intussusception in children, Surg., Gynec. & Obst., 116:398, 1963.

Perrin, W. S., and Lindsay, E. C. Intussusception; a monograph based on 400 cases, Brit. J. Surg., 9:46, 1921.

Randolph, J. G., Zollinger, R. M., Jr., and Gross, R. E. Mikulicz resection in infants and children: a 20-year survey of 196 patients., Ann. Surg., 158:481, 1963.

Ravitch, M. M., and McCune, R. M., Jr. Reduction of intussusception by barium enema; a clinical and experimental study, Ann. Surg., 128:904, 1948.

———— and McCune, R. M., Jr. Intussusception in infants and children, J. Pediat., 37:153, 1950.

———— Jonathan Hutchison and intussusception, Bull. Hist. Med., 25:342–353, 1951.

———— A consideration of errors in the diagnosis of intussusception, Am. J. Dis. Child., 84:17, 1952.

Rutherford, H. Irreducible intussuspection in the infant treated by ileo-colic anastomosis, Brit. J. Child. Dis., 6:405, 1909.

Santulli, T. V., and Ferrer, J. M., Jr. Intussusception: an appraisal of present treatment, Ann. Surg., 143:8, 1956.

———— Intussusception, Am. J. Surg., 107:443, 1964.

Snyder, W. H., Jr., Kraus, A. R., and Chaffin, L. Intussusception in infants and children, Ann. Surg., 130:200, 1949.

Strang, R. Intussusception in infancy and childhood: a review of 400 cases, Brit. J. Surg., 46:484, 1959.

Swenson, O., and Oeconomopoulos, C. T. The operative treatment of acute intussusception in infants and young children, Am. J. Surg., 103:599, 1961.

Ware, G. W., and Coffey, R. J. Intussusception in infancy and childhood, Surg., Gynec. & Obst., 91:173, 1950.

White, M., and Dennison, W. M. Irreducible intussusception in infants, Brit. J. Surg., 40:137, 1952.

RESECTION OF MECKEL'S DIVERTICULUM

Chaffin, L. Surgical emergencies during childhood caused by Meckel's diverticulum, Ann. Surg., 113:47, 1941.

Gross, R. E. The Surgery of Infancy and Childhood, Its Principles and Techniques, Philadelphia and London, W. B. Saunders Co., 1953.

Haber, J. J. Meckel's diverticulum: review of literature and analytical study of twenty-three cases with particular emphasis on bowel obstruction, Ann. Surg., 73:468, 1947.

Hunt, V. C., and Bonesteel, H. T. S. Meckel's diverticulum containing aberrant pancreas, Arch. Surg., 28:425, 1934.

Jay, G. D., III, Margolis, R. R., McGraw, A. G., and Northrip, R. R. Meckel's diverticulum: A survey of one hundred and three cases, Arch. Surg., 61:158, 1950.

Kittle, C. F., Jenkins, H. P., and Dragstedt, L. Patent omphalomesenteric duct and its relation to the diverticulum of Meckel, Arch. Surg., 54:10, 1947.

Mason, J. M., and Graham, G. S. Ulceration of aberrant gastric mucosa in Meckel's diverticulum as a source of intestinal hemorrhage, Tr. Am. S. A., 50:316, 1932.

Merritt, W. W., and Rabe, M. A. Meckel's diverticulum; review of the literature and report of an unusual case, Arch. Surg., 61:1083, 1950.

Michel, M. L., Field, R. S., and Ogden, W. W., Jr. Meckel's diverticulum, Ann. Surg., 141:819, 1955.

Miller, R. H., and Wallace, R. H. Meckel's diverticulum in acute abdominal emergencies, Ann. Surg., 98:713, 1933.

Thompson, J. E. Perforated peptic ulcer in Meckel's diverticulum; report of a case occurring intramesenteric, Ann. Surg., 105:44, 1937.

APPENDECTOMY

Barrow, W., and Ochsner, A. Treatment of appendical peritonitis, J.A.M.A., 115:1246, 1940.

Bower, J. O. A clinical pathologic classification of acute appendicitis and peritonitis complicating perforative appendicitis, Am. J. Surg., 45:66, 1939.

Bowers, W. F. Appendicitis, with especial reference to pathogenesis, bacteriology, and healing, Arch. Surg., 39:362, 1939.

Boyce, F. F. Acute Appendicitis and Its Complication, New York, Oxford University Press, 1949.

Commission on Acute Appendicitis Mortality: Report of the third statewide survey of acute

APPENDECTOMY (cont.)

appendicitis mortality, Pennsylvania M. J., 55: 449, 1952.

Crile, G., Jr. Peritonitis of appendiceal origin treated with massive doses of penicillin; report of 50 cases, Surg., Gynec. & Obst., 83:150, 1946.

DeLamotte, J. Observations made at the opening of a body of a person dead of tympanites, J. de méd., chir., pharm., etc., Par., 24:65–68, 1766.

Fitz, R. H. Perforating inflammation of the vermiform appendix with special reference to its early diagnosis and treatment, Am. J. M. Sc., 92:321, 1886.

Fowler, G. R. Diffuse septic peritonitis, with special reference to a new method of treatment, namely the elevated head and trunk posture, to facilitate drainage into the pelvis, with a report of 9 consecutively treated cases of recovery, M. Rec., 57:617, 1900.

Hanford, J. M. Indications for intraperitoneal drainage in operations for acute appendicitis, S. Clin. North America, 19:385, 1939.

Hawk, J. C., Jr., Becker, W. F., and Lehman, E. P. Acute appendicitis: III, analysis of 1003 cases, Am. Surg., 132:729, 1950.

Hodges, P. C., and Miller, R. E. Intestinal obstruction, Am. J. Roentgenol., 74:1015, 1955.

Kelly, H. A., and Hurdon, E. The Vermiform Appendix and Its Diseases, Philadelphia, W. B. Saunders Co., 1905.

Lahey, F. H. Technical procedures making appendectomy for gangrenous appendix safer, S. Clin. North America, 22:783, 1942.

Madden, J. L. Immediate complications following appendectomy, S. Clin. North America, 44:411, 1964.

McArthur, L. L. Choice of incisions of abdominal wall; especially for appendicitis, Chicago M. Rec., 7:289, 1894.

McBurney, C. The incision made in the abdominal wall in cases of appendicitis, with a description of a new method of operating, Ann. Surg., 20: 38, 1894.

McGraw, A. B. Factors contributing to the low mortality from appendectomy for acute appendicitis, Arch. Surg., 58:171, 1949.

Mèlier, F. Memoire et observation sur quelques maladies de l'appendice caecale, J. gén. de méd., chir., et pharm., Par., 100:317–345, 1827.

Mestivier, M. On a tumor situated near the umbilical region on the right side, produced by a large pin found in the vermiform appendix of the cecum, J. de méd., chir., pharm., etc., Par., 10:441, 1759.

Murphy, J. B. Acute appendicitis, S. Clin. North America, 2:107, 1913.

Ochsner, A., and Lilly, G. D. Technique of appendectomy with particular reference to treatment of appendiceal stump, Surgery, 2:532, 1937.

Parkinson, J. Case of diseased appendix vermiformis, Med. Chir. Tr., 3:57, 1812.

Ransom, H. K. Delayed intervention in appendiceal abscess and spreading peritonitis due to appendicitis; Collective Review Internat. Abstr. Surg., 68:359, 1939.

Schulinger, R. N. Observations on mortality from acute appendicitis at a university hospital, 1916–46, Ann. Surg., 126:448, 1947.

Shipley, A. M. The treatment of peritonitis complicating appendicitis, New England J. Med., 219:333, 1938.

Tashiro, S., and Zinninger, M. M. Appendicitis: a review of 936 cases at Cincinnati Hospital, Arch. Surg., 53:545, 1946.

Turner, G. G. Acute appendicitis, Brit. M. J., 2: 691, 1938.

Wakeley, C. P. G. The position of the vermiform appendix as ascertained by an analysis of 10,000 cases, J. Anat., 67:277, 1933.

Wangensteen, O. H., and Paine, J. R. Treatment of acute intestinal obstruction by suction with a duodenal tube, J.A.M.A., 101:1532, 1933.

———— and Bowers, W. F. Significance of the obstructive factor in the genesis of acute appendicitis; an experimental study, Arch. Surg., 34: 496, 1937.

———— Intestinal Obstruction, 3rd ed., Springfield, Ill., Charles C Thomas, 1955.

ILEOSTOMY AND SUBTOTAL COLECTOMY

Bacon, H. E., Yang, L. M. O., Carroll, P. T., Cates, B. A., Villalba, G., and McGregor, R. A. Non-specific ulcerative colitis, with reference to mortality, morbidity, complications and long-term survivals following colectomy, Am. J. Surg., 92:688, 1956.

Brooke, B. N. The management of an ileostomy —including its complications, Lancet, 2:102, 1952.

———— Cortisone and ulcerative colitis, Lancet, 2:1175, 1956.

———— The outcome of surgery for ulcerative colitis, Lancet, 2:532, 1956.

Bruce, D., and Cole, W. H. Complications of ulcerative colitis, Ann. Surg., 155:768, 1962.

Colcock, B. P., Bansant, J. H., and Contreras, O. Surgical treatment of co-existing regional enteritis and ulcerative colitis, Surg., Gynec. & Obst., 112:96, 1961.

Counsell, P., and Dukes, C. The association of chronic ulcerative colitis and carcinoma of the rectum and colon, Brit. J. Surg., 39:485, 1951.

Crile, G., and Thomas, C. Y. Treatment of acute, toxic ulcerative colitis by ileostomy and colectomy, Gastroenterol., 19:58, 1951.

Davidson, M. Management of ulcerative colitis in children, Am. J. Surg., 107:452, 1964.

Dennis, C. Ileostomy and colectomy in chronic ulcerative colitis, Surgery, 12:435, 1945.

———— and Karlson, K. E. Surgical measures as supplements to the management of idiopathic and ulcerative colitis; cancer, cirrhosis, and arthritis as frequent complications, Surgery, 32: 892–912, 1952.

———— and Karlson, K. E. Minimization of risk and disability in idiopathic ulcerative colitis, Am. J. Surg., 90:761, 1955.

———— Cancer risk in ulcerative colitis: Formidability per patient year of late disease, Surgery, 50:568, 1961.

Donovan, M., and O'Hara, E. Sexual function fol-

ILEOSTOMY AND SUBTOTAL COLECTOMY (cont.)

lowing surgery for ulcerative colitis, New England J. Med., 262:719, 1960.

Garlock, J. H., and Kirschner, P. A. The prevention of ileostomy dysfunction, Surgery, 40:678, 1956.

Goligher, J. C. Primary excisional surgery in the treatment of ulcerative colitis, Ann. Roy. Coll. Surg., 15:316, 1954.

Hickey, R. C., Tidrick, R. T., and Layton, J. M. Fulminating ulcerative colitis with colonic wall necrosis, Arch. Surg., 86:764, 1963.

Jackson, R. J., Bargen, J. A., and Helmholz, H. F. Life history of 95 children with chronic ulcerative colitis, Am. J. Dis. Child., 59:459, 1940.

Korelitz, B. I., and Gribetz, D. The prognosis of ulcerative colitis with onset in childhood, II. The steroid era, Ann. Int. Med., 57:592, 1962.

Lichtenstein, I. L., and Herzikoff, S. S. Recurrent ileostomy prolapse—an old problem, Ann. Surg., 141:95, 1955.

Lyons, A., and Garlock, J. The relationship of chronic ulcerative colitis to carcinoma, Gastroent., 18:170, 1951.

Mayo, C., Fly, O., Jr., and Connelly, M. Fate of the remaining rectal segment after subtotal colectomy for ulcerative colitis, Ann. Surg., 144:753, 1956.

Miller, G. G., Gardner, C. McG., and Ripstein, C. B. Primary resection of colon in ulcerative colitis, Canad., M.A.J., 80:584, 1945.

Noble, T. B., Jr. Plication of the small intestine as prophylaxis against adhesions, Am. J. Surg., 35:41–44, 1937.

Prohaska, J. V., Dragstedt, L. R., II, and Thompson, R. G. Ulcerative colitis: Surgical problems in corticosteroid treated patients, Ann. Surg., 154:408, 1961.

Ripstein, C. B. Primary resection of colon in acute ulcerative colitis, J.A.M.A., 152:1093, 1953.

Rowe, R. J. Dilatation of colon (toxic megacolon) in acute fulminating ulcerative colitis, Dis. Colon & Rectum, 6:23, 1963.

Slaney, G., and Brooke, B. Cancer in ulcerative colitis, Lancet, 2:694, 1959.

Warren, S., and Sommers, S. C. Pathogenesis of ulcerative colitis, Am. J. Path., 38:243, 1961.

Wilcox, H. R., and Beattie, J. L. Carcinoma complicating ulcerative colitis during childhood, Am. J. Clin. Path., 26:778, 1956.

COLOTOMY, COLOSTOMY, AND
EXCISION OF POLYP OF SIGMOID COLON

Bacon, H., and Peale, A. R. Appraisal of adenomatous polyps of the colon: their histopathology and surgical management, Ann. Surg., 144:9, 1956.

Castleman, B., and Krickstein, H. I. Do adenomatous polyps of colon become malignant? New England J. Med., 267:469, 1962.

Castro, A., Ault, G. W., and Smith, R. J. Adenomatous polyps of the colon and rectum, Surg., Gynec. & Obst., 92:164, 1951.

Cattell, R. B., and Swinton, N. W. The diagnosis and treatment of sigmoidal polyps, New England J. Med., 222:535, 1940.

Coffey, R. J., and Brinig, F. L. Symposium on diagnosis and treatment of pre-malignant conditions: polyps of large bowel, S. Clin. North America, 30:1749, 1950.

Deddish, M. R., and Hertz, R. E. Coloscopy, S. Clin. North America, 37:1287, 1957.

Enquist, I. F. The incidence and significance of polyps of the colon and rectum, Surgery, 42:681, 1957.

Gants, R. T., Raymond, B. A., and Pope, J. K. Extended colotomy incisions for intraluminal examination of colon, Ann. Surg., 144:865, 1959.

Helwig, E. B. The evolution of adenomas of the large intestine and their relation to carcinoma, Surg., Gynec. & Obst., 84:36, 1947.

Jackman, R., and Mayo, C. W. The adenoma-carcinoma sequence in cancer of the colon, Surg., Gynec. & Obst., 93:327, 1951.

Jeghers, H., McKusick, V. A., and Katz, K. N. Generalized intestinal polyposis and melanin spots of the oral mucosa, lips and digits, New England J. Med., 241,993, 1949.

Lillehei, R. C., and Wangensteen, O. H. Colectomy for cancer, polyps and diverticulitis, J.A.M.A., 159:163, 1955.

Morton, P. C. Adenomas of colon and rectum; diagnosis and treatment in relation to cancer prevention, Ann. Surg., 138:92, 1953.

Shackelford, R. T., and McGeehan, J. S. Improved technique of coloscopy, J.A.M.A., 167:280, 1958.

Spratt, J. S., Ackerman, L. V., and Moyer, C. A. Relationship of polyps of the colon to colonic cancer, Ann. Surg., 148:682, 1958.

Staley, C. J., and Schwartz, H., II. Gastrointestinal polyposis and pigmentation of the oral mucosa (Puetz-Jeghers Syndrome), Surg., Gynec. & Obst., International Abstracts of Surgery, 105:1, 1957.

Sunderland, D. A., and Binkley, G. E. Papillary adenomas of the large intestine: a clinical and morphological study of 48 cases, Cancer, 1:183, 1948.

Swinton, M. W., and Warren, S. Polyps of the colon and rectum and their relation to malignancy, J.A.M.A., 113:1927, 1939.

—— and Doane, W. A. The significance and treatment of polyps of the colon and rectum, New England J. Med., 249:673, 1953.

Turell, R. Diseases of Colon and Anorectum, Philadelphia, W. B. Saunders, 1959.

—— Adenomas of the colon and rectum in children—a recapitulation, S. Clin. North America, 40:985, 1960.

TRANSVERSE COLON COLOSTOMY

Albers, J. H., and Smith, L. L. A comparison of cecostomy and transverse colostomy in complete colon obstruction, Surg., Gynec. & Obst., 95:410, 1952.

Allen, A. W., and Welch, C. E. Cecostomy, Surg., Gynec. & Obst., 73:549, 1941.

Berry, R. E. L. Acute obstruction of the colon, S. Clin. North America, 35:1373 (Oct.) 1955.

TRANSVERSE COLON COLOSTOMY (cont.)

DeBakey, M., and Ochsner, A. A new clamp for the Devine colostomy, Surgery, 5:947, 1939.

Dennis, C. Treatment of large bowel obstruction: transverse colostomy—incidence of incompetency of ileocecal valve; experience at the University of Minnesota Hospitals, Surgery, 15:713, 1944.

Devine, H. B. Carcinoma of the colon, Brit. M. J., 2:1245, 1935.

——— Operation on a defunctioned distal colon, Surgery, 3:165, 1938.

Hunt, C. J. Surgical decompression of the colon for malignant obstruction, Arch. Surg., 61:131, 1950.

——— Surface cecostomy as a procedure for the decompression of the acutely obstructive colon, Am. Surgeon, 20:1062, 1954.

Lichtenstein, M. E. Colostomy, S. Clin. North America, 35:1347 (Oct.), 1955.

Maynard, A. De L., and Turell, R. Acute left colon obstruction with special reference to cecostomy versus transversostomy, Surg., Gynec. & Obst., 100:667, 1955.

Rack, F. J., and Clement, K. W. Cecostomy and colostomy in acute colon obstruction, J.A.M.A., 154:307, 1953.

Wangensteen, O. H. Complete fecal diversion achieved by simple loop colostomy, Surg., Gynec. & Obst., 84:409, 1947.

RADICAL RIGHT HEMICOLECTOMY

Cattell, R. B., and Colcock, B. P. Primary resection of the right colon, S. Clin. North America, 26:606, 1946.

Colcock, B. P. Carcinoma of the right colon, New England J. Med., 246:391, (Mar. 13) 1952.

Cole, W. H. Recurrence in carcinoma of the colon and proximal rectum following resection for carcinoma, Arch. Surg., 65:264, 1952.

——— Packard, D., and Southwick, H. W. Carcinoma of the colon with special reference to prevention and recurrence, J.A.M.A., 155:1549 (Aug. 22) 1954.

Fisher, E. R., and Turnbull, R. B., Jr. The cytologic demonstration and significance of tumor cells in the mesenteric venous blood in patients with colorectal carcinoma, Surg., Gynec. & Obst., 190:102, 1955.

Griffin, G. D. J., Judd, E. S., and Gage, R. P. Carcinoma of right side of colon: operability, resectability and survival rates, Ann. Surg., 143:330, 1956.

Jamieson, J. K., and Dobson, J. R. The lymphatic system of the cecum and appendix, Lancet, 1:1137, 1907.

Judd, E. S., Jr., and Merrill, J. G. Surgical treatment of carcinoma of the right portion of the colon, S. Clin. North America, 30:1025, 1950.

Kerr, H. H. The development of intestinal surgery, J.A.M.A., 81:641, (Aug. 25) 1923.

Lahey, F. H. Resection of the right colon and anastomosis of the ileum to the transverse colon after the plan of Mikulicz, Surg., Gynec. & Obst., 54:923, 1932.

——— A discussion of the modified Mikulicz operation for carcinoma of the colon and its technic, S. Clin. North America, 26:610, 1946.

——— and Colcock, B. P. A modified Mikulicz resection for cancer of the colon, S. Clin. North America, 22:773, 1942.

Martin, W. L., Veri, F. A., and Bower, R. Carcinoma of the cecum, Surgery, 36:814, 1954.

Mayo, C. W., and Lovelace, W. R., Jr. Malignant lesions of the cecum and ascending colon, Surg., Gynec. & Obst., 72:608, 1941.

——— and Schlicke, C. P. End-to-end ileocolostomy: indications for, and evaluation of, in resection of the right portion of the colon in one stage for malignant lesions, Surgery, 12:716, 1942.

McKittrick, L. S., and Wheelock, F. C., Jr. Carcinoma of the Colon, Springfield, Ill., Charles C Thomas, 1954.

Patterson, J. R., and Deaver, J. M. Carcinoma of the cecum, Am. J. Surg., 81:6, 618, 1951.

Philips, J. W., Waugh, M. J., and Dockerty, M. B. The surgical significance of regional lymphatic drainage of the hepatic flexure, Surg., Gynec. & Obst., 90:455, 1951.

Ransom, H. K. Carcinoma of the right colon, Surgery, 5:340, 1939.

Singleton, A. O. The blood supply of the large bowel with reference to resection, Surgery, 14:328, 1943.

Steward, J. A., and Rankin, F. W. Blood supply of the large intestine: its surgical considerations, Arch. Surg., 26:843, 1933.

Welch, C. E., McKittrick, J. B., and Behringer, G. Polyps of the rectum and colon and their relation to cancer, New England J. Med., 247:959, 1952.

Whipple, A. O. Use of Miller-Abbott tube in surgery of large bowel, Surgery, 8:289, 1940.

RESECTION FOR CANCER OF SPLENIC FLEXURE

Allen, A. W. The development of surgery for cancer of the colon, Ann. Surg., 134:785, 1951.

Black, W. A., and Waugh, J. M. The intramural extension of carcinoma of the descending colon, sigmoid and recto-sigmoid, Surg., Gynec. & Obst., 87:457–464, 1948.

Cheever, O. The choice of operation in carcinoma of the colon, Ann. Surg., 94:705, 1931.

Clogg, H. S. Cancer of the colon: a study of seventy-two cases, Lancet, 2:1007–1012, 1908.

Gilchrist, R. K., and David, V. C. A consideration of pathological factors influencing five-year survival in radical resection of the large bowel and rectum for carcinoma, Ann. Surg., 126:421, 1947.

Jamieson, J. K., and Dobson, J. F. The lymphatics of the colon with special reference to the operative treatment of carcinoma of the colon, Ann. Surg., 50:1077, 1909.

Madden, J. L., and McVeigh, G. J. The extension of operation in the treatment of carcinoma in

RESECTION FOR CANCER OF SPLENIC
FLEXURE (cont.)

the region of the splenic flexure, S. Clin. North America, 34:523, 1954.

McKittrick, L. S. Principles old and new of resection of the colon for carcinoma, Surg., Gynec. & Obst., 87:15, 1948.

Moynihan, Lord Berkely. Abdominal Operations, 4th ed., Revised, Philadelphia and London, W. B. Saunders Co., 1926, Vol. 2, p. 27.

Rankin, F. W. In discussion of paper by Gilchrist and David, Ann. Surg., 126:421, 1947.

Stone, H. B. The limitations of radical surgery in the treatment of cancer, Surg., Gynec. & Obst., 97:129, 1953.

RADICAL LEFT HEMICOLECTOMY

Allen, A. W., and Welch, C. E. Malignant disease of the colon, Am. J. Surg., 46:171, 1939.

——— Carcinoma of the colon, Surgery, 14:351, 1943.

——— The development of surgery for cancer of the colon, Ann. Surg., 134:785, 1951.

Ault, G. W., Castro, A. F., and Smith, R. S. Clinical study of ligation of the inferior mesenteric artery in left colon resections, Surg., Gynec. & Obst., 94:223, 1952.

Block, O. Om Extra-Abdominal Behandling of Cancer Intestinalis, Nord. med. Ark., 2:1, 1892.

Brunschwig, A. Radical surgical management of cancer of the colon spread to tissues and organs beyond the colon, Dis. Colon & Rectum, 4:83, 1961.

Castro, A. F. Surgical technique of ligation of inferior mesenteric artery and preaortic lymphadenectomy, Surg., Gynec. & Obst., 102:374, 1956.

Cheever, O. The choice of operation in carcinoma of the colon, Ann. Surg., 94:705, 1931.

Cohn, I., Jr., and Rives, J. D. Antibiotic protection of colon anastomoses, Ann. Surg., 141:707, 1955.

——— and Rives, J. D. Protection of colonic anastomoses with antibiotics, Ann. Surg., 144:738, 1956.

Colcock, B. P. Colostomy: historical role in surgery of colon and rectum, Surgery, 31:794, 1952.

Gibbon, J. H., Jr., and Hodge, C. C. Aseptic immediate anastomosis following resection of the colon for carcinoma, Ann. Surg., 114:635, 1941.

Grinnell, R. S. Lymphatic metastases of carcinoma of the colon and rectum, Ann. Surg., 131:494, 1950.

——— Results in the treatment of carcinoma of the colon and rectum: an analysis of 2,341 cases over a 35-year period with 5-year survival results in 1,667 patients, Surg., Gynec. & Obst., 96:31, 1953.

Hallenbeck, G. A. Operations for carcinoma of the colon, Proc. Staff Meet. Mayo Clinic, 36:470, 1961.

Jamieson, J. K., and Dobson, J. F. The lymphatics of the colon with special reference to the operative treatment of carcinoma of the colon, Ann. Surg., 50:1077, 1909.

Kerr, H. H. The development of intestinal surgery, J.A.M.A., 81:641 (Aug. 25), 1923.

Madden, J. L., and Amendola, F. H. Radical left hemicolectomy, Diseases of the Colon and Rectum, 1:81–89, 1958.

Maingot, R., Dukes, C. E., and Lloyd-Davies, O. V. Discussion on pathology and treatment of carcinoma of colon, Proc. Roy. Soc. Med., 38:377, 1945.

——— Abdominal Operations, 3rd ed., New York, Appleton-Century-Crofts, Inc., 1955.

Mayo, C. W., and Schlicke, C. P. Carcinoma of the colon and rectum: a study of metastasis and recurrences, Surg., Gynec. & Obst., 74:83–91, 1942.

McNealy, R. W., and Lands, V. G. Primary anastomosis in the treatment of carcinoma of the colon, Surgery, 21:283, 1947.

Meyer, K. A., Sheridan, A., and Kozoll, D. "One stage open" resection of the left colon without complementary colostomy, Surg., Gynec. & Obst., 81:507, 1945.

Morgan, C. N. Trends in treatment of tumours of the rectum, rectosigmoid and left colon, J. Roy. Coll. Surg., Edinburgh, 1:112–125, 1955.

Paul, F. T. Colectomy, Brit. M. J., 1:1136, 1895.

Poth, E. J., Jacobsen, L. W., and Dunlap, W. Control of tumor transplantation after primary anastomosis of the colon, Surgery, 49:723, 1961.

Raiford, T. S. Carcinoma of the large bowel, Part I: the colon, Ann. Surg., 101:1042, 1935.

Rankin, F. W. Resection and obstruction of the colon (obstructive resection), Surg., Gynec. & Obst., 50:594, 1930.

——— Modern management of cancer of the lower gastrointestinal tract, Surg., Gynec. & Obst., 74:905, 1942.

——— In discussion of paper by Gilchrist and David, Ann. Surg., 126:421, 1947.

Ravdin, I. S. The consideration of some problems of large bowel carcinoma, Surg., Gynec. & Obst., 102:257, 1956.

Schoemaker, J. Some technical points in abdominal surgery, Surg., Gynec. & Obst., 33:541, 1921.

Shaw, R. S., and Green, T. H., Jr. Massive mesenteric infarction following inferior mesenteric artery ligation in resection of the colon for carcinoma, New England J. Med., 248:890, 1953.

Southwick, H. W., and Cole, W. H. Prophylactic measures in local recurrence and venous metastases in carcinoma of the colon, S. Clin. North America, 35:1363, 1955.

Stone, H. B., and McLanahan, S. Surgical aspects of carcinoma of large bowel, J.A.M.A., 113:2282, 1939.

——— and McLanahan, S. Resection and immediate aseptic anastomosis for carcinoma of the colon, J.A.M.A., 120:1362, 1942.

——— The limitations of radical surgery in the treatment of cancer, Surg., Gynec. & Obst., 97:129, 1953.

RADICAL LEFT HEMICOLECTOMY (cont.)

von Mikulicz, J. Small contribution to the surgery of the intestinal tract, Boston M. & S. J., 148:608, 1903.

Wangensteen, O. H. Primary resection (closed anastomosis) of the colon and rectosigmoid, Surgery, 14:403, 1943.

Waugh, J. M., and Custer, M. D. Segmental resection of lesions occurring in the left half of the colon with primary end-to-end aseptic anastomosis, Surg., Gynec. & Obst., 81:593, 1945.

Wilkie, D. P. D. Surgery of malignant disease of the colon, Edinburgh M. J., 46:1, 1939.

COLON AND RECTUM

Ackerman, L. V., and Wheat, M. W. The implantation of cancer; an unavoidable surgical risk? Surgery, 37:341, 1955.

Babcock, W. W. The operative treatment of carcinoma of the recto-sigmoid with methods for elimination of colostomy, Surg., Gynec. & Obst., 55:627, 1932.

Bacon, H. E. Evaluation of sphincter muscle preservation and re-establishment of continuity in the operative treatment of rectal and sigmoidal cancer, Surg., Gynec. & Obst., 81:113, 1945.

———— and McGregor, R. A. Diverticulitis and its surgical management, Surgery, 49:676, 1961.

Baker, J. W., Margetts, L. H., and Schutt, R. P. The distal and proximal margin of resection in carcinoma of the pelvic colon and rectum, Ann. Surg., 141:693, 1955.

Beard, R. G., and Gazet, J. C. Perforated diverticulitis (of the colon) with generalized peritonitis, Guy's Hosp. Rep., 110:263, 1961.

Best, R. R. Selection of patients and anastomotic procedures for carcinoma of rectum and rectosigmoid, Am. J. Surg., 76:654, 1948.

Bevan, P. G. Acute diverticulitis, a review of emergency admissions, Brit. M. J., 5223:400, 1961.

Boehme, E. J., and Hanson, P. J. Carcinoma of the colon and rectum: site of growth of 1,457 lesions, S. Clin. North America, 26:551, 1946.

Broders, A. C. The grading of carcinoma, Minnesota Med., 8:726, 1925.

———— Practical points on the microscopic grading of carcinoma, New York State J. Med., 32:667, 1932.

Brooke, B. N. The management of an ileostomy—including its complications, Lancet, 2:102, 1952.

———— Simplified operative routine for carcinomatous obstruction of colon, Lancet, 1:945, 1955.

Brown, D. B., and Toomey, W. F. Diverticular disease of the colon; a review of 258 cases, Brit. J. Surg., 47:485, 1960.

Coller, F. A., Kay, E. B., and MacIntyre, R. S. Regional lymphatic metastasis of carcinoma of the rectum, Surgery, 8:294, 1940.

Davis, J. E., Seavey, P. W., and Sessions, J. T. Villous adenomas of the rectum and sigmoid colon with severe fluid and electrolyte depletion, Ann. Surg., 155:806, 1962.

Deddish, M. R., and Stearns, M. W., Jr. Anterior resection for carcinoma of the rectum and rectosigmoid area, Ann. Surg., 154:961–966, 1961.

Devine, H. B. Excision of the rectum, Brit. J. Surg., 25:351, 1937.

Dillard, B. M., Spratt, J. S., Jr., Ackerman, L. V., and Butcher, H. B., Jr. Epidermoid cancer of anal margin and canal: review of 79 cases, Arch. Surg., 86:772, 1963.

Dineen, P. The effect of neomycin bowel preparation on the susceptibility to systematic staphylococcal infection: an experimental study, Surgery, 49:727, 1961.

Dixon, C. F. Anterior resection for malignant lesion of upper part of rectum and lower part of sigmoid, Ann. Surg., 128:425, 1948.

Donaldson, G. A. The management of perforative carcinoma of the colon, New England J. Med., 258:201, 1958.

Dukes, C. E. The classification of cancer of the rectum, J. Path. & Bact., 35:323, 1932.

Dunphy, J. E., and Broderick, E. G. A critique of anterior resection in the treatment of cancer of the rectum and pelvic colon, Surgery, 30:106, 1951.

Findlay, C. W., Jr., and O'Connor, T. F. Villous adenomas of the large intestine with fluid and electrolyte depletion, J.A.M.A., 176:404, 1961.

Fitzgerald, M. G. Extreme fluid and electrolyte loss due to villous papilloma of the rectum, Brit. M. J., 1:831, 1955.

Fletcher, W. S., Krippaehne, W. W., and Dunphy, J. E. Current considerations in surgery of cancer of the colon and rectum, S. Clin. North America 42:1219, 1962.

Gabriel, W. B., Dukes, C. E., and Bussey, H. J. R. Lymphatic spread in cancer of the rectum, Brit. J. Surg., 23:395, 1935.

Garlock, J. H., and Ginsburg, L. An appraisal of the operation of anterior resection for carcinoma of rectum and rectosigmoid, Surg., Gynec. & Obst., 90:525–534, 1950.

———— Lerman, B., Klein, S. H., Lyons, A. S., and Kirschner, P. A. Twenty-five years experience with surgical therapy of cancer of the colon and rectum; An analysis of 1,887 cases, Dis. Colon & Rectum, 5:247, 1962.

Gerber, A., Thompson, R. P., Jr., Reiswig, O. K., and Vannix, R. S. Experience with primary resection for acute obstruction of the large intestine, Surg., Gynec. & Obst., 115:593, 1962.

Gilbertsen, V. A. Adenocarcinoma of the large bowel: 1,340 cases with 100 per cent follow-up, Surgery, 46:1027, 1959.

———— Adenocarcinoma of the rectum: a 15-year study with evaluation of the results of curative therapy, Arch. Surg., 80:135, 1960.

———— The results of the surgical treatment of cancer of the rectum, Surg., Gynec. & Obst., 114:313, 1962.

———— Results of treatment of bowel cancer, Ann. Surg., 157:198, 1963.

Gilchrist, R. K., and David, V. C. Lymphatic spread of carcinoma of the rectum, Ann. Surg., 108:621, 1938.

COLON AND RECTUM (cont.)

——— and David, V. C. A consideration of pathological factors influencing five-year survival in radical resection of the large bowel and rectum for carcinoma, Ann. Surg., 126:421, 1947.

Ginzburg, L., Freund, S., and Dreiling, D. A. Mortality and major complications following resection for carcinoma of the large bowel, Ann. Surg., 150:913, 1959.

Goligher, J. C. The blood supply to the sigmoid colon and rectum: with reference to the technic of rectal resection with restoration of continuity, Brit. J. Surg., 37:157, 1949.

——— Dukes, C. E., and Bussey, H. J. R. Local recurrence after sphincter-saving excision for carcinoma of the rectum and rectosigmoid, Brit. J. Surg., 39:199, 1951.

——— The adequacy of the marginal blood supply to the left colon after high ligation of the inferior mesenteric artery during excision of the rectum, Brit. J. Surg., 41:351, 1954.

——— and Smiddy, F. G. The treatment of acute obstruction or perforation with carcinoma of the colon and rectum, Brit. J. Surg., 45:270, 1957.

Graham, A. S. Current trends in surgery of the distal colon and rectum for cancer, Ann. Surg., 127:1022, 1948.

Gray, J. Evaluation of conservative resection with end-to-end anastomosis of carcinoma of the rectum and lower sigmoid colon, Arch. Surg., 57:361, 1948.

Gregg, R. O. The place of emergency resection in the management of obstructing and perforating lesions of the colon, Surgery, 37:754, 1955.

Grinnell, R. S. Lymphatic metastases of carcinoma of the colon and rectum, Ann. Surg., 131:494, 1950.

——— Results in the treatment of carcinoma of the colon and rectum: an analysis of 2,341 cases over a 35-year period with 5-year survival results in 1,667 patients, Surg., Gynec. & Obst., 96:31, 1953.

Hochenegg, J. Die Sacrale Methode des Extirpation von Mastoarmkrebsen nach Prof. Kraske, Wien. klin. Wchnschr., 1:254, 1888.

Jackman, R. J. Conservative management of selected patients with carcinoma of the rectum, J. Colon & Rectum, 4:429, 1961.

Jones, T. E., Newell, E. T., Jr., and Brubaker, R. E. The use of alloy steel wire in the closure of abdominal wounds, Surg., Gynec. & Obst., 72:1056, 1941.

——— Robinson, J. R., and Meade, G. B. One hundred and thirty-seven consecutive combined abdominoperineal resections without mortality, Arch. Surg., 56:109, 1948.

Kraske, P. Zur Extirpation Hochsitzender Mastoarmkrebse, Verhandl. d. deutsch. Gesellsch. f. Chir., 14:464, 1885.

Laufman, H. Management of diverticulitis, International Abstracts of Surgery (Surg., Gynec. & Obst.), 115:409, 1962.

Lockhart-Mummery, J. P. Perineal excision for cancer of the rectum, Surg., Gynec. & Obst., 67:655, 1938.

MacLaren, I. F. Perforated diverticulitis: a survey of 75 cases, J. Roy. Coll. Surg. Edin., 3:129, 1957.

Madden, J. L., and Tan, P. Y. Primary resection and anastomosis in the treatment of perforated lesions of the colon, with abscess or diffusing peritonitis, Surg., Gynec. & Obst., 113:646, 1961.

——— and Lee, B. Y. Cancer of the colon, Am. J. Surg., 107:346, 1964.

Mayo, C. W., and Schlicke, C. P. Carcinoma of the colon and rectum: a study of metastasis and recurrences, Surg., Gynec. & Obst., 74:83–91, 1942.

McSwain, B., Sadler, R. N., and Main, F. B. Carcinoma of the colon, rectum and anus, Ann. Surg., 155:782, 1962.

Mersheimer, W. L., and Miller, E. M. Diffuse peritonitis secondary to intestinal perforation complicating malignant lesions of the colon, Surg., Gynec. & Obst., 99:436, 1954.

Miles, W. E. A method of performing abdominoperineal resection of the rectum and of the terminal portion of the pelvic colon, Lancet, 2:1812, 1908.

——— The radical abdominoperineal operation for cancer of the rectum and of the pelvic colon, Brit. M. J., 2:941, 1910.

——— Technique of the radical operation for cancer of the rectum, Brit. J. Surg., 2:292, 1914.

——— Cancer of the Rectum, London, Harrison and Sons, Ltd., 1924.

Morgan, C. N. Trends in treatment of tumours of the rectum, rectosigmoid and left colon, J. Roy. Coll. Surg., Edinburgh, 1:112–125, 1955.

——— and Griffiths, J. D. High ligation of the inferior mesenteric artery during operations for carcinoma of the distal colon and rectum, Surg., Gynec. & Obst., 108:641, 1959.

Muir, E. G. Carcinoma of the Colon. London, Edward Arnold, 1961.

Nachlas, M. M., and Hannibal, M. J. Histochemical observations on the polyp-carcinoma sequence, Surg., Gynec. & Obst., 112:534, 1961.

Quan, S. H. Q., Deddish, M. R., and Stearns, M. W., Jr. The effect of pre-operative roentgen therapy upon the 10 and 5 year results of the surgical treatment of cancer of the rectum, Surg., Gynec. & Obst., 111:508, 1960.

Quenu, V. Technique operatoire pour l'amputation du rectum cancereux, Bull. et mém. Soc. d. chirurgiens de Paris, 23:163, 1897.

Ramsey, W. H. Treatment of inoperative cancer of rectum by fulguration, Dis. Colon & Rectum, 6:114, 1963.

Rosi, P. A., Cahill, W. J., and Carey, J. A ten-year study of hemicolectomy in the treatment of carcinoma of the left half of the colon, Surg., Gynec. & Obst., 114:15, 1962.

Ruff, C. C., Dockerty, M. B., Fricke, R. E., and Waugh, J. M. Pre-operative radiation therapy for adenocarcinoma of the rectum and rectosigmoid, Surg., Gynec. & Obst., 112:715, 1961.

Colon and Rectum (cont.)

Ryan, P. Emergency resection and anastomosis for perforated sigmoid diverticulitis, Brit. J. Surg., 45:611–616, 1958.

Sames, C. P. Resection of carcinoma of the colon in the presence of obstruction, Lancet, 2:948, 1960.

Sawyer, J. L., Herrington, J. L., and Main, F. B. Surgical considerations in treatment of epidermoid carcinoma of the anus, Ann. Surg., 157: 817, 1963.

Shnitka, T. K., Friedman, M. H. W., Kidd, E. G., and Mackenzie, W. C. Villous tumors of the rectum and colon characterized by severe fluid and electrolyte loss, Surg., Gynec. & Obst., 112: 609, 1961.

Smithwick, R. H. Experiences with the surgical management of diverticulitis of the sigmoid, Ann. Surg., 115:969, 1942.

———— Surgical treatment of diverticulitis of the sigmoid, Am. J. Surg., 99:192, 1960.

Spratt, J. S., Ackerman, L. V., and Moyer, C. A. Relationship of polyps of the colon to colonic cancer, Ann. Surg., 148:682, 1958.

Starr, A., Mueller, S., and McKittrick, J. R. Villous adenoma of the colon associated with severe hypopotassemia, Arch. Surg., 73:995, 1956.

State, D. Combined abdominoperineal excision of rectum—plan for standardization of proximal extent of dissection, Surgery, 30:349–354, 1951.

Thorlakson, R. H., and Ross, H. M. Leiomosarcoma of the rectum, Ann. Surg., 154:979, 1961.

Wangensteen, O. H. Primary resection (closed anastomosis) of rectal ampulla for malignancy with preservation of sphincteric function, Surg., Gynec. & Obst., 81:1, 1945.

Wheat, M. W., Jr., and Ackerman, L. V. Villous adenomas of the large intestine; clinicopathologic evaluation of 50 cases of villous adenomas with emphasis on treatment, Ann. Surg., 147:476, 1958.

End-to-Side Ureterosigmoidostomy

Bricker, E. M. Substitution for the urinary bladder by the use of isolated ileal segments, S. Clin. North America, 36:1117, 1956.

Butcher, H. R., Jr., Sugg, W. L., McAfee, C. A., and Bricker, E. M. Ileal conduit method of ureteral urinary diversion, Ann. Surg., 156: 682, 1962.

Coffey, R. C. Physiologic implantation of the severed ureter or common bile duct into the intestine, J.A.M.A., 56:397, 1911.

———— Transplantation of ureters into large intestine, Surg., Gynec. & Obst., 47:593, 1928.

———— Bilateral submucous transplantation of ureters into large intestine by tube technic; clinical report of twenty cases, J.A.M.A., 93:1529, 1929.

Cordonnier, J. J. Ureterosigmoid anastomosis, Surg., Gynec. & Obst., 88:441, 1949.

———— and Lage, W. J. An evaluation of uretero-

sigmoid anastomosis by mucosa-to-mucosa method after two and one-half years' experience, J. Urol., 66:565, 1951.

Dean, A. The upper urinary tract following uretero-intestinal anastomosis for bladder tumors, J. Urol., 63:858, 1950.

Foulds, G. S. Historical data on ureteral transplantation; Peters' operation, Am. J. Surg., 22: 217, 1933.

Gilbride, J. J. A new operation for ureteral anastomosis, J.A.M.A., 57:821, 1911.

Higgins, C. C. Transuretero-ureteral anastomosis; report of clinical cases, Tr. Am. A. Genito-Urin. Surgeons, 27:279, 1934.

———— Aseptic uretero-intestinal anastomosis, J. Urol., 31:791–802, 1934.

Mathisen, W. New method for ureterointestinal anastomosis: preliminary report, Surg., Gynec. & Obst., 96:255, 1953.

Moore, T. D. Transureteropyelostomy and transuretero-ureterostomy: the indications and operative technique, J. Urol., 60:859, 1948.

Murphy, J. J., and Mikuta, J. J. Urinary diversion in pelvic exenteration, Surg., Gynec. & Obst., 112:743, 1961.

Nesbit, R. M. Ureterosigmoid anastomosis by direct elliptical connection; a preliminary report, J. Urol., 61:728, 1949.

Sharpe, M. W. Transuretero-ureteral anastomosis, Am. Surg., 44:687, 1906.

Tan, P. Y., Taira, A., Arcilla, C., McCann, W. J., and Madden, J. L. Cross end-to-side ureteroureterostomy between normal ureters and between the unilateral obstructed and normal ureter. An experimental study, Surgical forum, Am. Coll. Surg., 13:504, 1962.

Weyrauch, H. M., and Young, B. W. Evaluation of common methods of uretero-intestinal anastomosis: an experimental study, J. Urol., 67: 880, 1952.

Congenital Megacolon (Hirschsprung's Disease)

Bodian, M., Carter, C. O., and Ward, B. C. H. Hirschsprung's disease, Lancet, 1:302, 1951.

Duhamel, B. A new operation for the treatment of Hirschsprung's Disease, Arch. Dis. Child., 35:38, 1960.

Ephrenpreis, T. H. Long term results of rectosigmoidectomy for Hirschsprung's Disease, with a note on Duhamel's operation, Surgery, 49:701, 1961.

Fisher, J. H., and Swenson, O. Aganglionic lesions of the colon, Am. J. Surg., 99:134, 1960.

Hallenbeck, G. A. The diagnosis of aganglionic disease of the bowel (Hirschsprung's Disease), S. Clin. North America, 41:935, 1961.

Hiatt, R. B. The pathologic physiology of congenital megacolon, Ann. Surg., 133:313, 1951.

———— The surgical treatment of congenital megacolon, Ann. Surg., 133:321, 1951.

———— The physiological bases for surgery in congenital megacolon, S. Clin. North America, 38: 561, 1958.

Congenital Megacolon (Hirschsprung's Disease) (cont.)

Hirschsprung, H. Stuhltragheit Neugeborener in Folge von Dilatation und Hypertrophie des Colons, Jahrb. f. Kinderh., 27:1, 1888.

———— Fortsatte Erfaringer Om den Medfodte Dilatation Og Hypertrofi of Tyktarmen, Hospitalstid., 43:165, 1900.

Lee, C. M., Jr. Megacolon with particular reference to Hirschsprung's disease, Surgery, 37:762, 1955.

Martin, L. W., and Altemeier, W. A. Clinical experience with a new operation (modified Duhamel procedure) for Hirschsprung's Disease, Ann. Surg., 156:678, 1962.

Potts, W. J., Riker, W. L., DeBoer, A., and Baffes, T. G. Intestinal obstruction in the newborn, Arch. Surg., 75:684, 1957.

State, D. Segmental colon resection in the treatment of congenital megacolon (Hirschsprung's Disease), Am. J. Surg., 105:93, 1963.

Swenson, O., and Bill, A. H., Jr. Resection of rectum and rectosigmoid with preservation of the sphincter for benign spastic lesions producing megacolon, Surgery, 24:212, 1948.

———— Neuhauser, E. B. D., and Pickett, L. K. New concepts of the etiology, diagnosis and treatment of congenital megacolon (Hirschsprung's disease), Pediatrics, 4:201, 1949.

———— Rheinlander, H. F., and Diamond, I. Hirschsprung's disease: a new concept of the etiology, New England J. Med., 241:551, 1949.

———— and Fisher, J. H. Resection of colon for Hirschsprung's disease, S. Clin. North America, 36:821, 1956.

———— and Fisher, J. H. Hirschsprung's disease during infancy, S. Clin. North America, 36:1511, 1956.

———— Follow-up on 200 patients treated for Hirschsprung's disease during a ten-year period, Ann. Surg., 146:706, 1957.

Tiffin, M. E., Chandler, L. R., and Faber, H. K. Localized absence of the myenteric plexus in congenital megacolon, Am. J. Dis. Child., 59:1071, 1940.

Whitehouse, F. R., and Kernohan, J. W. The myenteric plexus in congenital megacolon, Arch. Int. Med., 82:75, 1948.

Imperforate Anus

Arey, L. B. Developmental Anatomy, 6th ed., Philadelphia, W. B. Saunders Co., 1954.

Bacon, H. E., and Sherman, L. F. Surgical management of congenital malformation of the anus and rectum. Report of 3 cases, Arch. Surg., 64:331, 1952.

Berman, J. K. Congenital anomalies of the rectum and anus, Surg., Gynec. & Obst., 66:11, 1938.

Bill, A. H., Jr. Pathology and surgical treatment of "imperforate anus," J.A.M.A., 166:1429 (March 22) 1958.

———— Johnson, R. J., and Foster, R. A. Anteriorly placed rectal opening in the perineum (ectopic anus), Ann. Surg., 147:173, 1958.

Bradham, R. R. Delayed correction of type III imperforate anus in the male child, Ann. Surg., 154:972, 1961.

Brenner, E. C. Congenital defects of the anus and rectum, Surg., Gynec. & Obst., 20:579, 1915.

David, V. C. The treatment of congenital openings of the rectum into the vagina—atresia and vaginalis, Surgery, 1:163, 1937.

Donovan, E. J., and Stanley-Brown, E. G. Imperforate anus, Ann. Surg., 147:203, 1958.

Dunphy, J. E. Surgical anatomy of the anal canal, Arch. Surg., 57:791, 1948.

Gross, R. E. The Surgery of Infancy and Childhood: Its Principles and Technics, Philadelphia, W. B. Saunders Co., 1953, pp. 348–368.

Johnson, F. P. The development of the rectum in the human embryo, Am. J. Anat., 16:1, 1914.

Keith, A. Malformation of the hind end of the body, Brit. M. J., 2:1736, 1908.

Kiesewetter, W. B., Turner, C. R., and Sieber, W. K. Imperforate anus. Review of a sixteen-year experience with 146 patients, Am. J. Surg., 107:412, 1964.

———— and Turner, C. R. Continence after surgery for imperforate anus: a critical analysis and preliminary experience with sacroperineal pull-through, Ann. Surg., 158:498, 1963.

Koop, C. E. The management of imperforate anus, Pennsylvania M. J., 53:248, 1950.

Ladd, W. E., and Gross, R. E. Congenital malformations of anus and rectum, Am. J. Surg., 23:167, 1934.

Norris, W. J., Brophy, T. W., III, and Brayton, D. Imperforate anus: a case series and preliminary report on the one-stage abdominoperineal operation, Surg., Gynec. & Obst., 88:623, 1949.

Pohlman, A. G. The development of the cloaca in human embryos, Am. J. Anat., 12:1, 1911.

Potts, W. J., Riker, W. L., and De Boer, A. Imperforate anus with recto-vesical, urethro-vaginal and perineal fistula, Ann. Surg., 140:381, 1954.

Rhoads, J. E., Pipes, R. L., and Randall, J. P. A simultaneous abdominal and perineal approach in operations for imperforate anus with atresia of the rectum and recto-sigmoid, Ann. Surg., 127:552, 1948.

Rosenblatt, M. S., and May, A. Malformation of anus and rectum, Surg., Gynec. & Obst., 83:499, 1946.

Santulli, T. V. The treatment of imperforate anus and associated fistulas, Surg., Gynec. & Obst., 95:601, 1952.

———— In Benson, C. D., Mustard, W. T., Ravitch, M. M., Snyder, W. H., Jr., and Welch, K. J. Pediatric Surgery, Chicago, Year Book Publishers, 1962, p. 821.

Scott, J. E. S., Swenson, O., and Fisher, J. H. Some comments on the surgical treatment of imperforate anus, Am. J. Surg., 99:137, 1960.

Swenson, O., and Grana, L. Long term results of surgical treatment of imperforated anus. Dis. Col. & Rect., 5:13, 1962.

Trusler, G. A., and Wilkinson, R. H. Imperforate

IMPERFORATE ANUS (cont.)

anus: a review of 147 cases, Canad. J. Surg., 5:269, 1962.

Wallace, F. T., and Colvin, E. M. Complications of imperforate anus repair, Surgery, 24:832, 1948.

Wangensteen, O. H., and Rice, C. O. Imperforate anus, Ann. Surg., 92:77, 1930.

EXCISION OF FISSURE IN ANO

Blaisdell, P. C. Pathogenesis of anal fissure and implications as to treatment, Surg., Gynec. & Obst., 65:672, 1937.

Brossy, J. Anatomy and surgery of anal fissure. With special reference to internal sphincterotomy, Ann. Surg., 144:991, 1956.

Buie, L. A. Practical Proctology, Philadelphia, W. B. Saunders Co., 1937.

Hughes, E. S. R. Anal fissure, Brit. M. J., 2:803, 1953.

Turell, R. Surgical treatment of chronic anal fissure, Surg., Gynec. & Obst., 86:434, 1948.

EXCISION OF FISTULA IN ANO

Dunphy, J. E., and Pikula, J. Fact and fancy about fistula-in-ano, S. Clin. North America, 35:1469, 1955.

Fansler, W. A. Anal fistula and abscess, Am. J. Surg., 56:144, 1942.

Milligan, E. T. C., and Morgan, C. N. Surgical anatomy of the anal canal with special reference to anorectal fistulae, Lancet, 2:1150–1156, 1213–1217, 1934.

———— Morgan, C. N., Lloyd-Davies, O. V., and Thompson, H. R. Fistula in Ano, in British Surgical Practice, London, Thornton Butterworth, Ltd., 1948, Vol. 4.

HEMORRHOIDECTOMY

Bacon, H. E. Anus, Rectum, Sigmoid Colon, Philadelphia, J. B. Lippincott Co., 1949.

Baumeister, C. A., and Moon, L. A complete technique of hemorrhoidectomy, Surg., Gynec. & Obst., 71:360, 1940.

Ewing, M. R. The white line of Hilton, Proc. Roy. Soc. Med., 47:525, 1954.

Fansler, W. A., and Anderson, J. K. A plastic operation for certain types of hemorrhoids, J.A.M.A., 101:1064, 1933.

———— The surgical treatment of hemorrhoids, Minnesota Med., 17:254, 1934.

Fine, J., and Lawes, C. H. W. On the muscle-fibers of the anal submucosa with special reference to the pecten band, Brit. J. Surg., 27:723, 1940.

Gass, O. C., and Adams, J. Hemorrhoids, etiology and pathology, Am. J. Surg., 79:40, 1950.

Goligher, J. C., Leacock, A. G., and Brossy, J. J. The surgical anatomy of the anal canal, Brit. J. Surg., 43:51–61, 1955.

Granet, E. Plastic surgical procedure for extensive, complicated hemorrhoids, Dis. Colon & Rectum, 6:102, 1963.

Laufman, H. History of hemorrhoids, Am. J. Surg., 53:381, 1941.

Lewis, A. E. Anorectoplasty for hemorrhoidal surgery, Am. J. Surg., 90:767, 1955.

Milligan, E. T. C., Morgan, C. N., Jones, L. E., and Officer, R. Surgical anatomy of anal canal and operative treatment of hemorrhoids, Lancet, 2:1119, 1937.

Morgan, C. N. Hemorrhoids and their surgical treatment: a description of the St. Mark's Hospital operation for hemorrhoids, S. Clin. North America, 35:1457, 1955.

Parks, A. G. A note on the anatomy of the anal canal, Proc. Roy. Soc. Med., 47:997, 1954.

———— The surgical treatment of hemorrhoids, Brit. J. Surg., 43:23, 1956.

Rosser, C. The rational management of hemorrhoids, Texas State J. Med., 34:484, 1938.

Söderlund, S. Results of hemorrhoidectomy according to Milligan: a follow-up study of 100 patients, Acta, Chir. Scandinav., 124:444, 1962.

Swinton, N. W., and Mumma, J. F. The treatment of hemorrhoids, S. Clin. North America, 36:761, 1956.

Terrell, R. V., and Chewning, C. C., Jr. Present status of injection treatment of internal hemorrhoids, Am. J. Surg., 79:44, 1950.

Turell, R. Hemorrhoidectomy with special reference to open versus closed technics, S. Clin. North America, 32:677, 1952.

Whitehead, W. The surgical treatment of hemorrhoids, Brit. M. J., 1:148, 1882.

Wilde, F. R. Anal intermuscular septum, Brit. J. Surg., 36:779, 1949.

HEPATIC LOBECTOMY

Altman, W. A. Resection of the left lobe of liver for benign hemangioma, J.A.M.A., 146:254, 1951.

Bowden, L., and Murphy, A. I. Right hepatic lobectomy: report of a case complicated by homologous serum hepatitis, Gastroenterology, 28:288, 1955.

Brasfield, R. D. Right hepatic lobectomy for carcinoma of the gallbladder, Ann. Surg., 153:563, 1961.

Brunschwig, A. Surgery of hepatic neoplasms with special reference to secondary malignant neoplasms, Cancer, 6:725, 1953.

———— Observations on the surgical physiology of the human liver pertinent to radical partial hepatectomy for neoplasm, Cancer, 8:459, 1955.

Charache, H. Primary carcinoma of the liver: report of a case and review of the literature, Am. J. Surg., 43:96, 1939.

Cohn, I., and St. Raymond, A. H. Primary cancer of the liver, Surgery, 37:356, 1955.

Couinaud, C. Bases anatomiques des hépatectomies gauche et droite réglées techniques qui en découlent, J. chir., 70:933, 1954.

———— La Foie. Études anatomiques et chirurgicales. Paris, Masson & Cie, 1957.

HEPATIC LOBECTOMY (cont.)

Donovan, E. J., and Santulli, T. V. Resection of the left lobe of the liver for mesenchymoma, Ann. Surg., 124:90, 1946.

Duckett, J. W., and Montgomery, H. G. Resection of primary liver tumors, Surgery, 21:455, 1947.

Fineberg, C., Goldburgh, W. P., and Templeton, J. Y., III. Right hepatic lobectomy for primary carcinoma of the liver, Ann. Surg., 144:881, 1956.

Fishback, F. C. A morphologic study of regeneration of the liver after partial removal, Arch. Path., 7:955, 1929.

Goldsmith, M. A., and Woodburne, R. T. Surgical anatomy pertaining to liver resection, Surg., Gynec. & Obst., 105:310, 1957.

Greene, J. M. Primary carcinoma of the liver: ten year collective review, Surg., Gynec. & Obst., 69:231, 1939.

Hauch, E. W., and Lechstein, J. The clinical problem of primary carcinoma of the liver, Gastroenterology, 27:292, 1954.

Healey, J. E., Jr. Clinical and anatomic aspects of radical hepatic surgery, J. Internat. Coll. Surgeons, 22:542, 1954.

Hollinshead, W. H. Anatomy for Surgeons, Vol. 2, The Thorax, Abdomen and Pelvis, New York, Paul B. Hoeber, Inc., 1956.

Hoyne, R. M., and Kernohan, J. W. Primary carcinoma of the liver, Arch. Int. Med., 79:532, 1947.

Keen, W. W. Report of a case of resection of the liver for removal of a neoplasm with a table of seventy-six cases of resection of the liver for hepatic tumors, Ann. Surg., 30:267, 1899.

Lloyd-Davies, O. V., and Angell, J. C. Right hepatic lobectomy-operative technique, some anatomical points and an account of a case, Brit. J. Surg., 45:114, 1957.

Longmire, W. P., and Marable, S. A. Clinical experience with major hepatic resections, Ann. Surg., 154:460, 1961.

Lortat-Jacob, J. L., and Robert, H. G. Hépatectomie droite réglée, Presse méd., 60:549, 1952.

Love, R. J. M. Primary carcinoma of the liver, successful lobectomy, Brit. J. Surg., 22:387, 1934.

Mann, F. C. The portal circulation and restoration of the liver after partial removal, Surgery, 8:225, 1940.

Michels, N. A. Blood Supply and Anatomy of the Upper Abdominal Organs with a Descriptive Atlas, Philadelphia, J. B. Lippincott Co., 1955.

Nakayama, K. Simplified hepatectomy, Brit. J. Surg., 45:645, 1948.

Pack, G. T., and Baker, H. W. Total right hepatic lobectomy, Ann. Surg., 138:253, 1953.

——— and Miller, T. R. The Treatment of Hepatic Tumors, New York State J. Med., 53:2205, 1953.

Packard, G. B., and Palmer, H. D. Primary neoplasms of the liver in infants and children, Ann. Surg., 142:214, 1955.

Peck, C. H. Cavernous hemangioma of the left lobe of the liver, Surg., Gynec. & Obst., 33:277, 1921.

Pickrell, K. L., and Clay, R. C. Lobectomy of liver: report of three cases, Arch. Surg., 48:267, 1944.

Poulos, E. Hepatic resection for massive liver injuries, Ann. Surg., 157:525, 1963.

Quattlebaum, J. K. Massive resection of liver, Ann. Surg., 137:787, 1953.

——— and Quattlebaum, J. K., Jr. Technic of hepatic lobectomy, Ann. Surg., 149:648, 1959.

Rex, H. Beiträge zur Morphologie der Spügerleber, Morph. Jahrb., 14:517, 1888.

Schatzki, R. Roentgen diagnosis of primary cancer of the liver, Am. J. Roentgenol., 46:476, 1941.

Wallace, R. H. Resection of liver for hepatoma, Arch. Surg., 43:14, 1941.

CHOLECYSTECTOMY AND COMMON DUCT EXPLORATION

Arminski, T. C. Primary carcinoma of the gallbladder, Cancer, 2:379, 1949.

Baker, J. W. Operative cholangiography, Surg., Gynec. & Obst., 101:763–765, 1955.

Bartlett, M. K., and Quinby, W. C., Jr. Surgery of biliary tract. I. Mortality and complications of cholecystectomy and choledochostomy for chronic cholecystitis, New England J. Med., 254:154–156, 1956.

——— Quinby, W. C., Jr., and Donaldson, G. A. Surgery of the biliary tract. II. Treatment of acute cholecystitis, New England J. Med., 254:200–205, 1956.

——— and Waddell, W. R. Indication for common-duct exploration: Evaluation in 1,000 cases, New England J. Med., 258:164, 1958.

Borland, V. G., and Jaehnings, D. Acute cholecystitis; its early treatment: report of 108 cases, Surgery, 32:581–590, 1952.

Brewer, G. E. Some observations upon the surgical anatomy of the gallbladder and ducts, Contributions to the Science of Medicine, dedicated by his pupils to William H. Welch on the 25th anniversary of his doctorate, 1,076 pp., Baltimore, Johns Hopkins Press, 1900, 337–354.

Burdette, W. J. Carcinoma of the gallbladder, Ann. Surg., 145:832, 1957.

Burrows, H. Gall stones and cancer; problem of etiology with special reference to role of irritation, Brit. J. Surg., 27:166, 1939.

Buxton, R. W., Ray, D. K., and Coller, F. A. Acute cholecystitis, J.A.M.A., 146:301–307, 1951.

Cattell, R. B. Technic of cholecystectomy and choledochostomy, S. Clin. North America, 17:731–742, 1937.

——— The use of a long T-tube in surgery of the biliary tract, S. Clin. North America, 28:659, 1948.

——— and Colcock, B. P. Fibrosis of sphincter of Oddi, Ann. Surg., 137:797–806, 1953.

——— and Warren, K. W. Surgery of the biliary

CHOLECYSTECTOMY AND COMMON DUCT
EXPLORATION (cont.)

tract, New England J. Med., 255:698–704; 761–768, 1956.

Colcock, B. P., and McManus, J. E. Experiences with 1,356 cases of cholecystitis and cholelithiasis, Surg., Gynec. & Obst., 101:161–172, 1955.

———— Common duct stone, S. Clin. North America, 38:663, 1958.

Cole, W. H. Recent trends in gallbladder surgery, J.A.M.A., 150:631–637, 1952.

———— and Harridge, W. H. Diagnostic use of cholangiography in biliary tract, S. Clin. North America, 36:149–159, 1956.

———— Historical features of cholecystography. The Carman Lecture, Radiology, 76:354, 1961.

Comfort, M. W., Gray, H. K., and Wilson, J. M. Silent gall stones; a ten to twenty-five year follow-up study of 112 cases, Ann. Surg., 128:931, 1948.

Cooke, L., Jones, F. A., and Keech, M. K. Carcinoma of the gallbladder; a statistical study, Lancet, 2:585, 1953.

Cutler, E. C., and Zollinger, R. The surgical procedures for biliary calculi, Surg., Gynec. & Obst., 66:637, 1938.

DeCamp, P. T., Ochsner, A., Baffes, T. G., Bancroft, H., and Bendel, W. Timing in surgical treatment of acute cholecystitis, Ann. Surg., 135:734–745, 1952.

Donaldson, G. A., Allen, A. W., and Bartlett, M. K. Postoperative bile-duct strictures: their etiology and treatment, New England J. Med., 254:50–56, 1956.

Doubilet, H., Reed, G., and Mulholland, J. H. Delayed operative management of acute cholecystitis, J.A.M.A., 155:1570–1573, 1954.

———— and Mulholland, J. H. Eight-year study of pancreatitis and sphincterotomy, J.A.M.A., 160:521–528, 1956.

Dunphy, J. E., and Ross, F. P. Studies in acute cholecystitis. I. Surgical management and results, Surgery, 26:539–547, 1949.

Eisendrath, D. N. Anomalies of the bile ducts and blood vessels as the cause of accidents in biliary surgery, J.A.M.A., 71:864, 1918.

Glenn, F. Surgical treatment of acute cholecystitis, Surgery, 23:397, 1948.

———— Surgical treatment of acute cholecystitis, Surg., Gynec. & Obst., 90:643–648, 1950.

———— and Hays, D. M. Causes of death following biliary tract surgery for nonmalignant disease, Surg., Gynec. & Obst., 94:283–296, 1952.

———— Evans, J., Hill, M., and McClenahan, J. Intravenous cholangiography, Ann. Surg., 140:600–614, 1954.

———— and Hays, D. M. Age factor in mortality rate of patients undergoing surgery of biliary tract, Surg., Gynec. & Obst., 100:11–18, 1955.

———— The importance of technique in cholecystectomy, Surg., Gynec. & Obst., 101:201, 1955.

———— and Wantz, G. E. Acute cholecystitis following surgical treatment of unrelated diseases, Surg., Gynec. & Obst., 102:145–153, 1956.

———— and Thorbjarnarson, B. The surgical treatment of acute cholecystitis, Surg., Gynec. & Obst., 116:61, 1963.

Hallenbeck, G. A., Walters, W., Gray, H. K., Priestly, J. T., and Waugh, J. M. Report on surgery of biliary system and pancreas for 1954, Proc. Staff Meet., Mayo Clin., 30:640–646, 1955.

Hays, D. M., and Glenn, F. The fate of the cholecystostomy patient, Geriatrics, 3:21, 1955.

Hight, D., and Lingley, J. R. Value of cholangiograms during biliary-tract surgery, New England J. Med., 246:761–765, 1952.

Hoerr, S. O. Operative cholangiography as aid in surgery for jaundice, Arch. Surg., 69:432–443, 1954.

Holden, W. D., Cebul, F. A., and Loughry, C. W. Management of acute disorders of biliary tract, J.A.M.A., 148:879–884, 1952.

Hughes, E. S. R. Recurrent and residual stones in the common bile duct, Brit. J. Surg., 43:198, 1955.

Jackson, R. H. Avoidance of injury to the common bile duct, Surg., Gynec. & Obst., 67:769, 1938.

Johnston, E. V., and Anson, B. J. Variations in the formation and vascular relationships of the bile ducts, Surg., Gynec. & Obst., 91:271, 1950.

———— Waugh, J. M., and Good, C. A. Residual stones in common bile duct: question of operative cholangiogram, Ann. Surg., 139:293–301, 1954.

Jones, C. J. Carcinoma of the gallbladder; a clinical and pathologic analysis of 50 cases, Ann. Surg., 132:110, 1950.

Langenbuch, Carl. Ein Fall von Exstirpation der Gallenblase wegen chronischer Cholelithiasis Heilung, Berl. klin. Wchnschr., 19:725, 1882.

Large, A. M. On the formation of gallstones, Surgery, 54:928, 1963.

Maingot, R. Complications of cholecystectomy, Ann. Roy. Coll. Surgeons, 32:42, 1963.

Maki, T. Cholelithiasis in the Japanese, Arch. Surg., 82:599, 1961.

Masson, J. C. Exposure in gallbladder surgery, Ann. Surg., 69:422, 1919.

McClenahan, J. L., Evans, J. A., and Braunstein, P. M. Intravenous cholangiography in postcholecystectomy syndrome, J.A.M.A., 159:1353–1357, 1955.

McDonough, F. E., and Wise, R. E. Limitations to clinical application of intravenous cholangiography in determining disease of bile ducts after cholecystectomy, Gastroenterology, 29:771–784, 1955.

McKittrick, L. S., and Wilson, N. J. Indications for and results following exploration of the common bile duct for stones, California Med., 71:132, 1949.

Michels, N. A. Blood Supply and Anatomy of Upper Abdominal Organs, with Descriptive Atlas, 581 pp., Philadelphia, J. B. Lippincott Co., 1955.

Moore, T. C. Congenital atresia of the extrahepatic bile ducts; report of 31 proved cases,

CHOLECYSTECTOMY AND COMMON DUCT EXPLORATION (cont.)

Surg., Gynec. & Obst., 96:215, 1953.

Morton, C. B., II. Post-cholecystectomy symptoms from cystic duct remnants, Ann. Surg., 139: 679, 1954.

Mustard, R. L., and Custer, H. R. Management of acute cholecystitis, Surg., Gynec. & Obst., 95:59–62, 1952.

Orloff, T. L., Sklaroff, D. M., Cohn, E. M., and Gershon-Cohen, J. Intravenous choledochography with new contrast medium, "Cholografin," Radiology, 62:868–870, 1954.

Preston, D. J. Transduodenal ampullo-duodenostomy for treatment of common bile duct obstructions without T-tube drain, Surg., Gynec. & Obst., 100:498–502, 1955.

Pribram, B. O. C. Method for dissolution of common duct stones remaining after operation, Surgery, 22:806, 1947.

Roberts, B. Primary carcinoma of the gallbladder, Surg., Gynec. & Obst., 98:530, 1954.

Ross, F. P., and Dunphy, J. E. Studies in acute cholecystitis. II. Cholecystostomy: indications and technique, New England J. Med., 242:359, 1950.

—— Boggs, J. D., and Dunphy, J. E. Studies in acute cholecystitis. III. Pathological process in relation to clinical management of disease: Fallacy of "critical period," Surg., Gynec. & Obst., 91:271–276, 1950.

Saliba, N., Sawyer, K. C., and Sawyer, K. C., Jr. Traumatic hemobilia, Arch. Surg., 82:298, 1961.

Sethi, R. S. Surgical management of acute cholecystitis, Arch. Surg., 82:366, 1961.

Shingleton, W. W., and Peete, W. P. The post-cholecystectomy syndrome, Am. J. Surg., 28: 29, 1962.

Shieber, W. Duodenotomy with common duct exploration, Arch. Surg., 85:944, 1962.

Sterling, J. A. Common channel for bile and pancreatic ducts, Surg., Gynec. & Obst., 98:420–424, 1954.

Strohl, E. L., Diffenbaugh, W. G., Baker, J. H., and Cheema, M. H. Gangrene and perforation of the gallbladder, Surg., Gynec. & Obst., 114: 1, 1962.

Swedberg, J. Routine cholangiography at operations for gall stones, Acta chir. Scandinav., 103: 175–193, 1952.

Wallace, R. H., and Allen, A. W. Acute cholecystitis, Arch. Surg., 43:762–772, 1941.

Walters, W. Operative and postoperative cholangiography, Arch. Surg., 70:323–325, 1955.

—— Postcholecystectomy dyskinesia: with pancreatitis, sphincteritis, and choledocholithiasis as causes, J.A.M.A., 160:425–431, 1956.

Wapshaw, H. Radiographic and other studies of the biliary and pancreatic ducts, Brit. J. Surg., 43:132, 1955.

Warren, K. W. Technique of cholecystectomy and choledochostomy, S. Clin. North America, 36: 687–697, 1956.

Welch, C. E. Abdominal surgery, New England J. Med., 250:56–70, 1954.

—— Choledochotomy, Surg., Gynec. & Obst., 102:495, 1956.

Wise, R. E., and O'Brien, R. G. Intravenous cholangiography: preliminary report, Lahey Clin. Bull., 9:52–56, 1954.

—— and O'Brien, R. G. Interpretation of intravenous cholangiogram, J.A.M.A., 160:819–827, 1956.

—— Cholecystectomy for acute cholecystitis, Surgery, 49:284, 1961.

CHOLECYSTOJEJUNOSTOMY

Babcock, W. W. Cholecystogastrostomy and cholecystoduodenostomy, Am. Jour. Obst. & Gynec., 1:854, 1920–1921.

Coller, F., and Winfield, J. Evaluation of palliative operations for cancer of the pancreas, Am. J. Surg., 25:64, 1934.

DeBakey, M., and Ochsner, A. Simple technic for cholecystogastrostomy, Surgery, 6:126, 1939.

Gage, I. M. Cholecystogastrostomy and cholecystoduodenostomy, Proc. Soc. Exper. Biol. & Med., 28:693, 1931.

Gatewood, and Lawton, S. E. Effect of cholecystenterostomy on the biliary tract, Surg., Gynec. & Obst., 50:40, 1930.

Gentile, A. Cholecystogastrostomy and hepatitis: an experimental study, Arch. Surg., 30:449, 1935.

Lehman, E. P. Hepatitis following cholecystogastrostomy, Arch. Surg., 9:16, 1924.

Mallet-Guy, P. Biliary-intestinal anastomosis: late results, J. de chir., 55:303, 1940.

Mason, J. T. Technic of cholecystogastrostomy, J.A.M.A., 94:29, 1930.

Mirizzi, P. L. Cholecystduodenostomy valvular; technia personal, Bol. y. trab., Soc. de cir. de Buenos Aires, 18:1319, 1934.

Sandblom, P., Bergh, G. S., and Ivy, A. C. Cholecystoduodenostomy combined with pyloric exclusion, Ann. Surg., 104:702, 1936.

Trautman, M., Robbins, H. J., and Stewart, C. C. An experimental study of the operation of cholecystenterostomy, Surg., Gynec. & Obst., 44:612, 1927.

Wangensteen, O. H. Cholangitis following cholecystenterostomy, Ann. Surg., 87:54, 1928.

Zollinger, R. A method of valvular cholecystogastrostomy, Surg., Gynec. & Obst., 70:71, 1940.

PANCREATITIS

Abruzzo, J. L., Homa, M., Houck, J. C., and Coffey, R. J. Significance of the serum amylase determination, Ann. Sur., 147:921, 1958.

Campanale, R. P., and Gardner, B. "Fore and Aft" split pancreaticojejunostomy for chronic pancreatitis, Surgery, 50:618, 1961.

Comfort, M. W., Gambill, E. E., and Baggenstoss, A. H. Chronic relapsing pancreatitis;

PANCREATITIS (cont).

study of 29 cases without associated disease of biliary or gastrointestinal tract, Gastroenterol., 6:239, 1946.

Doubilet, H. Treatment of pancreatitis by sphincterotomy, Am. Surgeon, 24:205, 1958.

Howard, J., and Jordan, G. L., Jr. Surgical Diseases of the Pancreas. Philadelphia, J. B. Lippincott, 1960.

Mast, W. H., Telle, L. D., and Turek, R. O. Annular pancreas; errors in diagnosis and treatment of eight cases, Am. J. Surg., 94:80, 1957.

Saidi, F., and Donaldson, G. A. Acute pancreatitis following distal gastrectomy for benign ulcer, Am. J. Surg., 105:87, 1963.

Schlitt, R. J., and Perkoff, M. An analysis of one hundred twenty-two patients with pancreatitis, Am. J. Surg., 103:442, 1962.

Siler, V. E., Wulsin, J. H., and Carter, B. N. II. Important clinical factors of acute pancreatitis, Surg., Gynec. & Obst., 100:357, 1955.

Thal, A. P. A technique for drainage of the obstructed pancreatic duct, Surgery, 51:313, 1962.

Turner, G. G. Local discoloration of abdominal wall as a sign of acute pancreatitis, Brit. J. Surg., 7:394, 1919.

Warren, K. W. Surgery of the pancreas, Proc. Roy. Soc. Med., 54:119, 1961.

SPHINCTEROTOMY

Archibald, E. The experimental production of pancreatitis in animals as a result of the resistance of the common duct sphincter, Sur., Gynec. & Obst., 28:529, 1919.

Bowers, R. F. Surgical therapy for chronic pancreatitis, Surgery, 30:116, 1951.

——— and Greenfield, J. Choledochojejunostomy: its role in treatment of chronic pancreatitis, Ann. Surg., 134:99, 1951.

Boyden, E. A. The sphincter of Oddi, Surgery, 9:443, 1941.

Cattell, R. B., and Warren, K. W. The choice of therapeutic measures in the management of chronic relapsing pancreatitis and pancreatolithiasis, Gastroenterology, 20:1, 1952.

——— and Warren, K. W. Surgery of the Pancreas, Philadelphia, W. B. Saunders Co., 1953.

——— and Colcock, B. P. Fibrosis of the sphincter of Oddi, Ann. Surg., 137:797, 1953.

Colp, R. Chronic relapsing pancreatitis: treatment by subtotal gastrectomy and vagotomy, Ann. Surg., 131:145, 1950.

Doubilet, H., and Mulholland, J. H. The surgical treatment of recurrent acute pancreatitis by endocholedochal sphincterotomy, Surg., Gynec. & Obst., 86:295, 1948.

——— and Mulholland, J. H. Recurrent acute pancreatitis: observations on etiology and surgical treatment, Ann. Surg., 128:609, 1948.

——— and Mulholland, J. H. The surgical treatment of pancreatitis, S. Clin. North America, 29:339, 1949.

——— and Mulholland, J. H. Surgical treatment of calcification of the pancreas, Ann. Surg., 132:876, 1950.

——— Section of the sphincter of Oddi. Principles and technique, S. Clin. North America, 36:865, 1956.

——— and Mulholland, J. H. Eight-year study of pancreatitis and sphincterotomy, J.A.M.A., 160:521, 1956.

Du Val, M. K., Jr. Caudal pancreatico-jejunostomy for chronic relapsing pancreatitis, Ann. Surg., 140:775, 1954.

Edmondson, H. A., Bullock, W. K., and Mehl, J. W. Chronic pancreatitis and lithiasis: pathology and pathogenesis of pancreatic lithiasis, Am. J. Path., 26:37, 1950.

Gambill, E. E., Comfort, M. W., and Baggenstoss, A. H. Chronic relapsing pancreatitis; analysis of 27 cases associated with disease of the biliary tract, Gastroenterology, 11:1, 1948.

Haggard, W. D., and Kirtley, J. A., Jr. Pancreatic calculi: review of 65 operative and 139 non-operative cases, Ann. Surg., 109:809, 1939.

Hollinshead, W. H. The lower part of the common bile duct: a review, S. Clin. North America, 37:939, 1957.

Ivy, A. C., and Gibbs, G. E. Pancreatitis: a review, Surgery, 31:614, 1952.

Jones, S. A., Smith, L. I., and Gregory, G. Sphincteroplasty for recurrent pancreatitis. A second report, Ann. Surg., 147:180, 1958.

Lester, L. J., and Colp, R. Treatment of biliary dyskinesia with special reference to sphincterotomy, Arch. Surg., 64:168, 1952.

Long, H. Observations on the choledochoduodenal mechanism and their bearing on the physiology and pathology of the biliary tract, Brit. J. Surg., 29:422, 1942.

Longmire, W. P., Jr., Jordan, P. H., Jr., and Briggs, J. D. Experience with pancreatic resection for chronic relapsing pancreatitis, Ann. Surg., 144:681, 1956.

Mann, F. C., and Giordano, A. S. The bile factor in pancreatitis, Arch. Surg., 6:1, 1923.

Opie, E. L. Etiology of acute hemorrhagic pancreatitis, Bull. Johns Hopkins Hosp., 12:182, 1901.

Ray, B. S., and Console, A. D. Relief of pain in chronic (calcareous) pancreatitis by sympathectomy, Surg., Gynec. & Obst., 89:1, 1949.

Rhoads, J. E., Howard, J. M., and Moss, N. H. Clinical experiences with surgical lesions of the pancreas, S. Clin. North America, 29:1801, 1949.

Rich, A. R., and Duff, G. L. Experimental and pathological studies on the pathogenesis of acute hemorrhagic pancreatitis, Bull. Johns Hopkins Hosp., 58:212, 1936.

Reinhoff, W. F., Jr., and Pickrell, K. L. Pancreatitis: anatomic study of pancreatic and extrahepatic biliary systems, Arch. Surg., 51:205, 1945.

Snell, A. M., and Comfort, M. W. The incidence and diagnosis of pancreatic lithiasis, Am. J. Digest. Dis., 8:237, 1941.

SPHINCTEROTOMY (cont.)

Whipple, A. O. Radical surgery for certain cases of pancreatic fibrosis associated with calcareous deposits, Ann. Surg., 124:991, 1946.

———— Observations on radical surgery for lesions of pancreas, Surg., Gynec. & Obst., 82:623, 1946.

CHOLEDOCHODUODENOSTOMY

Allen, A. W. A method of re-establishing continuity between the bile ducts and the gastrointestinal tract, Tr. South. S. A., 56:28, 1944.

Branch, G. D., Bailey, D. T., and Zollinger, R. Consequences of instrumental dilatation of the papilla of Vater: an experimental study, Arch. Surg., 38:821, 1939.

Capper, W. M. External choledochoduodenostomy: an evaluation of 125 cases, Brit. J. Surg., 49:292, 1961–62.

Counseller, V. S., and McIndoe, A. H. Dilatation of the bile ducts (hydrohepatosis), Surg., Gynec. & Obst., 43:729, 1926.

del Valle, D., Jr. Patologia del esfinter der Oddi, Rev. Brasil Med., 4:479, 1928.

———— Patologia del esfinter de Oddi y sus relaciones con la litiasis biliar, Rev. Med. del Rosario, 28:362, 1930.

Finsterer, H. Die bedutenc der Choledocho-Duodenostonia externa für die dehandlung-des-gallensteinleidens, Arch. F. klin. Chir., 156:147, 1929.

———— Peut-on recommander la choledoco-duodénostomie pour le traitement des maladies des voies biliares? Mem. Acad. chir., 78:499, 1952.

Flörcken, H., and Steden, E. Die Nah- und Fern-Ergebnisse der Choledochoduodenostomie (ch d), Arch. f. klin. Chir., 124:59, 1923.

Fullerton, A. Anastomosis between the common bile duct and duodenum for obstructive jaundice, Brit. M. J., 2:1118, 1907.

Hartl, H., and Raindl, W. Ersahrungen mit der supraduodenalen Choledocho-Duodenostomie, Wien, Med. Wschr., 101:444, 1951.

Hayes, M. A., and Coller, F. A. Surgical decompression in biliary obstruction: a new operative procedure, Ann. Surg., 135:98, 1952.

Horgan, E. J. Reconstruction of the Biliary Tract; A Review of all the Methods that have been Employed, New York, The MacMillan Co., 1932.

Hunt, V. C. Reconstruction of the common duct, S. Clin. North America, 14:1389, 1934.

———— Obstructive jaundice. Its surgical consideration, Northwest Med., 39:358, 1940.

Jackson, R. H. Anterior choledochojejunostomy, Surg., Gynec. & Obst., 19:232, 1914.

Judd, E. S., and Parker, B. R. Biliary intestinal anastomosis for obstructive jaundice: analysis of 137 cases, Arch. Surg., 7:1, 1928.

Kehr, H. Wann soll man nach einer ektomie bei negativem palpationsbesund von steinen in choledochus diesen gang incidiren und drainiren

und wann nicht? Arch. f. klin. chir., 97:301, 1912.

Mallet-Guy, P., and Marion, P. La Cholédoco-duodénostomie d' Indication Relative, Paris, G. Doin & Cie., 1943.

———— and Descotes, J. Euquête sur les résultats éloignés de cent choledoco-duodénostomies d'indication relative, Lyon chir., 50:659, 1955.

Mason, J. T., and Baker, J. W. Choledochoduodenostomy: a modified technic, S. Clin. North America, 13:113, 1933.

Morton, D. R., Hathaway, E., and Brunschwig, A. Simultaneous cholecystenterostomy and choledochoenterostomy, Surgery, 20:820, 1946.

Moynihan, B. Abdominal Operations, 4th ed., Philadelphia, W. B. Saunders Co., 1926.

Peterman, J. Anastomotic operations between biliary tract and intestinal tract, Med. Klin., 35:464, 1939.

Pi-Figueras, J., personal communication, Barcelona, Spain, 1961.

Plenk, A., and Hartl, H. Erfahrungen mit der supraduodenalen Choledocho-Duodenostomie ais routine-operation bei Choledochusstein und seinen foigen, J. Internat. chir., 9:421, 1949.

Redell, G. Operative Anastomoses Between Biliary and Gastrointestinal Tracts. A Review of Earlier Literature and a Clinical Study of 809 Swedish Cases, Uppsala, Almqvist and Wiksels Boktr., 1940.

Riedel, H. Uber den zungenförmigen Fortsatz des rechten Leberlappens und seine pathognostische Bedeutung für die Erkrankung der Gallenblase nebst Bemerkungen über Gallensteinoperationen, Berl. klin. Wschr., 25:577, 602, 1888.

Sanders, R. L. Indications for and value of choledochoduodenostomy, Ann. Surg., 123:847, 1946.

Sasse, F. Ueber choledocho-duodenostomie, Arch. f. klin. chir., 100:969, 1913.

Schwartz, F., Benshimol, A., and Hurwitz, A. Choledochoduodenostomy in the treatment of stenosis of the lower portion of the common bile duct, Surgery, 46:1020, 1959.

Soupault, R., and Mallet-Guy, P. Technique de la cholédoco-duodénostomie (anastomose latero-latérale), J. de chir., 55:313, 1940.

Sprengel, O. Ueber einen Fall von Exstirpation der Gallenblase mit Anlegung einer communication zwischen Ductus Choledochus und Duodenum, Arch. f. klin. chir., 42:550, 1891.

Stoney, R. A. Choledochoduodenostomy, Irish J. M. Sc., 6th Series, 118:120, 1929.

Whipple, A. O. Sidetracking operations for bile duct obstruction, Ann. Surg., 86:540, 1928.

Zinninger, M. M. Some experiences with anastomosis of the common bile duct to the duodenum and repair of strictures of the common bile duct, Surgery, 23:337, 1948.

RECONSTRUCTION OF THE COMMON BILE DUCT

Boyd, D. P. Portal hypertension following stricture of common duct: report of 2 cases in which

RECONSTRUCTION OF THE COMMON BILE
DUCT (cont.)

splenectomy and splenorenal shunt were carried out, Lahey Clin. Bull., 8:217–220, 1954.

Cole, W. H., Ireneus, C., Jr., and Reynolds, J. T.
Strictures of common duct, Ann. Surg., 133:
684–696, 1951.

———— Precautions in treatment of strictures of
common duct, Am. Surgeon, 20:234–247, 1954.

———— Ireneus, C., Jr., and Reynolds, J. T. Strictures of common bile duct: studies in 122 cases,
Ann. Surg., 142:537–551, 1955.

———— Strictures of the common duct, Surgery,
43:320, 1958.

Colp, R. Repair of strictures of common and hepatic bile ducts, Bull. New York Acad. Med.,
22:300, 1946.

Donaldson, G. A., Allen, A. W., and Bartlett,
M. K. Post-operative bile-duct strictures: their
etiology and treatment, New England J. Med.,
254:50–56, 1956.

Douglass, T. C., Lounsbury, B. F., Cutter, W. W.,
and Wetzel, N. An experimental study of healing in the common bile duct, Surg., Gynec. &
Obst., 91:301, 1950.

Hooper, J. H., Jr., and Shackelford, R. T. Experimental replacement of the common bile duct,
Arch. Surg., 85:1016, 1962.

Horgan, E. J. Reconstruction of the Biliary Tract;
Review of All Methods that Have Been Employed, New York, The Macmillan Co., 1932.

Lahey, F. H. Strictures of common and hepatic
ducts, Ann. Surg., 105:765–786, 1937.

———— and Pyrtek, L. J. Experience with the operative management of 280 strictures of the bile
ducts, Surg., Gynec. & Obst., 91:25, 1950.

Lary, B. G., and Scheibe, J. R. Effect of rubber
tubing on healing of common duct anastomoses,
Surgery, 32:789–795, 1952.

Longmire, W. P., and Sanford, M. C. Intrahepatic
cholangiojejunostomy for biliary obstruction—
further studies, Ann. Surg., 130:455, 1949.

Madden, J. L., and McCann, W. J. Reconstruction
of the common bile duct by end-to-end anastomosis without the use of an internal splint or
stent support, Surg., Gynec. & Obst., 112:305,
1961.

McWhorter, G. L. Experimental suture of common bile duct with new methods of anastomosis,
S. Clin. North America, 12:163, 1932.

Pierce, F. R., and Marnane, J. P. Problems and
practices in community hospital. II. Postoperative stricture of biliary tract, New England J.
Med., 248:674–679, 1953.

Ravdin, I. S. Reconstruction of common bile duct,
Pennsylvania M. J., 53:807–810, 1950.

Sullivan, A. J. Reconstruction of the bile ducts,
J.A.M.A., 53:774, 1909.

Walton, J. Reconstruction of the common bile
duct, Surg., Gynec. & Obst., 79:57, 1944.

Wilson, H., and Storer, E. H. Strictures of the bile
ducts: Etiology, prevention, and management,
Arch. Surg., 82:171, 1961.

SPLENECTOMY

Ashby, W. B., and Ballinger, W. F. II. Indications
for splenectomy, Arch. Surg., 85:913, 1962.

Balfour, D. C. The technique of splenectomy,
Surg., Gynec. & Obst., 23:1, 1916.

Bevan, A. D. Surgical technique of splenectomy
with presentation of a new incision, Ann. Surg.,
88:347, 1928.

Calamel, P. M., Cleveland, H. C., and Waddell,
W. R. Ruptured spleen, S. Clin. North America,
43:445, 1963.

Carter, B. N. Combined thoraco-abdominal approach with particular reference to its employment in splenectomy, Surg., Gynec. & Obst.,
84:1019, 1947.

Cole, W. H., Walter, L., and Limarzi, L. R. Indications and results of splenectomy, Ann. Surg.,
129:702, 1949.

Coller, F. A., Blain, A., and Andrews, G. Indications for and Results of Splenectomy, American Lecture Series, Springfield, Ill., Charles C
Thomas, 1950.

Connors, J. F. Splenectomy for trauma, Ann.
Surg., 88:388, 1932.

Curtis, G. M., and Movitz, D. The surgical significance of an accessory spleen, Ann. Surg.,
123:276, 1946.

Davis, H. H., and Sharpe, J. C. Splenic vein
thrombosis following splenectomy, Surg., Gynec.
& Obst., 67:678, 1938.

Doan, C. A., and Wright, C. S. Primary congenital and secondary acquired splenic panhemato-
penia, Blood, 1:10, 1946.

Duckett, J. W. Splenectomy in treatment of secondary hypersplenism, Ann. Surg., 157:737,
1963.

Dunphy, J. E. Splenectomy for trauma, practical
points in surgical technic, Am. J. Surg., 71:
1450, 1946.

Elliott, R. H. E., Jr., and Turner, S. C. Splenectomy for purpura hemorrhagica, Surg., Gynec.
& Obst., 92:539, 1951.

Glenn, F., Cornell, G. N., Smith, C. H., and
Schulman, I. Splenectomy in children with idiopathic thrombocytopenic purpura, hereditary
spherocytosis, and Mediterranean anemia, Surg.,
Gynec. & Obst., 99:689, 1954.

Lahey, F. H., and Norcross, J. W. Splenectomy:
when is it indicated? Ann. Surg., 128:363, 1948.

Madden, J. L., and Appleberry, C. H. Splenectomy: removal of spleen weighing 5,450 grams,
Ann. Surg., 124:524, 1946.

Maughon, J. S., Geib, P. O., and Lenhardt, H. F.
Splenic trauma: an increasing problem, Surgery,
49:477, 1961.

Mayo, W. J. Surgical considerations of splenectomy, Ann. Surg., 62:172, 1915.

Moynihan, B. G. A. Removal of the spleen, Brit.
M. J., 2:701, 1932.

O'Neil, J. F., and Rousseau, J. P. Roentgenologic
examination of the abdomen as an aid in the
early diagnosis of splenic injury, Ann. Surg.,
121:111, 1945.

SPLENECTOMY (cont.)

Pemberton, J. de J., and Kiernan, P. C. Surgery of the spleen, S. Clin. North America, 25:880, 1945.

Pool, E. H., and Stillman, R. G. Surgery of the spleen. Surgical Monographs, New York, D. Appleton Co., 1923.

Rousselot, L. M. Present concepts of surgery of the spleen, S. Clin. North America, 29:368, 1949.

Schwegman, C. W., and Miller, L. D. Splenectomy: reduction of mortality and morbidity, S. Clin. North America, 42:1509, 1962.

Singleton, A. O. Splenectomy, Surg., Gynec. & Obst., 70:1051, 1940.

———— Splenectomy, Ann. Surg., 115:816, 1942.

Walton, A. J. Indications for and results of removal of spleen, Ann. Surg., 98:379, 1933.

Wilkie, D. P. D. Splenectomy; its indications and technique, Am. J. Surg., 14:340, 1931.

Wiseman, B. K., and Doan, C. A. A newly recognized granulopenic syndrome caused by excessive splenic leukolysis and successfully treated by splenectomy, J. Clin. Investigation, 18:473, 1939.

Zollinger, R. M., Martin, M. M., and Williams, R. D. Surgical aspects of hypersplenism, J.A.M.A., 149:24, 1952.

ANNULAR PANCREAS

Anderson, J. R., and Wapshaw, H. Annular pancreas, Brit. J. Surg., 39:43, 1951.

Baldwin, W. M. A specimen of annular pancreas, Anat. Rec., 4:299, 1910.

Bickford, B. J., and Williamson, J. C. F. Annular pancreas, Brit. J. Surg., 39:49, 1951.

Brines, O. A. Annular pancreas, involved in acute hemorrhagic pancreatitis, Ann. Surg., 92:241, 1930.

Brown, M., Bingham, D. L. C., and Cronk, L. B. Annular pancreas, Gastroenterology, 11:367, 1948.

Castleton, K. B., Morris, R. P., and Kukral, A. J. Annular pancreas, Am. Surgeon, 19:38, 1953.

Conroy, C. F., and Woelfel, G. F. Annular pancreas. A report of two cases, Surgery, 29:902, 1951.

Custer, M. D., Jr., and Waugh, J. M. Annular pancreas with secondary dilatation of the duodenum: report of a case, Proc. Staff Meet., Mayo Clin., 19:388, 1944.

Ecker, A. Malformation of pancreas and heart, Ztschr. f. rat. Med., 16:354, 1862.

Gillette, L., and Lynch, B. Annular pancreas, Ann. Surg., 139:374, 1954.

Goldyne, A. J., and Carlson, E. Annular pancreas causing duodenal obstruction, Am. J. Surg., 71:429, 1946.

Gross, R. E., and Chisholm, T. C. Annular pancreas producing duodenal obstruction, Surgery, 119:759, 1944.

Howard, N. J. Annular pancreas, Surg., Gynec. & Obst., 50:533, 1930.

Kiesewetter, W. B., and Koop, C. E. Annular pancreas in infancy, Surgery, 36:146, 1954.

Lecco, T. M. Sur morphologie des pancreas annulaire, Sitzungsb. d. Wein Akad. d. Wissensch., 119:391, 1910.

Lehman, E. P. Annular pancreas as a clinical problem, Ann. Surg., 115:574, 1942.

MacPhee, I. W. Annular Pancreas, Brit. J. Surg., 40:510, 1953.

McGee, A. M., Black, L. W., and Beattie, H. Annular pancreas, Radiology, 60:532, 1953.

McNaught, J. B. Annular pancreas: a compilation of forty cases with a report of a new case, Am. J. M. Sc., 185:249, 1933.

———— and Cox, A. J., Jr. Annular pancreas: reports of a case, with simple method for visualizing duct system, Am. J. Path., 11:179, 1935.

Payne, R. L., Jr. Annular pancreas, Ann. Surg., 133:754, 1951.

Ravitch, M. M., and Woods, A. C., Jr. Annular pancreas, Ann. Surg., 132:1116, 1950.

Shapiro, D. J., Dzurik, F. J., and Gerrish, E. W. Obstruction of duodenum in newborn infant due to annular pancreas, Pediatrics, 9:764, 1952.

Silvis, R. S. Annular pancreas, Ann. Surg., 135:276, 1952.

Stofer, B. E. Annular pancreas. A tabulation of the recent literature and report of a case, Am. J. M. Sc., 207:430, 1944.

Swynnerton, B. F., and Tanner, N. C. Annular pancreas, Brit. M. J., 7:1028, 1953.

Tendler, M. J., and Ciuti, A. The surgery of annular pancreas. A summary of sixty patients operated upon, Surgery, 38:298, 1955.

Tieken, T. Annular pancreas, Am. Med., 2:826, 1901.

Truelsen, F. Annular pancreas, Nord. med (Hospitalstid.), 8:2226, 1940.

Wakeley, J. C. N. Annular pancreas, Lancet, 2:811, 1951.

Warren, K. W. The surgical treatment of uncommon lesions of the duodenum, S. Clin. North America, 32:877, 1952.

Whelan, T. J., Jr., and Hamilton, E. B. Annular pancreas, Ann. Surg., 146:252, 1957.

Whipple, A. O., and Frantz, V. K. Adenoma of the islet cells with hyperinsulinism: a review, Ann. Surg., 101:1299, 1935.

Wilson, H., and Bushart, J. H. Annular pancreas producing duodenal obstruction, Ann. Surg., 137:818, 1953.

PSEUDOCYSTS OF THE PANCREAS

Adams, R., and Nishijima, R. A. Surgical treatment of pancreatic cysts, Surg., Gynec. & Obst., 83:181, 1946.

Bozeman, N. Removal of a cyst of the pancreas weighing 20½ pounds, Med. Rec., 21:46–47, 1882.

Brunschwig, A. The Surgery of Pancreatic Tu-

PSEUDOCYSTS OF THE PANCREAS (cont.)

mors, St. Louis, C. V. Mosby Co., 1942, Chap. 10.

Carter, R. F., and Slattery, L. R. Factors influencing the management of pancreatic cysts, S. Clin. North America, 27:411, April, 1947.

Cattell, R. B., and Warren, K. W. Surgery of the pancreas, Philadelphia and London, W. B. Saunders Co., 1953, Chap. 5.

Chesterman, J. T. Treatment of pancreatic cysts, Brit. J. Surg., 30:234, 1943.

Chollet, H. A., and James, P. M. Massive hemorrhage following cystogastrostomy for a pancreatic cyst; with a case report, Ann. Surg., 154:931, 1961.

Collins, D. C. Pseudocysts of the pancreas; total excision. Report of a case, Arch. Surg., 61:524, 1950.

Doubilet, H., and Mulholland, J. H. Pancreatic cysts. Principles of treatment, Surg., Gynec. & Obst., 96:683, 1953.

Gussenbauer, C. Zur operativen Behandlung der Pancreas-Cysten, Arch. f. klin. Chir., 29:355, 1883.

Hahn, A. Beitrag zur Behandlung der Pankreascysten, Zentrabl. f. Chir., 54:585, 1927.

Hillis, W. The surgical management of pseudocysts of the pancreas, Am. J. Surg., 105:651, 1963.

Jedlicka, R. Eine neue Operationsmethode der Pankreascysten (Pancreato-gastrostomie) (Abst.) Zentrabl. f. Chir., 50:132, 1923.

Judd, E. S., Mattson, H., and Mahorner, H. R. Pancreatic cysts, Arch. Surg., 22:838, 1931.

Jurasz, A. Zur Frage der operativen Behandlung der Pankreascysten, Arch. f. klin. Chir. 164:272, 1931.

Kerschner, F. Transduodenale Anastomosierung einer Pankreascyste mit dem Duodenum. Ein Beitrag zur Operation der Pankreascysten, Beitr. z. klin. Chir., 147:28, 1929.

Koucky, J. D., Beck, W. C., and Todd, M. C. Perforation of pseudocysts: report of 6 cases, Surg., Gynec. & Obst. 73:103, 1941.

Kunc, Z. Direct anastomosis between pancreatic cyst and intestinal tract (pancreaticoduodenostomy and pancreaticogastrostomy), J. Internat. Coll. Surgeons, 10:529, 1947.

Mahorner, H. R., and Mattson, H. The etiology and pathology of cysts of the pancreas, Arch. Surg., 22:1018, 1931.

Mercadier, M. Cystoduodenal anastomosis for cephalic cyst of the pancreas, Ann. Surg., 153:81, 1961.

Neuffer, H. Zur operativen Behandlung der Pankreascysten, Arch. f. klin. Chir., 170:488, 1932.

Pinkham, R. D. Pancreatic collections (pseudocysts) following pancreatitis and pancreatic neurosis: review and analysis of 10 cases, Surg., Gynec. & Obst., 80:225, 1945.

Poer, D. H., and Stephenson, R. H. Late results in treatment of pancreatic cysts by internal drainage, Surg., Gynec. & Obst., 89:257, 1949.

Reinhoff, W. F. An evaluation of pancreatic cysts treated at the Johns Hopkins Hospital, Surgery, 47:188, 1960.

Walzel, P. Innere Drainage einer Pankreascyste unter Ausnutzung des Resorptions vermögens der Gallenblase, Mitt. a.d. Grenzgeb. d. Med. u. Chir., 40:171, 1927.

Warren, K. W. Pancreatic cysts, S. Clin. North America, 28:753, 1948.

Zaoussis, A. L. Pancreatic cysts: surgical treatment especially by the use of internal drainage: report of 6 cases, Ann. Surg., 138:13, 1953.

TRANSDUODENAL EXCISION OF TUMOR ABOUT THE PAPILLA OF VATER

Aronsohn, H. G. Pathogenesis of "white bile," Proc. Soc. Exper. Biol. & Med., 32:695, 1935.

Baggenstoss, A. H. Major duodenal papilla: variations of pathological interest and lesions of the mucosa, Arch. Path., 26:853, 1938.

Baker, H. I., and Caldwell, D. W. Lesions of the ampulla of Vater, Surgery, 21:523, 1947.

Bazzocchi, G., and Pezzani, R. Carcinoma of ampulla of Vater, J.A.M.A., 152:1164, 1953.

Brink, A. J., and Barnard, P. J. J. Primary periampullary carcinoma of duodenum, South African M.J., 24:161, 1950.

Brooks, A., and Weinstein, A. Cyst of the ampulla of Vater, Ann. Surg., 117:728, 1943.

Brunschwig, A. Resection of head of pancreas and duodenum for carcinoma—pancreatoduodenectomy, Surg., Gynec. & Obst., 65:681, 1937.

——— and Childs, A. Resection of carcinoma (carcinoid?) of the infrapapillary portion of the duodenum involving the ampulla of Vater, Am. J. Surg., 45:320, 1939.

——— The Surgery of Pancreatic Tumors, St. Louis, C. V. Mosby Co., 1942.

——— Pancreatoduodenectomy: "curative" operation for malignant neoplasms in pancreatoduodenal region; report of three over-five-year survivors, Ann. Surg., 136:610, 1952.

Cattell, R. B. Technique of pancreatoduodenal resection, S. Clin. North America, 28:761, 1948.

——— and Pyrtek, L. J. Premalignant lesions of the ampulla of Vater, Surg., Gynec. & Obst., 90:21, 1950.

——— and Warren, K. W. Surgery of the Pancreas, Philadelphia, W. B. Saunders Co., 1953.

Child, C. G., III. Radical one-stage pancreaticoduodenectomy, Surgery, 23:492, 1948.

——— Advances in management of pancreaticoduodenal cancer in Advances in Surgery, Andrus, W. D., Ed., New York, Interscience Publishers, Inc., 1949, Vol. 2, p. 495.

——— and Ellis, J. T. Radical pancreaticoduodenectomy. Report of two autopsies performed five and four years after operation, Ann. Surg., 134:80, 1951.

Christopher, F. Andenoma of the ampulla of Vater, Surg., Gynec. & Obst., 56:202, 1933.

Chu, P. T. Benign neoplasms of the extra hepatic biliary ducts: review of the literature and report of a case of fibroma, Arch. Path., 50:84, 1950.

Clifton, E. E. Carcinoma of pancreas: symptoms,

TRANSDUODENAL EXCISION OF TUMOR ABOUT THE
PAPILLA OF VATER (cont.)

signs and results of treatment in 122 cases, Arch. Surg., 65:290, 1952.

Cooper, W. A. Carcinoma of the ampulla of Vater, Ann. Surg., 106:1009, 1937.

Dennis, C., and Varco, R. L. Neoplastic biliary obstruction: an improved type of radical pancreaticoduodenostomy for ampullary and pancreatic cancers, Surgery, 20:72, 1946.

Dragstedt, L. R., and Woodward, E. R. Transduodenal reconstruction of the bile ducts, Surg., Gynec. & Obst., 94:53, 1952.

Glenn, F., and Hays, D. M. Carcinoma of the extra hepatic biliary tract, S. Clin. North America, 33:479, 1953.

Gray, H. K., and Sharpe, W. S. Carcinoma of the gall bladder, extra hepatic bile ducts and major duodenal papilla, S. Clin. North America, 14:717, 1934.

Grove, L., and Rasmussen, E. A. Benign papilloma of the ampulla of Vater, Am. J. Surg., 64:141, 1944.

Halsted, W. S. Contributions to the surgery of the bile passages, especially of the common bile duct, Bull. Johns Hopkins Hosp., 11:1, 1900.

Haunz, E. A., and Baggenstoss, A. H. Carcinoma of head of pancreas: the effects of obstruction on the ductal and acinar systems, Arch. Path., 49:367, 1950.

Henry, C. K. P. Benign papillomata of the gall bladder and biliary ducts, Canad. M.A.J., 28:300, 1933.

Horsley, J. Resection of duodenum for tumor of ampulla of Vater, Ann. Surg., 113:802, 1941.

Hunt, V. C., and Budd, J. W. Transduodenal resection of the ampulla of Vater for carcinoma of the distal end of the common duct, Surg., Gynec. & Obst., 61:651, 1935.

————— Surgical management of carcinoma of the ampulla of Vater and of the periampullary portion of the duodenum, Ann. Surg., 114:570, 1941.

Kausch, W. Das Carcinom der Papilla duodeni und seine radicale Entfernung, Beitr. z. Klin. Chir., 78:439, 1912.

Kirsteins, A., Govostis, M. C., and Van Prohaska, J. Benign tumors of the ampulla of Vater, Arch. Surg., 67:708, 1953.

Knight, W. A., Jr., and Muether, R. O. Carcinoma of the pancreas; the comparison of clinical and laboratory findings of carcinoma of the pancreas and chronic pancreatitis, South. M. J., 46:660, 1953.

Kyle, L. H., Sparling, H. J., and Jeghers, H. Carcinoma of the ampulla of Vater of minute size, Arch. Surg., 61:357, 1950.

Landry, R. M., and Walters, W. Obscure malignant obstructions of the ampullary portion of the common bile duct, Proc. Staff Meet., Mayo Clin., 25:179, 1950.

Lieber, M. M., Stewart, H. L., and Lund, H. Carcinoma of the peripapillary portion of the duodenum, Ann. Surg., 109:219, 1939.

Logan, P. B., and Kleinsasser, L. J. Surgery of the pancreas: results of pancreaticoduodenal resections reported in the literature, Surg., Gynec. & Obst., 93:521, 1951.

Lyday, R. O. Benign neoplasms of the extra hepatic bile ducts: case report of cyst causing obstruction, Ann. Surg., 137:807, 1953.

Marshall, J. M. Tumors of the bile ducts, Surg., Gynec. & Obst., 54:6, 1932.

Miller, E. M., Dockerty, M. B., Wollaeger, E. E., and Waugh, J. M. Carcinoma in the region of the papilla of Vater: a study of cases in which resection was performed, Surg., Gynec. & Obst., 92:172, 1951.

Miller, J. R., Baggenstoss, A. H., and Comfort, M. W. Carcinoma of the pancreas: effect of histologic type and grade of malignancy on its behavior, Cancer, 4:233, 1951.

Mirizzi, P. L. Remocion del calculo encajado en la ampolla de Vater; papilotomía transduodenal mínima, Bol. y trab., Acad. argent. de cir., 29:492, 1945.

Orr, T. G. Resection of duodenum and head of pancreas for carcinoma of ampulla, Surg., Gynec. & Obst., 73:240, 1941.

————— Pancreaticoduodenectomy for carcinoma of the ampulla and ampullary region, Surgery, 18:144, 1945.

————— Surgical treatment of carcinoma of the pancreas and ampulla of Vater: analysis of 82 cases, Texas State J. Med., 42:183, 1946.

————— Some observations on the treatment of carcinoma of the pancreas, Surgery, 32:933, 1952.

Outerbridge, G. W. Carcinoma of the papilla of Vater, Ann. Surg., 57:402, 1913.

Pack, G. T., and Booher, R. J. Surgical problem of periampullary surgery, Arch. Surg., 57:71, 1948.

Pearse, H. E. A simplified anastomosis for resection of the duodenum and head of pancreas, Surg., Gynec. & Obst., 75:333, 1942.

Riegel, C., Ravdin, I. S., Johnston, C. G., and Morrison, P. J. Study of the gall bladder function XII: the composition of "white bile," Am. J. M. Sc., 190:655, 1935.

Sharpe, W. S., and Comfort, M. W. Carcinoma of the papilla of Vater: clinical features in forty cases, Am. J. M. Sc., 202:238, 1941.

Sterling, J. A. The Biliary Tract, Baltimore, The Williams & Wilkins Co., 1955.

Trimble, I. R., Parsons, J. W., and Sherman, C. P. A one-stage operation for the cure of carcinoma of the ampulla of Vater and of the head of the pancreas, Surg., Gynec. & Obst., 73:711, 1941.

van Weel, M. W. The importance of pancreaticoduodenectomy in the treatment of tumors in the region of the head of the pancreas and Vater's papilla, Arch. Chir., Neerl., 5:31, 1953.

Vaughn, A. M. Primary carcinoma of the ampulla of Vater, Am. J. Surg., 52:489, 1941.

Walters, W. Resections of the common and hepatic bile ducts and ampulla of Vater for obstructing lesions, Surg., Gynec. & Obst., 56:235, 1933.

TRANSDUODENAL EXCISION OF TUMOR ABOUT THE
PAPILLA OF VATER (cont.)

——— Successful resection of the ampulla of Vater including a portion of the duodenum with choledochoduodenostomy for carcinoma of ampulla of Vater, Surg., Gynec. & Obst., 55:648, 1949.

Waugh, J. M. Radical resection of head of pancreas and total pancreatectomy, J.A.M.A., 137: 141, 1948.

——— and Giberson, R. G. Radical resection of the head of the pancreas and of the duodenum for malignant lesions, S. Clin. North America, 37:965, Aug., 1957.

Whipple, A. O., Parson, W. B., and Mullins, C. R. Treatment of carcinoma of the ampulla of Vater, Ann. Surg., 102:763, 1935.

——— Surgical treatment of carcinoma of the ampullary region and head of the pancreas, Am. J. Surg., 40:260, 1938.

——— The rationale of radical surgery for cancer of the pancreas and ampullary region, Ann. Surg., 114:612, 1941.

RADICAL PANCREATICODUODENECTOMY

Benson, R. E. Primary carcinoma of the duodenum; with a report of four cases treated surgically, Ann. Surg., 157:204, 1963.

Brown, D. B., Strang, R., Gordon, J., and Hendry, E. B. Primary carcinoma of the extrahepatic bile ducts, Brit. J. Surg., 49:22, 1961.

Cattell, R. B., Warren, K. W., and Au, F. T. C. Periampullary carcinomas: Diagnosis and surgical management, S. Clin. North America, 39:781, 1959.

Dennis, C., and Varco, R. L. Survival for more than five years after pancreatoduodenectomy for cancers of the ampulla and pancreatic head, Surgery, 39:92, 1956.

Duff, G. L. The clinical and pathological features of carcinoma of the body and tail of the pancreas, Bull. Johns Hopkins Hosp., 65:69, 1939.

Guynn, V. L., Overstreet, R. J., and Reynolds, J. T. Reduction of mortality and morbidity in pancreatoduodenectomy, Arch. Surg., 85:260, 1962.

Hartenstein, P. E., Ziperman, H. H., and Smith, M. L. Infrapapillary obstruction of the duodenum, Ann. Surg., 154:125, 1961.

Higgins, D. C., Judd, E. S., and Dockerty, M. B. Surgical aspects of infrapapillary duodenal tumors, Surgery, 49:149, 1961.

Howard, J. M., Moss, N. H., and Rhoads, J. E. Collective review: hyperinsulinism and islet cell tumors of pancreas with 398 recorded tumors, Internat. Abst. Surg., Surg., Gynec. & Obst., 90:417, 1950.

Hubbard, T. B., Jr. Carcinoma of the head of the pancreas: resection of the portal vein and portocaval shunt, Ann. Surg., 147:935, 1958.

Markowitz, A. M., Slanetz, C. A., Jr., and Frantz, V. K. Functioning islet cell tumors of the pancreas; 25 year follow up, Ann. Surg., 154:877, 1961.

Monge, J. J., Dockerty, M. B., Wolleager, E. E., Waugh, M. J., and Priestley, J. T. Clinicopathologic observations on radical pancreatoduodenal resection for peripapillary cancer, Surg., Gynec. & Obst., 118:275, 1964.

Porter, M. R. Carcinoma of the pancreatico-duodenal area, operability and choice of procedure, Ann. Surg., 148:711, 1958.

Rhoads, J. E., Zintel, H. A., and Helwig, J., Jr. Results of operations of the Whipple type in pancreaticoduodenal carcinoma, Ann. Surg., 146:661, 1957.

Salti, I. G., and Walker, T. H. Islet-cell tumors of the pancreas, Arch. Surg., 85:238, 1962.

Stanislaw, J. J., and Zwemer, F. L. Periampullary carcinoma, Surg., Gynec. & Obst., 115:342, 1962.

Warren, K. W., Cattell, R. B., Blackburn, J. P. and Nora, P. F. A long term appraisal of pancreaticoduodenal resection for peri-ampullary carcinoma, Ann. Surg., 155:653, 1962.

Whipple, A. O., and Frantz, V. K. Adenoma of islet cells with hyperinsulinism; a review, Ann. Surg., 101:1299, 1935.

ADRENALECTOMY

Adrenalectomy and hypophysectomy in disseminated mammary carcinoma: preliminary statement by the Joint Commission on Endocrine ablative procedures in disseminated mammary carcinoma, J.A.M.A., 175:787, 1961.

Aird, I., and Helman, P. Bilateral anterior transabdominal adrenalectomy, Brit. M. J., 2:708, 1955.

Albright, F. Cushing's Syndrome, Harvey Lectures, 38:123, 1942.

Anson, B. J., Cauldwell, E. W., Pick, J. W., and Beaton, L. E. The blood supply of the kidney, suprarenal gland, and associated structures, Surg., Gynec. & Obst., 84:313, 1947.

Atkins, H. J., Falconer, M. A., Hayward, J. L., MacLean, K. S., Schurr, P. H., and Armitage, P. Adrenalectomy and hypophysectomy for advanced cancer of the breast, Lancet, 1:1148, 1960.

Beatson, G. T. On the treatment of inoperable cancer of the mamma: suggestions for a new method of treatment, with illustrative cases, Lancet, 2:104, 1896.

Block, G. E., Vial, A. B., McCarthy, J. D., Porter, C. W., and Coller, F. A. Adrenalectomy in advanced mammary cancer, Surg., Gynec. & Obst., 108:651, 1959.

Brady, F. C., and Flandreau, R. H. Transabdominal approach to the adrenal glands, Am. Surg., 148:919, 1958.

Brostner, L. R., and Vines, H. W. C. The Adrenal Cortex, London, H. K. Lewis, 1933.

Cade, S. Adrenalectomy for hormone dependent cancers: breast and prostate, Roy. Coll. Surgeons, 15:71, 1954.

Cahill, G. F., Loeb, R. F., Kurzrok, R., Stout, A. P., and Smith, F. W. Adrenal cortical tumors, Surg., Gynec. & Obst., 62:287, 1936.

Adrenalectomy (cont.)

Cope, O., and Raker, J. W. Cushing's disease: the surgical experience in the care of 46 cases, New England J. Med., 253:119, 253:165, 1955.

Cushing, H. Pituitary Body, Hypothalmus and Parasympathetic Nervous System. Springfield, Ill., Charles C Thomas, 1932.

———— The basophil adenomas of the pituitary body and their clinical manifestations (pituitary basophilism), Bull. Johns Hopkins Hosp., 50: 137, 1932.

Donnellan, W. L. Surgical anatomy of the adrenal glands, Ann. Surg., 154 (Suppl.):298, 1961.

Evans, J. A., and Poker, N. Newer roentgenographic techniques in the diagnosis of retroperitoneal tumors, J.A.M.A., 161:1128, 1956.

Franksson, C., and Hellstrom, J. Bilateral adrenalectomy with particular references to operative technique, Acta. Chir. Scand., 111:54, 1956.

Galante, M., and McCorkle, H. J. Clinical evaluation of bilateral adrenalectomy and oophorectemy for advanced mammary carcinoma, Am. J. Surg., 90:180, 1955.

Glenn, F., Karl, R. C., and Horwith, M. The surgical treatment of Cushing's syndrome, Ann. Surg., 148:365, 1958.

Herrera, M. G., Cahill, G. F., Jr., and Thorn, G. W. Cushing's Syndrome: diagnosis and treatment, Amer. J. Surg., 107:144, 1964.

Hollinshead, W. H. Anatomy of endocrine glands, S. Clin. North America, 32:1115, 1952.

Holmes, G. A case of virilism associated with a suprarenal tumor: recovery after its removal, Quart. J. Med., 18:143, 1924.

Huggins, C., and Scott, W. W. Bilateral adrenalectomy in prostatic cancer: Clinical features and urinary excretion of 17 ketosteroids and estrogen, Ann. Surg., 122:1031, 1945.

———— and Bergenstal, D. M. Surgery of the adrenals, J.A.M.A., 147:101, 1951.

———— and Dao, T. L-Y. Adrenalectomy for mammary cancer, Ann. Surg., 136:595, 1952.

Hume, D. M. Pheochromocytoma in the adult and in the child, Am. J. Surg., 99:458, 1960.

Johnstone, F. R. C. The suprarenal veins, Am. J. Surg., 64:615, 1957.

Lapides, J. An operative technique for adrenalectomy, Bull. N. Y. Acad. M., 34:303, 1958.

Luttwak, E. M., and Saltz, N. J. Studies on postoperative antidiurosis in adrenalectomized patient, Surg., Gynec. & Obst., 115:312, 1962.

MacDonald, I. Endocrine ablation in disseminated mammary carcinoma, Surg., Gynec. & Obst., 115:215, 1962.

McKeown, K. C., and Ganguli, A. Anterior approach for bilateral adrenalectomy, Brit. M. J., 1:1466, 1956.

Miles, R. M. Cushing's Syndrome: experiences with adrenalectomy, Ann. Surg., 153:887, 1961.

Nelson, D. H., Meakin, J. W., and Thorn, G. W. ACTH—producing pituitary tumors following adrenalectomy for Cushing's Syndrome, Ann. Int. Med., 52:560, 1960.

Priestley, J. T., Sprague, R. G., Walters, W., and

Salassa, R. M. Subtotal adrenalectomy for Cushing's Syndrome: a preliminary report of 29 cases, Ann. Surg., 134:464, 1951.

———— Lesions of the adrenal glands, S. Clin. North America, 32:1053, 1952.

———— Kvale, W. F., and Gifford, R. W., Jr. Pheochromocytoma: clinical aspects and surgical treatments, Arch. Surg., 86:778, 1963.

Pyrah, L. N., and Smiddy, F. G. Mammary cancer treated by bilateral adrenalectomy, Lancet, 1:1041, 1954.

Scott, H. W., Liddle, G. W., Harris, A. P., and Foster, J. H. Diagnosis and treatment of Cushing's syndrome, Ann. Surg., 155:697, 1962.

Tobin, C. E. The renal fascia and its relations to transversalis fascia, Anat. Rec., 89:295, 1944.

Walters, W., Wilder, R. M., and Kepler, E. J. Suprarenal cortical syndrome with presentation of 10 cases, Ann. Surg., 100:670, 1934.

Young, H. H. A technique for simultaneous exposure and operation on the adrenals, Surg., Gynec. & Obst., 63:179, 1936.

Hysterectomy

Aldridge, A. H., and Meredith, R. J. Complete abdominal hysterectomy; a simplified technique and end results in 500 cases, Am. J. Obst. & Gynec., 59:748, 1950.

Donnelly, G. G., and Bauld, W. A. G. Total hysterectomy and carcinoma of the cervical stump, J. Obst. & Gynec., Brit. Emp., 56:971, 1949.

Meigs, J. V. Carcinoma of the cervix—the Wertheim Operation, Surg., Gynec. & Obst., 78: 195, 1944.

———— The Wertheim Operation for carcinoma of the cervix, Am. J. Obst. & Gynec., 49:542, 1945.

Munnell, E. W. Total hysterectomy, Am. J. Obst. & Gynec., 54:31, 1947.

Pearse, R. L. Supravaginal and total hysterectomy, Am. J. Obst. & Gynec., 42:22, 1941.

Richardson, E. H. A simplified technic for abdominal panhysterectomy, Surg., Gynec. & Obst., 48:248, 1929.

Schauta, F. Die operation des Gebärmutterkrebses mittels des Schuchardt'schen Paravaginalschnittes, Monatsschr. Geburtsh. u. Gynäk., 15:133, 1920.

Siddal, R. S., and Mack, H. C. Subtotal versus total hysterectomy, Surg., Gynec. & Obst., 60: 102, 1935.

Taussig, F. J. Iliac lymphaderectomy for group II cancer of the cervix: technique and 5 years' results in 195 cases, Am. J. Obst. & Gynec., 45: 733, 1943.

Ward, G. G. Cancer of the cervix following supravaginal hysterectomy, Am. J. Obst. & Gynec., 41:660, 1941.

Weir, W. C. A statistical report of 1,914 cases of hysterectomy, Amer. J. Obst. & Gynec., 42: 285, 1941.

Wertheim, E. Zur Frage der Radikaloperation beim uteruskrebs, Arch. f. Gynäk., 61:627, 1900.

SALPINGO-OOPHORECTOMY FOR OVARIAN TUMOR

Allan, M. S., and Hertig, A. T. Carcinoma of the ovary, Am. J. Obst. & Gynec., 58:640, 1949.

Cullen, T. S. Adeno-myoma of the round ligament, Bull. Johns Hopkins Hosp., 7:112, 1896.

———— Adenomyoma of the Uterus. Philadelphia, W. B. Saunders, 1908.

———— The distribution of adenomyomata containing uterine mucosa, Am. J. Obst., 86:130, 1919.

Dannreuther, W. T. The treatment of pelvic endometriosis, Am. J. Obst. & Gynec., 41:461, 1941.

Meigs, J. V. Endometriosis—its significance, Ann. Surg., 114:866, 1941.

Sampson, J. A. Perforating hemorrhagic (chocolate) cysts of the ovary. Their importance and especially their relation to pelvic adenomas of endometrial type (adenomyoma of the uterus, rectovaginal septum, sigmoid, etc.), Arch. Surg., 3:245, 1921.

———— The development of the implantation theory for the origin of peritoneal endometriosis, Am. J. Obst. & Gynec., 40:549, 1940.

Shaw, W. Ovarian carcinomata, J. Obst. & Gynec., Brit. Emp., 39:816, 1936.

TENDON GRAFT

Allen, H. S. Flexor tendon grafting to the hand, Arch. Surg., 63:362, 1951.

———— Symposium on techniques and procedures in surgery; management of lacerations of flexor tendons within digits, S. Clin. North America, 35:189, 1955.

Boyes, J. H. Flexor tendon grafts in the fingers and thumb. An evaluation of end results, J. Bone & Joint Surg., 32–A:489, 1950.

———— Evaluation of results of digital flexor tendon grafts, Am. J. Surg., 89:116, 1955.

Bunnell, S. Repair of nerves and tendons of the hand, J. Bone & Joint Surg., 10:1, 1928.

———— Treatment of tendons in compound injuries of the hand, J. Bone & Joint Surg., 23:240, 1941.

———— Primary and secondary repair of flexor tendons of hand, J. Am. Soc. Plastic & Joint Surg., 12:65, 1943.

———— Surgery of the Hand, 3rd ed., Philadelphia, J. B. Lippincott Co., 1956, pp. 474–597.

Couch, J. H. Principles of tendon suture in hands, Canad. M. A. J., 41:27, 1939.

Coventry, M. B., and Beck, N. R. Posteroperative results in primary tendon suture of hand and wrist, J.A.M.A., 135:80, 1947.

Flynn, J. E. Flexor-tendon grafts in the hand, New England J. Med., 241:807, 1949.

Graham, W. C. Flexor-tendon grafts to the finger and thumb, J. Bone & Joint Surg., 29:553, 1947.

Harmer, T. W. Tendon suture, S. Clin. North America, 1:809, 1921.

Jennings, E. R., Mansberger, A. R., Jr., Smith, E. P., Jr., and Yeager, G. H. New technic in primary tendon repair, Surg., Gynec. & Obst., 95:597, 1952.

Kinmonth, J. B. Cut flexor tendon: experiences with free grafts and steel wire fixation, Brit. J. Surg., 35:29, 1947.

Koch, S. L. Division of flexor tendons within digital sheath, Surg., Gynec. & Obst., 78:9, 1944.

Koth, D. R., and Sewell, W. H. Freeze-dried arteries used as tendon sheaths, Surg., Gynec. & Obst., 101:615, 1955.

Kyle, J. B., and Eyre-Brook, A. L. Surgical treatment of flexor tendon injuries in the hand: results obtained in a consecutive series of 57 cases, Brit. J. Surg., 41:592, 1954.

Littler, J. W. Free tendon grafts in secondary flexor tendon repair, Am. J. Surg., 74:315, 1947.

Mason, M. L., and Shearon, C. G. Process of tendon repair, experimental study of tendon suture and tendon graft, Arch. Surg., 25:615, 1932.

———— Primary and secondary tendon suture; discussion of significance of technique in tendon surgery, Surg., Gynec. & Obst., 70:392, 1940.

———— and Allen, H. S. Rate of healing of tendons; experimental study of tensile strength, Ann. Surg., 113:424, 1941.

Mayer, L. Repair of severed tendons, Am. J. Surg., 42:714, 1938.

Miller, H. Repair of severed tendons of hand and wrist; statistical analysis of 300 cases, Surg., Gynec. & Obst., 75:693, 1942.

Peacock, E. E., Jr., and Hartrampf, C. R. The repair of flexor tendons in the hand, Internat. Abst. Surg., Surg., Gynec. & Obst., 113:411, 1961.

Posch, J. L. Secondary tenorrhaphies and tendon grafts in injuries to the hand, Am. J. Surg., 85:306, 1953.

Pulvertaft, R. G. Tendon grafts for flexor tendon injuries in the finger and thumb. A study of technique and results, J. Bone & Joint Surg., 38B:175, 1956.

Rank, B. K., and Wakefield, A. R. The repair of flexor tendons in the hand, Brit. J. Plastic Surg., 4:244, 1952.

Stewart, D. Experimental study of return of function after tendon section, Brit. J. Surg., 24:388, 1936.

Strandell, G. Tendon grafts in injuries of flexor tendons in fingers and thumb: end results in consecutive series of 74 cases, Acta chir. Scandinav., 111:124, 1956.

Watson, A. B. Some remarks on repair of flexor tendons in the hand, with particular reference to technic of free grafting, Brit. J. Surg., 43:35, 1955.

White, W. L. Secondary restoration of finger flexion by digital tendon grafts, Am. J. Surg., 91:662, 1956.

STENOSING TENDOVAGINITIS (DE QUERVAIN'S DISEASE)

Bunnel, S. Surgery of the Hand. Philadelphia, Lippincott, 1948, p. 450.

STENOSING TENDOVAGINITIS (DE QUERVAIN'S DISEASE) (cont.)

Burman, H. Stenosing tendovaginitis of dorsal and volar compartments of the wrist, A.M.A. Arch. of Surg., 65:752, 1952.

Conklin, J. E., and White, W. L. Stenosing tenosynovitis, S. Clin. North America, 40:531, 1960.

Finkelstein, H. Stenosing tendovaginitis at the radial styloid process, J. Bone & Joint Surg., 12:509, 1930.

Keon-Cohen, B. de Quervain's disease, J. Bone & Joint Surg., 33B:96, 1951.

Lamphier, T. A., Long, N. G., and Dennehy, T. de Quervain's disease. An analysis of 52 cases, Ann. Surg., 138:832, 1953.

Lapidus, P. W., and Fenton, R. Stenosing tendovaginitis at the wrist and fingers. Report of 423 cases in 369 patients with 354 operations, A.M.A. Arch. Surg., 64:475, 1952.

de Quervain, F. Über eine form von chronischer tendovaginitis, Cor-Bl. Schweiz Aerzte, 25:389, 1895.

Winterstein, O. Zur tendovaginitis stenosans an processus styloideus radii (de Quervain: "styloidalgia radii"), München Med. Wchnschr, 74:12, 1927.

SUPRACONDYLAR AMPUTATION

Allredge, R. H. Major amputations, Surg., Gynec. & Obst., 84:751, 1947.

Batch, J. W., Spittler, A. W., and McFaddin, J. G. Advantages of the knee disarticulation over amputations through the thigh, J. Bone & Joint Surg., 36A:921, 1954.

Callander, C. L. A new amputation in the lower third of thigh, J.A.M.A., 105:1746, 1935.

———— Tendoplastic amputation through femur at knee; further studies, J.A.M.A., 110:113, 1938.

Dale, W. A., and Jacobs, J. K. Lower extremity amputations: results in Nashville, 1956–1960, Ann. Surg., 155:1011, 1962.

Grodinsky, M. Modification of the Callander amputation, Surg., Gynec. & Obst., 76:337, 1943.

Kendrick, R. R. Below-knee amputation in arteriosclerotic gangrene, Brit. J. Surg., 44:13, 1956.

Kirk, N. T. Amputation stumps of the lower extremity, J. Bone & Joint Surg., N.S., 15:101, 1933.

———— Amputations, Dean Lewis Practice of Surgery. Hagerstown, Md., Prior, 1942.

———— and McKeever, F. M. Guillotine amputation, J.A.M.A., 124:1027, 1944.

Macey, H. B., and Bickel, W. H. Amputation of the lower extremities in occlusive arterial diseases; A ten year review, Surg., Gynec. & Obst., 74:821, 1942.

McKeever, F. M. A discussion of controversial points in amputation surgery, Surg., Gynec. & Obst., 82:495, 1946.

———— Amputations, in Cole, W. Operative Technic, New York, Appleton-Century-Crofts, Inc., 1955, Vol. 1, pp. 140–252.

McKittrick, L. S., McKittrick, J. B., and Risley, T. S. Transmetatarsal amputation for infection or gangrene in patients with diabetes mellitus, Ann. Surg., 30:826, 1949.

Orr, T. G. Modern methods of Amputation. St. Louis, Mosby, 1926.

Pearl, F. L. Atraumatic amputation through the lower thigh (Callander): modified technique, Surg., Gynec. & Obst., 73:381, 1941.

Perlow, S. Amputation for gangrene because of occlusive arterial disease, Amer. J. Surg., 103:569, 1952.

Reeves, M. M., and Quattlebaum, F. W. Lateral flap technique in supracondylar amputations, Surg., Gynec. & Obst., 102:751, 1956.

Rogers, B. P. Amputations at the knee joint, J. Bone & Joint Surg., 22:974, 1940.

Slocum, D. D. An atlas of Amputations. St. Louis, Mosby, 1949.

Symposium on amputations, S. Clin. North America, 18:267, 1938.

Thompson, T. C., and Allredge, R. H. Amputations; surgery and plastic repair, J. Bone & Joint Surg., 26:639, 1944.

Veal, J. R. High ligation of femoral vein in amputations of lower extremities, J.A.M.A., 114:1616, 1940.

White, J. C. Pain after amputation and its treatment, J.A.M.A., 124:1030, 1944.

INDEX